○ **Describe the landmarks for performing ulnar, median, and superficial ra_____**

Ulnar: radial to the flexor carpi ulnaris tendon, at the level of proximal wrist crease and in the direction of the pisiform bone. (Can also be injected dorsally at the same point to block the dorsal ulnar cutaneous nerve.)

Median: between the palmaris longus and flexor carpi radialis tendons at the level of the proximal wrist crease.

Superficial branch of radial nerve: base of the extensor pollicis longus tendon and across the anatomical snuffbox lateral to the radial artery.

○ **How many nerve branches supply the digits?**

Four nerve branches supply digital sensation: two volar and two dorsal branches along the respective sides of each digit.

○ **How does the ulnar nerve distribution differ from the median nerve distribution distal to the DIP joint?**

In the small finger, the dorsal digital nerve extends up to the end of the finger, whereas in the median nerve distribution the volar digital nerve supplies a dorsal branch that comes off distal to the PIP joint. Dorsal branches need also to be blocked for complete finger anesthesia.

○ **What kind of approaches can be used for a digital nerve block?**

1. Volar approach:
   a. Common digital nerve
   b. Proximal to the common digital arterial communications
   c. Skin wheal made over the flexor tendon proximal to the distal palmar crease, and 2- to 3-mL lidocaine without epinephrine is injected on each side of the flexor tendons
   d. More painful than the dorsal approach

2. Dorsal approach:
   a. Less painful
   b. Allows simultaneous blockade of dorsal branches without a second stick
   c. Injection to the side of the extensor tendons proximal to the web and then palmar to block the volar digital nerves

3. Intrathecal or flexor tendon sheath approach:
   a. Single injection of 2 mL into the flexor tendon sheath at the level of the distal palmar crease or metacarpophalangeal flexion crease
   b. Rapid onset

○ **What should be avoided during digital blockade?**

1. Circumferential ring blocks
2. Excessive or prolonged digital tourniquet
3. Excessive local anesthetic volume injection

○ **Is epinephrine injection into the finger safe?**

Generally yes, there are no cases of finger death associated with high-dose epinephrine (1:1,000) in spite of hundreds of case reports. In patients who have poor perfusion to the fingertips, and slow capillary refill epinephrine should still be avoided.

○ **How do you reverse the effects of epinephrine in the finger?**

1 mg of phentolamine is diluted in 20 cc of saline, and injected subcutaneously at the same site as the epinephrine.

○ **What is the acidity of 1% lidocaine with 1:100,000 epinephrine?**

pH = 4.2, which is 1,000 times more acidic than physiologic pH.

○ **How does bicarbonate quicken the onset time of lidocaine?**

Local anesthetics work by blocking nerve transduction, but first must diffuse into the nerve. Buffering the local anesthetic accelerates the passage of more uncharged molecules through the cell membrane, which is lipophilic.

○ **What is minimally invasive anesthesia for wide awake hand surgery?**

The only medications given are lidocaine and epinephrine infiltrated at the surgical site. The local anesthetic results in an extravascular "bier block." The other term used to describe this approach is tumescent local anesthesia.

○ **What are the advantages of wide awake hand surgery?**

1. No tourniquet is required for the procedure
2. Procedure can be done in a minor care setting at where there is no sedation
3. Active mobility can be used intraoperatively to determine:
   a. The strength of a tendon repair
   b. The degree of release with a tenolysis
   c. Adjust the tension on a tendon transfer accurately
   d. The amount of malrotation on a fracture

○ **When is this approach contraindicated?**

1. Patients with high anxiety
2. Patients with PTSD
3. Patients with cognitive impairment

○ **When does maximum vasoconstriction occur after injecting lidocaine with 1:100,000 epinephrine?**

Maximum vasoconstriction occurs 26 minutes post injection.

○ **What are nine principles of decreasing pain during local anesthetic injections?**

1. Buffer lidocaine 10:1 with 8.4% bicarbonate
2. Warm the local anesthetic
3. Distract the patient (touch, pressure, pinch, ice)
4. Use a 27-gauge needle
5. Stabilize the syringe to avoid needle wobble
6. Inject 0.5 cc perpendicularly and sub-dermally, then pause until the patient states that the needle pain is gone
7. Inject an additional 2 cc before moving the needle, then move antegrade slowly
8. Reinsert needles within 1 cm of blanched areas
9. Learn from patients, by asking them to score the number of times they felt pain during the injection

○ **What does a stellate ganglion block interrupt?**

Sympathetic innervation of the upper extremity.

○ **What are the two types of central nerve blockade available?**

1. Epidural anesthesia: this occurs when a local anesthetic is injected into the epidural space and generally requires a large volume of anesthetic. Mostly used to block sensory function, not motor function, and often performed as a continuous block; for example, obstetrics.

2. Spinal anesthesia: this occurs when a local anesthetic is injected into the subarachnoid space cerebrospinal fluid (CSF) and requires smaller volumes of anesthetic compared to epidural anesthesia. Used to block sensory **and** motor functions.

○ **List five potential complications from central nerve blockade.**

1. Hypotension: results from vasodilation; risk: patients who are hypovolemic
2. High spinal: spinal anesthetic migrates cephalad; T1–4: blocks sympathetic innervation to heart (bradycardia, decreased cardiac output), above C4 (phrenic nerve, apnea)
3. Spinal headache: because of continued CSF leak through the dura; treatment: caffeine, fluids, blood patch.
4. Urinary retention: common
5. Spinal cord injury

● ● ● **GENERAL ANESTHESIA** ● ● ●

○ **What is balanced anesthesia?**

Uses several different categories of drugs to achieve desired anesthesia, results in less of each drug and less toxicity.

○ **What are the different stages of anesthesia?**

Stage 1: amnesia (from induction to loss of consciousness)

Stage 2: delirium (most dangerous stage, can have injurious pain response, e.g., N&V, laryngospasm, hypertension, tachycardia, uncontrolled movements)

Stage 3: surgical anesthesia (target point, no pain response)

Stage 4: overdose (shallow or absent respirations, hypotension, dilated and nonreactive pupils)

○ **Which muscle relaxant is not recommended for induction in burn patients and why?**

Succinylcholine. An increase in the number of muscle receptor sites for acetylcholines has been documented in burn patients. Succinylcholine is an agonist of acetylcholine and can be responsible for a large and sometimes fatal release of potassium up to 2 years after the initial burn injury. Nondepolarizing muscle relaxants as well as careful monitoring with a nerve stimulator are recommended.

○ **Describe the patient American Society of Anesthesiologists (ASA) classification for anesthesia.**

The ASA scale is the following:

ASA1: patient is a healthy individual with no major systemic disease

ASA 2: patient has a one-system, well-controlled disease

ASA 3: patient with multisystem disease or well-controlled major system disease

ASA 4: patient with severe, incapacitating, poorly controlled, or end-stage disease

ASA 5: patient with imminent danger of death with or without surgery

"E": patient who qualifies for emergency surgery

○ **Which general anesthetic is most commonly associated with cardiac arrhythmias?**

Halothane.

○ **What are the features of sleep apnea?**

STOP

S. Snoring Loudly

T. Tiredness or daytime hypersomnolence

O. Observed pauses in breathing during sleep

P. Pressure = history of hypertension

○ **What can be done to minimize the risk to patients with known sleep apnea who are undergoing plastic surgery procedures?**

1. Preoperative anesthesiologist evaluation

2. Bring CPAP or BIPAP machine to the hospital, for use in the PACU and overnight

3. Consider 23 hours observation post op, with oxygen saturation monitoring

4. minimize opioids and sedatives

5. Use NSAIDs

6. Use local or regional anesthesia, if possible

○ **What are the clinical effects of clonidine?**

1. Analgesia

2. Sedation

3. Hypotension

○ **What is the mechanism of action of clonidine?**

It acts centrally, and stimulates the alpha-2 adrenergic receptors to treat hypertension. The sedating and analgesic effects are not fully understood, but are likely related to action in the prefrontal cortex.

○ **Under what circumstances is clonidine used in plastic surgery procedures?**

It is primarily used as an adjuvant in patients undergoing facial plastic surgery, such as a facelift. The analgesic and sedating aspects of the medication complement the local anesthesia and sedation approach. Also, the mild hypotension decreases intraoperative bleeding, and reduces the risk of a postoperative hematoma.

○ **What is the dose of clonidine?**

The recommended dose for hypertension is 0.1 to 0.3 mg po BID as a starting dose. For operative procedures typically 0.1 to 0.2 mg po is given immediately prior to the procedure.

● ● ● **NEW DEVELOPMENTS** ● ● ●

○ **What are the advantages of local aesthetics delivered via elastomeric pumps?**

1. Reduced narcotic use

2. Reduced hospital stay

3. Reduced post-op nausea and vomiting

4. High patient satisfaction rate for a variety of procedures

○ **What are the potential complications from local aesthetics delivered via elastomeric pumps?**

1. Inconsistent infusion rates

2. Clogging or leaking

3. Premature emptying of medication

4. Technical pump failure

○ **What is the trade name for liposomal bupivacaine for infiltration anesthesia?**

EXPAREL

○ **What is the mechanism of action for EXPAREL?**

The bupivacaine is encapsulated in multi-vesicular liposomal particles which then releases the drug over a desired period of time.

○ **What is the dosage of EXPAREL?**

The drug is supplied as 1.3% in 20 cc vial. This is 266 mg of medication, and is the maximum dosage.

○ **What are the precautions with EXPAREL?**

1. Lidocaine can cause an immediate release of bupivacaine from EXPAREL. Therefore, if administered together, wait 20 minutes before administering EXPAREL after lidocaine.

2. Bupivacaine HCl may affect the pharmacokinetics of EXPAREL when the bupivacaine dose is >50% of the EXPAREL dose in milligrams.

3. Surfactant containing topical anesthetics (betadine and chlorhexidine) should be allowed to dry prior to administration of EXPAREL as the surfactant can destabilize the liposomes.

○ **What is the duration of action of standard bupivacaine, compared to liposomal bupivacaine?**

Standard bupivacaine has a duration of action of 6 to 8 hours, while liposomal bupivacaine has a duration of action of up to 24 to 72 hours.

● ● ● **REFERENCES** ● ● ●

Ben-David B. Complications of regional anesthesia: an overview. *Anesthesiol Clin North America.* 2002;20(3):665–667.

Gerancher JC. Upper extremity nerve blocks. *Anesthesiol Clin North America.* 2000;18(2):297–317.

Lalonde D. Minimally invasive anesthesia in wide awake hand surgery. *Hand Clin.* 2014;30(1):1–6.

Lin YC, Krane EJ. Regional anesthesia and pain management in ambulatory pediatric patients. *Anesthesiol Clin North America.* 1996;14(4):803–816.

Morales R Jr, Mentz H, Newall G, Patronella C, Masters O. Use of abdominal field block injections with liposomal bupivacaine to control postoperative pain after abdominoplasty. *Aesth Surg J.* 2013;33(8):1148–1153.

Ramamurthy S, Hickey R. Anesthesia. In: Green DP, Hotchkiss RN, Pederson WC, eds. *Green's Operative Hand Surgery.* 4th ed. Philadelphia, PA: Churchill Livingstone; 1999:22–47.

Richards BG, Schleicher WF, Zins JE. Putting it all together: recommendations for improving pain management in plastic surgical procedures: surgical facial rejuvenation. *Plast Reconstr Surg.* 2014;134(4S-2):108S–112S.

Stephan PJ, Mercier D, Coleman J, Rohrich RJ. Obstructive sleep apnea: implications for the plastic surgeon and ambulatory surgery centers. *Plast Reconstr Surg.* 2009;124(2):652–655

Tetzlaff JE. The pharmacology of local anesthetics. *Anesthesiol Clin North America.* 2000;18(2):217–233.

CHAPTER 31 Hand Tumors

Trenton M. Morton, MD and
Jeffrey B. Friedrich, MD, FACS

○ **What is the role of computed tomography (CT) in assessing upper extremity tumors?**

CT is used to evaluate extent of bone destruction as well as calcified lesions.

○ **What is the role of magnetic resonance imaging (MRI) in assessing upper extremity tumors?**

MRI is used for evaluation of lesions involving bone and soft tissue.

○ **How is clonality used to differentiate between neoplasms and benign tissue growths (i.e., Dupuytren disease)?**

Benign and inflammatory conditions are typically polyclonal, whereas neoplasms are monoclonal.

○ **In which direction should the incision be oriented when obtaining a biopsy of an upper extremity mass?**

Orient the incision longitudinal (rather than transverse or zigzag) so as to incorporate the biopsy site within the definitive excision or amputation.

○ **When performing a biopsy on a lesion, should one dissect around muscle planes or split the muscle sharply?**

Split the muscle sharply (to avoid seeding other muscle compartments).

○ **Should drains be placed after performing an open biopsy?**

No, drains can seed tumor cells along their tracts. Thus, use diligent hemostasis to prevent hematoma formation.

○ **Should a tourniquet be used when operating on a neoplasm of the upper extremity?**

Yes, a tourniquet should be used, but exsanguination of the arm should be done through elevation. Do not use an Esmarch bandage.

● ● ● BENIGN TUMORS ● ● ●

○ **What is the usual etiology of epidermal inclusion cysts?**

Epidermal cells become embedded in the dermis, which is usually the result of trauma.

○ **Where do epidermal inclusion cysts usually occur?**

In the glabrous, non–hair-bearing skin of the palms and fingertips (especially perionychium).

○ **What is the treatment of epidermal inclusion cysts?**

Complete excision along with the skin puncture wound (or punctum, if present).

○ **What is a glomus tumor?**

A glomus tumor is a benign hamartomatous neoplasm formed from the thermoregulatory neuromyoarterial apparatus in the stratum reticulare.

○ **What are the clinical findings seen with a subungual glomus tumor?**

Severe pain, cold sensitivity, tenderness, nail deformity, or discoloration.

○ **What is the treatment of a subungual glomus tumor?**

Removal of nail plate and complete excision of the tumor.

○ **What is the most likely diagnosis in a patient with a subcutaneous elevation just proximal to the eponychial fold and associated nail grooving?**

Mucous cyst. Mucous cysts are fluid-filled ganglia of the distal interphalangeal joint associated with bony spurs and nail grooving.

○ **What is the treatment of mucous cysts?**

Cyst excision and removal of bone spurs.

○ **What is a pyogenic granuloma? What demographic does it affect most commonly?**

Pyogenic granuloma is a rapidly growing vascular, friable nodule. It is frequently seen on fingertips in young adults, and notably most common after pregnancy.

○ **What is a Keratoacanthoma?**

Keratoacanthoma is a lesion commonly found on the dorsal hand that is round, elevated, and usually has a central crater. This lesion usually resolves spontaneously and only occasionally progresses to squamous cell carcinoma.

○ **What is the natural history of keratoacanthomas?**

They undergo three phases:

1. Proliferation

2. Maturation

3. Involution

The history and clinical presentation will usually include the rapid growth of a pre-existing lesion that then gradually gets smaller as the central crater expels a keratin plug.

○ **What is the recommended treatment for keratoacanthomas?**

Surgical excision or intralesional injection using 5-fluorouracil (5-FU) or methotrexate.

○ **What are the first and second most common tumors or masses of the hand?**

Ganglions and giant cell tumors (GCTs), respectively.

○ **What is the predominant cell type in GCTs (aka localized nodular synovitis)?**

Histiocytes.

○ **What is the usual site of origin of GCTs?**

Flexor tendon sheath.

○ **What is the treatment of GCTs?**

Complete excision along with stalk (if present).

○ **How is a lipoma diagnosed?**

Physical examination demonstrating a soft, mobile, nontender mass that does not transilluminate along with a consistent clinical history of slow growth.

○ **What is the difference between a neurofibroma and a neurilemmoma?**

Neurofibroma: tumor arising within the nerve fascicles. Neurilemmoma (also known as schwannoma): tumor of Schwann cells on the nerves surface.

○ **How does this difference impact treatment?**

Neurilemmoma can be "shelled out" easily leaving the nerve intact, while neurofibroma requires transection at the proximal and distal fascicles.

○ **Are these common tumors?**

Neurilemmomas are the <u>most common benign nerve tumors</u> in the upper extremity.

○ **A patient presents with multiple neurofibromas of the upper extremity and cutaneous café-au-lait spots. What is your diagnosis?**

Von Recklinghausen disease or neurofibromatosis type 1.

○ **A patient presents with bilateral acoustic schwannomas. What is the likely diagnosis?**

Neurofibromatosis type 2. Of note, these patients rarely have neurofibromas.

○ **What diagnostic studies can be used to differentiate between neurofibroma and neurilemmoma?**

Magnetic resonance (MR) and nerve conduction studies.

○ **What is the treatment of fibromatosis and juvenile aponeurotic fibromas?**

Treatment involves wide excision with skin grafting or free tissue transfer. Despite this approach there remains a high potential for recurrence.

○ **What is infantile digital fibromatosis (IDF)?**

IDF is a benign condition presenting in children between 5 months and 6 years in which broad-based, firm, and nontender nodule(s) develop on the dorsal or lateral aspects of the fingers.

○ **What are the histologic findings associated with IDF?**

Histologic examination demonstrates interlacing fibroblasts and intracytoplasmic eosinophilic inclusion bodies. These inclusion bodies distinguish IDF from other fibromatosis.

○ **What is the recommended treatment for IDF?**

Wide excision of the lesion(s) with full-thickness skin grafting if the defect warrants.

○ **What is the chief problem seen with desmoid tumors?**

High rate of recurrence (especially in female patients).

○ **In general, what is the treatment for upper extremity arteriovenous malformations (AVM)?**

AVMs are treated with ligation of feeding vessels and complete excision of the malformation. Preoperative embolization of the malformation may be performed prior to excision.

○ **Are vascular malformations considered neoplasms?**

No, they are simply an abnormal collection of blood vessels.

○ **What is the most common benign bone tumor?**

Enchondroma.

○ **What are the common locations of enchondromas?**

The most common location of an enchondroma is in the proximal phalanx, followed second by the metacarpal, and third by the middle phalanx (as per 2010 In-service examination question).

○ **What is Ollier's disease?**

A nonhereditary disease of multiple enchondromas that usually presents unilaterally.

○ **What is Maffucci syndrome?**

A condition characterized by multiple enchondromas and hemangiomas.

○ **What is the lifetime chance of a solitary enchondroma undergoing malignant transformation?**

Less than 5%.

○ **What can enchondromas degenerate into?**

Chondrosarcomas.

○ **How do enchondromas frequently present?**

Enchondromas are often discovered as the cause of a pathologic fracture presenting with pain.

○ **What is the treatment of enchondromas?**

Curettage and bone grafting. In cases of pathologic fracture, it is optimal to allow fracture healing prior to definitive resection.

○ **What is a periosteal chondroma?**

Periosteal chondroma is a benign cartilaginous tumor that is similar to an enchondroma and most commonly found at the metaphyseal–diaphyseal junction of the phalanges.

○ **What is the peak age range of unicameral bone cysts (UBCs)?**

5 to 10 years. In fact, it is seen almost exclusively in children.

○ **What is the typical presentation of UBC?**

An incidental finding on radiography or a pathologic fracture through the cyst.

○ **What nonsurgical treatment is used for UBCs?**

Intralesional corticosteroid injection.

○ **What is the name of a blood-filled cyst that typically occurs in the metaphysis of a metacarpal and then grows toward the physis?**

Aneurysmal bone cyst (ABC).

○ **What is the peak age range of ABC?**

Second decade of life.

○ **What is the typical presentation of ABC?**

Swelling and pain, often following an injury.

○ **What is the treatment of ABCs?**

Curettage and bone grafting is recommended as ABCs are erosive, although benign, lesions that must be removed.

○ **What is the usual structure of an osteochondroma?**

Osteochondromas have a bone stalk and cartilaginous cap growing from the metaphysis in skeletally immature patients.

○ **Is excision necessary for osteochondromas?**

Excision is not necessary unless they are symptomatic as osteochondromas rarely undergo malignant degeneration.

○ **What are the symptoms of an osteoid osteoma?**

Pain at night that is generally relieved by nonsteroidal anti-inflammatory drugs.

○ **How do osteoid osteomas present on imaging studies?**

Sclerotic nidus with a lucent halo, less than 1.0 cm in diameter (by definition).

○ **What is the histology of osteoid osteomas?**

Hypervascular nidus of osteoblasts with surrounding cortical reactive bone formation.

○ **What is the treatment of osteoid osteomas?**

Curettage and bone grafting.

○ **What is an osteoblastoma?**

Same as an osteoid osteoma, but these are larger than 1 cm in diameter. They have unlimited growth potential and all should be resected.

○ **What is the clinical presentation of a GCT of bone?**

Gradual swelling, pain, sometimes with pathologic fracture, most often in the distal radius.

○ **Why do some classify GCTs as low-grade malignancies?**

They are capable of metastasizing.

○ **Where do GCTs of bone typically metastasize?**

The lungs (2%).

○ **How do GCTs look on radiographs?**

Lytic lesion without new bone formation; the lesion encroaches on, but does not penetrate joint surface.

○ **What is the surgical treatment of GCTs?**

Wide excision and joint reconstruction, if necessary.

○ **What is the pathophysiology of fibrous dysplasia?**

Bone marrow of involved bone(s) filled with noncalcified collagen.

○ **What is the x-ray appearance of fibrous dysplasia?**

Ground-glass opacity.

○ **Is treatment of fibrous dysplasia of the hands required?**

Not usually. Surgical treatment is only performed for pathologic fractures, or "impending" fractures.

○ **What are some other common soft-tissue masses in the upper extremity?**

Ganglia, lipomas, foreign-body granulomas, retinacular cysts, palmar fibromatosis, or nodules (Dupuytren).

• • • MALIGNANT TUMORS • • •

○ **What is the staging system for <u>malignant</u> musculoskeletal tumors?**

Stage	Grade	Site	Metastasis
IA	Low (G1)	Intracompartmental (T1)	M0
IB	Low (G1)	Extracompartmental (T2)	M0
IIA	High (G2)	Intracompartmental (T1)	M0
IIB	High (G2)	Extracompartmental (T2)	M0
III	Any	Any	M1 (regional or distant)

Known as the Enneking Classification and originally described in 1980 by WF Enneking.

○ **What is the most common malignant tumor of the hand?**

Squamous cell carcinoma.

○ **What is the most common type of melanoma among African Americans and Asians?**

Acral lentiginous melanoma, generally presenting on hands and feet.

○ **When treating melanoma of the hand, how is the amputation level determined?**

Amputate proximal to the nearest joint (i.e., for a subungual melanoma, amputation would be through the middle phalanx).

○ **What role does sentinel node biopsy play in the treatment of subungual melanoma, and why?**

Sentinel node biopsy is useful with subungual melanoma because depth of the tumor is difficult to determine in the nail bed.

○ **What is Dermatofibrosarcoma protuberans (DFSP)?**

A soft-tissue neoplasm arising in the dermis that presents as a purple-red plaque or nodule.

○ **Has Mohs surgery been shown to be an effective treatment of DFSP?**

Yes.

○ **Name a strong risk factor associated with malignant peripheral nerve sheath tumor?**

Neurofibromatosis type 1 (Von Recklinghausen disease).

○ **What is a synovial cell sarcoma?**

Synovial cell sarcoma is a high-grade sarcoma that grows in proximity to (but not in) joints. Size of the lesion is proportional to the mortality.

○ **What is the treatment of synovial cell sarcoma?**

Synovial cell sarcoma is treated with wide excision with lymph node sampling (and dissection if nodes involved), and consideration of adjuvant radiation therapy.

○ **What other sarcoma is similar to synovial cell sarcoma and usually arises from muscle?**

Epithelioid sarcoma.

○ **What pattern of spread does epithelioid sarcoma demonstrate that makes it particularly dangerous?**

It spreads proximally along fascial planes, tendons, and lymphatics.

○ **Where is malignant fibrohistiocytoma usually found in upper extremities?**

Malignant fibrohistiocytomas are found on the deep muscle mass of adductor pollicis or within flexor muscles.

○ **What is the most common malignant primary bone tumor of the hand seen in children and teens?**

Osteogenic sarcoma.

○ **How does osteogenic sarcoma look on plain radiograph?**

Bone growth outside normal skeletal boundaries with hazy "cloud-like" bone formation into soft tissues.

○ **Is there a role for external beam radiation in treatment of osteogenic sarcoma?**

There is no role for external beam radiation in the treatment of osteogenic sarcoma, but chemotherapy has greatly improved survival and limb salvage.

○ **What is the most common malignant primary bone tumor of the hand in adults?**

Chondrosarcoma.

○ **Is chondrosarcoma sensitive to chemotherapy or radiation?**

No.

○ **What is the benign predecessor that can rarely degenerate into a chondrosarcoma?**

Enchondroma.

○ **What is a rare bone tumor of the metacarpals and phalanges that consists of abnormal endothelial cells?**

Angiosarcoma.

○ **What is a typical presentation of a Ewing sarcoma of the hand?**

Pain, swelling, soft-tissue mass; generalized symptoms such as fever, elevated WBC and/or ESR may also be present.

○ **What is the radiographic presentation of Ewing sarcoma?**

Large lytic lesion of bone with a soft-tissue component.

○ **What is the periosteal reaction on radiographs called in Ewing sarcoma?**

"Onion skin" appearance or "sunburst" pattern.

○ **What are the common sites of Ewing sarcoma of the hand?**

Metacarpals, phalanges.

○ **What is the treatment of Ewing sarcoma?**

Treatment of Ewing sarcoma includes surgical excision, systemic chemotherapy, and/or external beam radiation.

○ **What percentage of patients with primary cancers in other parts of the body will develop a metastasis to the hands or feet?**

0.3%.

○ **What is the most common primary carcinoma that metastasizes to the hand?**

Bronchogenic carcinoma (followed by breast and kidney).

○   **When primary carcinoma metastasizes to the hand, where does it go?**

The distal phalanx.

• • • REFERENCES • • •

Altay M, Bayrakci K, Yildiz Y, Erekul S, Saglik Y. "Secondary chondrosarcoma in cartilage bone tumors: report of 32 patients." *J Orthop Sci*. 2007;12(5):415–423.

Athanasian EA. Bone and soft tissue tumors. In: Green DP, Hotchkiss RN, Pederson WC, eds. *Green's Operative Hand Surgery*. 4th ed. Philadelphia, PA: Churchill Livingstone; 1993:2223–2253.

Athanasian EA, Wold LE, Amadio PC. Giant cell tumors of the bones of the hand. *J Hand Surg Am*. 1997;22(1):91–98.

Bednar MS, Weiland AJ, Light TR. Osteoid osteoma of the upper extremity. *Hand Clin*. 1995;11:211–221.

Enneking WF, Spanier SS, Goodman MA. Current concepts review. The surgical staging of musculoskeletal sarcoma. *J Bone Joint Surg Am*. 1980;62(6):1027–1030.

Falco NA, Upton J. Infantile digital fibromas. *J Hand Surg Am*. 1995;20(6):1014–1020.

Floyd WE 3rd, Troum S. Benign cartilaginous lesions of the upper extremity. *Hand Clin*. 1995;11:119–132.

Mankin HJ, Lange TA, Spanier SS. The hazards of biopsy in patients with malignant primary bone and soft tissue tumors. *J Bone Joint Surg Am*. 1982;64(8):1121–1127.

O'Leary JA, Berend KR, Johnson JL, Levin LS, Seigler HF. Subungual melanoma. A review of 93 cases with identification of prognostic variables. *Clin Orthop Relat Res*. 2000;(378):206–212.

Scaglietti O, Marchetti PG, Bartolozzi P. The effects of methylprednisolone acetate in the treatment of bone cysts. Results of three years follow-up. *J Bone Joint Surg Br*. 1979;61-B(2):200–204.

Simon MA, Finn HA. Diagnostic strategy for bone and soft tissue tumors. *J Bone Joint Surg Am*. 1993;75(4):622–631.

Trumble TE, Berg D, Bruckner JD, et al. Benign and malignant neoplasms of the upper extremity. In: Trumble TE, ed. *Principles of Hand Surgery and Therapy*. 1st ed. Philadelphia, PA: WB Saunders; 2000:529–578.

CHAPTER 32 Infections of the Hand

Emily Cushnie, MD, PhD and
César J. Bravo, MD

○ **What organism is found in all the hand infections?**

Staphylococcus aureus. Seen in 50% to 80% of infections.

○ **What are the most common bacteria involved in acute hand infections?**

Staphylococcus aureus (up to 60%) and beta-hemolytic streptococci.

○ **What proportion of hand infections are polymicrobial?**

Over half.

○ **What is the basic treatment principle when dealing with infections of the hand?**

DICE. **D**rainage and **D**ebridement. **I**mmobilization. **C**hemotherapy (antibiotics). **E**levation.

○ **What is the most common site of hand infections?**

Dorsal subcutaneous tissue. Followed by tendon, joint, bone, and the subfascia.

○ **What is the most common mechanism of hand infections?**

Trauma, such as penetrating injuries or bites.

○ **How do superficial hand infections tend to be treated? Exception?**

With antibiotics, which can be supplemented with splinting depending on severity. Typical course if 14 to 21 days. Exception is necrotizing fasciitis, which requires early surgical intervention.

○ **How do deep hand infections tend to be treated?**

Surgical irrigation and debridement in conjunction with antibiotics and splinting as indicated.

○ **What patient risk factors predispose them to hand infections?**

Immunocompromised state, Intravenous (IV) drug abuse, diabetes mellitus, and steroid use. Microvascular disease and damage to blood supply, as in trauma, also impairs host immune response.

○ **What are the common pathogens found in diabetic patients with hand infections?**

Gram–negative and polymicrobial infections. Subepidermal abscesses are unique to this patient population.

○ **How do hand infections in immunocompromised patients behave?**

Hand infections in this population tend to run a virulent course; for example, herpetic whitlow will not resolve spontaneously and require antiviral agents.

○ **What characterizes cellulitis in the hand?**

Characterized by erythema, swelling, and tenderness. Associated lymphangitis may indicate a more severe infection.

○ **What is the most commonly involved organism in cellulitis of the hand?**

Group A β-hemolytic *Streptococcus*.

○ **What other organism is also involved, specifically in less severe cases of cellulitis?**

S. aureus.

○ **What are the oral antibiotics of choice in cellulitis of the hand?**

Nafcillin, dicloxacillin, and cephalexin; erythromycin, if allergic to penicillin.

○ **How do subcutaneous abscesses typically occur in the hand?**

After a puncture wound or as a response to a retained foreign body.

○ **What are the most commonly isolated pathogens in human-bite infections?**

α-Hemolytic *Streptococcus and S. aureus*.

○ **What is the area most commonly involved in human bites?**

The metacarpophalangeal joint, commonly referred to as "fight bites."

○ **Where is the most common topography for occurrence of hand infections?**

Flexor tendon zone injury II.

○ **What organism is commonly isolated in one-third of human bite wounds?**

Eikenella corrodens. Cultured in 7% to 29% of human bites. Must be cultured in 10% carbon dioxide. Destroys articular cartilage quickly.

○ **What is the recommended treatment of a human bite injury?**

Surgical extension and debridement with arthrotomy and culture acquisition. The wound is left open.

○ **What organism commonly infects animal bites and scratch wounds?**

Pasteurella multocida.

○ **Why do you need an x-ray if the patient had a simple animal bite?**

To rule out a retained foreign body like a broken tooth.

○ **How should animal bites be treated?**

Irrigation and oral amoxicillin-clavulanate, or IV ampicillin-sulbactam.

○ **What are the common cultures requested in hand infections?**

Aerobic cultures, anaerobic cultures, cultures Löwenstein–Jensen medium for atypical *Mycobacterium* (*Mycobacterium marinum* at 32°C, *Mycobacterium tuberculosis* at 37°C).

○ **What are the common stains needed in hand infections?**

Gram stain, Ziehl–Neelsen stain (atypical *Mycobacteria*), Tzanck smear (*herpes simplex* virus).

○ **When evaluating a hand infection and a fungus is suspected, what preparation should be done for examination?**

Potassium hydroxide preparation.

○ **What is the most common infection in the hand in human immunodeficiency virus (HIV)–positive patients?**

Herpes simplex infection.

○ **When using an aminoglycoside (e.g., gentamicin) for gram-negative coverage, what adverse effects are commonly overlooked?**

Nephrotoxicity and ototoxicity.

○ **What is the drug of choice for methicillin-sensitive *S. aureus* (MSSA) infections of the hand?**

Cephalexin, amoxicillin clavulanate (orally).

○ **What is the drug of choice for methicillin-resistant *S. aureus* (MRSA) infections of the hand?**

Vancomycin.

○ **What is the current reported incidence of MRSA hand infections, and is it rising?**

34–73% of all hand infections, Yes.

○ **What is the recommended empirical oral antibiotic for MRSA?**

Sulfamethoxazole/trimethoprim (Bactrim) covers 90% community-acquired MRSA, current recommendation is for 2 double-strength Bactrim tablets twice a day. Clindamycin and ciprofloxacin are also appropriate, however they have 50% and 40% resistance to community-acquired MRSA, respectively. The *mecA* gene, which codes for penicillin-binding protein 2A, provides its resistance to methicillin.

○ **Which is the most common hand infection?**

Paronychia. It is an infection beneath the eponychial fold or along the paronychial fold and nail plate. Not to be confused with perionychium, which is the skin around the nail margin (see Fig. 32-1).

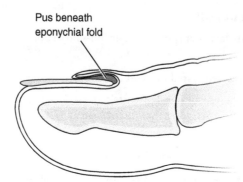

Pus beneath
eponychial fold

Figure 32-1 Paronychial infection.

○ **Which is the area around the fingertip most resistant to infection?**

The hyponychium is the most resistant area to infection.

○ **How do you treat an acute paronychia without abscess?**

Warm water soaks with or without povidone or chlorhexidine and oral antibiotics. With and abscess in place, incision and drainage is recommended, routinely with removal of the nail plate.

○ **What is a runaround abscess?**

A paronychial infection that forms an abscess that tracks around beneath the entire nail fold superficial to the nail plate.

○ **In what type of patient population is chronic paronychial infection often seen?**

Patients exposed to constant moisture such as dishwashers, swimmers, or medical professionals. Also, children who frequently dig in dirt.

○ **What organism is commonly implicated in chronic paronychial infection and how is it treated?**

Candida albicans. Marsupialization and nail removal.

○ **What adjunct treatment for chronic paronychial infections is recommended?**

Topical corticosteroid—antifungal ointment (3% clioquinol in a triamcinolone-nystatin ointment). (Mycolog)

○ **In what subset of diabetic patients with hand infections is morbidity particularly high?**

Renal transplant patients.

○ **What is a felon?**

Closed-space infection of the digital pulp.

○ **What is the most common organism found in felons?**

S. aureus, with MRSA being more common.

○ **What are the preferred incisions for draining a felon?**

Midvolar and high lateral incisions (see Fig. 32-2). Longitudinal incisions from distal flexion crease to pulp apex allows for incision of septal compartments while protecting neurovascular bundles.

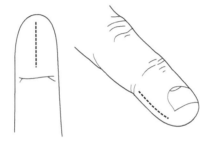

Figure 32-2 Midvolar and high lateral incision for drainage of felon.

○ **What type of incision used for draining a felon is associated with vascular compromise of the digital pad?**

Fish-mouth incisions.

○ **What are the consequences of untreated felons?**

Deep-space infections, septic arthritis, osteomyelitis, amputation, acute flexor tenosynovitis, and painful/insensate pulp scars.

○ **How long does viral shedding and ability to infect others persist in people with herpetic whitlow?**

Until lesion epithelialization is complete.

○ **What is the natural course of herpetic whitlow?**

A self-limiting disease resolving over a period of 3 to 4 weeks. Presents initially with prodromal throbbing pain, tingling, swelling, and erythema of the affected finger (first 48–72 hours). This is followed by erythema and tenderness around clear vesicles which coalesce to form ulcers over 10 to 14 days. Twenty percent recurrence rate reported.

○ **Is surgical irrigation and debridement indicated?**

No, this could cause a bacterial superinfection to develop, surgical intervention is contraindicated.

○ **What is pyogenic flexor tenosynovitis of the hand?**

A bacterial infection of the flexor sheath between the visceral epitenon layer and the outer parietal layer. *S. aureus* is the most common causative organism.

○ **What are the four cardinal signs described by Kanavel characteristic of pyogenic flexor tenosynovitis?**

1. Flexed resting position of the involved digit.

2. Tenderness over the flexor sheath.

3. Severe pain of passive extension (commonly proximally along the finger tendon sheath).

4. Fusiform swelling of the finger.

All signs may not be present, especially early in the course of infection.

○ **What laboratory values are helpful in diagnosis of flexor tenosynovitis?**

White blood cell count, erythrocyte sedimentation rate, and C-reactive protein. Elevation of at least one of these markers, plus a positive clinical examination was shown to be 100% specific (although not nearly as sensitive) in diagnosing flexor tenosynovitis.

○ **What type of bacterial flexor tenosynovitis usually results from hematogenous spread?**

Gonococcal infections.

○ **Which two digital flexor sheaths communicate with bursae in the palm and thus can propagate proximal extension of tenosynovial infections?**

The flexor sheath of the thumb (radial bursa) and the small finger (ulnar bursa). The ulnar and radial bursae extend proximally in 50% to 80% of persons into carpal tunnel.

○ **What is a horseshoe abscess?**

Infection of either small finger or thumb flexor sheath with contiguous spread through communication of the radial and ulnar bursae.

○ **What has happened if a patient with suppurative flexor tenosynovitis of the small finger suddenly develops acute carpal tunnel symptoms?**

Extensive proximal spread of infection into Paronas space (the quadrilateral potential space at the wrist bordered by the pronator quadratus, digital flexors, pollicis longus, and flexor carpi ulnaris).

○ **Can contiguous spread from the index-finger sheath cause infection of thenar space?**

Yes.

○ **How do you treat early infections of suppurative flexor tenosynovitis (within 24 hours)? Late?**

Elevation, splinting, and intravenous antibiotics. Surgical irrigation of the tendon sheath and IV antibiotics.

○ **If limited incision and catheter irrigation are used, why is it important to make sure catheter is within digital sheath?**

Digital compartment syndrome can occur. The presence of fluid in the interstitial tissue.

○ **What is the favored exposure for severe tenosynovitis infections with subcutaneous purulence or necrotic tendon?**

Open exposure of the sheath and irrigation through windows sparing the A2 and A4 pulleys, midaxial approach is preferred over Bruner to limit postoperative tendon exposure.

○ **What is the recommended empiric choice and duration of treatment for antibiotics in pyogenic flexor tenosynovitis?**

Vancomycin and piperacillin/tazobactam for 2 to 3 weeks.

○ **What deep spaces of the hand can be involved in infection?**

Dorsal subaponeurotic, thenar, midpalmar, Parona's quadrilateral, and interdigital subfascial web spaces (see Fig. 32-3).

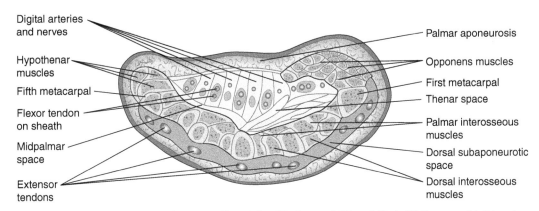

Figure 32-3 Reproduced, with permission, from Tintinalli JE, Kelen GD, Stapczynski JS, et al. *Tintinalli's Emergency Medicine: A Comprehensive Study Guide*. 6th ed. New York, NY: McGraw-Hill; 2004. Fig. 268–8.

○ **Name the fascial spaces of the hand and its possible pertinent infecting area.**

Fascial Space	Infected Area
Middle palmar space	Infection of ring- or middle-finger flexor tendon sheath
Thenar space	Infection of index flexor tendon sheath
Dorsal subaponeurotic space	Aponeurosis of extensor tendons (deep)
Dorsal subcutaneous space	Entire dorsum of hand

○ **What are the most common infectious agents in deep-space hand infections?**

Streptococcus, S. aureus, and coliform organisms.

○ **What is the name used when the interdigital subfascial web space is infected?**

Collar button abscess. Treated with incision and drainage/broad-spectrum antibiotics.

○ **Why are they called collar button abscesses?**

They typically form two swellings—one volarly and one dorsally with each on one end of a narrower stalk. The shape is like a dumbbell or the collar buttons used on shirts years ago. Tuxedos still come with collar buttons frequently.

○ **In contrast to a simple dorsal subcutaneous abscess, a collar button abscess is characterized by:**

Abducted resting posture of the adjacent digits.

○ **An infection of the thenar space, first web space, and dorsoradial aspect of the hand is known as?**

Dumbbell or pantaloon infection.

○ **The boundaries of the thenar space are:**

Volar: Index-finger flexor tendon.

Dorsal: Adductor pollicis musculature.

Radial: Insertion of adductor pollicis into the proximal phalanx of thumb and thenar muscle fascia.

Ulnar: Midpalmar space or oblique septum extending from palmar fascia to the volar ridge to the third metacarpal (midpalmar septum).

○ **Why is the thumb held in marked abduction in thenar-space infections?**

This posture reduces pressure (and thus pain) within the thenar space.

○ **What are the mimickers of hand infection?**

Gout, pseudogout, pyogenic granuloma, pyoderma gangrenosum, and neoplasia.

○ **What is the most common algae infection seen in fishermen?**

Prototheca wickerhamii (Tx: Tetracycline).

○ **What are the recommended incisions for drainage of thenar-space infections?**

Combined volar and dorsal incisions (see Fig. 32-4).

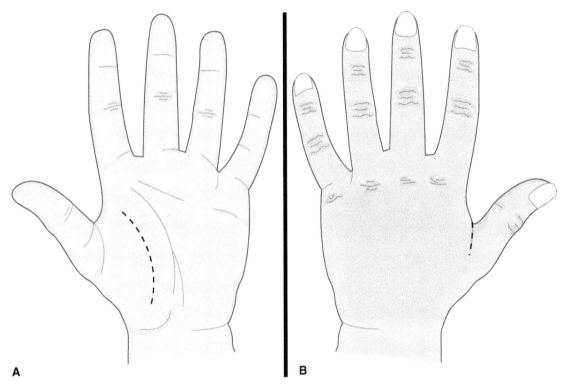

Figure 32-4 Incisions for thenar-space hand infections.

○ **Why are incisions that parallel the first-web commissure not recommended in thenar-space infection?**
To avoid web space contracture.

○ **What is the only infection resulting in loss of palmar concavity?**
Midpalmar space infection.

○ **What are the boundaries of the midpalmar space?**
Volar: Flexor tendons and lumbricals
Dorsal: Middle- and ring-finger metacarpals and second and third palmar interosseous muscles
Radial: Midpalmar septum
Ulnar: Hypothenar muscles

○ **Exposure to what virus causes milker's node in the hand (or granuloma)?**
Poxvirus. Handling a cow's udder.

○ **What is an interdigital pilonidal cyst?**
When a foreign piece of hair enters the web space and becomes secondarily infected. Seen in barbers and sheep shearers.

○ **What is the usual rate of infections after elective hand surgery?**

1% to 7%; 0.47% deep infection rate after carpal tunnel release.

○ **What are the recommended incisions for midpalmar space infections?**

Figure 32-5.

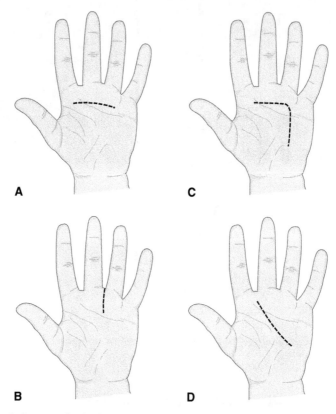

Figure 32-5 Incisions for midpalmar space hand infections.

○ **Name organisms found in hand infections associated with river or seawater?**

Vibrio vulnificus—coastal and brackish water (Tx: tetracycline, chloramphenicol)

Mycobacterium marinum—fresh water (Tx: rifampin, ethambutol trimethoprim-sulfamethoxazole)

Aeromonas hydrophila—fresh water (Tx: ciprofloxacin, tetracycline, trimethoprim-sulfamethoxazole)

○ **What is sporotrichosis?**

A chronic granulomatous infection caused by the saprophytic fungus *Sporothrix schenckii*. Most common subcutaneous fungal lesion in North America seen mostly in the upper extremities.

○ **What is the treatment of choice for sporotrichosis? If allergic to iodine?**

Oral potassium iodide. Itraconazole.

○ **What organisms are commonly found in septic arthritis of the hand? Cause?**

S. aureus and *Streptococcus. Haemophilus influenzae* (young). *Gonococcus* (young adult with <u>monoarticular nontraumatic</u> septic arthritis). Penetrating trauma.

○ **What is the most common cause of osteomyelitis in the hand?**

Open fractures.

○ **Where is the most common location of osteomyelitis in the hand?**

Distal phalanx.

○ **What is necrotizing fascitis? What is it usually caused by?**

Liquefaction necrosis of the fascia with selective spread along fascial planes with involvement of skin and muscle during later stages of infection with bullae formation, myonecrosis, and skin slough. Group A *Streptococcus*.

○ **Gas gangrene is frequently caused by?**

Clostridium perfringens.

○ **Are there pathognomonic physical findings in mycobacterial infections of the hand?**

No, but deep infections are frequently associated with abundant tenosynovitis or joint synovitis.

○ **What unique infection can occur in the hands of a patient receiving Taxol?**

Subungual abscess of multiple digits (including the toes) with painful onycholysis or nail plate separation.

○ **How is septic arthritis of the hand transmitted?**

Commonly by penetrating trauma or spread of infection from contiguous structures

○ **What are the physical findings in hand septic arthritis?**

Fusiform swelling of the joint with erythema and pain upon active or passive motion.

○ **How is septic arthritis diagnosed?**

Joint aspiration for definitive diagnosis, with analysis of cultures, cell count, and crystal content. Cell count of 50,000 cells with >75% polymorphonuclear leukocytes is traditionally thought to be diagnostic of septic arthritis, however more recent studies suggest lower cell count values as being more accurate.

○ **What is the treatment for hand septic arthritis?**

Irrigation and debridement with antibiotics.

1. Wrist septic arthritis can be addressed either open through longitudinal incisions between the third and fourth extensor compartments, or via arthroscopy.

2. MCP joints should be entered through a longitudinal, dorsal incision with at least partial preservation of the sagittal bands to prevent extensor tendon subluxation.

3. IP joints approached through midaxial incisions.

○   **What duration of antibiotics is recommended for septic arthritis of the hand?**

Between 1 and 4 weeks of IV antibiotics.

● ● ● **REFERENCES** ● ● ●

Abrams RA, Botte MJ. Hand infections: treatment recommendations for specific types. *J Am Acad Orthop Surg.* 1996;4:219–230.

Arons MS, Fernando L, Polayes IM. Pasteurella multocida—the major cause of hand infections following domestic animal bites. *J Hand Surg Am.* 1982;7:47–52.

Bishop GB, Born T. Kakar S, Jawa A. The diagnostic accuracy of inflammatory blood markers for purulent flexor tenosynovitis. *J Hand Surg Am.* 2013;38(11):2201–2211.

Burkhalter WE. Deep space infections. *Hand Clin.* 1989;5(4):553–559.

Canales FL, Newmeyer WL 3rd, Kilgore ES Jr. The treatment of felons and paronychias. *Hand Clin.* 1989;5:515–523.

Chuinard RG, D'Ambrosia RD. Humanbite infections of the hand. *J Bone Joint Surg Am.* 1977;59:416–418.

Draeger RW. Bynum DK Jr. Flexor tendon sheath infections of the hand. *J Am Acad Orthop Surg.* 2012;20(6):373–382.

Fowler JR. Viral infections. *Hand Clin.* 1989;5:613–627.

Freeland AE, Senter BS. Septic arthritis and osteomyelitis. *Hand Clin.* 1989;5:533–552.

Glickel SZ. Hand infections in patients with acquired immunodeficiency syndrome. *J Hand Surg Am.* 1988;13:770–775.

Goldstein EJ, Citron DM, Wield B, et al. Bacteriology of human and animal bite wounds. *J Clin Microbiol.* 1978;8:667–672.

Hausman MR, Lisser SP. Hand infections. *Orthop Clin North Am.* 1992;23:171–185.

Hitchcock TF, Amadio PC. Fungal infections. *Hand Clin.* 1989;5:599–611.

Houshian S, Seyedipour S, Wedderkopp N. Epidemiology of bacterial hand infections. *Int J Infect Dis.* 2006;10(4):315–319.

Hurst LC, Amadio PC, Badalamente MA, Ellstein JL, Dattwyler RJ. Mycobacterium marinum infections of the hand. *J Hand Surg Am.* 1987;12:428–435.

Kanavel AB. *Infections of the Hand.* 7th ed. Philadelphia, PA: Lea & Febiger; 1939.

Mann RJ, Hoffeld TA, Farmer CB. Humanbites of the hand: twenty years of experience. *J Hand Surg Am.* 1977;2:97–104.

Neviaser RJ. Infections. In: Green DP, ed. *Operative Hand Surgery.* Vol 1. 3rd ed. New York, NY: Churchill Livingstone; 1993: 1021–1038.

Osterman M, Draeger R, Stern P. Acute hand infections. *J Hand Surg Am.* 2014;39(8):1628–1635.

Ritting AW, O'Malley MP, Rodner CM. Acute paronychia. *J Hand Surg Am.* 2012;37(5):1068–1070.

Schecter W, Meyer A, Schecter G, Giuliano A, Newmeyer W, Kilgore E. Necrotizing fasciitis of the upper extremity. *J Hand Surg Am.* 1982;7:15–20.

Siegel DB, Gelberman RH. Infections of the hand. *Orthop Clin North Am.* 1988;19:779–789.

Stern P, Staneck J, McDonough J, Neal H, Tyler G. Established hand infections: a controlled, prospective study. *J Hand Surg Am.* 1983;8(5):553–559.

Tosti R, Ilyas A. Emperic antibiotics for acute infections of the hand. *J Hand Surg Am.* 2010;35(1):125–128.

CHAPTER 33 Dupuytren Contracture

Pieter G.L. Koolen, MD,
John B. Hijjawi, MD, FACS, and
Samuel J. Lin, MD, MBA, FACS

○ **What is the cause of Dupuytren disease?**

It is usually familial disease with multifactorial causes. The tissue-level problem is a proliferative fibroplasias.

○ **What are the diseases associated with Dupuytren disease?**

1. Diabetes mellitus
2. Anti-convulsant therapy and epilepsy
3. Chronic alcoholism
4. HIV infection
5. Tobacco consumption

○ **Is the disease related to work or trauma?**

The disease has been noticed to increase in heavy manual workers or following injury to the hand.

○ **Who gets this disease?**

Typically Scandinavian or Northern European men (10:1 prevalence over women).

○ **Where do they get it?**

The most common fingers to get Dupuytren are the ring and small fingers.

○ **What is Ledderhose disease?**

Plantar fibromatosis.

○ **What is Peyronie disease?**

Penile fibromatosis.

○ **Do these have anything to do with Dupuytren diathesis?**

Yes. Dupuytren diathesis is the presence of a <u>strong family history</u> of Dupuytren disease associated with <u>knuckle pads, Ledderhose or Peyronie disease.</u> The patient often develops <u>aggressive disease</u> at a young age with a high likelihood of <u>recurrence</u> following surgery.

○ **What are the risk factors in developing Dupuytren disease?**

1. Family history
2. Other type of fibromatosis
3. Early and aggressive onset
4. Severe bilateral disease

○ **What is Luck's classification of the disease?**

Three phases:

1. proliferative phase
2. involutional phase
3. residual phase

○ **What is the difference between the collagen in normal fascia and that of the disease?**

Normal fascia contains mostly type I collagen, whereas collagen in Dupuytren disease contains mostly type III collagen.

○ **What cell type is implicated in Dupuytren disease?**

The myofibroblast.

○ **What other molecules may play a role in the development of Dupuytren disease?**

Transforming growth factors (TGF-B), platelet-derived growth factor, fibroblast growth factor.

○ **Cytokines, which are hormone-like peptides, may be responsible for which process in humans that can lead to Dupuytren disease?**

Signaling the transformation of fibroblasts into myofibroblasts.

○ **Name the normal fascia and their pathological forms in Dupuytren disease.**

• Pretendinous band becomes pretendinous cord.
• Lateral digital sheet becomes lateral cord.
• Natatory ligament becomes natatory cord.

○ **What other cords contribute to the disease?**

Central and spiral cords.

○ **What forms the spiral cord?**

It is formed by the pretendinous band, spiral band, lateral digital sheet, and Grayson ligament.

○ **What other ligaments in the hand are not affected by the disease?**
- Superficial transverse ligament
- Deep transverse ligament
- Cleland ligament
- Landsmeer ligament

○ **What causes metacarpophalangeal (MCP) joint flexion contracture in Dupuytren disease?**
Pretendinous cord.

○ **What causes proximal interphalangeal (PIP) joint flexion contracture in Dupuytren disease?**
Spiral cord, lateral cord, and central cord.

○ **What causes MCP adduction contracture in Dupuytren disease?**
Natatory cords and the termination of the transverse fibers of the palmar aponeurosis.

○ **Does the distal interphalangeal (DIP) get involved in Dupuytren disease? If so, how?**
Yes, essentially by the retrovascular cord and to some extent by the lateral cord.

○ **What is the key thing to remember about natatory cords?**
They prevent abduction of the fingers at the MCP joints.

○ **What causes neurovascular displacement in the disease?**
The spiral cord.

○ **What is the histological hallmark of the disease?**
The high cellularity. Notably, polyclonal in nature suggesting that the tissue is not truly neoplastic.

○ **What could it be caused by?**
Local ischemia and production of free radicals.

○ **What are the two forms of the diseased fascia?**
Cord and nodule.

○ **What is the histological feature of the nodule?**
Dense collection of myofibroblasts.

○ **What are Garrod nodes?**
An associated finding in Dupuytren disease: knuckle pads over the dorsum of the PIP joint.

○ **How should Garrod nodes be treated?**
Local steroid injection or oral nonsteroidal anti-inflammatory drugs.

○ **What are the histological features of the cord?**

Contains no myofibroblasts but highly organized collagen as seen in tendons.

○ **What causes cord contracture?**

Myofibroblasts in the nodules account for active contraction.

○ **Where are nodules usually located?**

Usually just distal or just proximal to the distal palmar crease.

○ **What can an area of skin dimpling alert the surgeon of in a patient with Dupuytren disease?**

A spiral cord may exist, and the possibility that a digital nerve may be located in the immediate subcutaneous position.

○ **What is the differential diagnosis for Dupuytren disease (including isolated nodules)?**

1. Ganglion
2. Inclusion cyst
3. Epithelioid sarcoma
4. Camptodactyly
5. Trigger finger
6. Boutonniere deformity

○ **How does one differentiate a Boutonniere deformity from a severe PIP joint flexion contracture?**

Hyperextension of the DIP joint may indicate that a Boutonniere deformity is present. If there is resistance to passive DIP joint when the PIP is passively extended, the oblique retinacular ligament is contracted and the lateral bands are held palmar to the PIP joint axis.

○ **If a patient has carpal tunnel syndrome and Dupuytren disease, can the two conditions be treated surgically at the same time?**

Controversy exists. Nissenbaum and Kleinert believe that the conditions should be treated at separate times, while Michon, Gonzalez, and Watson advocated for simultaneous surgical treatment.

○ **What are the nonsurgical treatments for the Dupuytren disease?**

1. Steroid injections
2. Splinting and skeletal traction
3. Ultrasound therapy
4. Laser therapy
5. Collagenase and enzymatic fasciotomy

○ **How successful is the nonsurgical treatment?**

Recent evidence has shown collagenase injections to be a promising alternative to surgery. In early trials, the safety profile is promising and the recurrence rates after injections appear to be low. At the time of this writing, collagenase therapy is Food and Drug Administration approved for Dupuytren contractures of both the MP and PIP joints.

○ **What are the indications for surgery?**

1. MCP contracture of 30 degrees or more

2. Any PIP contracture

3. Severe adduction contracture

○ **What is the tabletop test?**

Described by Hueston, it simply tests the patient's ability to place the palm flat on a tabletop. Once they cannot, some surgeons recommend surgery.

○ **What are some of the functional tasks that a patient with Dupuytren contractures may complain of?**

Retrieving an object from a pocket, wearing a glove.

○ **What are the three aspects to be considered in the surgical treatment of Dupuytren disease?**

1. Management of the skin.

2. Management of the fascia.

3. Management of the wound.

○ **What does management of the skin involve?**

It involves the skin incision either transverse or longitudinal (linear, zigzag, or lazy S).

○ **What does management of the fascia involve?**

Either can be used:

1. incision (fasciectomy)

2. local excision (regional fasciectomy)

3. wide excision (extensive radical fasciectomy)

○ **What does management of the wound involve?**

The wound is sutured, left open, or skin grafted.

○ **What is percutaneous needle fasciotomy (PNF)?**

A technique first described by Cooper, it involves performing an aponeurotomy of the diseased fascia using a needle. Several percutaneous stab incisions are made in the cord using the needle to "cut" or puncture the cord in the palm and/or digit, while passive extension of the finger assists in releasing the contractures (Figs. 33-1 to 33-4).

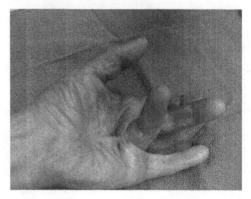

Figure 33-1 A 90-degree MP joint flexion contracture.

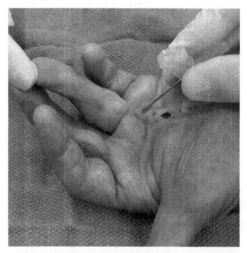

Figure 33-2 Percutaneous needle fasciotomy.

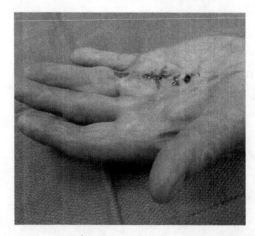

Figure 33-3 Full extension following percutaneous release.

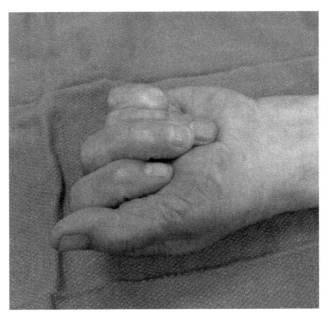

Figure 33-4 Full flexion following percutaneous release.

○ **What are the results of PNF?**

van Rijssen treated 88 rays by PNF and 78 rays by open-limited fasciectomy. Follow-up was 6 weeks. The total passive extension deficit improved by 63% in the PNF group, and 79% in the limited fasciectomy group. The results favored the limited fasciectomy group with larger preoperative flexion contractures. The rates of major complications were 5% in the limited fasciectomy group, and 0% in the PNF group. The authors concluded that in cases of total passive extension deficit of 90 degrees or less, PNF is a very good treatment option.

○ **What is dermatofasciectomy?**

Wide excision of the involved palmar and digital skin and fascia combined with skin grafting.

○ **What are possible indications for skin grafting?**

1. Patients with Dupuytren diathesis.
2. Patients with recurrent PIP joint contracture.
3. Patients with primary, severe PIP contracture resulting in skin deficiency at closure once the joint has been restored to extension.

○ **What is the difference between extension and recurrence of the disease?**

Extension refers to the postoperative appearance of the disease in an area of the hand not involved in the surgery. Recurrence refers to postoperative appearance of the disease in the area of previous surgery.

○ **Mention some complications of the surgery.**

1. Neurovascular bundle injury

2. Hematoma and skin necrosis

3. Joint stiffness

4. Reflex sympathetic dystrophy

5. Recurrent or uncorrected deformity

○ **What is the postoperative management?**

1. Operated hand usually splinted in extension.

2. Wound care and frequent dressing changes.

3. Active and passive range-of-motion exercises postoperatively.

4. Splinting varies depending on the surgical technique used.

5. PIP joint usually need 6 weeks of full-time splinting and at least 3 months of night splinting.

● ● ● REFERENCES ● ● ●

Benson LS, Williams CS, Kahle M. Dupuytren's contracture. *J Am Acad Orthop Surg.* 1998;6(1):24–35.

Budalamente MA, Hurst LC. Efficacy and safety of injectable mixed collagenase subtypes in the treatment of Dupuytren's contracture. *J Hand Surg Am.* 2007;32:767–774.

Foucher G, Medina J, Navarro R. Percutaneous needle aponeurotomy: complications and results. *J Hand Surg Br.* 2003;28:427–431.

Gonzalez F, Watson HK. Simultaneous carpal tunnel release and Dupuytren's fasciectomy. *J Hand Surg Br.* 1991;16:175–178.

Hurst LN. Dupuytren's contracture. In: Achauer BM, Ericksson E, Guyuron B, et al., eds. *Plastic Surgery Indications, Operations and Outcomes.* Vol 4. St Louis, MO: Mosby; 2000:2057–2071.

Lubahn JD. Dupuytren's disease. In: Trumble TE, ed. *Hand Surgery Update 3 Hand, Elbow and Shoulder.* Rosemont: American Society for Surgery of the Hand; 2003:393–401.

Lubahn JD. Dupuytren's disease. In: Trumble TE, Budoff JE, Cornwall R, eds. *Hand, Elbow and Shoulder: Core Knowledge in Orthopaedics.* Philadelphia, PA: Mosby; 2006:279–287.

Macfarlane RM, Ross DC. Dupuytren's disease. In: Weinzweig J, ed. *Plastic Surgery Secrets.* Philadelphia, PA: Hanley and Belfus; 1999:554–559.

McGrouther DA. Dupuytren's contracture. In: Green DP, Hotchkiss RN, Pederson WC, eds. *Green's Operative Hand Surgery.* Vol 1. 4th ed. New York, NY: Churchill Livingstone; 1999:563–591.

Michon J. Serious postoperative complications in Dupuytren's disease. *J Hand Surg.* 1977;2:238.

Nissenbaum M, Kleinert HE. Treatment considerations in carpal tunnel syndrome with coexistent Dupuytren's disease. *J Hand Surg Am.* 1980;5:544–547.

Short WH, Watson HK. Prediction of the spiral nerve in Dupuytren's contracture. *J Hand Surg Am.* 1982;7:84–86.

van Rijssen AL, Gerbrandy FS, Tinden HT, Klip H, Werker PM. A comparison of the direct outcomes of percutaneous needle fasciotomy and limited fasciectomy for Dupuytren's disease: a six-week follow-up study. *J Hand Surg Am.* 2006;31:717–725.

Zachariae L. Dupuytren's contracture. The aetiological role of trauma. *Scan J Plast Reconstr Surg.* 1971;5:116–119.

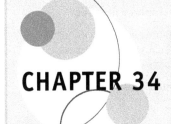

CHAPTER 34
Nerve Compression Syndromes

Trenton M. Morton, MD and
Jeffrey B. Friedrich, MD, FACS

○ **How is nerve conduction in the carpal tunnel reported?**

Nerve conduction is reported as "latency" in milliseconds (ms).

○ **What is "latency"?**

Latency is the time it takes for an electrical stimulus to travel along a nerve from the site of stimulation to a recording electrode in a target muscle.

○ **What is the normal value for motor latency at the carpal tunnel?**

Less than 4.0 ms.

○ **How is nerve conduction at the elbow reported?**

Nerve conduction is reported as velocity in meters per second (m/s).

○ **What is a clinically significant decrease in velocity at the elbow?**

A decrease in velocity of 10 m/s or more is considered clinically significant.

○ **What is the difference between compressive neuropathies and peripheral neuropathies?**

In peripheral (systemic) neuropathies, the nerve conduction is decreased diffusely both proximally and distally in multiple nerves. In compressive neuropathies nerve conduction is decreased distal to the site of compression.

○ **What are typical electromyography (EMG) findings for long-standing nerve compression and axonal damage?**

EMG will demonstrate wide biphasic fibrillation potentials in the presence of long-standing nerve compression with axonal damage.

○ **What is double crush syndrome?**

The double crush syndrome hypothesizes that a site of proximal nerve compression in series with a site of distal compression of the same nerve results in clinical neuropathy; whereas independently, neither site of compression is severe enough to result in clinical neuropathy.

○ **What is the treatment of choice for an ulnar neuroma-in-continuity with intact motor function?**

The current optimal therapy involves micro-dissection of the neuroma using electrostimulation to identify and preserve motor fascicles. En bloc resection of the neuroma is inappropriate, as this would sacrifice intact nerve fascicles.

○ **What are some nonsurgical modalities that can be used to desensitize an amputation stump neuroma?**

Vibration, massage, and transcutaneous nerve stimulation.

○ **What is complex regional pain syndrome?**

Complex regional pain syndrome (CRPS) is recognized as a constellation of symptoms including pain at rest, vasomotor instability, and swelling that results in functional impairment of the affected hand or limb. It is usually the result of previous limb trauma or surgery.

○ **What diagnostic study can help establish the diagnosis of CRPS?**

Three-phase bone scintigraphy has been shown to be highly specific for the diagnosis of CRPS in the upper limb.

● ● ● **ULNAR NERVE** ● ● ●

THORACIC OUTLET SYNDROME

○ **What nerve is affected with thoracic outlet syndrome (TOS)?**

Lower trunk of brachial plexus with symptoms mimicking cubital tunnel syndrome.

○ **What are the contents of the "thoracic outlet"?**

Subclavian vein, subclavian artery, and brachial plexus.

○ **In what gender is TOS more prevalent?**

Female (3.5:1).

○ **Among the population of patients with cervical ribs, how many are bilateral?**

50%.

○ **When do patients with TOS typically get their symptoms (ulnar-sided numbness)?**

Patient's symptoms worsen when their hands are elevated above their head.

○ **What is Adson maneuver?**

Dampening of radial pulse with inhalation, neck extension, and head rotation to the affected side in patients with TOS. There are varying descriptions of how to perform this maneuver.

○ **How accurate is an Adson maneuver?**

False positives are very common and thus the Adson maneuver is valued in terms of historical interest only.

○ **What is Wright maneuver?**

The Wright maneuver is reproduction of TOS symptoms and/or dampening of radial pulse with arm hyper-abducted with the patient's head positioned in neutral or turned contralateral.

○ **How accurate is Wright maneuver?**

The Wright maneuver is positive in 7% of normal patients thus should be used only to support a diagnosis of compression in patients with arterial symptoms.

○ **What is Roos maneuver?**

The Roos maneuver involves placing both arms into 90 degrees of abduction and external rotation and the patient is asked to open and close the hands for 3 minutes. Patients with TOS have reproduction of their symptoms, while those without TOS generally experience forearm fatigue.

○ **How accurate is Roos maneuver?**

Of the three maneuvers described, the Roos is the most accurate. However, some patients with carpal tunnel syndrome (CTS) and no TOS will develop symptoms limited to the median nerve distribution.

○ **What are the electrodiagnostic testing results seen with TOS?**

Negative EMG for ulnar nerve, positive somatosensory-evoked potentials with arm in offending position.

○ **What is the first-line therapy for TOS?**

Conservative treatment with exercises to strengthen the shoulder girdle, weight loss, and occasionally breast reduction in women are first line.

○ **Name the two approaches to the thoracic outlet.**

Supraclavicular and transaxillary.

○ **What is similar and what is different about the presentation of TOS and cubital tunnel syndrome?**

Both TOS and cubital syndrome can present with ulnar distribution numbness, although TOS also presents with medial forearm numbness whereas cubital tunnel syndrome does not.

CUBITAL TUNNEL COMPRESSION

○ **How do you tell the difference between ulnar nerve compression at the cubital tunnel from compression at the wrist (Guyon canal)?**

Diminished sensation on the dorsoulnar hand is present with cubital tunnel syndrome. This is due to the fact that the dorsal sensory branch of the ulnar nerve exits the ulnar nerve approximately 7 cm proximal to the pisiform, to provide sensation to the dorsoulnar hand.

○ **What is the distribution of motor weakness seen with cubital tunnel syndrome?**

Motor weakness is seen in the flexor digitorum profundus (FDP) of ring and small fingers, as well as the ulnar intrinsic muscles.

○ **Describe Froment sign.**

With ulnar nerve palsy, patients compensate for lack of adductor pollicis (ulnar innervated) function by flexing the thumb interphalangeal (IP) joint (pinch power is then provided entirely by the median-innervated flexor pollicis longus [FPL]).

○   **What are potential sites of ulnar nerve compression?**

See Figure 34-1.

1. <u>Arcade of Struthers</u>—an upper arm fascial arcade through which the nerve passes. Present in 70% of patients.

2. <u>Intermuscular septum</u> between the brachialis and medial head of triceps. Can cause compression even in the absence of arcade of Struthers so they are distinct.

3. <u>Medial head of triceps</u>—can cause compression by triceps hypertrophy (bodybuilders) or anterior subluxation of the ulnar nerve over medial epicondyle.

4. <u>Osborne ligament</u>—Most common site of ulnar nerve compression. This is a fascial arcade formed between the two heads of the flexor carpi ulnaris (FCU).

5. <u>Flexor-pronator aponeurosis</u>—a fascial band between the flexor digitorum superficialis (FDS) and the FDP.

6. <u>Guyon canal</u>—Second most common site of ulnar nerve compression. Located at the wrist (see Fig. 34-1).

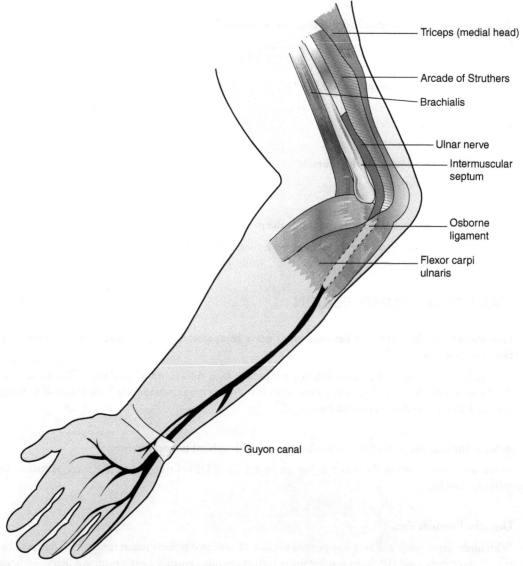

Figure 34-1 Potential sites of ulnar compression.

○ **Where is the arcade of Struthers?**

Located 8 cm proximal to the medial epicondyle of the elbow.

○ **What are the boundaries of the cubital tunnel?**

Floor—medial collateral ligament of elbow (spans from medial epicondyle to olecranon).
Roof—Osborne ligament.
Sides—medial epicondyle and olecranon (to which the above two structures attach).

○ **Explain why the elbow hyperflexion test elicits symptoms of cubital tunnel syndrome?**

Elbow flexion increases the distance the ulnar nerve has to travel to traverse the elbow.

Try it yourself: Palpate your own olecranon and medial epicondyle with your elbow extended. Now flex your elbow and notice how the distance between them grows, tightening Osborne ligament and compressing the nerve.

○ **How sensitive is electrodiagnostic testing at the elbow?**

Electrodiagnostic testing has a 50% false-negative rate for nerve compression at the elbow.

○ **What is a Martin–Gruber anastomosis, and what is its significance in relation to cubital tunnel syndrome?**

Naturally occurring anatomic variant involving an interconnection between the median and ulnar nerves at the level of the forearm. The presence of this anomalous interconnection can result in spared intrinsic muscle function with cubital tunnel syndrome (because the median nerve innervates the intrinsics in this situation).

○ **What is a Riche–Cannieu anastomosis?**

Naturally occurring anatomic variant involving an interconnection between the median and ulnar nerve in the hand, typically the deep or motor branch of the ulnar nerve. Again, there may be confusion for the examiner as muscles usually innervated by the ulnar nerve continue to function.

○ **What are the key steps involved in anterior submuscular ulnar nerve transposition?**

Release of FCU origin, transposition of ulnar nerve anterior to medial epicondyle, resuturing of FCU to epicondyle.

○ **Must you do a submuscular transposition of the nerve when performing a cubital tunnel release?**

Maybe not. In 1957, Geoffrey Osborne, a British orthopedic surgeon, reported 13 cases of cubital tunnel syndrome in which he released the ligament or band that now bears his name noting that it was tight in elbow flexion but lax in extension. These patients did no differently than those patients having a formal transposition. Several studies since then have supported this finding.

○ **What is the other common ulnar nerve transposition method?**

The ulnar nerve may be transposed subcutaneously.

○ **What is a common postoperative complication of ulnar nerve surgery at the cubital tunnel that generally results in a painful incision?**

Injury to the medial antebrachial cutaneous nerve can result in painful neuroma formation.

○ **What are the boundaries of the Guyon canal?**

Roof: volar carpal ligament proximally and palmaris brevis distally.

Floor: transverse carpal ligament.

Ulnar wall: pisiform.

Radial wall: less well established, although some consider the hamate hook the radial border despite the fact that in many specimens the ulnar neurovascular bundle lies palmar or even radial to the hamate hook.

○ **What are the usual causes of ulnar tunnel syndrome?**

Ganglions, trauma (hamate fractures), tumors, vascular anomalies, arthritis.

○ **What is the distribution of numbness with ulnar tunnel syndrome?**

Small and ring fingers, but not dorsum of hand (because dorsal sensory branch originates proximal to the Guyon canal).

○ **How does the motor examination differ between ulnar nerve compression at the wrist and the elbow?**

Ulnar nerve compression at the wrist affects pinch strength but not grip strength; compression at the elbow affects both pinch and grip strength.

○ **In general, what is the treatment for ulnar tunnel syndrome?**

Exploration of the Guyon canal, decompression of nerve, removal of space-occupying lesion(s), and ulnar artery reconstruction (if necessary). It is important to palpate for masses intraoperatively as they are responsible for 30% to 45% of all cases of ulnar tunnel syndrome.

○ **What ligaments must be released when surgically treating ulnar tunnel syndrome?**

Release the pisohamate ligament and volar carpal ligament.

○ **In what portion of the ulnar nerve cross-section is the motor fascicle at the level of the wrist?**

Ulnar and dorsal.

● ● ● **MEDIAN NERVE** ● ● ●

○ **What are the syndromes associated with median nerve compression?**

1. Pronator syndrome
2. Anterior interosseous syndrome
3. CTS

○ **What conditions are associated with an increased incidence of CTS?**

Most cases of CTS are idiopathic, but it can be associated with pregnancy, diabetes, alcoholism, arthritis, amyloidosis, or thyroid disorders.

○ **How often is CTS bilateral?**

60% of cases of CTS are bilateral.

○ **What are the borders of the carpal tunnel?**

1. Roof—transverse carpal ligament
2. Floor—carpal bones and their ligaments
3. Radial wall—trapezium and scaphoid tubercle
4. Ulnar wall—hook of hamate

○ **Describe the classic symptoms of CTS.**

Classic symptoms of CTS are numbness in the median nerve distribution (index, middle, radial side of ring finger), weakness, nocturnal pain, and relief of symptoms while wearing a wrist brace.

○ **What are the structures thought to cause effort-associated CTS (i.e., symptoms seen with repetitive gripping)?**

Lumbrical muscles. They originate from the FDP tendons and reside within the carpal tunnel during gripping activities which can exacerbate CTS.

○ **What is Phalen's test?**

Wrist is passively dropped into flexion. If symptoms are seen within 30 seconds, the test is positive.

○ **What is the most sensitive physical examination maneuver for diagnosis of CTS?**

Carpal compression test.

○ **How are results of the carpal compression test reported?**

Report the result of the carpal compression test in number of seconds from initiation of thumb pressure over the carpal tunnel (pressure should only be hard enough to make examiner's thumb blanch).

○ **What electrodiagnostic study results signify median nerve conduction changes?**

Median nerve latency increase of 10% or more above that of the ulnar nerve.

○ **What electrodiagnostic study result signifies muscle denervation with CTS?**

Fibrillation potentials in the abductor pollicis brevis signify muscle denervation.

○ **What is the earliest one might expect to see electromyographic changes after suspected nerve damage?**

EMG studies will typically be altered around 2 to 3 weeks after the nerve injury.

○ **What is the success rate of steroid injections for CTS?**

Only approximately 20% to 22% of patients get long-term (>18 months) relief.

○ **Where is the median nerve located in the proximal forearm?**

Between the superficial (humeral) and deep (ulnar) heads of the pronator teres muscle.

○ **Where is the motor fascicle of the median nerve cross-section at the wrist?**

Radial and volar. This should be easy to remember since the recurrent motor branch of the median nerve comes off of the main nerve radially and palmarly. In addition, remember that the median nerve motor fascicle (radial, volar) is the direct opposite of the ulnar nerve motor fascicle (ulnar, dorsal).

○ **What is Kaplan's line and how is it used to determine the position of the motor branch of the median nerve?**

Kaplan's line is a line drawn as an extension along the ulnar border of the abducted thumb. The intersection of Kaplan's line and one drawn longitudinally from the index–middle finger web space is the rough approximation of the entrance of the recurrent motor branch of the median nerve into the thenar musculature.

○ **What are the patterns of the route of the motor branch to the thenar musculature in relation to the transverse carpal ligament?**

Extraligamentous (approximately 50%), subligamentous (30%), and transligamentous (20–25%).

○ **Which muscles are innervated by the motor branch of the median nerve in the hand?**

1. Opponens pollicis
2. Flexor pollicis brevis
3. Abductor pollicis brevis
4. Two radial lumbrical muscles

○ **What are the advantages of endoscopic carpal tunnel release when compared with the open technique?**

Early postoperative differences include decreased scar tenderness, and earlier restoration of grip and pinch strength. After 3 months postoperatively, there are no differences.

○ **What has been demonstrated as the chief disadvantage of endoscopic carpal tunnel release when compared to open?**

Endoscopic carpal tunnel release carries a slightly higher incidence of reversible nerve injury like neuropraxia and numbness.

○ **Which outcomes between endoscopic and open carpal tunnel release have been found to be equivocal?**

Pain and return to work.

○ **Is internal neurolysis indicated during routine carpal tunnel decompression?**

No.

○ **During secondary surgery for recurrent CTS, where should the incision be made?**

A new incision should be made more ulnar to the previous scar because the median nerve is adherent to or within the transverse carpal ligament.

○ **What are sites of median nerve compression in the elbow/forearm?**

1. Ligament of Struthers—ligament located between humeral supracondylar process and medial epicondyle
2. Lacertus fibrosis—aka bicipital aponeurosis—a fascial band between the biceps tendon and the fascia of the flexor pronator mass
3. Two heads of the pronator teres
4. FDS fibrous arch

○ **How can one specifically test for median nerve compression at the ligament of Struthers?**

The symptoms are exacerbated when flexing the elbow against resistance.

○ **How can one specifically test for median nerve compression at the pronator teres?**

Have the patient fully extend their elbow and pronate their forearm while the examiner introduces resistance to patient pronation. With resisted pronation, symptoms are exacerbated. The elbow must be fully extended to avoid confusion with compression by the bicipital aponeurosis.

○ **How can one specifically test for median nerve compression at the FDS arch?**

Long finger flexion test: with resisted flexion of the long finger, the FDS arch compresses the median nerve, and symptoms are exacerbated.

○ **What is a Gantzer muscle?**

An accessory head of the FPL originating from the medial humeral epicondyle and possibly the coronoid process of the ulna. This muscle is found in up to 45% of specimens and can contribute to compression of the median nerve.

○ **What is the chief difference between the pronator syndrome and the anterior interosseous nerve (AIN) syndrome?**

Deficits in pronator syndrome are sensory, whereas AIN syndrome demonstrates motor deficits.

○ **What are the symptoms of the pronator syndrome?**

Pain in forearm, numbness in median nerve sensory distribution (thumb, index, and middle fingers).

○ **What muscles are innervated by the AIN?**

1. FPL
2. Pronator quadratus
3. FDP to index finger
4. FDP to middle finger (this varies between the AIN and ulnar nerve depending on the patient)

○ **What are the symptoms of AIN syndrome?**

Loss of precision pinch (cannot flex thumb IP or index DIP) and pain in the forearm relieved by rest are the classic symptoms of AIN syndrome.

○ **What can patients with AIN syndrome NOT do?**

Make an "OK" sign. They cannot flex their thumb IP or index DIP joints.

○ **Is there a difference in the surgical treatment of AIN syndrome and pronator syndrome?**

No. In both cases the nerve is explored completely and released from all compressing structures from the elbow to the distal forearm.

• • • RADIAL NERVE • • •

○ **What are possible sites of radial nerve compression?**

See Figure 34-2.

1. The lateral humeral intermuscular septum

2. The radial head

3. Supinator fascia—aka arcade of Fröhse (posterior interosseous nerve [PIN] syndrome)

4. Vascular Leash of Henry—radial recurrent vessels at the elbow

5. Extensor carpi radialis brevis (ECRB) origin

6. Between brachioradialis and extensor carpi radialis longus (ECRL)—Wartenberg syndrome (involves the superficial sensory branch of the radial nerve only)

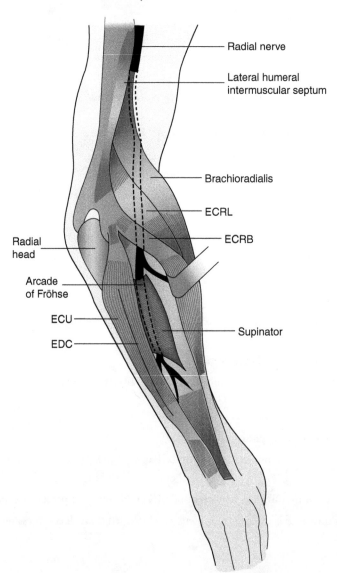

Figure 34-2 Potential sites of radial nerve compression.

○   **What is the most common site of radial nerve compression?**

Supinator muscle fascia (aka the arcade of Fröhse).

○   **Where is the radial tunnel?**

It runs from the radial head to the distal edge of the supinator; the biceps tendon is the medial wall, and the ECRL and ECRB origins form the lateral wall.

○   **How is the radial nerve approached in the dorsal forearm?**

The radial nerve can be approached between the ECRB and the extensor digitorum communis.

○   **What are the symptoms of radial tunnel syndrome?**

Lateral elbow pain, especially with repetitive elbow extension. Motor findings are usually absent.

○   **What physical examination finding differentiates radial tunnel syndrome from lateral epicondylitis?**

Tenderness 4 cm distal to lateral epicondyle (between brachioradialis and ECRL) is seen with radial tunnel syndrome.

○   **Is there typically a sensory component to PIN syndrome?**

No. The PIN innervates the extensors, and therefore results in weakness and pain, but not sensory deficits.

○   **What is the difference between radial tunnel syndrome and PIN compression?**

In radial tunnel syndrome symptoms involve pain over the dorsoradial forearm near the elbow. There is rarely weakness.

In PIN compression symptoms include weakness of the thumb and finger extensors AS WELL AS pain.

○   **Is it common to see electrodiagnostic changes with radial nerve compression?**

Often the EMG/NCS is normal, thus electrodiagnostic studies are of little use in evaluating radial nerve compression. Diagnosis is often based solely on history and physical examination.

○   **What is the role for surgery in PIN syndrome and radial tunnel syndrome?**

Radial tunnel syndrome should be initially managed nonoperatively (muscle palsy is not seen with this syndrome); PIN syndrome should be treated operatively to prevent permanent muscle palsy.

○   **What is the vascular leash of Henry?**

The vascular leash of Henry is a network of radial recurrent vessels at the elbow that can compress the PIN, the radial sensory nerve, or both.

○   **What is Wartenberg syndrome?**

Wartenberg syndrome is a compression neuropathy of the radial sensory nerve due to entrapment between the brachioradialis and ECRL. Other names include superficial radial neuritis or "cheiralgia paresthetica."

○ **What can cause Wartenberg syndrome?**

It is generally caused by external compression (handcuffs), tight watch, surgical scarring, or repetitive activities.

○ **What is Wartenberg sign?**

Wartenberg sign indicates <u>ulnar</u> neuropathy and is seen when the small finger is unable to adduct. The patient is unable to hold the small finger against the ring finger with the fingers in extension due to the unopposed action of the <u>radially innervated</u> extensor digiti minimi. The <u>ulnarly innervated</u> palmar interossei is weak and unable to adduct the small finger.

○ **How does one differentiate radial sensory nerve compression from de Quervain extensor tenosynovitis in the presence of a positive Finkelstein sign?**

Resisted thumb extension with the wrist held in neutral causes <u>pain</u> in tendinitis but not in nerve entrapment.

○ **What is Volkmann's contracture?**

Volkmann's contracture is the sequelae of forearm compartment syndrome generally following a supracondylar humerus fracture that results in a severely contracted forearm and hand. Generally the forearm is fixed in pronated, the wrist is flexed, MCP joints are hyperextended and the IP joints are flexed forming a nonfunctional claw hand.

○ **How high must forearm compartment pressures be and for how long in order to develop Volkmann's contracture?**

Compartment pressures >30 mm Hg for at least 6 to 12 hours generally are necessary to result in sequelae of Volkmann's contracture.

○ **What muscles are most at risk of ischemic sequelae with forearm compartment syndrome?**

The FDP muscle within the deep muscle compartment is most at risk of the sequelae of ischemia.

○ **What is the treatment of Volkmann's contracture?**

Moderate Volkmann's contractures are treated with operative exploration of the forearm with neurolysis of the median and ulnar nerves as well as a muscle slide tendon-lengthening procedure.

• • • REFERENCES • • •

Botte MJ, Keenan MA, Gelberman RH. Volkmann's ischemic contracture of the upper extremity. *Hand Clin*. 1998;14(3):483–497

Botte MJ. Nerve anatomy. In: Doyle JR, Botte MJ, eds. *Surgical Anatomy of the Hand and Upper Extremity*. 1st ed. Philadelphia, PA: Lippincott Williams & Wilkins; 2003:185–236.

Durkan JA. A new diagnostic test for carpal tunnel syndrome. *J Bone Joint Surg Am*. 1991;73(4):535–538.

Fitzgerald BT, Dao KD, Shin AY. Functional outcomes in young, active duty military personnel after submuscular ulnar nerve transposition. *J Hand Surg Am*. 2004;29(4):619–624.

Heithoff SJ. Cubital tunnel syndrome does not require transposition of the ulnar nerve. *J Hand Surg Am*. 1999;24(5):898–905.

Lowe JB III, Mackinnon SE. Management of secondary cubital tunnel syndrome. *Plast Reconstr Surg*. 2004;113(1):1e-16e.

Lowry WE Jr, Follender AB. Interfascicular neurolysis in the severe carpal tunnel syndrome. A prospective, randomized, double-blind, controlled study. *Clin Orthop Relat Res*. 1988;227:251–254.

Nath RK, Mackinnon SE. Management of neuromas in the hand. *Hand Clin.* 1996;12(4):745–756.

Posner MA. Compressive ulnar neuropathies at the elbow: I. Etiology and diagnosis. *J Am Acad Orthop Surg.* 1998;6(5):282–288.

Szabo RM. Entrapment and compression neuropathies. In: Green DP, Hotchkiss RN, Pederson WC, eds. *Green's Operative Hand Surgery.* 4th ed. Philadelphia, PA: Churchill Livingstone; 1993:1404–1447.

Thoma A, Veltri K, Haines T, Duku E. A meta-analysis of randomized controlled trials comparing endoscopic and open carpal tunnel decompression. *Plast Recon Surg.* 2004;114(5):1137–1146.

Thoma A, Veltri K, Haines T, Duku E. A systematic review of reviews comparing the effectiveness of endoscopic and open carpal tunnel decompression. *Plast Reconstr Surg.* 2004;113(4):1184–1191.

Trumble TE. Compressive neuropathies. In: Trumble TE, ed. *Principles of Hand Surgery and Therapy.* 1st ed. Philadelphia, PA: WB Saunders; 2000:324–341.

Wüppenhorst N Maier C, Frettlöh J, Pennekamp W, Nicolas V. Sensitivity and specificity of 3-phase bone scintigraphy in the diagnosis of complex regional pain syndrome of the upper extremity. *Clin J Pain.* 2010;26(3):182–189.

Żyluk A, Puchalski P. Complex regional pain syndrome of the upper limb: a review. *Neurol I Neurochir Pol.* 2014;48:200–205.

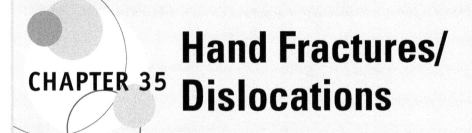

CHAPTER 35
Hand Fractures/ Dislocations

Pieter G.L. Koolen, MD,
John B. Hijjawi, MD, FACS, and
Samuel J. Lin, MD, MBA, FACS

○ **What three structures provide the greatest stability to the proximal interphalangeal (PIP) joint?**

The three-sided box configuration of the medial and lateral collateral ligaments and the volar plate.

○ **What is the classification of Mallet fractures of the finger?**

Type 1: closed tendon avulsion with or without fracture

Type 2: laceration with extensor tendon disruption

Type 3: open injury with loss of skin and tendon substance

Type 4: physeal fracture in children

○ **What is the treatment of choice for a displaced fracture of the dorsal base of the distal phalanx comprising over 25% of the articular surface?**

Operative intervention with closed or open reduction and internal fixation.

○ **What is the treatment of choice for a volar base fracture of the distal phalanx with loss of the flexor digitorum profundus insertion?**

Open reduction and internal fixation.

○ **What is the acceptable angulation for metacarpal shaft fractures (index, middle, ring, and little)?**

1. Index metacarpal: 10 to 15 degrees

2. Middle metacarpal: 10 to 15 degrees

3. Ring metacarpal: 30 to 35 degrees

4. Small metacarpal: 40 to 45 degrees

○ **What is the most likely direction of angulation of an unstable transverse metacarpal shaft fracture?**

Apex dorsal angulation due to the volar directed pull of the interosseous muscles.

○ **What are some indications for operative fixation of phalangeal and metacarpal fractures?**

- Malrotation
- Irreducible fractures
- Intra-articular fractures
- Open fractures
- Fractures with bone loss
- Fractures with associated tendon, vascular or nerve injury
- Polytrauma patients

○ **How does one assess for malrotation in phalangeal and metacarpal fractures?**

The hand is assessed with the fingers in extension and flexion. In extension the fingers should be parallel and in flexion they should all point toward the scaphoid tuberosity. Malrotation would present as subtle overlap or scissoring of the fingers.

○ **What is the number one complication of operatively treated phalangeal fractures?**

Digital stiffness.

○ **What is the most likely block to reduction in a complex dorsal dislocation of the metacarpophalangeal (MCP) joint?**

Volar plate.

○ **What two structures act as a noose around the metacarpal head in an irreducible (complex) dorsal dislocation of the index MCP joint?**

The flexor tendons (ulnarly) and the lumbricals (radially) maintain a tight encirclement around the narrow neck of the metacarpal preventing reduction.

○ **In a Bennett fracture, what is the deforming force that causes proximal migration of the thumb metacarpal?**

Abductor pollicis longus.

○ **What is a Stener lesion?**

A Stener lesion is formed when the distally avulsed ulnar collateral ligament of the thumb MCP joint comes to lie dorsal to the leading edge of the adductor aponeurosis.

○ **What are the most reasonable treatment options for a fracture/dislocation of the PIP joint with a severely comminuted volar base fracture of the middle phalanx involving 40% of the joint surface?**

Volar plate arthroplasty or Suzuki-type dynamic external fixation/traction.

○ **In volar dislocation of the PIP joint, what commonly associated injury must be examined for?**

Rupture or avulsion of the extensor tendon central slip.

○ **What is the treatment for a fifth metacarpal neck fracture (Boxer fracture) with 40 degrees of apex dorsal angulation?**

40 degrees is the maximal angulation acceptable; however, some would suggest attempted closed reduction to improve angulation and ulnar gutter splinting.

○ **What is the most common carpal bone fractured?**

Scaphoid fractures account for 80% of all carpal bone fractures.

○ **Describe the anatomy of the major blood supply to the scaphoid.**

The major blood supply is from branches of the radial artery that enter the dorsal ridge of the scaphoid (distal to the scaphoid waist). This blood supply accounts for 70% to 80% of the total blood supply of the scaphoid and 100% of the blood supply to the proximal pole.

○ **What is snuffbox tenderness?**

Tenderness on palpation of the anatomic snuffbox (interval between the tendons of the first and third dorsal compartments distal to the radial styloid), which may indicate fracture of the scaphoid.

○ **What is a scaphoid humpback deformity?**

The apex dorsal angulation seen with a scaphoid waist nonunion or malunion. The distal scaphoid fragment angulates volarly and the proximal scaphoid fragment extends with the lunate.

○ **What type of carpal instability is seen most commonly with a malunited scaphoid (humpback deformity)?**

Dorsal intercalated segment instability is visualized on a lateral radiograph as the proximal scaphoid fragment extends with the lunate.

○ **What is the definition of scaphoid fracture displacement or instability?**

- Presence of a fracture gap of greater than 1 mm on any radiographic projection
- Scapholunate angle of greater than 60 degrees
- Radiolunate angle of greater than 15 degrees
- Intrascaphoid angle of greater than 30 degrees

○ **What is the space of Poirier?**

A palmar area of inherent capsular weakness between the capitate and lunate, which is torn in perilunate injuries creating a capsular rent across the midcarpal joint.

○ **What is Mayfield's progressive sequence of perilunate disruption or dislocation?**

Stage I: disruption of the scapholunate interosseous ligament complex

Stage II: disruption through the space of Poirier and the lunocapitate interval

Stage III: disruption of the lunotriquetral ligament complex and resultant separation of the entire carpus from the lunate

Stage IV: dislocation of the lunate from its fossa in to the carpal tunnel

○ **What is a "lesser arc" injury?**

This type of injury refers to a purely ligamentous disruption around the lunate.

○ **What is a "greater arc" injury?**

This type of injury refers to disruption around the lunate that involves fractures of some or all of the carpal bones.

○ **What is the most common "greater arc" injury?**

A trans-scaphoid perilunate fracture—dislocation.

○ **What is the normal intracarpal angle between the scaphoid and lunate (scapholunate angle)?**

Between 30 and 60 degrees.

○ **What is the most sensitive and specific test for assessment of posttraumatic avascular necrosis of the scaphoid?**

Magnetic resonance imaging—MRI with gadolinium.

○ **What is scaphocapitate syndrome?**

Fracture of the neck of the capitate with rotation of the proximal fragment in association with a scaphoid waist fracture.

○ **What is carpal instability dissociative?**

Refers to intrinsic ligament disruptions that occur between carpal bones of the same carpal row (i.e., scapholunate dissociation caused by a scapholunate ligament tear).

○ **What is carpal instability nondissociative?**

Refers to extrinsic ligament disruptions that occur between carpal rows (i.e., midcarpal instability).

○ **What is Watson scaphoid shift test?**

The test assesses for scapholunate ligament dissociation. The examiner applies dorsally directed thumb pressure over the patient's distal scaphoid tubercle. If the SL ligament is torn, pain is elicited when the proximal pole of the scaphoid subluxates dorsally out of the scaphoid fossa of the radius as the patient's hand is passively moved from ulnar deviation to radial deviation.

○ **What is a Terry-Thomas sign?**

Increased gap between the scaphoid and lunate, greater than 3 mm, indicative of a scapholunate dissociation.

○ **On a PA wrist radiograph, what are findings of scapholunate dissociation?**

- Terry-Thomas sign
- Cortical ring sign
- Reduced carpal height
- Triangular shaped lunate
- Foreshortened scaphoid

○ **What are Gilula lines?**

Gilula et al. described three smooth curved lines on a PA projection of the carpus. The first line represents the proximal cortical surfaces of the proximal carpal row. The second line represents the distal cortical surfaces of the proximal carpal row and the third line represents the proximal cortical surfaces of the distal carpal row. A step-off or disruption in any of these lines may indicate carpal malalignment or instability.

○ **What radiographic projection would best visualize a hook of hamate fracture?**

Carpal tunnel profile view.

○ **What is the treatment of choice for a symptomatic hook of hamate nonunion?**

Excision of the hamate hook.

○ **What is the "safe" position of immobilization for the hand?**

The "safe" position or the intrinsic-plus position of James is 70 degrees of MCP joint flexion and full IP joint extension.

○ **What is the Salter–Harris classification of physeal injuries?**

Salter–Harris classification:

Type I: transverse fracture through the physis

Type II: fracture through the physis with a metaphyseal fragment

Type III: fracture through the physis and in to the epiphysis (intra-articular)

Type IV: fracture through the physis, epiphysis, and metaphysis

Type V: crush injury of the physis

○ **What radiographic projections would best visualize the position of a screw in the proximal pole of the scaphoid?**

To best visualize the proximal pole, an ulnar-deviated posteroanterior view and a true lateral radiograph.

○ **What is the treatment of choice for a scaphoid fracture that is 1.5 mm displaced?**

Open reduction and internal fixation with a compression screw.

○ **What is an important factor to consider, other than the degree of intra-articular step, when deciding to operate on a bony mallet finger?**

Distal phalanx subluxation.

○ **What is the most likely direction of a CMC dislocation of the thumb?**

Dorsal.

○ **What is the most likely direction of angulation of an unstable transverse proximal phalanx shaft fracture?**

Proximal phalangeal fractures, typically angulated apex volar.

○ **What is the structure at risk when treating a hook of hamate nonunion?**

Motor branch of the ulnar nerve.

○ **Trans-trapezium, trans-hamate peri-pisiform, and peri-hamate trans-triquetrum are all examples of which carpal instability pattern?**

Longitudinal or axial carpal instability.

○ **What is the "Jahss maneuver"?**

The maneuver used for reduction of metacarpal neck fractures with MP and PIP joints flexed to 90 degrees.

● ● ● REFERENCES ● ● ●

Amadio PC, Taleisnik J. Fractures of the carpal bones. In: Green DP, ed. *Operative Hand Surgery*. 4th ed. New York, NY: Churchill Livingstone; 1999:809–864.

Garcia-Elias M. Carpal instabilities and dislocations. In: Green DP, ed. *Operative Hand Surgery*. 4th ed. New York, NY: Churchill Livingstone; 1999:865–928.

Glickel SZ, Barron OA, Eaton RG. Dislocations and ligament injuries in the digits. In: Green DP, ed. *Operative Hand Surgery*. 4th ed. New York, NY: Churchill Livingstone; 1999:772–808.

Henry M. Fractures and dislocations of the hand. In: Bucholz RW, Heckman JD, eds. *Rockwood and Green's Fractures in Adults*. 5th ed. Philadelphia, PA: Lippincott Williams and Wilkins; 2001:655–748.

Seitz WH, Papandrea RF. Fractures and dislocations of the wrist. In: Bucholz RW, Heckman JD, ed. *Rockwood and Green's Fractures in Adults*. 5th ed. Philadelphia, PA: Lippincott Williams and Wilkins; 2001:749–814.

Stern PJ. Fracture of the metacarpals and phalanges. In: Green DP, ed. *Operative Hand Surgery*. 4th ed. New York, NY: Churchill Livingstone; 1999:711–771.

CHAPTER 36 Tendon Injuries

Steven L. Henry, MD, FACS

• • • ANATOMY AND PHYSIOLOGY • • •

○ **From where do tendons receive their nourishment?**

In the forearm, from vessels in the paratenon.

In the hand, from the vincular vessels (intrinsic system) and from the synovial fluid (extrinsic system) within the tendon sheath.

○ **Which source is more important to the tendons in the hand?**

Synovial fluid.

○ **What are the vincula?**

Folds of mesotendon containing blood vessels. Each tendon (Flexor digitorum superficialis [FDS] and Flexor digitorum profundus [FDP]) has two vincula, a short vinculum distally and a long vinculum proximally, that enter the dorsal surface of the tendons.

○ **What are the source vessels of the vincula?**

The transverse digital arteries, which enter the fibro-osseous tunnel at the levels of the cruciate pulleys.

○ **How is the short vinculum of the superficialis tendon related to the long vinculum of the profundus tendon?**

They cross each other at the distal P1 level.

○ **How many pulleys are there in the fingers?**

Eight (five annular and three cruciate).

○ **What effect do the pulleys have?**

They prevent bowstringing of the flexor tendons in flexion, increasing the effective excursion of the tendons and thus the degree of finger flexion. Theoretically, a finger with bowstringing flexor tendons will actually flex with greater strength because the force vector is farther from the joint axis, but will not be able to flex fully.

○ **Which pulleys are the most important in the fingers, and where are they located?**
- A2, at the proximal part of the proximal phalanx
- A4, at the middle part of the middle phalanx

○ **The interval between which annular ligaments has no cruciate ligament?**
Between A1 and A2. The first cruciate ligament lies between A2 and A3.

○ **How many pulleys are there in the thumb?**
Three:
- A1 at the MP level
- Oblique at the P1 level
- A2 at the IP level

The oblique and A2 pulleys are the most important in the thumb.

○ **What comprises the floor of the fibro-osseous tunnel?**
The periosteum of the phalanges and the volar plates of the MP and PIP joints.

○ **What lies immediately volar to the volar plate of the PIP joint?**
FDS tendon.

○ **Describe the orientation of the FDS tendons within the carpal tunnel.**
The tendons of the index and small fingers are dorsal to the tendons of the long and ring fingers.

● ● ● **FLEXOR TENDONS** ● ● ●

○ **Describe the boundaries of the five flexor zones of the fingers.**
Zone I: Distal to the insertion of FDS on P2.
Zone II: Within the fibro-osseous tunnel (from the A1 pulley to the FDS insertion).
Zone III: The area of the palm between the carpal tunnel and the fibro-osseous tunnel.
Zone IV: Within the carpal tunnel.
Zone V: Proximal to the carpal tunnel.

○ **What are the two main deficits resulting from zone I tendon laceration?**
Loss of DIP flexion and diminution of grip strength.

○ **What provides the stronger repair in zone I injuries—suturing of tendon ends together or anchoring of tendon end directly to bone?**
Anchoring directly to bone.

○ **What is the farthest the FDP tendon should be advanced to achieve direct anchoring to bone?**

1 cm.

○ **What is a jersey finger?**

Avulsion of the FDP tendon from its insertion on P3 (an injury that might occur when a football player reaches out to grab an opponent's jersey).

○ **What finger is most commonly affected, and why?**

The ring finger, because:

1. It has the weakest FDP insertion.

2. It is the most protruding finger when the hand is in the grasping position.

3. The juncturae tendinae prevent independent extension of the ring finger (much more so than the other fingers).

4. The common muscle belly of FDP prevents independent relaxation of the FDP tendon.

○ **Describe the four types of FDP avulsion injuries.**

Type I: Tendon retracts into palm.

Type II: Tendon retracts to level of PIP.

Type III: Tendon avulsed with large bony fragment, which catches at A4.

Type IV: Large bony fragment, with avulsion and retraction of tendon from fragment.

○ **Which type of FDP avulsion is most common? Which has the best prognosis? The worst?**

Most common: type II.

Best prognosis: type III.

Worst prognosis: type I and type IV.

○ **What is the lumbrical plus deformity?**

If an injured FDP tendon retracts into the palm (type I avulsion), the lumbrical (which originates on the FDP tendon) will be under tension, creating an extension force on the IP joints. When one attempts to make a fist, the FDP tendon will place even greater tension on the lumbrical, paradoxically extending the finger. This can also happen if an FDP tendon in the finger is reconstructed with a tendon graft that is too long.

○ **Why must type I FDP avulsion be repaired without significant delay?**

Because both the vincular and synovial nutritional supplies have been disrupted.

○ **What holds the FDP tendon at the level of the PIP in a type II FDP avulsion?**

The vincula.

○ **A heavy laborer sustained a type I FDP avulsion 1 month ago. What treatment should be considered?**

DIP fusion, if the joint is symptomatically unstable or painful. Attempt at repair would likely result in worse stiffness.

○ **Where is a zone II flexor tendon laceration usually located with respect to the skin laceration?**

Distal (the finger is usually flexed at the time of injury).

○ **If the vinculum is ruptured in a zone II injury, to where will the tendon usually retract?**

To the palm, held in place by the lumbrical.

○ **How can the tendon be retrieved from the palm?**

A rubber catheter or infant feeding tube is guided down the tendon sheath from the site of injury in retrograde manner. An incision is made at the distal palmar crease, and the catheter is retrieved from the proximal end of the fibro-osseous tunnel. The tendon is attached to the catheter and pulled back into the tunnel.

○ **What can happen if the FDP tendon is repaired but the FDS is not?**

Higher risk of rupture of the FDP repair, loss of dexterity and grip strength, and hyperextension deformity at the PIP.

○ **When should flexor tendon lacerations be repaired?**

Flexor tendons should be repaired within a few days, if reasonably possible. Successful tendon healing may be possible after a delay of several weeks if the vincular or synovial nutritional supplies are intact; however, scarring within the tendon sheath and/or myostatic contracture of the muscle belly may preclude primary repair if surgery is delayed beyond 10 to 14 days.

○ **How many core suture strands are ideal?**

Good question! It depends on the suture technique and the size/material of the suture. In general, more strands are stronger, but many strands can increase the bulk at the repair site and can be difficult to place in small tendons. In the author's opinion, a locking technique using 4-0 Fiberwire suture with 4 core strands is adequate to permit early active motion.

○ **How far from the cut edge of the tendon should the core suture purchase be?**

Roughly 1 cm. Placing the suture closer to the edge weakens the repair, while placing it farther from the edge causes excessive bunching at the repair site.

○ **What percentage of the total strength of a tendon repair is attributable to the epitendinous suture?**

Approximately 20%.

○ **Following repair, when does tendon rupture most commonly occur?**

Around the 10th postoperative day.

○ **How should the patient be splinted immediately following flexor tendon repair?**

The wrist should be held in approximately 30 degrees of flexion, the MPs in 50 to 70 degrees of flexion, and the IPs in full extension.

○ **When should passive range-of-motion exercises be initiated following flexor tendon repair? Active range of motion?**

Passive: as soon as possible.
Active: depends on the strength of the repair. If a strong repair is achieved (i.e., at least four core suture strands), active motion can be started immediately. If not, about 4 weeks.

○ **How is a splint constructed to permit active extension and passive flexion?**

A rubber band is attached to the nail of the involved finger and to the splint in the region of the distal volar forearm. The wrist is held in neutral and the MP is blocked at 60 to 70 degrees of flexion. The rubber band passively pulls the finger into flexion, and provides resistance against active IP extension. (The finger flexors are reflexively inhibited when the finger extends against resistance.)

○ **What are the most important prerequisites to flexor tendon grafting?**

Full passive range of motion and intact flexor sheath.

○ **What are the most common donor sites for flexor tendon grafts?**

Palmaris longus, plantaris, and the long toe extensors.

○ **Where is plantaris with respect to the Achilles tendon?**

Anterior and medial.

○ **In reconstructing a zone II FDP injury with a graft, how can the appropriate length of the graft be determined?**

By matching the cascade of the injured digit with its uninjured neighbors. Additionally, performing the surgery under local anesthesia allows assessment of tendon balance with active flexion.

○ **What can happen if the graft is too long?**

Lumbrical plus deformity, in which attempts to flex the finger cause paradoxical extension of the interphalangeal joints.

○ **What is quadriga syndrome?**

If one FDP is tethered or shortened following a repair, the others cannot shorten enough to achieve full flexion. Try flexing your ring finger DIP while holding your long finger in extension with the other hand. Named by Verdan for the Roman charioteers who controlled teams of four horses with four sets of reins slung over their backs.

○ **What is the most common complication of tendon grafting?**

Adhesions (and thus, stiffness).

○ **Following a zone II flexor tendon repair, a patient has limited active range of motion and has made little progress in therapy. When is the earliest that flexor tenolysis should be considered?**

At least 3 months of therapy should be attempted prior to performing tenolysis.

○ **What is a Hunter rod?**

A Hunter rod is a flexible silicone implant that is placed within a scarred flexor tendon bed. Formation of a capsule around this implant will create a pseudosheath within which a tendon graft can later be placed.

● ● ● EXTENSOR TENDONS ● ● ●

○ **At what level do the extensor tendons lie within a synovial sheath?**

At the level of the extensor retinaculum. The extensor tendons are surrounded only by paratenon at all other levels.

○ **What tendons are present within each of the six extensor compartments?**

First	APL, EPB
Second	ECRL, ECRB
Third	EPL
Fourth	EDC, EIP
Fifth	EDQ
Sixth	ECU

○ **Which tendon inserts on the second MC? On the third? On the fifth?**

- ECRL on the second
- ECRB on the third
- ECU on the fifth

○ **What is the relationship of the proprius tendons (EIP and EDQ) to the communis tendons at the level of the MPs?**

The proprius tendons lie <u>ulnar</u> to the communis tendons.

○ **The EDC tendon is often missing from which finger?**

The small finger. In these instances, there are often two slips of EDC to the ring finger. There may also be two slips of EDQ to the small finger.

○ **What muscles extend the MP joints?**

The extrinsic extensors (EDC, EIP, and EDQ) are the only muscles that extend the MP joints.

○ **What muscles flex the MP joints?**

Primarily the intrinsic (lumbricals and interossei). The extrinsic flexors (FDP and FDS) have a relatively weak effect at the MP joints.

○ **What muscles extend the IP joints?**

When the MPs are flexed, the extrinsics extend the IPs. When the MPs are extended, the intrinsics extend the IPs. Remember that muscles can create little force if they are not under stretch. When the MPs are extended, the intrinsics are under stretch and can thus extend the IPs. When the MPs are flexed, it is the extrinsics that are under stretch.

○ **What is the intrinsic minus deformity?**

Extension of the MPs and flexion of the IPs, as in the claw deformity seen with low ulnar nerve palsies. This is a good way to remember the function of the intrinsics (i.e., to flex the MPs and extend the IPs).

○ **A patient sustains a dorsal hand laceration at the mid-metacarpal level, completely transecting the EDC tendon to the long finger. Yet he is still able to extend the MP joint of the long finger. How is this possible?**

The juncturae tendinae are interconnections between the extensor tendons at the level of the distal metacarpals. The juncturae extend in a distal-oblique direction from the EDC tendon of the ring finger to those of the small finger and long finger, and from the EDC tendon of the long finger to that of the index finger. In this case, the tendon was lacerated proximal to the junctura, which transmits extensile force from the ring finger tendon to the long finger tendon.

○ **Which extensor tendons do not have juncturae?**

The proprius tendons (EIP and EDQ).

○ **What is a relative motion splint?**

A yoke splint (think of brass knuckles, except made from Thermoplast) that allows motion at all joints, but holds the affected finger's MP in relative extension or flexion, thereby unloading tension on the extensor or flexor tendon, respectively. The most common use is for rehabilitation of an EDC repair at the dorsal hand, in which case the affected finger is held in relative extension. It works because the EDC tendons have a common muscle belly, so tension is borne by the other fingers' tendons rather than the finger held in relative extension.

○ **What are the sagittal bands?**

The sagittal bands are transverse ligamentous structures that pass from the extensor tendon to the volar plate of the MP. Their function is to hold the extensor tendon in place over the MP. They also transmit force from the extensor tendon to the proximal phalanx, thus extending the MP joint. They are somewhat analogous to the A1 pulley of the flexor system, except that the sagittal bands undergo proximal and distal excursion with extension and flexion of the MP, much like a bucket handle.

○ **What holds the extensor mechanism in place over the PIP?**

Transverse retinacular ligament.

○ **Where is the extensor trifurcation?**

Proximal to the PIP, the extensor tendon trifurcates into a central slip and two lateral bands. The central slip inserts on the dorsal base of P2, while the lateral bands bypass the PIP and insert on P3.

○ **Where is the triangular ligament? What does it do?**

The triangular ligament spans the dorsal surface of the middle phalanx, <u>connecting the lateral bands to each other</u>. It helps to prevent the lateral bands from migrating volarly.

○ **What deformity results from laceration of the central slip with preservation and volar migration of the lateral bands?**

Boutonnière deformity.

○ **What is the oblique retinacular ligament of Landsmeer?**

A ligament extending from the volar aspect of the PIP to the dorsal aspect of the DIP. It functions to coordinate flexion and extension of the IP joints—if the PIP flexes, the ligament relaxes, permitting the DIP to flex; if the PIP extends, the ligament tightens, helping the DIP to extend. In a long-standing boutonnière deformity, this ligament gradually contracts, potentially making the deformity permanent. Thus, resistance to passive flexion of the DIP (Boyes test) is a hallmark of a boutonnière.

○ **How do you splint a patient with a Boutonnière deformity?**

Splint the PIP in extension (either with a static splint if the PIP is passively supple, or a static progressive [spring-loaded] splint if the PIP has a flexion contracture), keeping the DIP free. The patient should then actively flex the DIP, which encourages dorsal migration of the lateral bands and stretching of the ligament of Landsmeer. Alternatively, a relative motion splint can be used, keeping the affected MP in relative flexion compared to the other fingers, also encouraging dorsal migration of the lateral bands.

○ **A patient has sustained a complete laceration of the EPL tendon, yet can still extend the IP joint of the thumb. How is this possible?**

The intrinsics of the thenar eminence insert on the extensor hood and can provide weak extension of the IP. In addition, the EPB can have a superficial division that inserts on the extensor hood. However, only the EPL can extend the entire first ray. Thus, if the patient places the palm flat on a table, he or she will be unable to lift the thumb off the table in the presence of a complete EPL laceration.

○ **Describe the zones of injury of the extensor tendons of the fingers.**

Odd zones are over joints.

Zones I, III, V, and VII overlie the DIP, PIP, MP, and carpal joints, respectively. Zones II, IV, VI, and VIII overlie the P2, P1, MC, and distal forearm, respectively.

○ **What can be done to prevent adhesions in the repair of a zone VII extensor tendon laceration?**

Excision of the portion of the extensor retinaculum that overlies the repair site.

○ **What is a mallet finger?**

Flexion deformity of the DIP resulting from loss of continuity of the extensor mechanism.

○ **Describe the classification of mallet finger injuries.**

Type I: Closed, with or without a small chip fracture.

Type II: Open laceration.

Type III: Deep abrasion of skin and tendon substance.

Type IV: P3 fracture. This type includes transepiphyseal fracture in children (type IV-A), hyperflexion injuries (type IV-B), and hyperextension injuries (type IV-C). Note that these fractures involve significant portions of the articular surface and are not to be confused with the largely irrelevant chip fractures seen in type I injuries.

○ **How are various types of mallet injuries treated?**

Type I: Splinting of the DIP in slight hyperextension (no more than 5 degrees) for 6–8 weeks, followed by night splinting for 2 weeks.

Type II: Repair of skin and tendon with a single figure-of-eight suture, followed by splinting as above.

Type III: Skin coverage and tendon graft.

Type IV-A: Closed reduction of the fracture, followed by extension splinting for 3–4 weeks.

Type IV-B: Extension splinting, with ORIF reserved for cases in which the fragment is significantly displaced or the distal phalanx has subluxated volarly.

Type IV-C: As above.

○ **What can happen if a mallet injury is left unrepaired?**

Hyperextension at the PIP (i.e., swan neck deformity). This is because the force of the extensor tendon is concentrated only at the PIP, creating PIP hyperextension.

⬤ ⬤ ⬤ **REFERENCES** ⬤ ⬤ ⬤

Britton EN, Kleinert JM. Acute flexor tendon injury: repair and rehabilitation. In: Peimer CA, ed. *Surgery of the Hand and Upper Extremity*. New York, NY: McGraw-Hill; 1996:1113–1132.

Doyle JR. Extensor tendons–acute injuries. In: Green DP, ed. *Operative Hand Surgery*. 2nd ed. New York, NY: Churchill Livingstone; 1988:2045–2072.

Henry SL, Katz MA, Green DP. Type IV FDP avulsion: lessons learned clinically and through review of the literature. *Hand(N Y)*. 2009;4(4):357–361.

Lee SK, Goldstein RY, Zingman A, Terranova C, Nasser P, Hausman MR. The effects of core suture purchase on the biomechanical characteristics of a multistrand locking flexor tendon repair: a cadaveric study. *J Hand Surg Am*. 2010;35(7):1165–1171.

Lee WAP, Gan BS, Harris SU. Flexor tendons. In: Russell RC, ed. *Plastic Surgery: Indications, Operations, and Outcomes, Vol. IV: Hand Surgery*. St Louis, MO: Mosby; 2000:1961–1982.

Merritt WH. Relative motion splint: Active motion after extensor tendon injury and repair. *J Hand Surg Am*. 2014;39(6):1187–1194.

Pederson WC. Extensor tendons. In: Russell RC, ed. *Plastic Surgery: Indications, Operations, and Outcomes, Vol. IV: Hand Surgery*. St Louis, MO: Mosby; 2000:1983–1994.

Schneider LH, Hunter JM. Flexor tendons-late reconstruction. In: Green DP, ed. *Operative Hand Surgery*. 2nd ed. New York, NY: Churchill Livingstone; 1988:1969–2044.

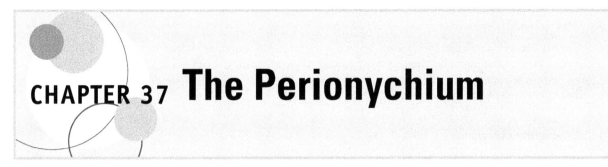

CHAPTER 37 The Perionychium

Dipan Das, MD, FACS and
James R. Sanger, MD, FACS

• • • ANATOMY • • •

○ **Name the labeled structures in Figure 37-1.**

1. Nail plate
2. Lunula
3. Eponychium
4. Nail fold

5. Distal phalanx
6. Germinal matrix
7. Sterile matrix
8. Hyponychium

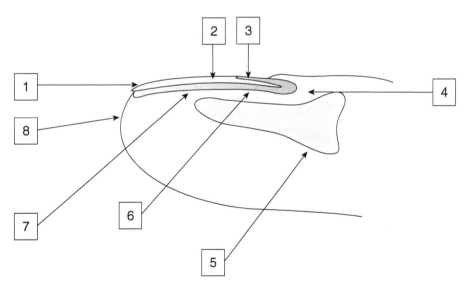

Figure 37-1 Anatomy of the perionychium.

○ **What is the perionychium?**

The nail bed (composed of the sterile and germinal matrix) and surrounding soft tissues (paronychium).

○   **What is the hyponychium?**

The junction of the nail bed (sterile matrix) and the fingertip skin, beneath the distal free margin of the nail. It consists of a keratinous plug that prevents debris from getting under the nail plate. The hyponychium also contains large numbers of leukocytes and lymphocytes and is the first barrier of defense to prevent bacteria and fungi from invading the subungual area.

○   **What is the eponychium?**

The distal portion of the nail fold where it attaches to the surface of the nail.

○   **What is the paronychium?**

Soft tissue around the nail and the nail folds comprises the paronychium.

○   **What is the nail bed?**

The nail bed consists of (a) the germinal matrix on the proximal ventral floor of the nail fold and (b) the sterile matrix extending from the lunula to the hyponychium.

○   **What is the germinal matrix?**

The germinal matrix comprises the ventral floor of the nail fold. Highly vascular and composed of germinal cells near the periosteum, the germinal matrix produces 90% of the nail volume. As the germinal cells duplicate, previously formed cells are forced toward the nail and the pressure causes the cells to flatten, elongate, and stream distally into the nail.

○   **What is the sterile matrix?**

Part of the nail bed that extends from the lunula to the hyponychium.

○   **What is the nail fold? Why is it important?**

The nail fold houses the proximal nail plate and is composed of the germinal matrix on the **ventral floor** and the portion of the nail bed that forms the cells which makes the nail shine on the **dorsal roof**. The patency of the nail fold is crucial for normal nail growth; hence, either the nail plate or a temporary stent should be placed to keep the nail fold open.

○   **What is the lunula?**

The curved white opacity representing the visible, distal portion of the germinal matrix.

○   **What is the nerve supply to the perionychium?**

Dorsal branches from the volar digital nerves.

○   **What is the arterial supply to the nail?**

Two dorsal branches of the volar digital arteries.

○   **What makes up the nail plate?**

Flattened sheets of anuclear keratinized epithelium densely adherent to one another.

○ **What changes occur in the nail plate distal to the lunula?**

The cell nuclei degenerate distal to the lunula. This is the junction of the sterile and germinal matrix.

○ **What lies beneath the sterile matrix?**

Periosteum of the distal phalanx; hence fracture of the distal phalanx is associated with a high incidence of nail bed injury.

● ● ● **PHYSIOLOGY** ● ● ●

○ **What produces the nail plate?**

The germinal matrix produces 90% of the nail plate volume.

○ **What contributes to nail plate adherence?**

The sterile matrix produces keratin, which thickens the nail and allows adherence of the nail plate to the bed as it migrates distally.

○ **What contributes to the smooth shiny surface of the nail plate?**

The dorsal roof of the nail fold.

○ **How is the nail produced?**

The nail plate is a multilayered stacked sheet of cornified cells derived from anucleate onychocytes that arise from the germinal matrix epithelium of the nail bed.

The epithelium of the germinal matrix, sterile matrix, and eponychial fold contributes to the production of the nail plate through three modes of keratinization.

The germinal matrix epithelium undergoes onychokeratinization, forming the main substance of the hardened nail plate, which is composed of stratified layers of cornified onychocytes.

The sterile matrix epithelium produces a semirigid keratin through a process known as onycholemmal keratinization. This semirigid keratin increases the overall thickness of the nail and also acts as superglue adhesive for the nail plate to maintain its adherence to the nail bed.

The eponychial fold (dorsal roof) is responsible for the external sheen of the healthy nail plate by epidermoid keratinization. The cuticle, hyponychium, and lateral nail folds also contribute, in a minor degree, to the surface epidermoid keratinization of the nail plate.

○ **Name five functions of the fingernail.**

1. Protection of the fingertip

2. Improved pulp tactile sensation through provision of counterforce to the pulp

3. Assistance in picking up objects

4. Self-defense (scratching)

5. Regulation of peripheral circulation

○ **What area of the body has the highest concentration of lymphatics?**

The hyponychium.

○ **At what rate does the nail grow?**

An average of 0.1 mm/day or 100 days for complete nail growth; however, after an injury, distal growth is halted for 21 days as the proximal nail thickens.

● ● ● MEDICAL PATHOLOGY ● ● ●

○ **What is clubbing?**

Exaggerated convex curvature of the nail plate.

○ **What conditions are thought to cause clubbing?**

- Familial clubbing (idiopathic)
- Pulmonary disease—pulmonary fibrosis, sarcoidosis, cystic fibrosis
- Cardiac disease—cyanotic congenital heart disease, bacterial endocarditis
- Gastrointestinal disease—ulcerative colitis, Crohn disease, liver cirrhosis
- Cancer—thyroid, thymus, disseminated chronic myelogenous leukemia
- Other—acromegaly, pregnancy

○ **What is chromonychia?**

Changes in nail color.

○ **What causes this?**

Chromonychia can be induced by renal failure, subungual hemorrhage, or medications. Antineoplastic drugs frequently cause melanonychia. Drugs most commonly involved are adriamycin, cyclophosphamide, and vincristine. Chromonychia is also associated with AIDS.

● ● ● SURGICAL PATHOLOGY ● ● ●

○ **What is onycholysis?**

Premature separation of the nail bed and nail plate.

○ **What causes this?**

Abnormalities of the sterile matrix, often secondary to posttraumatic scarring.

○ **What medications are strongly associated with onycholysis?**

Taxane chemotherapeutics including paclitaxel and docetaxel.

○ **What causes longitudinal splitting of the nail plate?**

Abnormalities of the germinal matrix (ventral nail fold), often secondary to posttraumatic scarring between the nail roof and nail floor.

○ **What causes longitudinal grooving in the nail plate?**

Abnormalities of the nail fold (tumor, bony change, or posttraumatic deformities).

○ **What are nail spikes or remnants?**

Small, often painful, volumes of nail plate that grow through the overlying skin. These usually occur after incomplete removal of the nail matrix following fingertip amputations.

○ **How are these treated?**

Definitive excision.

○ **Which is the most commonly injured fingernail?**

The long finger followed in order of descending length, by the ring, index, small, and thumb.

○ **What is the most common mechanism of injury?**

Doors.

○ **What is the significance of a subungual hematoma?**

There is an underlying nail bed injury.

○ **How are these treated?**

Trephination, if the hematoma covers less than 50% of the nail plate. Removal of the nail plate and direct repair of the nail bed is required if the hematoma is more than 50% of the nail plate.

○ **What is trephination?**

Creation of a hole in the nail plate to allow drainage of the hematoma, done with a large bore needle. The nail plate should be surgically scrubbed prior to trephination to avoid infection.

○ **When should nail bed injuries be treated and why?**

Acutely because secondary repair will rarely provide satisfactory results.

○ **Key steps in nail bed repair (to be carried out under loupe magnification):**

1. Adequate anesthesia to the finger in the form of a digital block.
2. Use of digital tourniquet for optimal visualization.
3. Careful removal of the nail plate using sharp scissors or a periosteal elevator to prevent further iatrogenic injury to nail bed.
4. Repair of laceration using fine absorbable suture such as 6-0 chromic.
5. Replacement of nail plate, or if absent, placement of a substitute material to protect the repair and maintain the nail fold.
6. Alignment and approximation of lacerated edges to avoid ridging.

○ **Do you need an x-ray of the fingertip?**

Yes, to evaluate the distal phalanx.

○ **What percent of nail bed injuries are associated with a distal phalanx fracture?**

50%.

○ **How are nondisplaced fractures treated?**

Repair the nail bed if necessary and replace the nail plate, to act as a splint.

○ **How are unstable displaced fractures treated?**

Fracture reduction, bony fixation with crossed K-wires, repair of the nail bed, and replacement of the nail plate.

○ **What is the treatment for an avulsed nail plate?**

Find the nail plate, replace it with any attached portions of sterile matrix. If this is not available, splint the nail fold open with a piece of Adaptic, the back of a suture pack, or portion of a Penrose drain.

○ **After nail plate removal, why is it important to replace the nail plate (or use a substitute replacement)?**

To splint the repair and prevent scarring between the roof and floor of the nail fold.

○ **With severe crush injuries, what is done with the nail bed tissue attached to the nail plate after the nail plate is removed?**

Replaced onto the nail bed as free grafts.

○ **What is a Seymour Fracture?**

Displaced distal phalangeal fracture that involves the physis with an associated nail bed laceration. Technically these are open fractures and may have the nail bed incarcerated with the fracture. The nail bed needs to be delivered from the fracture to get reduction.

○ **When are split-free nail bed grafts used?**

To replace large defects in the nail bed.

○ **Where is a split-free nail bed graft harvested from?**

Ideally from an undamaged area on the injured finger or from an amputated digit.

○ **What is alternative source for split nail bed grafts?**

The great toe.

○ **What is a hook nail deformity?**

Nail that curves volar sharply at the fingertip.

○ **What causes this?**

Inadequate tip support, usually due to traumatic loss of bone.

○ **What is pincer nail deformity?**

Referred to as omega nail deformity or trumpet nail deformity, it is a relatively rare condition in which there is a transverse overcurvature of the nail plate.

○ **What is the etiology?**

The exact etiology is obscure, but a loss of the lateral integrity of the distal phalanx may occur, allowing a greater curvature of the nail plate.

○ **What is the treatment?**

Restoration of the normal contour and shape of the nail plate is achieved with the aid of dermal grafts under the lateral edges of the nail bed.

○ **What causes nail ridges?**

Scar beneath the nail bed or an irregularly healed distal phalanx fracture.

○ **What is the treatment?**

Excision of the scar and/or smoothing out the irregularity.

○ **What causes a split nail deformity?**

A ridge or longitudinal scar in the germinal matrix.

○ **What is the treatment?**

Resection of the scar and replacement with a FULL-thickness germinal matrix graft (typically from the second toe).

○ **What causes nonadherence of the nail plate?**

A transverse scar in the sterile matrix.

○ **What is the treatment?**

Scar resection and replacement with a split-thickness sterile matrix graft.

○ **What are nail cysts or nail spikes?**

A spike of nail plate growing out from an amputation stump.

○ **What causes this?**

Failure to remove all of the germinal matrix from the nail fold when performing an amputation at the proximal portion of the distal phalanx.

○ **What is the treatment?**

Complete resection of the nail cyst and its wall.

● ● ● **INFECTIOUS DISEASES** ● ● ●

○ **What is an acute paronychia?**

Infection of the skin surrounding the nail plate.

○ **What is the most common cause?**

Staphylococcus aureus infection.

○ **What is the treatment?**

Drainage with or without partial nail plate removal.

○ **What is chronic paronychia?**

Chronic paronychia is characterized by persistent, indurated infections of the eponychium, typically seen in people whose hands are chronically exposed to water with detergents and alkali, such as cleaning workers, bartenders, and kitchen staff. The etiology is thought to be initial bacterial infection, typically followed by superinfection and colonization of the eponychium with a <u>fungus</u> such as *Candida albicans.*

○ **How is it treated?**

Systemic antifungals or antibiotics with or without nail plate removal. Eponychial marsupialization has been described and has been highly effective at clearing persistent infections.

○ **What is onychomycosis?**

Chronic fungal infections of the nail.

○ **How does it present?**

Nail plate discoloration, thickening, and onycholysis.

○ **How is this treated?**

Topical antifungals alone are typically unsuccessful. Topical antifungal with nail plate removal or systemic antifungal is recommended.

○ **What is the most common cause of paronychial infections?**

Chronic fungal infections.

○ **What is the most common bacterial infection of the nail?**

S. aureus paronychium.

○ **What is the treatment?**

Drain any abscesses by lifting the paronychium with or without partial nail plate removal using a number 11 or 15 blade, followed by soapy water soaks 3 to 4 times a day.

○ **What is herpetic whitlow?**

Self-limited viral infection of the fingertips caused by the herpes simplex virus. It is transmitted by skin-to-skin contact and is often seen in medical and dental personnel, as well as in children. Herpetic whitlow may also present with swelling and erythema, though typically patients have disproportionately greater pain than in the case of bacterial infections. Vesicles are also seen, containing fluid that may be clear or turbid, but is never purulent.

○ **How do you diagnose herpetic whitlow?**

The diagnosis is usually made clinically, though it is possible to confirm it by use of a Tzanck preparation or viral culture. It is important to distinguish herpetic whitlow from bacterial infections, as a surgical incision for the former can lead to complications involving the entire digit or systemic spread, and is contraindicated.

○ **How do you treat herpetic whitlow?**

Herpetic whitlow should generally be treated conservatively and typically runs a self-limited course of approximately 21 days. Treatment most often is directed toward symptomatic relief.

In primary infections, topical acyclovir 5% has been demonstrated to shorten the duration of symptoms and viral shedding. Oral acyclovir may prevent recurrence. Doses of 800 mg twice daily initiated during the prodrome may abort the recurrence. Antibiotic treatment should only be used in cases complicated by bacterial superinfection.

Tense vesicles may be unroofed to help ameliorate pain.

● ● ● **ONCOLOGY** ● ● ●

○ **Name three common benign periungual tumors.**

Mucous cyst, glomus tumor, and pyogenic granuloma.

○ **What is a mucous cyst?**

A dorsal ganglion of the DIP, they are usually associated with an osteophyte.

○ **How does it present?**

Dorsal swelling of the DIP with or without longitudinal grooving of the nail plate.

○ **How are they treated?**

Excision of the ganglion and removal of the osteophyte.

○ **What is the key to the treatment of a mucous cyst?**

Removal of the osteophyte.

○ **How do glomus tumors present?**

These are 1 to 2 mm in size and have a classic triad of tenderness, pain, and <u>cold sensitivity</u>.

○ **How can they be diagnosed?**

MRI.

○ **How are they treated?**

Resection with an approach that includes removal of the nail plate.

○ **What is a pyogenic granuloma?**

Exuberant mass of granulation tissue that forms after a relatively minor trauma.

○ **How are they treated?**

Complete excision through curettage or ablation with silver nitrate sticks. Incomplete excision will lead to recurrence.

○ **Differential diagnosis of a pigmented subungual lesion?**

Posttraumatic hemorrhage (most common), benign nevus, subungual melanoma.

○ **What is the differential diagnosis of pigment deposition within the nail plate?**

Melanonychia striate longitudinalis (benign lesions common in black patients), a benign subungual nevus, and a malignant melanoma.

○ **What is Hutchinson sign?**

Broad pigmented streaks of variegated color with cuticular pigmentation within the nail plate. It is associated with a subungual melanoma.

○ **How is a subungual hematoma differentiated from a subungual melanoma?**

Mark the nail plate and watch. If it is a hematoma, it will migrate distally. Ultimately, a nail bed biopsy is recommended if even minor suspicion of melanoma exists.

• • • REFERENCES • • •

Abzug JM, Kozin SH. Seymour fractures. *J Hand Surg Am*. 2013;38:2267–2270.

Baden HP. Regeneration of the nail. *Arch Dermatol*. 1965;91:619–620.

Fleegler EJ, Ziewonwicc RJ. Tumors of the perionychium. *Hand Clin*. 1990;6:113–134.

Hijjawi JB, Dennison DG. Acute felon as a complication of systemic paclitaxel therapy: case report and review of the literature. *Hand (N Y)*. 2007;2:101–103.

Kleinert HE, Kutz JE, Fishman JH, McGraw LH. Etiology and treatment of the so-called mucous cyst of the finger. *J Bone Joint Surg Am*. 1972;54:1455–1458.

Newmeyer WL, Kilgore ES Jr. Common injuries of the fingernail and nail bed. *Am Fam Physician*. 1977;16:93–95.

Quitkin HM, Rosenwasser MP, Strauch RJ. The efficacy of silver nitrate cauterization for pyogenic granuloma of the hand. *J Hand Surg Am*. 2003;28:435–438.

Schiller C. Nail replacement in finger tip injuries. *Plast Reconstr Surg*. 1957;19:521–530.

Seaberg DC, Angelos WJ, Paris PM. Treatment of subungual hematomas with nail trephination: a prospective study. *Am J Emerg Med*. 1991;9:209–210.

Sorene ED, Goodwin DR. Magnetic resonance imaging of a tiny glomus tumour of the fingertip: a case report. *Scand J Plast Reconstr Surg Hand Surg*. 2001;35:429–431.

Wong CH, Chow L, Yen CH, Ho PC, Yip R, Hung LK. Uncommon hand tumours. *Hand Surg*. 2001;6:67–80.

Zook EG, Brown RE. The perionychium. In: Green DP, ed. *Green's Operative Hand Surgery*. Vol 2. 4th ed. New York, NY: Churchill Livingstone; 1999:1353–1380.

Zook EG, Russell RC. Reconstruction of a functional and esthetic nail. *Hand Clin*. 1990;6:59–68.

Zook EG, Van Beek AL, Russell RC, Beatty ME. Anatomy and physiology of the perionychium: a review of the literature and anatomic study. *J Hand Surg Am*. 1980;5:528–536.

CHAPTER 38 Rheumatoid Hand

Emily Cushnie, MD, PhD and
César J. Bravo, MD

○ **What are the three primary goals in treating the rheumatoid hand?**

PRC:

1. **P**ain relief.

2. **R**estoration of function.

3. **C**osmetic improvement of the hand.

○ **What are the three basic principles in rheumatoid hand surgery?**

1. Synovectomy/soft-tissue reconstruction done early in disease.

2. Highly erosive disease (arthritis mutilans) treated early with fusion before bone loss.

3. Correction of deformity that causes loss of motion and may severely compromise hand function.

○ **What surgical sequence should be followed in a rheumatoid patient?**

1. Lower extremity addressed first.

2. Proximal joints before distal joints (e.g., elbow before wrist, wrist before metacarpophalangeal joint [MCPJ] and proximal interphalangeal joint [PIPJ]).

○ **What is an essential part of the preoperative evaluation in a rheumatoid patient?**

Cervical spine evaluation. 25% to 50% of patients can have atlantoaxial instability (plain cervical radiographs including flexion and extension views are standard).

○ **What is the pathogenesis in rheumatoid arthritis (RA) of the hand?**

Autoimmune disorder resulting in erosive synovitis of the hand and wrist secondary to injury to synovial microvascular endothelial cells triggering an inflammatory reaction causing influx of polymorphonuclear leukocytes (PMNs), monocytes, and macrophages.

○ **Inflammatory cells/mediators produced by macrophages, monocytes, PMNs stimulate which cell type in the rheumatoid hand?**

Osteoclast. These are responsible for subchondral osteopenia.

○ **What three classes of drugs are used to treat RA medically?**

Nonsteroidal anti-inflammatory agents (NSAIDs), corticosteroids, and disease-modifying anti-rheumatic drugs (DMARDs).

○ **Which of these medications can help to change the disease course?**

Only DMARDs are found to alter the course of RA and improve associated radiographic outcomes. They have both anti-inflammatory effects as well as structural-modifying properties.[1,2]

○ **What are the two classes of biologic agents that exist to treat RA?**

Tumor necrosis factor (TNF) inhibitors and interleukin-1 (IL-1) receptor antagonists. These agents act to neutralize cytokines that mediate the inflammatory pathogenesis in RA.[1]

○ **What are the extra-articular manifestations seen in RA? Which one is most common?**

Vasculitis, pericarditis, pulmonary nodules, episcleritis, and subcutaneous nodules. Subcutaneous nodules (25% of patients with RA).

○ **Manifestation of accumulated inflammatory cells around capillaries of the synovium and tenosynovium is known as:**

Synovitis and tenosynovitis.

○ **What cellular processes are responsible for cartilage damage in RA?**

Cytokine-activated neutrophils release lysosomal enzymes and free oxygen radicals, which destroy cartilage in the affected joint.[3]

○ **Is pattern of joint involvement in RA different from osteoarthritis (OA) of the hand?**

Yes. In RA, MCPJ and PIPJ are commonly involved. In OA, distal interphalangeal joint and basilar joint of thumb are involved.

○ **What are Bouchard's nodes?**

Enlargement of PIPJ seen mainly in RA. **Heberden's nodes are seen in OA and refer to DIP enlargement.

○ **What is the most commonly affected joint in RA?**

The wrist.[4]

○ **What is the most frequently affected area about the wrist in RA patients?**

Distal radioulnar joint (DRUJ).

○ **Why is the DRUJ affected early in the disease course?**

There is a greater degree of vascularity at the prestyloid recess of the distal ulna, which allows for early synovial infiltration.[3]

○ **What are other commonly affected areas of the wrist in RA?**

Palmar side of distal radius, waist of scaphoid, triquetrum.[3]

○ **What is the typical presentation of RA early in the disease?**

Insidious onset of morning stiffness and polyarthropathy involving most commonly the hands and feet.

○ **Decreased active digital flexion in a patient with RA is usually caused by what?**

Synovial nodules within flexor tendons. These nodules within retinacular system reduce active flexion of finger.

○ **What is the natural course of rheumatoid disease with articular involvement at the MCPJ?**

Progressive joint erosion and collapse with palmar displacement.

○ **How do tendon ruptures of the hand and wrist occur in patient with RA?**

By attrition (abrasion over bony prominences), infiltration (synovitis), and ischemia (external pressure by compressive synovium).

○ **What is the more common direction of sagittal band rupture in RA?**

Radial sagittal band, results in ulnar displacement of the extensor tendons.

○ **How is the wrist affected in patients with RA?**

Synovitis begins in ulnar aspect of the wrist with the DRUJ and radiocarpal joint first affected, usually sparing the midcarpal joint. Erosive changes seen at the prestyloid recess of the ulnar styloid, sigmoid notch of radius, insertion of radioscapholunate ligament, and the scaphoid waist. The carpus subluxes ulnarly and volarly with supination relative to radius. This carpal alignment leads to radial deviation of the metacarpals.

○ **What is the natural course of wrist deformities with rheumatoid disease?**

Supination, palmar dislocation, radial deviation, and volar–ulnar dislocation of the carpus on the radius (see Fig. 38-1).

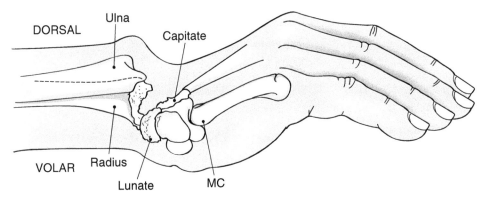

Figure 38-1 Natural course of wrist deformities with rheumatoid disease.

○ **What are the treatment options available for the rheumatoid DRUJ/wrist?**

Treatment/Procedure	Benefit
Synovectomy of radiocarpal joint and DRUJ	Pain relief, done after 6 months of medical treatment and no radiographic changes
Partial arthrodesis (radiolunate and scaphoradiolunate fusions)	Prevents progression of collapse. Radiolunate preserves function in patients with ulnocarpal translocation.
Resection hemiarthroplasty of DRUJ	Preserves length of ulna and TFCC attachments. No DRUJ contact on pronation/supination—pain relief
Darrach procedure (resection of distal ulna)	Easy. Can have radioulnar impingement/instability.
Sauvé–Kapandji (fusion of DRUJ, osteotomy of ulna at radial metaphyseal flare)	Less cosmetic defect than Darrach. Can have radioulnar impingement. Good for younger patients.
Total wrist arthrodesis	90–95% good to excellent results (fused in 10–20 degrees extension and neutral deviation)
Wrist arthroplasty	Motion-preserving procedure (good bone stock, minimal deformity, intact extensors)

DRUJ, distal radioulnar joint; TFFC, triangular fibrocartilage complex.

○ **What is the total wrist arthroplasty experience in the United States?**

1. 1967: Swanson. Silicone hinge.
2. 1972: Meuli. Ball and trunnion.
3. 1973: Volz. Dorsopalmar tracking.
4. 1977: Figgie and Ranawat. Trispherical (hinge).
5. 1982: Beckenbaugh. Biaxial (ellipsoidal).
6. 1990: Mennon. Universal (anatomic).
7. 2002: Adams. Universal 2 (uncemented).

○ **What are current accepted indications for total wrist arthroplasty?**

1. Painful pancarpal (diffuse) and advance arthritis.
2. Progressive deformity with advanced arthritis.
3. Patients who do not use walking aids with affected hand.
4. Other joints of same extremity have significant limitations.
5. Personal factors (low-demand activities that require wrist motion).
6. Contralateral wrist fused.

○ **What are current accepted contraindications for total wrist arthroplasty?**

1. Previous sepsis.

2. Rupture and not fully reconstructible wrist extensors.

3. Resorption of distal carpal row.

4. Previous wrist arthrodesis (autofusion not a contraindication).

5. Failed silicone wrist implant with fragmentation and particulate synovitis.

6. Progressive deformity with advanced arthritis.

○ **What is the recommended treatment for RA patients with bilateral wrists that require surgical intervention?**

Arthroplasty of the dominant wrist and arthrodesis of the nondominant wrist with fusion in neutral or 10 to 15 degrees of extension.4

○ **In the rheumatoid hand, are women affected more than men?**

Yes. 2.5:1.

○ **What is a painless dorsal wrist mass distal to the extensor retinaculum typically in RA patients?**

Typical presentation of extensor tenosynovitis. Tenosynovectomy indicated after 4 to 6 months of medical treatment to prevent rupture of extensor tendon.

○ **What is the differential diagnosis of a patient with a rheumatoid hand and with inability to extend his fingers?**

1. Ulnar subluxation of extensor tendon over the MP joints due to failure of the radial sagittal band.

2. Posterior interosseous nerve (PIN) palsy because of synovitis at the elbow.

3. MP joint subluxation/dislocation.

4. Extensor tendon attritional rupture.

○ **When should PIN palsy at the elbow be a prime consideration in RA patients?**

Inability to extend all four fingers and IP joint of thumb. Also, unable to deviate the wrist ulnarly secondary to extensor carpi ulnaris (ECU) paralysis.

○ **Does a patient with an extensor tendon rupture have the ability to maintain a digit extended if passively placed in that position?**

No. They also lose the tenodesis effect of the hand (e.g., finger extension with wrist flexion and vice versa).

○ **Why might a patient with a ruptured extensor digiti quinti (EDQ) minimi still be able to partially extend the small finger?**

The juncturae tendinum between the ring and the small finger is still intact.[4]

○ **How might one clinically test the EDQ tendon in isolation?**

Hold all other digits in flexion and ask the patient to extend just the small finger.

○ **In decreasing incidence, which extensor tendons are affected by RA?**

Extensor digiti minimi (EDM), extensor digitorum communis (EDC) 5, EDC 4, EPL, EDC 3.

○ **What anatomical landmark contributes to extensor pollicis longus rupture in patients with RA?**

Lister's tubercle. Contributes to attritional rupture while acting as a bone pulley.

○ **What is Vaughn–Jackson syndrome?**

Ischemic rupture of ulnar extensor tendons secondary to prominent irregular ulnar head. Most common cause of tendon rupture in RA patients.

○ **What is caput ulnae syndrome?**

Failure of the ulnar aspect of the wrist and DRUJ secondary to RA resulting in:

1. dorsal dislocation of distal ulna

2. supination of carpus on the radius

3. volar subluxation of ECU

○ **What is the "piano keyboard sign"? What does it signify?**

Elicited when the prominent ulnar head is volarly depressed and rebounds as pressure is released. DRUJ instability, seen in a third of patients with RA.

○ **What is the scallop sign in patients with RA?**

Erosion of the radial sigmoid notch with formation of a sclerotic border. It is an ominous sign of impending extensor tendon ruptures.

○ **When is extensor tendon surgery indicated in patients with RA?**

1. Refractory to medical treatment

2. Dorsal dislocation of the ulnar head

3. A positive scallop sign

4. Recurrent dorsal tenosynovitis

○ **Is surgery needed after an extensor tendon rupture in RA patients to prevent damage to intact tendons?**

Yes. Unchecked tenosynovitis damages outer surfaces of underlying tendons, leads to tendon adhesions and eventual attritional rupture.

○ **What is referred to as a *pseudotendon* in patients with RA?**

A thin strand of opaque tissue situated between healthy appearing tendinous material proximally and distally.

○ **Attritional rupture of flexor pollicis longus (FPL) is known as?**

Mannerfelt–Norman syndrome. Most common flexor tendon rupture in RA.

○ **Where is the most common location for rupture of FPL?**

Scaphoid. Secondary to a spur at the level of STT joint. If spur is not excised, it will lead to tendon ruptures of the FDP tendons in a radial to ulnar progression.

○ **What is the most common location of flexor tenosynovitis?**

The palm. Seen as pain, triggering, and tendon rupture with passive finger flexion that is greater than active flexion.

○ **Should the A1 pulley be preserved in rheumatoid patients?**

<u>Yes.</u> Avoid increasing the lever arm of the tendon and thus potentiating flexion deformity at the MP joints.

○ **Triggering secondary to digital flexor tenosynovitis usually locks the digit in flexion. What is happening if locked in extension?**

Profundus tendon nodule distally at the A2 pulley is the cause of locking.

○ **What are the commonly used extensor tendon transfers used after rupture?**

Ruptured Tendon	Transfer Recommended
EPL	EIP to EPL or EPB to EPL at metacarpal level
EDM and EDC5, or EDM alone	EIP to EDC5 or EDM, side–to-side to EDC4
EDM, EDC5, EDC4	EDC4 side to side to EDC3, EIP to EDM or EDC5, tendon grafts
EDC5/EDM, EDC4, EDC3	FDS (long) to EDC4 and EDC5, EDC3 side to side to EDC2/EIP
EDC5/EDM, EDC4, EDC3, EDC2	FDS (long) to EDC2 and EDC3, FDS (ring) to EDC4 and EDC5

EPL, extensor pollicis longus; EDM, extensor digiti minimi; EDC, extensor digitorum communis; FDS, flexor digitorum superficialis.

○ **How is tension adjusted in extensor tendon reconstruction/transfer in patients with RA?**

Tenodesis of the wrist established. Wrist extension produces finger flexion and wrist flexion produces finger extension.

○ **What is associated with extension loss for all four fingers with the absence of all digital extensor and proprius tendon function at surgery?**

Palmar dislocation of the carpus on the radius rather than extensor tenosynovitis.

○ **What is a contraindication in using the superficialis flexor tendon for extensor tendon transfer in RA?**

Presence of swan neck deformity and significant flexor tenosynovitis.

○ **What is the recommended treatment for loss of wrist extensors in RA?**

Arthrodesis of the wrist.

○ **What is Clayton procedure in the rheumatoid hand? Prevents what?**

Transfer of the ECRL to ECU. Redistributes wrist forces, diminishing radial rotation and volar subluxation of carpus at the wrist.

○ **What are the eight steps leading to MCPJ ulnar drift?**

1. Synovitis leading to stretching of radial sagittal bands.
2. Extrinsic extensors subluxate into intermetacarpal sulcus, become ulnar deviators.
3. Lax MP collateral ligaments from joint synovitis allow ulnar deviation.
4. Synovitis causing further damage to cartilage and bone—destabilizes MCPJ.
5. Ulnar intrinsics contract and become ulnar and volar deforming forces.
6. Radial deviation of wrist alters vector pull on the extrinsic extensors toward ulnar direction.
7. Flexor sheath synovitis distends retinaculum allowing the flexors to shift in an ulnar direction.
8. Resultant forces during pinch are in volar and ulnar directions.

○ **What is the Nalebuff classification of MCPJ in a rheumatoid hand?**

Stage I: only synovial proliferation.

Stage II: recurrent synovitis without deformity.

Stage III: moderate articular degeneration, ulnar and palmar drift of digits that is passively correctable.

Stage IV: severe joint destruction with fixed deformities.

○ **What is the treatment recommendation based on the Nalebuff classification of MCPJ?**

Stage I: medical management and splinting.

Stage II: synovectomy (after 6 months of medical treatment).

Stage III: synovectomy plus extensor tendon relocation, intrinsic releases, crossed intrinsic transfers, and radial collateral ligament imbrication.

Stage IV: silicone spacer combined with relocation of extensors and radial collateral ligament imbrication.

**Surgical intervention reserved for patients with pain and functional disability.

○ **If you have MCPJ disease and tendon rupture, which do you treat first?**

MCPJ. Multiple authors recommend treating both at same time.

○ **What is the reported arc of motion usually achieved after silicone interposition arthroplasty for MCPJ in patients with RA?**

40 to 60 degrees. Regression of digits ulnarly commonly seen, typically <10 degrees.

○ **What is a swan neck deformity? Causes?**

PIP hyperextension and DIP flexion. DIP mallet, synovitis attenuating volar plate, FDS rupture, and intrinsic tightness from MCPJ disease.

○ **What is the recommended treatment and classification for rheumatoid swan neck deformity?**

**Classification based on severity of PIP deformity, stiffness, and arthritis (radiographic findings).

Type	Description	Treatment
I	PIP flexible in all MCPJ positions	**Proximal** Fowler tenotomy, flexor PIP tenodesis, SORL reconstruction
II	PIP joint flexion position-dependent on MCPJ	Intrinsic release and/or realignment or arthroplasty MCPJ
III	PIP flexion limited in all MCPJ positions	Open capsular release, dorsal skin releases, closed manipulation with/without pinning, lateral band mobilization
IV	Radiographic joint destruction with minimal PIP joint motion	Arthrodesis and arthroplasty

PIP, proximal interphalangeal; SORL, spiral oblique retinacular ligament; MCPJ, metacarpophalangeal joint.

○ **What is a boutonnière deformity? Causes?**

Hyperflexion of PIP joint and hyperextension DIP joint. Synovitis leading to attenuated central slip, volar subluxation of lateral bands, tight transverse retinacular ligament, and volar plate contracture.

○ **What is the recommended treatment and classification for rheumatoid boutonnière deformity?**

**Classification based on PIP motion and severity of arthritis.

Type	Description	Treatment
I	Mild loss of PIP active extension, full passive PIP extension	Synovectomy, inject PIP and splints, lateral band, or **distal** Fowler's tenotomy
II	Moderate loss of PIP extension, full passive PIP extension	Synovectomy, central slip reconstruction, lateral band reconstruction, or **distal** Fowler's tenotomy
III	PIP not passively correctable, no arthritic changes	PIP injection, serial extension casting, consider type II treatment if motion restored
IV	Fixed PIP contracture, arthritic changes	Objective is to reduce PIP, PIP fusion or arthroplasty

PIP, proximal interphalangeal.

○ **What is the most common rheumatoid thumb deformity?**

Boutonnière deformity (MP joint flexion and IP joint hyperextension).

○ **What is the tendon most commonly responsible for the deformity and in what direction is it displaced?**

EPL. It subluxes ulnarly and volarly, producing flexion at the MCP joint and weakening extension. This deformity can also occur with MCP volar capsule laxity and/or FPL tendon rupture, with the deformity occurring secondary to IP hyperextension.[5]

○ **What is the Nalebuff classification of rheumatoid thumb?**

Type I: Boutonnière deformity.

Type II: Boutonnière deformity with CMC involvement

Type III: Swan neck deformity (stage 1: CMC synovitis, stage 2: CMC joint synovitis, MP joint extension deformity correctable, stage 3: CMC joint destruction, MP joint extension deformity fixed)

Type IV: Gamekeeper deformity

Type V: Swan neck deformity with MP joint and CMC unaffected

Type VI: Arthritis mutilans

○ **What is the recommended treatment for the first four stages of the rheumatoid thumb?**

	Early Disease	*Moderate Disease*	*Advanced Disease*
Type I	MP synovectomy and EPL rerouting	MP fusion or arthroplasty	IP fusion and MP arthroplasty
Type II	MP synovectomy and EPL rerouting	MP joint fusion and CMC hemiarthroplasty	MP joint fusion and CMC hemiarthroplasty
Type III	CMC partial trapezial/metacarpal base resection CMC implant arthroplasty	MP fusion CMC partial trapezial/metacarpal base resection	MP fusion CMC partial trapezial/ metacarpal base resection CMC implant arthroplasty Release first web space contracture
Type IV	MP synovectomy, UCL reconstruction	MP fusion	MP fusion Release first web space contracture

MP, metacarpophalangeal; EPL, extensor pollicis longus; CMC, carpometacarpal; UCL, ulnar collateral ligament.

○ **What is the recommended treatment for the stages V and VI of the rheumatoid thumb?**

Stage V:

a. No articular degeneration of MCPJ—volar capsulodesis.

b. Articular degeneration—MCPJ fusion.

Stage VI: Fusion and soft-tissue balancing when possible.

○ **What are the three major types of juvenile rheumatoid arthritis (JRA)?**

(**Based on presentation at onset of diagnosis and during first 6 months of disease.)

1. Systemic onset (25%)

2. Polyarticular onset (30%)

3. Pauciarticular onset (45%)

○ **What are the characteristics of pauciarticular onset JRA?**

1. Involvement of fewer than five joints in an asymmetric pattern.

2. Involvement of large joints.

3. Male	Female
Onset 10 years old	Onset <6 years old
ANA and RF negative	ANA and RF positive
HLA–B27 association	Predominance of iridocyclitis
Lower-extremity involvement	
Risk for sacroiliitis	

○ **Name five clinical differences found in JRA not found in the rheumatoid hand?**

1. Ulnar deviation of wrist and metacarpals.

2. Radial deviation of MCP J.

3. Abnormal ring and small finger metacarpals secondary to long bone epiphyseal accelerated maturation.

4. Shortened ulna.

5. Narrow small tubular bones of the hand (hand size is small).

○ **What is Still disease?**

It is the systemic onset of 20% JRA cases. Clinical findings consist of:

1. intermittent high fevers

2. transient arthritis with associated fevers

3. hepatosplenomegaly, lymphadenitis, uveitis

4. leukocytosis and anemia

5. rheumatoid factor not present

6. severe, chronic arthritis in only 25% of patients

• • • **REFERENCES** • • •

1. Gibofsky A. Combination therapy for rheumatoid arthritis in the era of biologicals. *HSS J.* 2006;2:30–41.

2. Schett G, Stach C, Zwerina J, Voll R, Manger B. How antirheumatic drugs protect joints from damage in rheumatoid arthritis. *Arthritis Rheum* 2008;58:2936–2948.

3. Papp SR, Athwal GS, Pichora DR. The Rheumatoid Wrist. *J Am Acad Orthop Surg* 2006;14:65–77.

4. Chung K, Pushman, A. Current Concepts in the Management of the Rheumatoid Hand. *J Hand Surg.* 2011;36:736–747.

5. Rozental TD, Reconstruction of the Rheumatoid Thumb. *J Am Acad Orthop Surg.* 2007;15:118–125.

● ● ● **ADDITIONAL BIBLIOGRAPHY** ● ● ●

Freiberg RA, Weinstein A. The scallop sign and spontaneous rupture of finger extensor tendons in rheumatoid arthritics. *Clin Orthop Relat Res.* 1972;83:128–130.

Herren DB, Simmen BR. Limited and complete fusion of the rheumatoid wrist. *J Hand Surg Am.* 2002;2:21–32.

Lipsky PE. Rheumatoid arthritis. In: Braunwald E, Fauci AS, Kasper DL, Hauser SL, Longo DL, Jameson JL, eds. *Harrison's Principles of Internal Medicine.* 15th ed. New York, NY: McGraw-Hill; 2001:1928–1937.

Millender LH, Nalebuff EA, Holdsworth DE. Posterior interosseous nerve syndrome secondary to rheumatoid synovitis. *J Bone Joint Surg.* 1973;55:753–757.

Millender LH, Nalebuff EA, Albin R, Ream JR, Gordon M. Dorsal tenosynovectomy and tendon transfer in the rheumatoid hand. *J Bone Joint Surg Am.* 1974;56:601–609.

Moore JR, Weiland AJ, Valdata L. Tendon ruptures in the rheumatoid hand: analysis of treatment and functional results in 60 patients. *J Hand Surg Am.* 1987;12:9–14.

Nalebuff EA. Diagnosis, classification and management of rheumatoid thumb deformities. *Bull Hosp Joint Dis.* 1968;29:119–137.

Nalebuff EA. Surgical treatment of tendon rupture in the rheumatoid hand. *Surg Clin North Am.* 1969;49:811–822.

Richards RA, Wilson RL. Management of extensor tendons and the distal radioulnar joint in rheumatoid arthritis. *J Hand Surg Am.* 2003;3:132–144.

Sauerbier M, Hahn ME, Fujita M, Neale PG, Berglund LJ, Berger RA. Analysis of dynamic distal radioulnar convergence after ulnar head resection and endoprosthesis implantation. *J Hand Surg Am.* 2002;27:425–434.

Stuart PR, Berger RA, Linscheid RL, An KN. The dorsopalmar stability of the distal radioulnar joint. *J Hand Surg Am.* 2000;25:689–699.

Terrono AL. The rheumatoid thumb. *J Am Soc Surg Hand.* 2001;1:81–90.

Wadstein T. Spontaneous rupture of the long extensor tendon of the extensor pollicis longus. Transplantation of the extensor indicis proprius. *Acta Orthop Scand.* 1946;16:194–202.

Wilson RL. Rheumatoid arthritis of the hand. *Orthop Clin North Am.* 1986;17:313–342.

Obstetrical Brachial Plexus Injuries

CHAPTER 39

Dennis S. Kao, MD and
Hani S. Matloub, MD

○ **What is the cause of obstetric brachial plexus palsy?**

Traction injury to the brachial plexus during the birth process due to excessive lateral flexion of the neck. When the fetus is delivered in cephalic presentation, shoulder dystocia can cause excessive lateral flexion of the neck. When the fetus is delivered in breech presentation, difficulty with delivery of the head after the body has emerged, can cause the same problem.

○ **What is the estimated incidence of obstetric brachial plexus palsy?**

0.2% to 4% of live births globally, with higher incidence in underdeveloped countries with poor obstetrical care.

○ **What maternal factors may be associated with obstetric brachial plexus palsy?**

1. Diabetes
2. Preeclampsia
3. Long duration of labor
4. History of delivery problem or fetus brachial plexus injury with prior pregnancy

○ **What fetal factors may be associated with obstetric brachial plexus palsy?**

1. Large fetus for gestational age
2. History of humeral fracture or clavicle fracture during birth

○ **What factors during birth may be associated with obstetric brachial plexus palsy?**

1. Difficult arm or head extraction in breech deliveries
2. Shoulder dystocia in vertex deliveries
3. Forceps or vacuum use during delivery

○ **Does Cesarean section (C-section) protect against obstetric brachial plexus palsy?**

C-section helps to lower, but not completely eliminate the risk of obstetric brachial plexus injury. There is a reported ~1% rate of obstetric brachial plexus injury associated with C-section.

○ **What are the common types and incidence of obstetric brachial plexus injuries?**

1. Erb palsy (~60%), involving C5 and C6.
2. Extended Erb palsy (~20%), involving C5, C6, and C7.
3. Total brachial plexus palsy (~20%), involving C5, C6, C7, C8, and T1
4. Klumpke palsy (<1%), involving C8 and T1.

○ **What is the typical posture of Erb palsy (Figure 39-1)?**

The features of upper plexus palsy ("waiter's tip" position) involving C5, C6, ±C7 are:

1. shoulder adduction and internal rotation
2. elbow extension
3. forearm pronation
4. wrist flexion
5. finger flexion

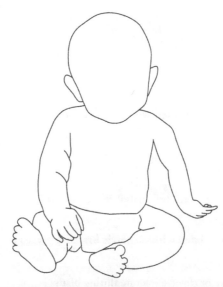

Figure 39-1 Typical posture of Erb palsy ("waiter's tip" position). Reproduced with permission from Stead LG, Kaufman MS, Waseem M. *First Aid for the Pediatrics Clerkship*. 3rd ed. New York: McGraw-Hill, 2010. Fig. 2-5.

○ **Which is the most useful classification system for management and prognosis of obstetric brachial plexus?**

The classification system proposed by Gilbert/Tassin (later refined by Narakas) provides a simple and reliable way of assessing obstetric brachial plexus palsy.

Group	Affected Nerve Roots	Physical Findings	Spontaneous Recovery Rate (%)
I	C5, C6	Lack of shoulder motion and elbow flexion, (+) elbow extension and wrist/hand function	~90
II	C5, C6, C7	Lack of shoulder and elbow motion, (+) wrist/hand function	~65
III	C5, C6, C7, C8, T1	Flail arm	<50
IV	C5, C6, C7, C8, T1, with Horner's syndrome	Flail arm, with ipsilateral ptosis, meiosis, and anhydrosis	~0

○ **What is the significance of Horner's syndrome in a patient with brachial plexus injury?**

It indicates disruption of sympathetic fibers proximal to where the preganglionic fibers arise and suggests severe brachial plexus avulsion injury (usually avulsion of T1 root, with disruption of communicating branch supplying sympathetics to the stellate ganglion).

○ **What is the significance of phrenic nerve palsy in a patient being evaluated for brachial plexus injury?**

The presence of phrenic nerve palsy suggests severe avulsion injury of the upper trunk. It also eliminates phrenic nerve as a potential donor nerve for neurotization.

○ **What studies can be ordered to evaluate obstetric brachial plexus injury?**

1. CXR (look for elevated hemidiaphragm as an indication of ipsilateral phrenic nerve palsy)
2. MRI (evaluate for signs of nerve root avulsion)
3. EMG/NCS (assess the function of each nerve and the muscles it innervates)

○ **What is the most reliable method of assessing the level and severity of obstetric brachial plexus injury?**

Physical examination to assess motor and sensory function. EMG/NCS may be helpful but lacks accuracy.

○ **What is the controversy regarding use of EMG/NCS in evaluation of obstetric brachial plexus palsy?**

Denervation changes occur and disappear much faster in infants than adults. There is also early massive collateral sprouting of denervated muscles. Therefore, EMG/NCS overestimates the clinical recovery, and may provide false hope to the parents and delay timely surgical intervention.

○ **What is the modified Mallet classification system used for?**

It is used to assess and document the recovery of upper trunk function in obstetric brachial plexus palsy. However, it cannot be used to assess forearm/wrist/hand function.

○ **What is the most common indication for surgery in obstetric brachial plexus palsy patients?**

Absence of elbow flexion (biceps function) by 3 to 6 months of age. Further delay results in poorer outcome, especially in hand function.

○ **What are the common primary surgical treatments for obstetric brachial plexus palsy?**

1. Neurolysis
2. Neurotization (with neuroma resection and nerve grafting, vs. nerve transfer)

○ **In avulsion injuries, innervation must be provided by alternative sources. This can be accomplished from remaining roots (intraplexal neurotization) or donor nerve outside the plexus (extraplexal neurotization). What are the options for extraplexal neurotization?**

1. Spinal accessory nerve
2. Intercostal nerves
3. Contralateral C7 root

○ **What secondary surgical procedures are used to correct internal rotation contracture of the shoulder due to obstetric brachial plexus injury?**

1. Early release of the subscapularis muscle/subscapularis tendon lengthening.
2. Anterior release of the pectoralis major tendon and transfer of the latissimus dorsi/teres major tendon (conjoined tendon).
3. Humeral derotational osteotomy (if advanced glenohumeral joint deformity).

● ● ● **REFERENCES** ● ● ●

Abzug JM, Kozin SH. Evaluation and management of brachial plexus birth palsy. *Orthop Clin North Am.* 2014;45:225–232.

Al-Qattan M. Obstetric brachial plexus injuries. *J Am Soc Surg Hand.* 2003;3(1):41–53.]

Capek L, Clarke HM, Curtis CG. Neuroma-in-continuity resection: early outcome in obstetric brachial plexus palsy. *Plast Reconstr Surg.* 1998;102:1555–1562.

Chuang DC, Mardini S, Ma HS. Surgical strategy for infant obstetrical brachial plexus palsy: experiences at Chang Gung Memorial Hospital. *Plast Reconstr Surg.* 2005;116:132–142.

Gilbert A, Brockman R, Carlioz H. Surgical treatment of brachial plexus birth palsy. *Clin Orthop Relat Res.* 1991;264:39–47.

Gilbert A. Long-term evaluation of brachial plexus surgery in obstetrical palsy. *Hand Clin.* 1995;11:583–594.

Michelow BJ, Clarke HM, Curtis CG, Zuker RM, Seifu Y, Andrews DF. The natural history of obstetric brachial plexus palsy. *Plast Reconstr Surg.* 1994;93:675–680.

Vredeveld JW. Clinical neurophysiologic investigations. In: Gilbert A, ed. *Brachial Plexus Injuries.* London, United Kingdom: Martin-Dunitz, 2001:42.

CHAPTER 40 Brachial Plexus

Pieter G.L. Koolen, MD,
John B. Hijjawi, MD, FACS, and
Samuel J. Lin, MD, MBA, FACS

• • • DEMOGRAPHICS • • •

O **What is the most common mechanism for brachial plexus injuries?**
Closed injury (traction, compression, or combination of the two).

O **What is the most common location of brachial plexus injuries?**
Supraclavicular, root, and trunks.

O **What is the typical mechanism of a C8–T1/lower trunk traction injury?**
Forceful abduction of the arm overhead.

O **What brachial plexus injury is typically produced by violent lateral bending of the head and neck?**
Traction injury of C5, C6/upper trunk.

O **What is a common site for brachial plexus compression injuries?**
Between clavicle and first rib, near the coracoid process.

O **What are the demographics of the majority of patients with brachial plexus injuries?**
Male, aged 15 to 25.

O **What proportion of brachial plexus injuries occur in motor vehicle accidents?**
70%.

O **What type of vehicle is most commonly implicated in brachial plexus injuries?**
The motorcycle (70% of motor vehicle accidents). Snow mobiles in colder climates.

○   **At what level do most root avulsions occur?**
Lower roots (C7, C8, T1).

• • • **ANATOMY** • • •

○   **How many nerve roots form the brachial plexus?**
Five (C5–8, T1).

○   **What term describes a contribution of the C4 nerve root to the brachial plexus?**
Prefixed plexus.

○   **What phenomenon is described by the term "postfixed" brachial plexus?**
T2 contribution to the plexus.

○   **What are the five separate sections of the brachial plexus?**
Roots, trunks, divisions, cordserminal branches.
(Robert Taylor Drinks Coffee Black)

○   **What structure is formed by coalescence of the ventral and dorsal rootlets?**
The nerve root.

○   **What vascular structure is associated with the C7 root in the exposure of the cervical region of the brachial plexus?**
Transverse cervical artery.

○   **The medial cord of the brachial plexus receives contributions from which nerve roots?**
C8 and T1.

○   **Where does the nerve root leave the spinal canal?**
Through the neuroforamen.

○   **What is contained in the dorsal root ganglion?**
The cell bodies of the sensory nerves.

○   **Where do the motor nerves travel?**
In the volar root ganglion. (V volar, Vroom!!)

○   **What is described by the term preganglionic brachial plexus lesion?**
1. Lesion proximal to the dorsal root ganglion
2. Intradural rupture of the rootlets
3. Avulsion from spinal cord

○ **How are the upper, middle, and lower trunk typically formed?**

Upper trunk by C5 and C6.

Middle trunk by C7.

Lower trunk by C8 and T1.

○ **What is Erb's point?**

Point where C5 and C6 merge to form <u>upper trunk</u>.

○ **What structures join to become the posterior cord?**

All three posterior divisions.

○ **What is formed by the anterior divisions of the upper and middle trunk?**

The lateral cord.

(Imagine a football announcer, "Number 34 runs <u>up</u> [upper trunk] the <u>middle</u> [middle trunk] and throws a <u>lateral</u> [lateral cord]!")

○ **What continues as the medial cord?**

The anterior division of the lower trunk.

○ **The cords are named after their location in relation to which structure?**

The axillary artery.

○ **What part of the brachial plexus crosses underneath the clavicle?**

The divisions.

○ **What muscles are innervated by the dorsal scapular nerve?**

Rhomboid major/minor and levator scapulae.

○ **What are the terminal branches of the posterior cord?**

Proximal to distal:

1. upper subscapular n.

2. thoracodorsal n.

3. lower subscapular n.

4. axillary n.

5. radial n.

○ **What branches originate at the C5 root level?**

1. Phrenic n. contribution

2. Long thoracic n. contribution

3. Dorsal scapular n. (levator scapulae, rhomboids)

○ **What are the terminal branches of the medial cord?**

Four "medial (or median)" structures and the ulnar nerve.

<u>Medial</u> pectoral n.

<u>Medial</u> brachial cutaneous n.

<u>Medial</u> antebrachial cutaneous n.

Contribution to the <u>median</u> n.

Ulnar n.

○ **What are the branches of the lateral cord?**

1. Lateral pectoral n.

2. Contribution to the median n.

3. Musculocutaneous n.

○ **What branches originate from the upper trunk?**

Suprascapular n. nerve to the subclavius.

○ **Where is the inferior cervical sympathetic ganglion located?**

In proximity of the T1 nerve root.

● ● ● **PHYSICAL EXAMINATION** ● ● ●

○ **What is Horner syndrome?**

1. Ptosis

2. Miosis

3. Anhydrosis

4. Enophthalmos

This constellation indicates a lesion of the cervicothoracic sympathetic ganglion (adjacent to C8, T1) disrupting the oculosympathetic pathway.

○ **How is muscle strength graded?**

By the British Medical Research Council grading system:

M0: no evidence of contractility

M1: evidence of contractility <u>but no motion</u>

M2: complete range of motion with gravity eliminated

M3: complete range of motion against gravity

M4: complete range of motion against some resistance

M5: normal power

○ **Examination of which upper extremity functions will test for the condition of the posterior cord?**
1. Wrist extension (radial n.)
2. Elbow extension (radial n.)
3. Shoulder abduction (axillary n. via deltoid)

○ **How can the condition of the suprascapular n. be tested?**
1. Shoulder elevation (supraspinatus)
2. External rotation (infraspinatus)

○ **What is a strong indicator for a preganglionic lesion at the C8 and T1 nerve roots?**
Presence of a Horner syndrome (indicating a lesion of the cervicothoracic sympathetic ganglion [adjacent to C8, T1]).

○ **Dysfunction of which nerve will result in scapular winging with forward elevation of the shoulder?**
Long thoracic nerve via serratus anterior (SALT—serratus anterior long thoracic).

• • • RADIOLOGY • • •

○ **What is the significance of transverse process fractures on the cervical spine x-rays in brachial plexus patients?**
May indicate root avulsion.

○ **What findings on a chest x-ray may point toward a brachial plexus lesion?**
Fractures of the first and second rib.

○ **What is the significance of pseudomeningoceles on a cervical CT myelogram?**
Indicates root-level injury.

○ **What finding would be expected on the chest x-rays of patients with phrenic nerve injury?**
Elevation of ipsilateral hemidiaphragm.

• • • ELECTRICAL STUDIES • • •

○ **What do fibrillation potentials in the EMG indicate?**
Denervation of the tested muscles (just like the heart fibrillates when it is dying).

○ **After acute brachial plexus injury, how soon would muscles exhibit fibrillations in the EMG?**
10 to 14 days for proximal muscles and 3 to 4 months for distal muscles.

○ **What evidence can be found in electrodiagnostic studies of preganglionic lesions?**
Preservation of sensory nerve action potentials (SNAPs).

○ **What is the significance of the appearance of nascent potentials in follow-up EMGs?**
Early sign of reinnervation.

○ **What does the presence of intraoperative nerve action potentials (NAPs) across a lesion indicate?**
Intact axons.

○ **How many patients with detectable NAPs across a lesion will make a clinically useful recovery?**
90%.

○ **What pattern of NAPs would be expected in a preganglionic plexus lesion?**
Accelerated conduction velocity with increased amplitude.

○ **What do motor evoked potentials assess?**
Integrity of motor pathway via the ventral root (remember Vroom).

○ **How can the integrity of the sensory pathway via the dorsal roots be tested?**
Somatosensory evoked potentials.

● ● ● TREATMENT PRINCIPLES ● ● ●

○ **When is immediate exploration and primary repair of brachial plexus injuries indicated?**
Sharp, open injuries.

○ **What is the preferred treatment for low-velocity gunshot wounds of the brachial plexus?**
Observation, local wound management.

○ **What type of nerve injury is typically associated with low-velocity gunshot wounds?**
Neuropraxia.

○ **What is the recommended time frame for brachial plexus exploration in stretch injuries that fail to recover?**
3 to 6 months.

○ **What is the order of priority for restoration of function to the flail extremity?**
1. Elbow flexion
2. Shoulder abduction/stability
3. Hand sensibility
4. Wrist extension/finger flexion
5. Wrist flexion and finger extension

○ **What type of injury is preferably addressed with primary nerve repair?**

Sharp laceration, not possible in stretch injuries.

○ **What procedure needs to be performed to facilitate intraoperative nerve conduction studies?**

External neurolysis.

○ **What is the treatment for electrically silent ruptures or neuromas of the brachial plexus that are electrically silent?**

Interpositional nerve grafting (e.g., sural cable graft).

○ **What upper extremity function should be targeted if interpositional nerve grafting from a functioning C5 nerve root is performed?**

Shoulder abduction (suprascapular, axillary nerves).

○ **What nerve root (when available) should be used to restore elbow flexion by interpositional sural nerve grafting?**

C6 (musculocutaneous n.).

○ **How can triceps function be restored in a patient with a brachial plexus injury at the trunk level?**

By interpositional grafting from C7 across the zone of injury.

○ **What is the likely etiology of neuropathic pain after brachial plexus reconstruction?**

Regenerating axons from nonavulsed nerve roots.

● ● ● NERVE TRANSFER ● ● ●

○ **What type of brachial plexus injuries requires the use of nerve transfer (neurotization) to restore function?**

Preganglionic injuries.

○ **How can a nerve transfer accelerate recovery of function?**

By decreasing the distance between the nerve repair site and the end organ (muscle).

○ **What is the Oberlin transfer?**

Transfer of selected ulnar nerve fascicles in the upper arm to motor branches of the musculocutaneous nerve to the biceps to restore elbow flexion.

○ **What nerve has been used successfully to neurotize the serratus anterior muscle to address scapular winging?**

Thoracodorsal nerve.

○ **What function can be restored by neurotizing the suprascapular nerve with spinal accessory or phrenic nerve?**

Shoulder abduction/external rotation.

○ **What nerve can be targeted in addition to suprascapular nerve to further improve shoulder abduction?**
Axillary nerve.

○ **What nerve transfers are commonly used for restoration of biceps function after upper trunk disruption?**
Medial pectoral nerve to musculocutaneous nerve or the biceps motor branch Oberlin transfer.

○ **What is the advantage of the Oberlin transfer over interpositional nerve grafts from C6 to regain biceps function?**
Faster and more predictable recovery of function.

○ **In the Oberlin transfer fascicles of the ulnar nerve transmitting which function should preferably be used?**
Fascicles that stimulate wrist flexion (FCU).

○ **What modification of the Oberlin transfer is available to improve recovery of elbow flexion strength?**
Double fascicular nerve transfer described by MacKinnon, et al.

○ **What additional muscle is targeted in the double fascicular nerve transfer of the Oberlin transfer?**
Brachialis muscle.

○ **What donor fascicles are used to neurotize the brachialis muscle in the double fascicular nerve transfer?**
FCR or FDS fascicles of the median nerve.

○ **What donor nerves are available for neurotization to restore elbow flexion in a "panbrachial" plexopathy without signs of recovery?**
1. Intercostal nerves
2. Spinal accessory via nerve grafts
3. Phrenic nerve with interpositional grafts

○ **Comparing intercostal and partial ulnar nerve transfers to the biceps branch of the musculocutaneous nerve, which restores elbow flexion more successfully?**
Partial ulnar nerve (Oberlin).

○ **What is the advantage of a vascularized nerve graft?**
Reinnervation at a faster rate (theoretically).

○ **What <u>contralateral</u> nerve root can be used as a donor of large amounts of motor axons?**
C7—usually half of it.

○ **What function is addressed by contralateral C7 transfer via vascularized ulnar nerve to the median nerve?**
Finger flexion.

○ **What overall success rate can be expected with nerve transfers to the musculocutaneous nerve?**

71% flexion strength >M3, 37% >M4.

○ **What is the success rate of the Oberlin transfer?**

97% for >M3, 94% >M4.

○ **How much shoulder abduction can be expected in a good result after nerve transfer?**

45 degrees.

○ **What options are available for restoration of elbow flexion in patients that present late (>12 months after injury)?**

1. Free functioning muscle transfer
2. Tendon transfer of available, expendable muscles
3. Steindler flexorplasty (transposition of flexor-pronator origin to anterior humerus)
4. Pectoralis major transfer
5. Latissimus dorsi transfer
6. Triceps transfer

● ● ● OBSTETRICAL BRACHIAL PLEXUS INJURY ● ● ●

○ **What are the risk factors for obstetrical brachial plexus palsy?**

1. Increased birth weight
2. Vertex presentation
3. Births that require instrumentation for delivery
4. Shoulder dystocia

○ **What are causes for obstetric brachial plexus injury (birth palsy)?**

Traction injury secondary to:

Fetal malposition

Cephalopelvic disproportion

Forceps use

○ **What are the three distributions observed in obstetric brachial plexus palsy?**

1. Erb palsy
2. Panplexus palsy
3. Klumpke palsy

○ **What nerve roots are involved in <u>Erb palsy</u>?**

C5-6—upper roots.

○ **What nerve roots are involved in <u>Klumpke</u> palsy?**

C5-T1—lower roots.

○ **What is considered an indication for surgery in obstetric brachial plexus injuries?**

Absent biceps recovery at age 3 months.

○ **What does the Mallet classification assess?**

Upper extremity function

○ **Which root levels are more likely to be affected by root avulsions?**

Lower levels C8, T1.

○ **What is the mainstay for treatment of children with partial lesions?**

1. Conservative treatment
2. ROM exercises
3. Prevention of contractures

○ **What is the typical pattern of contracture of the shoulder in children with brachial plexus birth palsy?**

Internal rotation.
Adduction.

○ **What is a common complication due to the internal rotation contracture in children with brachial plexus birth palsy?**

Posterior shoulder dislocation.

○ **What nonsurgical treatment can be used to treat early posterior shoulder dislocation due to internal rotation contracture?**

Closed reduction and Botulinum toxin A injection into the shoulder internal rotators.

○ **What tendon transfer can be used to improve external rotation of the shoulder and prevent the development of internal rotation contracture?**

Transfer of latissimus dorsi and teres major to the humeral greater tuberosity.

○ **What deformity of the elbow will frequently develop in children with obstetric brachial plexus palsy?**

Posterior radial head dislocation. Typically by age 5 to 8 years.

○ **What is a typical finding in the forearm of children with obstetric palsy?**

Supination contracture.

● ● ● REFERENCES ● ● ●

Bertelli JA, Ghizoni MF. Brachial plexus avulsion injury repairs with nerve transfers and nerve grafts directly implanted into the spinal cord yield partial recovery of shoulder and elbow movements. *Neurosurgery.* 2003;52:1385–1390.

Bertelli JA, Ghizoni MF. The possible role of regenerating axons in pain persistence after brachial plexus grafting. *Microsurgery.* 2010;30(7):532–536.

Brandt KE, Mackinnon SE. A technique for maximizing biceps recovery in brachial plexus reconstruction. *J Hand Surg Am.* 1993;18(4):726–733.

Brunelli G, Monini L. Direct muscular neurotization. *J Hand Surg Am.* 1985;10:993–997.

Carvalho GA, Nikkhah G, Matthies C, Penkert G, Samii M. Diagnosis of root avulsions in traumatic brachial plexus injuries: value of computerized tomography myelography and magnetic resonance imaging. *J Neurosurg.* 1997;86:69–76.

Coulet B, Boretto JG, Lazerges C, Chammas M. A comparison of intercostal and partial ulnar nerve transfers in restoring elbow flexion following upper brachial plexus injury (C5-C6+/−C7). *J Hand Surg Am.* 2010;35(8):1297–1303.

Doi K, Muramatsu K, Hattori Y, et al. Restoration of prehension with the double free muscle technique following complete avulsion of the brachial plexus. indications and long-term results. *J Bone Joint Surg Am.* 2000;82(2):652–666.

Ezaki M, Malungpaishrope K, Harrison RJ, et al. OnabotulinumtoxinA injection as an adjunct in the treatment of posterior shoulder subluxation in neonatal brachial plexus palsy. *J Bone Joint Surg Am.* 2010;92(12):2171–2177.

Narakas AO. The treatment of brachial plexus injuries. *Int Orthop.* 1985;9:29–36.

Oberlin C, Beal D, Leechavengvongs S, Salon A, Dauge MC, Sarcy JJ. Nerve transfer to biceps muscle using a part of ulnar nerve for C5-C6 avulsion of the brachial plexus: anatomical study and report of four cases. *J Hand Surg Am.* 1994;19:232–237.

Ruch DS, Friedman AH, Nunley JA. The restoration of elbow flexion with intercostal nerve transfers. *Clin Orthop Relat Res.* 1995;314:95–103.

Terzis JK, Kostopoulos E. Our experience with secondary reconstruction of external rotation in obstetrical brachial plexus palsy. *Plast Reconstr Surg.* 2010;126(3):951–963.

Tung TH, Mackinnon SE. Nerve transfers: indications, techniques, and outcomes. *J Hand Surg Am.* 2010;35(2):332–341.

Uerpairojkit C, Leechavengvongs S, Witoonchart K, Malungpaishorpe K, Raksakulkiat R. Nerve transfer to serratus anterior muscle using the thoracodorsal nerve for winged scapula in C5 and C6 brachial plexus root avulsions. *J Hand Surg Am.* 2009;34(1):74–78.

CHAPTER 41 Tendon Transfers

Pieter G.L. Koolen, MD,
John B. Hijjawi, MD, FACS, and
Samuel J. Lin, MD, MBA, FACS

• • • PRINCIPLES • • •

○ **What should the patient's joints be assessed for prior to considering a tendon transfer?**

1. Mobility
2. Contracture

○ **What is a prerequisite for successful outcome of tendon transfers?**

Flexibility of the joint to be moved by transferred tendons.

○ **What are the goals of preoperative therapy?**

Maintain passive mobility.

Prevent joint contractures.

○ **What factors need to be considered when selecting a donor muscle for tendon transfer?**

1. Adequate strength
2. Tendon excursion
3. Straight line of pull
4. Synergism of action between the donor and recipient muscles
5. Expendable donor
6. Tissue equilibrium

○ **What geometric feature correlates with the strength of a muscle?**

Cross-sectional area of the muscle.

○ **What does the work capacity of a muscle correlate with?**
Muscle volume.

○ **What does muscle excursion correlate with?**
Muscle-fiber length.

○ **How much tendon excursion can be found in wrist flexors and extensors?**
30 mm.

○ **What is the amplitude of tendon excursion for finger extensors and flexors, respectively?**
1. 50 mm
2. 70 mm
Thus, when wrist tendons are used to restore finger function, there is usually incomplete correction.

○ **How can the effective amplitude of tendon excursion be increased?**
1. Increasing the number of joints the muscle tendon unit crosses.
2. Dissection of the muscle from its surrounding fascial attachments.

• • • RADIAL NERVE • • •

○ **What is the most significant limb dysfunction after radial nerve palsy?**
Inability to extend the wrist and stabilization for all other hand activities.

○ **What is the effect of restoring active wrist extension on grip strength?**
Grip strength will increase three to fivefold.

○ **What is the advantage of maintaining active wrist motion?**
Tenodesis effect.

○ **What is the tenodesis effect?**
Finger extension with wrist flexion. Try this on yourself.

○ **What are the indications for tendon transfer?**
Insufficient recovery of function after nerve injury that has been observed for an appropriate length of time.

○ **What is often considered as an early tendon transfer within weeks after nerve injury?**
Single tendon for wrist extension (e.g., pronator teres to ECRB) as an internal splint.

○ **What is the advantage of the early tendon transfer?**
Facilitates power grip by wrist extension, and finger extension through tenodesis effect.

○ **What is the preferred timing for the delayed tendon transfers?**

6 to 18 months.

○ **In general what are the available donor muscles for tendon transfers in radial nerve palsy?**

All extrinsic median and ulnar nerve innervated muscles.

○ **What muscle tendon transfers are included in the Brand transfer for radial nerve palsy?**

1. PT to ECRB
2. FCR to EDC
3. PL to EPL

Thus, wrist, finger, and thumb extension, the critical deficits in radial nerve palsy, are restored.

○ **What is the Boyes tendon transfer?**

A tendon transfer for radial nerve palsy includes:

1. PT to ECRB
2. FDS III to EDC
3. FDS IV to EIP and EPL
4. FCR to APL and EPB

○ **What is the advantage of the Boyes transfer?**

It can be used in patients who do not have a palmaris longus.

○ **What is the disadvantage of the FDS III and IV tendon transfer?**

Bowing of the donor digits.

○ **What tendon transfers are included in the FCU transfer for radial nerve palsy?**

1. PT to ECRB
2. FCU to EDC
3. PL to EPL

○ **What is the preferred tendon transfer to restore active wrist extension in a radial nerve palsy?**

PT to ECRB.

○ **What muscle tendon transfers can be used for restoration of MPJ extension?**

1. FCR to EDC
2. FCU to EDC
3. FDS III to EDC

○ **What is the theoretical advantage of the FDS III to EDC transfer in restoration for MPJ extension?**

1. Straight line of pull
2. Expendable donor
3. Sufficient strength
4. Sufficient excursion
5. Synergism

○ **What are potential disadvantages of the FCU to ECRB transfer?**

Weakness of wrist flexion with wrist radial deviation deformity and unnecessary strength of wrist extension.

○ **What is the primary choice for restoration of finger extension?**

FCR to EDC transfer.

○ **Why does the FDS III transfer not interfere with the flexor power of the other three FDS muscles?**

Because the FDS III has a separate muscle belly.

○ **What are the two functions of the functioning EPL?**

1. Thumb IP extension
2. Thumb adduction

○ **How can the PL to EPL transfer restore thumb abduction in addition to thumb extension?**

Rerouting the EPL from the third dorsal compartment and allowing it to lie along the first dorsal compartment will convert its adduction moment into an abduction moment.

○ **Which anatomic route is used for the FDS III to EDC tendon transfer?**

FDS III tendon is rerouted through a large window in the interosseous membrane of the forearm.

○ **What is the position of immobilization after tendon transfers for wrist extension, finger extension, and thumb extension?**

1. 90-degree elbow flexion
2. Neutral forearm rotation
3. 45-degree wrist extension
4. Full extension of MPJ
5. Thumb abduction and full extension of IP and MPJ

○ **When should dynamic splinting be initiated?**

After 3 weeks of initial immobilization.

○ **What does the dynamic splint after tendon transfer for radial nerve palsy entail?**

1. Dynamic extension outrigger
2. 30-degree wrist extension
3. MP flexion block at 30 degrees increased at weekly intervals
4. Active ROM initiated at 5 weeks postoperation

○ **How is extensor lag at the MPJ postoperatively addressed?**

1. Delay of passive ROM and dynamic splinting
2. Extension splinting

• • • MEDIAN NERVE • • •

○ **What is the major deficit associated with low median nerve palsy?**

Loss of thumb opposition and sensation of palmar surfaces of thumb, index, long, and radial half of ring finger.

○ **What muscles facilitate thumb opposition?**

1. Abductor pollicis brevis
2. Opponens pollicis
3. Superficial head of flexor pollicis brevis

○ **What are conditions leading to loss of thumb opposition?**

1. Median nerve laceration
2. Chronic carpal tunnel syndrome
3. Congenital deficiency of thenar musculature (thumb hypoplasia)
4. Polyneuropathy
5. Thenar trauma

○ **What trapeziometacarpal joint motions constitute thumb opposition?**

1. Abduction
2. Flexion
3. Pronation—opposes the volar surfaces of the thumb and fingers

○ **What explains maintained ability of thumb opposition after complete median nerve laceration at the wrist?**

Variable ulnar nerve innervation of the superficial head of the flexor pollicis brevis.

○ **What are four reliable options for opponensplasty?**

1. EIP
2. ADM (Huber)
3. Palmaris longus (Camitz)
4. FDS of the ring finger

○ **What are the landmarks of the vector line of pull for the most common tendon transfers to restore thumb opposition?**

1. Os pisiforme

2. APB insertion

○ **What is the most common tendon transfer used for low median nerve palsy?**

EIP to APB transfer.

○ **Where can the EIP tendon be located at the dorsum of the second MPJ?**

Ulnar to the EDC tendon to the index.

○ **How is proper tensioning of the opponensplasty assessed?**

1. Full thumb adduction with passive wrist flexion.

2. Appropriate thumb opposition with passive wrist extension.

○ **What is the Huber transfer?**

Abductor digiti minimi transfer for thumb opposition.

○ **What is the classic indication for the Huber transfer?**

Congenital hypoplastic thumb.

○ **What is the advantage of the Huber transfer?**

Cosmesis—the muscle bulk restores the hypoplastic thenar eminence.

○ **What is the disadvantage of the Huber transfer in thumb hypoplasia?**

Insufficient tendon for thumb MCP reconstruction. The long or ring finger FDS transfer does not have this limitation although it lacks bulk.

○ **What is the position of immobilization after opponensplasty?**

1. Thumb spica with opposition of thumb.

2. Slight wrist extension for EIP and ADM transfers.

3. Slight wrist flexion for FDS and PL transfers.

○ **What additional deficits distinguish the high from the low median nerve palsy?**

1. Inability to bend the thumb IP joint (FPL).

2. Inability to bend the index and long finger (FDS, FDP).

○ **What progressive deformity may develop after chronic high median nerve palsy?**

Swan neck deformity of the small and ring finger (absent FDS function).

○ **How is the variability in loss of finger flexion particularly of the long finger explained?**

Variable innervation of the FDP of the long finger by the ulnar nerve.

○ **What is the preferred procedure to restore a normal finger flexion cascade in high median nerve palsy?**

Side-to-side tenodesis of long and index finger FDP to the ring and small finger FDP.

○ **What donor muscle is most commonly used for restoration of FPL function?**

Brachioradialis.

○ **How can the available excursion of the brachioradialis muscle be maximized?**

1. Mobilization of the muscle.

2. Freeing it from its fascial envelope up to the proximal forearm.

3. Excursion up to 5 cm can be accomplished.

○ **What is the appropriate tension of the BR to FPL transfer?**

1. Full IP extension with 20 degrees of wrist flexion.

2. Adequate IP flexion with wrist extension.

○ **How can lack of active forearm rotation be addressed?**

Rerouting of the biceps tendon insertion to the lateral aspect of the proximal radius.

○ **What is the significance of sensory deficits?**

1. Limit the usefulness of tendon transfers.

2. Every effort to restore sensation should be made prior to tendon transfer via:

   i. Nerve repair/grafting

   ii. Nerve decompression

   iii. Nerve transfers

   iv. Neurovascular island flaps

• • • ULNAR NERVE • • •

○ **What is low ulnar nerve palsy as opposed to high ulnar nerve palsy?**

Lesion of ulnar nerve distal to innervation of FDP.

○ **Which fingers will typically be clawing in low ulnar nerve palsy?**

Small and ring fingers.

○ **What is the reason for the claw deformity?**

Absent intrinsic muscle function (remember that the ulnar innervated lumbricals extend the ring and small finger PIP joints).

○ **Why do index and long finger typically not develop clawing in isolated ulnar nerve palsy?**

Persistent function of the radial two lumbrical muscles that are median innervated.

○ **What does the claw deformity involve?**

1. Hyperextension of the MPJ
2. Inability to fully extend the PIP and DIP

○ **Which type of ulnar nerve palsy will demonstrate more significant clawing?**

1. Low ulnar nerve palsy.
2. Persistent function of ulnar two FDP in low ulnar nerve palsy will produce deforming force on the PIP joints. These FDPs are not functional in high ulnar nerve palsy.

○ **What eponym describes the clawing of ring and small fingers?**

Duchenne sign.

○ **What is the Bouvier maneuver?**

Blocking of MP hyperextension that will allow the EDC to fully extend the PIP and DIP.

○ **What is the Wartenberg sign?**

Inability to adduct the extended small finger.

○ **What is the deforming force for the Wartenberg sign?**

Unopposed pull of the radially innervated EDQ (absent fourth dorsal IO muscle).

○ **What is the Froment sign?**

Hyperflexion of the thumb IP joint with key pinch to compensate for the deficient thumb adductor.

○ **What is the Jeanne sign?**

Hyperextension of the MPJ of the thumb with attempted key pinch.

○ **What tendon transfers are available to restore thumb adduction?**

1. ECRB to thumb adductor via intercalated tendon graft
2. FDS of long or ring to thumb adductor insertion

○ **Which route is used for the ECRB transfer for thumb adduction?**

1. Subcutaneously extracompartmental
2. Around the second or third metacarpal neck
3. Volar to adductor pollicis
4. Deep to flexor tendon and neurovascular structures

○ **What additional function can be restored to improve the power of key pinch?**

Index finger abduction.

○ **What transfers are available for restoration of index finger abduction?**

Accessory slip of abductor pollicis longus or EIP (EIP transfer may lead to unacceptable amount of abduction).

○ **What are the general two types of tendon transfers that are performed for correction of claw deformity?**

1. Static transfer
2. Dynamic transfer

○ **What is involved in a static anti-claw transfer?**

Tenodesis of the lateral bands with a tendon graft around the deep transverse metacarpal ligaments providing an internal splint that prevents hyperextension of the MPJ.

○ **What does the Zancolli lasso procedure effectively treat?**

Claw deformity.

○ **What does the Zancolli Lasso procedure consist of?**

1. FDS is looped back to itself around the A1 pulley.
2. Providing a dynamic flexion moment at the MPJ.

○ **What tendon transfer to correct claw deformity originates from the dorsal side of the wrist?**

The Bunnell–Stiles tendon transfer.

○ **What are the steps of the Bunnell–Stiles tendon transfer?**

1. ECRL transected distally and rerouted dorsally.
2. Two slips of palmaris longus or plantaris graft extension sewn into the ECRL.
3. Tendons rerouted through the lumbrical canal (volar to the deep transverse metacarpal ligament).
4. Graft tails attached to radial lateral bands of the ring and small fingers or alternatively to radial side of proximal phalanx (see next question).

○ **What deformity can occur after the Bunnell–Stiles transfer to the radial lateral bands?**

Swan neck deformity.

○ **How can the development of swan neck deformity after the Bunnell–Stiles tendon transfer prevented?**

Transfer of the tendon to the proximal phalanx rather than the lateral band.

○ **What patient factors lead to a higher likelihood of swan neck deformity after the Bunnell–Stiles transfer into the lateral bands?**

PIP joint hyperextensibility.

○ **What additional function is lost in a high ulnar nerve palsy?**

Absent small and ring finger FDP.

○ **What tendon transfer reliably restores ring and small finger DIP joint flexion?**

Side-to-side transfer of small and ring finger FDP to median innervated index and long finger FDP tendon.

• • • COMBINED PALSIES • • •

○ **What is the most common mechanism for combined nerve palsies?**

Lacerations—particularly at the wrist.

○ **What is the most common combined nerve palsy?**

Low median-ulnar nerve palsy.

○ **What are the requirements for restoration of wrist and hand function in low median and ulnar nerve palsy?**

1. Improve key pinch.
2. Thumb abduction (to improve opposition).
3. Tip pinch (increase index strength in pinch which has been compromised by first dorsal interosseous palsy).
4. Power finger flexion with coordinated MP and PIP motion.
5. Sensibility in the distribution involved in key pinch.

○ **What is the preferred thumb opposition transfer in combined median-ulnar nerve palsy?**

1. EIP transfer
2. Second choice: PL, FDS

○ **What muscles are preferred for restoration of thumb adduction?**

1. ECRB
2. Long finger FDS

○ **How can the last two transfers use the FDS if these are for combined ulnar-median nerve palsies?**

Because they are for low (wrist level) combined palsies.

○ **What procedures can help to improve thumb-index tip pinch?**

1. Thumb IP fusion.
2. Transfer of APL with graft extension to first dorsal interosseous.

○ **What type of procedure will help with integration of MP and IP joint motion?**

Intrinsic transfers (e.g., Bunnell–Stiles).

● ● ● **REFERENCES** ● ● ●

Anderson GA, Lee V, Sundararaj GD. Opponensplasty by extensor indicis and flexor digitorum superficialis tendon transfer. *J Hand Surg Br.* 1992;17:611–614.

Friden J, Lieber RL. Tendon transfer surgery: clinical implications of experimental studies. *Clin Orthop Relat Res.* 2002;(403 Suppl): S163–S170.

Goldfarb CA, Stern PJ. Low ulnar nerve palsy. *J Am Soc Surg Hand.* 2003;3:14–26.

Green DP. Radial nerve palsy. In Green DP, Hotchkiss RN, Pederson WC, eds. *Green's Operative Hand Surgery.* Vol 2. 4th ed. New York, NY: Churchill Livingstone; 1999:1481–1496.

Krishnan KG, Schackert G. An analysis of results after selective tendon transfers through the interosseous membrane to provide selective finger and thumb extension in chronic irreparable radial nerve lesions. *J Hand Surg Am.* 2008;33(2):223–231.

Mc Carroll HR. Tendon transfers. In: Light TR, ed. *Hand Surgery Update.* 2nd ed. Rosemont, IL: American Academy of Orthopaedic Surgeons; 1999:161–169.

Omer G. Combined nerve palsies. In: Green DP, Hotchkiss RN, Pederson WC, eds. *Green's Operative Hand Surgery.* Vol 2. 4th ed. New York, NY: Churchill Livingstone; 1999:1542–1555.

Ratner JA, Peljovich A, Kozin SH. Update on tendon transfers for peripheral nerve injuries. *J Hand Surg Am.* 2010;35(8):1371–1381.

Sammer DM, Chung KC. Tendon transfers: part II. transfers for ulnar nerve palsy and median nerve palsy. *Plast Reconstr Surg.* 2009; 124(3):212e–221e.

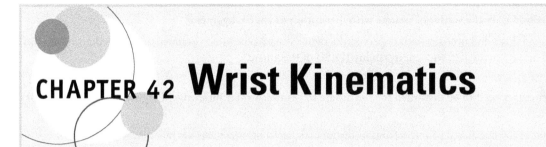

CHAPTER 42 Wrist Kinematics

Sanjeev Kakar, MD, MRCS and
Bassem T. Elhassan, MD

○ **What is the carpal height ratio?**

It is the distance defined from the base of the third metacarpal to the distal subchondral bone of the radius divided by the length of the third metacarpal. The normal ratio is 0.54 ± 0.03.

○ **What are the *main* muscles primarily responsible for wrist motion?**

They include the flexor carpi radialis, flexor carpi ulnaris, extensor carpi radialis longus and brevis, and extensor carpi ulnaris (ECU).

○ **What is the only muscle that inserts into the carpus?**

Flexor carpi ulnaris attaches into the pisiform.

○ **How many degrees of freedom are there pertaining to wrist range of motion?**

There are six degrees of freedom: flexion, extension, radial deviation, ulnar deviation, pronation, and supination.

○ **What is the intercalated segment within the wrist?**

The proximal row (scaphoid, lunate, and triquetrum) is the intercalated segment within the wrist. The bones of the proximal row are less tightly bound together than the distal row and there is approximately three times more motion between the scaphoid and lunate compared to the lunotriquetral joint.

○ **How does the position of the proximal row change with wrist range of motion?**

During wrist flexion, the bones of the proximal row go into flexion and ulnar deviation whereas with wrist extension, they go into extension and radial deviation. Similar motion is noted within the distal carpal row albeit with less radial and ulnar deviation as noted with the proximal carpal row during wrist extension and flexion, respectively.

○ **What are the different regions within the scapholunate (SL) ligament called?**

There are three regions that comprise the SL ligament: the dorsal, the membranous or proximal, and palmar regions. In cadaveric studies, disruption of the dorsal SL ligament resulted in a significant change in the spatial relationship between the scaphoid and lunate.

○ **What position does the scaphoid assume with disruption of the SL ligament?**

The scaphoid flexes and pronates with respect to the radius whereas the lunate assumes an extended position. This is termed dorsal intercalated segment instability (DISI) of the lunate.

○ **What structures need to be disturbed for the lunate to assume a volar intercalated segment instability (VISI) position?**

Disruption of the dorsal and palmar regions of the lunotriquetral ligament *does not* manifest with VISI static instability. For VISI to be noted, disruption of the dorsal radiotriquetral or dorsal scaphotriquetral must also occur.

○ **What is the normal force transmission through the wrist?**

In neutral position and neutral ulnar variance, approximately 80% to 85% of axial load is transmitted through the radiocarpal joint and 15% to 20% through the ulnocarpal joint.

○ **What are the components of the triangular fibrocartilaginous complex (TFCC)?**

The TFCC comprises an articular disc, superficial and deep dorsal and palmar radioulnar ligaments, ulnotriquetral, ulnolunate, ulnocapitate ligaments, and the ECU within its subsheath.

○ **What is the function of the TFCC?**

The primary responsibility of the TFCC is to maintain stability of the distal radioulnar joint (DRUJ). In addition, it plays an important role in force transmission across the wrist with studies showing that removal of two-thirds or more of complex having an effect on force transmission.

○ **What is the stable bone of the DRUJ?**

The ulnar is the fixed bone of the DRUJ around which the radius rotates.

○ **What are the dynamic and static stabilizers of the DRUJ?**

The dynamic stabilizers of the DRUJ include the ECU and pronator quadratus whereas the static restraints include the DRUJ capsule, ulnotriquetral and ulnolunate ligaments, interosseous membrane, and TFCC. In terms of the latter, the primary stabilizers of the DRUJ are the palmar and dorsal radioulnar ligaments. They originate from the distal margins of the DRUJ and appear as thickenings at the junction of the TFCC, DRUJ, and ulnocarpal capsule. The cartilaginous disc is located centrally between these ligaments. As the radioulnar ligaments pass toward the ulna, they divide into a superficial limb, which inserts into the ulna styloid, and a deep limb that attaches to the fovea. They remain in a relaxed position until terminal pronation and supination, thereby permitting palmar and dorsal translation of the ulna head over several millimeters.

○ **What is the name of the articular surface of the radius that articulates with the ulnar?**

The sigmoid notch. The sigmoid notch has a radius of curvature that is greater than that of the ulnar head. Increased stability to this articulation is provided by the DRUJ ligaments and palmar/dorsal fibrocartilaginous projections from the sigmoid notch.

○ **What changes are seen in relation of the ulnar head to sigmoid notch of the radius during pronation and supination?**

In full pronation, the ulnar head rests against the dorsal lip of the sigmoid notch. In supination, the ulnar head rests against the palmar surface of the sigmoid notch.

○ **What position of the forearm reduces dorsal dislocation of the ulna with respect to the radius?**

These dislocations are reduced with the forearm in a supinated position.

○ **What is the eponym commonly given to ipsilateral radial head fractures and concomitant DRUJ injuries?**

Essex-Lopresti lesions represent ligament injury at the distal DRUJ combined with elements of attenuation or disruption of the interosseous membrane. Its importance is related to the observation that the radius can migrate proximally if the radial head is excised and not replaced given disruption of its distal tether at the wrist.

○ **What happens to force transmission across the wrist with changes in ulnar length?**

In patients with a short ulnar (ulnar negative variance), as often seen in Kienbock disease, there is a decrease in force transmission across the ulnar with corresponding increase across the radiocarpal joint.

○ **What is the blood supply to the proximal pole of the scaphoid?**

The main blood supply is from the radial artery and enters through small foramina in the dorsal ridge. Fractures proximal to this area may result in avascular necrosis of the proximal pole.

○ **Which extrinsic wrist ligament is felt to be the strongest support in the wrist?**

The radioscaphocapitate ligament is felt to be the most important ligament for wrist support.

○ **As the wrist moves from ulnar deviation to radial deviation, what happens to the scaphoid?**

The scaphoid moves from an extended position into a palmar-flexed position.

○ **What are the major extrinsic ligaments of the dorsal wrist?**

The dorsal radiocarpal ligament and the dorsal intercarpal ligament are the major dorsal extrinsic wrist ligaments.

○ **What does DISI stand for?**

DISI stands for dorsal intercalary segment instability and is related to tears of the SL ligament.

○ **What is the Terry Thomas sign?**

The Terry Thomas sign is an abnormal gap between the scaphoid and lunate that occurs in SL ligament tears. It is named after the gap-toothed British comedian.

○ **The spilled tea-cup sign is seen in which carpal instability pattern?**

The spilled tea-cup sign is seen in volar intercalary segment instability (VISI).

○ **What is meant by "progressive perilunate instability"?**

Progressive perilunate instability is a progression of injury, beginning at the SL joint and progressing in severity to total perilunate injury.

○ **What is Stage I perilunate instability?**

Stage I perilunate instability is scaphoid fracture or a SL interosseous ligament tear.

○ **What is Stage II perilunate instability?**

Stage II perilunate instability is a SL ligament injury with lunocapitate dislocation and a tear through the space of Poirier.

○ **What is Stage III perilunate instability?**

Stage III perilunate instability is associated with a lunotriquetral ligament tear or triquetrum fracture.

○ **What is Stage IV perilunate instability?**

Stage IV perilunate instability is a lunate dislocation.

○ **How does one differentiate a perilunate dislocation from a lunate dislocation?**

In a perilunate dislocation, the lunate remains seated in the lunate fossa of the radius and all other carpal bones are sitting dorsal to their typical position. In a lunate dislocation the lunate is dislocated palmarly into the carpal tunnel and the other carpal bones are in their typical location.

○ **What is the most common fracture in carpal bones?**

The scaphoid is the most commonly fractured carpal bone.

○ **What differentiates a perilunate dislocation and a trans-scaphoid perilunate dislocation?**

In a trans-scaphoid perilunate dislocation, the scaphoid bone is fractured and the SL interosseous ligament remains intact.

○ **What radiographic lines in the wrist are used to help determine normal anatomy from certain pathologic states including lunate and perilunate dislocations?**

Gilula lines show continuity of the radiocarpal and midcarpal joints.

○ **What is the scaphoid shift test?**

The scaphoid shift test is a test looking for SL ligament injury. With the wrist held in ulnar deviation, and the examiner's thumb holding pressure on the scaphoid tubercle, the wrist is passively brought into radial deviation. In patients with SL dissociation, the scaphoid, being held extended by the thumb, shifts dorsally causing pain and a clunk as the scaphoid moves back into the scaphoid fossa.

○ **What is the current treatment for the acute static SL dissociation?**

Most surgeons are currently performing SL ligament repair, supplemented by some form of dorsal wrist capsulodesis.

○ **What is the current treatment for lunate and perilunate dislocations?**

The recommended treatment is ORIF with both volar capsular repair and dorsal ligament repair.

○ **What is the current recommendation for proximal pole fractures of the scaphoid?**

Owing to the high rate of nonunion ORIF with screw fixation, using a dorsal approach is recommended.

○ **What is ulnar translocation of carpus?**

In individuals where there is tearing of the radioscaphocapitate and long radiolunate ligaments, the carpus will sometimes migrate ulnarly and volarly following the slope of the radius. Translocation can also occur in certain rheumatologic conditions of the wrist.

○ **Which fractures of the radius are frequently associated with SL ligament tears?**

Intra-articular fractures of the radius that are in the vicinity of the SL ligament are frequently associated with SL ligament tears.

○ **What is the appropriate initial treatment for an individual who after a fall onto an outstretched hand has pain in the snuffbox and negative radiographs?**

The appropriate initial treatment is short arm thumb spica splinting or casting with follow-up in 2 weeks. Continued pain in the snuffbox in the absence of x-ray findings required additional studies to rule out scaphoid fracture (bone scan/MRI/CT scan).

○ **Scaphoid fractures in which location have the best prognosis?**

Fractures of the distal pole of the scaphoid have the best prognosis. These fractures can be managed by short arm thumb spica splint or short arm thumb spica cast.

○ **What is the second most commonly fractured carpal bone?**

The triquetrum is the second most commonly fractured carpal bone. Most triquetral fractures are dorsal marginal fractures.

○ **What is the most common mechanism for fractures of the hook of the hamate?**

Most fractures of the hook of the hamate occur as a result of a direct blow.

○ **If one suspects a hook of the hamate fracture clinically, what is the best confirmatory study?**

The best confirmatory for hook of hamate fractures study is a CT scan.

○ **In a patient with a hook of hamate nonunion, what is the best treatment?**

The best treatment for a hook of hamate nonunion is excision of the hook of the hamate.

○ **What imaging modality is used to stage Kienbock disease?**

Plain radiographs are used to stage Kienbock disease. MRI is helpful in diagnosing Kienbock disease.

○ **What are the x-ray findings in Stage I Kienbock disease?**

X-rays are either normal or you may see linear fractures in the lunate.

○ **What are the x-ray findings in Stage II Kienbock disease?**

The lunate shows increased density in Stage II Kienbock disease.

○ **What are the x-ray findings in Stage III Kienbock disease?**

The lunate shows collapse and/or fragmentation in Stage III Kienbock disease.

○ **What are the x-ray findings in Stage IV Kienbock disease?**

Arthritis is present in Stage IV Kienbock disease.

○ **What x-ray finding of the bones of the forearm is associated with Kienbock disease?**

Ulnar negative variance has been associated with Kienbock disease.

○ **What are the measurements of carpal height used for?**

Measurements of carpal height are used as a means of diagnosing SL dissociation. The normal ratio is 0.54. Smaller ratios are indicative of the carpal collapse seen in SL dissociation.

○ **What does the term SLAC wrist refer to?**

The term SLAC refers to SL advanced collapse.

○ **What is the SLAC procedure and what must be normal to consider this procedure?**

The SLAC procedure is a four-corner (C-L-H-T) fusion with excision of the scaphoid and radial styloidectomy. The lunate fossa and proximal articular surface of the lunate must be intact to consider this procedure.

○ **What radiographic findings are usually present in patients with a lunatotriquetral ligament tear?**

Plain radiographs are usually normal in patients with isolated lunatotriquetral ligament tears. VISI deformities can be seen in more complex LT ligament injuries.

○ **What are the components of the triangular fibrocartilage complex?**

The components are the TFC proper, the ulnar collateral ligament, the ECU subsheath, the meniscus homologue, the ulnolunate and ulnotriquetral ligaments, and the dorsal and palmar radioulnar ligaments.

○ **What parts of the SL ligament are responsible for the biomechanical behavior of the joint?**

The thick dorsal and volar portions of the ligament are 3 mm thick and give strength and integrity to the joint.

○ **What is a Geisler Stage I SL instability?**

This is where attenuation or hemorrhage of the SL ligament can be seen from the radiocarpal joint. The SL joint appears to be congruent when viewed from the midcarpal portal.

○ **What is a Geisler Stage II SL instability?**

Similar findings are noted within the radiocarpal joint as seen with Geisler Stage I. The SL joint appears to be incongruent when viewed from the midcarpal portal and a gap less than the width of a probe may be present between the scaphoid and the lunate.

○ **What is a Geisler Stage III instability?**

Incongruency/step-off between the scaphoid and the lunate can be seen from both the radiocarpal and midcarpal spaces and the probe can be passed between the carpal bones.

○ **What is a Geisler Stage IV instability?**

Geisler Stage IV instability occurs when the arthroscope (2.7 mm) can be passed through the midcarpal joint to the radiocarpal joint. This is also known as the drive-through sign.

○ **What percent of arthrograms will show a SL ligament tear in an asymptomatic patient?**

27% of arthrograms will show an SL tear in asymptomatic patients.

○ **What is the reported accuracy of MR arthrogram for determining SL ligament tears?**

The reported accuracy of MR arthrography is 95%.

○ **What is the definitive diagnostic test for intercarpal pathology?**

Wrist arthroscopy is the definitive test for intercarpal pathology.

○ **What is the average radial inclination of the distal radius?**

22 degrees.

○ **What is the average volar tilt of the distal radius?**

11 degrees.

○ **How many millimeters of intra-articular displacement within a distal radius fracture is considered to be acceptable with nonoperative management?**

Up to 1 mm of displacement.

○ **What is a "Colles" fracture?**

This is a distal radius fracture with dorsal angulation, dorsal comminution, dorsal displacement, and radial shortening.

○ **What is a "Smith" fracture?**

This is a distal radius fracture with apex dorsal angulation with volar subluxation of the carpus (this is opposite to a Colles fracture that has apex volar angulation with dorsal displacement of the carpus). This is an important recognition as the mold placed within the cast for each fracture differs.

○ **What is a "Barton" fracture?**

This is an intra-articular distal radius fracture.

○ **Why is the assessment of median nerve function important in the examination of patients with a distal radius fracture?**

Patients with acute distal radius fractures can experience paresthesias within the median nerve distribution secondary to an acute carpal tunnel syndrome. After fracture reduction, these symptoms should improve and nerve compression can be treated with observation alone. Should they progress, an emergent release of the carpal tunnel is indicated.

○ **What is the most common tendon susceptible to spontaneous rupture in undisplaced distal radius fracture?**

The EPL tendon is susceptible to rupture and is more likely in undisplaced compared to displaced distal radius fractures. Postulated theories for the etiology include tendon attrition and impaired blood supply to the tendon.

○ **What is the most common tendon rupture seen with volar plating of distal radius fracture?**

The FPL tendon is susceptible to rupture as it runs over the volar lip of the distal radius. For this reason, it is of vital importance that the plate NOT be placed to distal.

● ● ● **REFERENCES** ● ● ●

Andrews JG, Youm Y. A biomechanical investigation of wrist kinematics. *J Biomech.* 1979:12:83–93.

Adolfsson L. Arthroscopy for the diagnosis of post-traumatic wrist pain. *J Hand Surg Am.* 1992;17:46–50.

Barber H. The interosseous arterial anatomy of the adult human carpus. *Orthopedics.* 1972;5:1–19.

Beckenbaugh RD. Accurate evaluation and management of the painful wrist following injury. An approach to carpal instability. *Orthop Clin North Am.* 1984;15:289–306.

Berger RA, Crowninschield RD, Flatt AE. The three dimensional rotational behaviours of the carpal bones. *Clin Orthop Relat Res.* 1982;167:303–310.

Berger RA, Garcia-Elias M. General anatomy of the wrist. In: An KN, Berger RA, Cooney WP, eds. *Biomechanics of the Wrist Joint.* New York, NY: Springer; 1991.

Berger RA. The gross and histologic anatomy of the scapholunate interosseous ligament. *J Hand Surg Am.* 1996;21:170–178.

De Lange ALH. *A kinematic study of the human wrist joint.* the Netherlands: Doctoral thesis; 1987.

Dobyns JH, Linscheid RL, Chao EYS, et al. Traumatic instability of the wrist. *AAOS Instructional Course Lectures.* 1975;24:182–199.

Fisk GR. Carpal instability and the fractured scaphoid. *Ann R Coll Surg Engl.* 1970;46:63–76.

Fisk GR. The wrist. *J Bone Joint Surg.* 1984;66:396–407.

Garcia-Elias M, Dobyns JH, Cooney WP, Linscheid RL. Traumatic axial dislocations of the carpus. *J Hand Surg Am.* 1989;14:446–456.

Garcia-Elias M, Horii E, Berger RA. Individual carpal bone motion. In: An KN, Berger RA, Cooney WP, eds. *Biomechanics of the Wrist Joint.* New York, NY: Springer; 1991.

Gilula LA, Destout JM, Weeks PM, Young LV, Wray RC. Roentgenographic diagnosis of the painful wrist. *Clin Orthop Relat Res.* 1984;187:52–64.

Green DP, O'Brien ET. Classification and management of carpal dislocations. *J Bone Joint Surg.* 1980;149:55–72.

Horii E, Garcia-Elias M, An KN, et al. A kinematic study of lunotriquetral dissociations. *J Hand Surg Am.* 1991:16:355–362.

Johnson RP. The acutely injured wrist and its residuals. *Clin Orthop Relate Res.* 1980;149:33–44.

Kihara H, Short WH, Werner FW, Fortino MD, Palmer AK. The stabilizing mechanism of the distal radioulnar joint during pronation and supination. *J Hand Surg Am.* 1995;20(6):930–936.

Kirschenbaum D, Sieler S, Solonick D, Loeb DM, Cody RP. Arthrography of the wrist. assessment of the integrity of the ligaments in young asymptomatic adults. *J Bone Joint Surg Am.* 1995;77:1207–1209.

Lavernia CJ, Cohen MS, Taleisnik J. Treatment of scapholunate dissociation by ligamentous repair and capsulodesis. *J Hand Surg Am.* 1992;17:354–359.

Lichtman DM, Schneider JR, Swafford AR, Mack GR. Ulnar midcarpal instability—clinical and laboratory analysis. *J Hand Surg Am.* 1981;6:515–523.

Linscheid RL, Dobyns JH. The unified concept of carpal injuries. *Ann Chir Main.* 1984;3:35–42.

Lynched RL, Dobbins JH, Beabout JW, Bryan RS. Traumatic instability of the wrist. *J Bone Joint Surg.* 1972;54:1612–1632.

Mayfield JK, Johnson RP, Kilcoyne RK. Carpal dislocations: pathomechanics and progressive perilunar instability. *J Hand Surg Am.* 1980;5:226–241.

Moneim MS. Management of greater arc carpal fractures. *Hand Clin.* 1988;4:457–467.

Panagis JS, Gelberman RH, Taleisnik J, Baumgaertner M. The arterial anatomy of the human carpus. Part II: the interosseous vascularity. *J Hand Surg Am.* 1983;8:375–382.

Palmer AK, Werner FW, Glisson RR, Murphy DJ. Partial excision of the triangular fibrocartilage complex. *J Hand Surg Am.* 1988;13:391–394.

Ruby LK, Cooney WP 3rd, An KN, Linscheid RL, Chao EY. Relative motion of selected carpal bones: a kinematic analysis of the normal wrist. *J Hand Surg Am.* 1988;13:1–10.

Schuind F, An KN, Berglund L, et al. The distal radioulnar ligaments: a biomechanical study. *J Hand Surg Am.* 1991;16(6):1106–1114.

Smith DK, An KN, Cooney WP 3rd, Linscheid RL, Chao EY. Effects of a scaphoid waist osteotomy on carpal kinematics. *J Orthop Res.* 1989;7:590–598.

Smith DK, An KN, Cooney WP 3rd, Linscheid RL, Chao EY. The effects of simulated unstable scaphoid fractures on carpal motion. *J Hand Surg Am.* 1989;14:283–291.

Taleisnik J. Current concepts review. Carpal instability. *J Bone Joint Surg Am.* 1988;70:1262–1268.

Viegas SF. Midcarpal arthroscopy: anatomy and technique. *Arthroscopy.* 1992;8:385–390.

Ward LD, Ambrose CG, Masson MV, Levaro F. The role of the distal radioulnar ligaments, interosseous membrane, and joint capsule in distal radioulnar joint stability. *J Hand Surg.* 2000;25(2):341–351.

Watson HK, Ashmead D 4th, Maklouf MV. Examination of the scaphoid. *J Hand Surg Am.* 1988;13:657–660.

Watson HK, Ballet FL. The SLAC wrist: scapholunate advanced collapse pattern of degenerative arthritis. *J Hand Surg Am.* 1984;9:358–365.

Wiedrich TA. The use of suture anchors in the hand and wrist. *Oper Tech Plast Reconstr Surg.* 1997;4:42–48.

Zlatkin MB, Chao PC, Osterman AL, Schnall MD, Dalinka MK, Kressel HY. Chronic wrist pain: evaluation with high resolution MR imaging. *Radiology.* 1989;173:723–729.

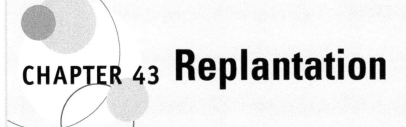

CHAPTER 43 Replantation

Sarosh N. Zafar, MD and
Scott L. Hansen, MD, FACS

● ● ● **DIGITAL REPLANTATION** ● ● ●

○ **What is the goal of digital replantation?**

Equivalent or improved function when compared to revision amputation and prosthesis.

○ **What are the current indications for digital replantation?**

- Thumb
- Multiple digits
- Single digit distal to sublimis
- Hand at the wrist or forearm (sharp amputation)
- Any level amputation in a child

○ **What is the appropriate preoperative workup for a patient with an amputated digit?**

- Evaluate and stabilize the patient using ATLS protocol.
- Do not complete partial amputations until fully examined in operating room.
- Wrap amputated part in moist gauze and place in plastic bag, then place on ice. Avoid direct contact with ice which can result in irreversible damage to microvascular system.
- Administer intravenous antibiotics, and tetanus prophylaxis.
- Radiographs of the involved hand and the amputated part.
- Appropriate preoperative counseling and consent (include possible nerve/vein/skin graft as well as possible amputation).

○ **What is the order for a single digit replant?**

BEFANV:

- Bone
- Extensors
- Flexors
- Arteries
- Nerves
- Veins

○ **What is the order for multiple digit replantations—digit by digit or structure by structure?**

Structure by structure, systemically repairing as above.

○ **What are the potential advantages to skeletal shortening in digital replantation?**

- May enable more secure bone fixation
- May minimize the need for vessel or nerve grafting

○ **What are the options for skeletal stabilization in digit replantation?**

- Kirschner wires
- 90–90 wiring
- Miniplates and screw
- Intramedullary bone pegs

○ **What are the functional deficits associated with ray amputation of the index finger?**

Loss of power grip and key pinch.

○ **What is the lumbrical plus deformity?**

The FDP tendon and lumbrical muscle migrate proximally after division of the tendon in trauma. With flexion, tension is exerted on the lumbrical via the radial lateral band causing paradoxical extension of the PIP during flexion of the MP joint.

○ **Treatment?**

Division of the lumbrical insertion.

○ **What is the most common cause of digital replantation failure?**

Arterial insufficiency.

○ **What is the treatment of arterial insufficiency after digital replantation?**

1. If any concern about arterial patency **RETURN to OR**
2. Loosen dressings
3. Heparin
4. Anti-vasospastic medications (Thorazine)
5. Sympathetic blocks

○ **What is the treatment of venous congestion after digital replantation?**
1. Removal of dressings
2. Leech therapy
3. Heparin
4. Nail bed bleeding with heparin-soaked sponges
5. Revision of the venous anastomosis

○ **Which tissue is most sensitive to warm ischemia?**
Skeletal muscle.

○ **What is the maximal cold ischemia time reported for digital replantation?**
30 to 40 hours.

○ **When should prophylactic fasciotomies be performed in upper extremity replantation?**
With any replantation proximal to the wrist prophylactic fasciotomies should be performed because of the increased amount of skeletal muscle present.

○ **What is the quadriga effect?**
Weakness in flexion of fingers secondary to excess pull of one FDP tendon of the amputated finger.

○ **What is the maximum nerve gap for use of a neural tube (PGA)?**
2.5 cm.

○ **What nerves are available for use as donors for nerve grafting?**
• Posterior interosseous nerve
• Sural nerve
• Superficial radial nerve
• Superficial peroneal nerve

○ **What is the treatment of choice for a tip amputation through the nail bed without bone exposure?**
Local dressing changes (i.e., healing by secondary intention).

○ **What is a good option for a failed thumb replantation at the MCP level?**
Revision amputation followed by toe-to-thumb transfer at a later date.

○ **What donor vessel is the toe-to-thumb transfer based on?**
First dorsal metatarsal artery from dorsalis pedis artery or plantar digital artery from lateral plantar artery.

○ **What is a good option for a thumb-tip amputation with exposed bone?**
Moberg flap.

○ **How much advancement can be obtained from a Moberg flap?**

1.5 cm.

○ **What are contraindications to digital replantation?**

- Severe concomitant injuries
- Severely crushed or mangled
- Multilevel amputations
- Significant comorbidities
- Prolonged warm ischemia time
- Mentally unstable/self-mutilation
- Single finger proximal to FDS insertion

○ **How many arteries and veins are needed for a digital replantation?**

One artery and one vein (two are preferred).

○ **Is an artery only digital replantation possible?**

Yes. Leeching and/or bleeding of the nail bed can be used to relieve venous congestion.

○ **How many places can you find a digital vein?**

Two. Dorsal and volar.

○ **What is the concern in avulsion amputation versus guillotine amputation?**

Zone of injury is much greater in avulsion injuries.

○ **What is the red stripe sign?**

A red streak along the artery indicating severe intimal injury along the length of the vessel.

○ **What is the best method for treating the zone of injury of an artery or vein in cases of crush or avulsion injuries?**

Resection of compromised vessel and vein grafting.

○ **Where can veins be reliably found on the hand dorsum?**

Proximal to each web space.

○ **What vascular pattern exists in a finger that was crushed and has the appearance of venous congestion and slow capillary refill?**

Loss of proper digital artery inflow, intact venous flow.

○ **Eight months post digital replantation, what operation would you offer to the patient with minimal passive or active ROM?**

Extensor tenolysis and open capsulotomy.

○ **What operation would you offer for someone with good passive but minimal active ROM?**

Flexor tenolysis.

○ **What is the greatest danger in digital reoperation after replantation?**

Injury to the neurovascular bundle embedded in scar.

○ **What is fluorimetry?**

A method of monitoring tissue perfusion by injecting fluorescein dye intravenously and using a fluorometer to quantitatively measure rise and fall of fluorescein in tissue.

○ **What if there is a two to threefold rise but no fall in the numbers?**

Sign of venous congestion.

○ **What if the absolute number is very low and remains low, but the digit clinically looks viable?**

Thick skin or heavily contaminated skin can alter the numbers.

○ **When is the highest likelihood of a thrombotic event at the microanastomosis?**

Within 24 to 48 hours of microanastomosis.

○ **At the microanastomosis, what is the predominant layer on day 3?**

Platelets.

○ **On days 4 to 14?**

Pseudointima.

○ **On day 14 onward?**

Intima.

○ **One year postreplantation at the PIPJ level with severe arthritis or fusion at the PIPJ. What surgery can you offer the patient?**

PIP joint arthroplasty.

○ **Which Urbaniak class of ring avulsion injury is considered a relative contraindication to replantation?**

III—complete degloving or complete amputation.

○ **What type of flap can be used if there is a soft-tissue defect in a Type II ring avulsion injury?**

Venous flow-through flap.

○ **What is the average 2PD of a replanted thumb?**

9 to 11 mm.

○ **What is the average 2PD of a replanted digit?**

8 to 15 mm—depending on sharp versus avulsion.

○ **What is the "No-reflow phenomenon"?**

Inability to maintain perfusion to the replanted tissue despite restoration of blood flow through a technically acceptable anastomosis. Thought to be the result of ischemia-induced endothelial injury.

○ **What is a common long-term sequelae of digit replantation?**

Cold intolerance. This occurs more commonly in the adult population but can also affect the pediatric population.

○ **How much time should you tell a patient he will have to wait for cold intolerance symptoms to resolve?**

At least 2 years, possibly a lifetime.

● ● ● LEECHES AND ANTICOAGULANTS ● ● ●

○ **Scientific name for medical leeches?**

Hirudo medicinalis.

○ **Action of hirudin?**

- Binds activated thrombin (1:1).
- Inhibits conversion of fibrinogen to fibrin.
- Blocks activation of factors V, VIII, XI, vWF.
- Decreases activation of TPA, protein C, plasmin.
- Prolongs thrombin-dependent coagulation tests (PTT, TT, ACT, ECT).
- There is no direct effect on platelets or endothelial cells.
- Can monitor by thrombin time and PTT.

○ **Excretion of hirudin?**

Renal excretion.

○ **Organism to cover while patient is on leech therapy?**

<u>Aeromonas hydrophila</u>—enteric organism that can cause severe soft-tissue infection. Can cover with third-generation cephalosporin (Cefizox) or aminoglycosides (tobramycin, gentamycin) in adults. For pediatric patients, bactrim or ciprofloxacin can be safely used.

○ **What is the mechanism of heparin?**

Action is primarily via activation of serum <u>antithrombin III</u> and lowering of blood viscosity; increases AT III activity.

○ **What is the mechanism of dextran?**

- Polysaccharide—molecular weights of 40,000 and 70,000.
- Decreases platelet aggregation by imparting a negative charge on the platelets, inactivating vWF.
- Modifying structure of fibrin.
- Altering rheologic property of blood.
- Possible complications: antigenic test dose of less than 5 mL must be given prior to administration of a full dose.
- Renal failure—volume expansion.
- Noncardiogenic pulmonary edema.

○ **What is the mechanism of aspirin?**

- Acetylates <u>cyclooxygenase enzyme</u>
- Decreases arachidonic acid, thromboxane, prostacyclin
- Decreases platelet aggregation and vasoconstriction

○ **What is the mechanism of Thorazine?**

Potent vasodilator.

○ **What is the mechanism of papaverine?**

Salt of an opium alkaloid. Smooth muscle relaxant especially with cerebral and peripheral ischemia associated with arterial spasm.

○ **What is the mechanism of Lidocaine?**

Potent local vasodilatation. Commonly used as a 2% solution.

○ **What is the definitive role of anticoagulation in microsurgery?**

Controversial. Not enough randomized controlled trials to definitively characterize its role. Common uses: high-dose heparin irrigation during the microanastomosis. Intravenous heparin after a thrombotic event with anastomotic revision.

● ● ● **HYPERCOAGULABLE STATES** ● ● ●

○ **What percentage of venous thrombotic events in the human body are caused by genetic factors?**

Inherited deficiencies account for 5% to 15% of venous thrombosis.

○ **Is the antiphospholipid antibody associated with arterial or venous thrombosis?**

It is associated with both.

○ **What is activated protein C resistance (APC/factor V Leiden)?**

- One of the most common hereditary causes of thrombophilia.
- 4% frequency in European population, extremely uncommon in Africans, Asians, and Australians.
- APC inactivates factors V and VIII—keeps thrombosis in check.

○ **What is a prothrombin 2021A mutation?**

- Relative risk of thrombosis with this mutation is 2.8
- Prevalence—2%
- Extremely uncommon in nonwhite population
- Treatment: Coumadin 3 to 6 months; recurrence—indefinitely

○ **What is hyperhomocysteinemia?**

- Usually an enzyme deficiency in states of chronic renal disease, hypothyroid, malignancy.
- Can be associated with medications.
- Strong correlation between elevated homocysteine levels and arterial and venous disease.
- Arterial—increased cardiac, cerebral vascular disease; 3× risk.
- Venous—increased risk of thrombosis

○ **How much does an elevated factor VIII cause a hypercoagulable state?**

Levels greater than 1,500 IU/L lead to a 5× increase of thrombosis.

○ **Does an elevated factor XI cause an increased rate of thrombosis?**

Yes. Relative risk 2.2.

○ **What is the workup for hypercoagulable states?**

Be suspicious when patient has a thrombotic event early in life (age <45), family history, recurrence or multiple spontaneous abortions.

Laboratory studies to order: Antithrombin III, proteins C and S, antiphospholipid antibody, factor V Leiden, prothrombin 2021 A mutation, homocysteinemia. Involve a hematology oncologist early.

Note: Proteins C and S and antithrombin III are decreased in acute thrombosis; antithrombin III decreased during heparin.

• • • SCALP REPLANTATION • • •

○ **What is the typical history of a scalp amputation?**

Young female factory worker with long hair, with avulsion of scalp along the supraorbital rim extending to the ears laterally and to the nape of the neck posteriorly.

○ **Which vessels are commonly used for replantation?**

- Superficial temporal
- Posterior auricular
- Occipital
- Supraorbital
- Usually a single artery and vein can be used to replant the scalp. Vein grafts are commonly used.

○ **What is a common complication after scalp replantation?**

Hematoma.

• • • **EAR REPLANTATION** • • •

○ **Which vessels are commonly used in ear replantation?**

Superficial temporal or posterior auricular.

○ **Venous drainage?**

Veins are extremely difficult to find and most often, the ear has to be leeched.

○ **What options exist if the amputated part is not replantable?**

Banking of ear cartilage for future ear reconstruction.

○ **What is the "pocket principle"?**

The epidermis is removed from the severed part, leaving the cartilage covered by a thick layer of dermis. The part is then attached to its original position. A retroauricular incision is made and a subcutaneous pocket is created large enough to accommodate the ear. The ear is removed in 2 to 4 weeks.

• • • **LIP REPLANTATION** • • •

○ **Which arteries to look for in a lip replantation?**

Labial arteries.

○ **Veins in lip replantation?**

Extremely difficult, usually requires leeching.

○ **Most common cause of lip amputation?**

Dog bite.

○ **Can the tongue be replanted?**

Yes. Three have been reported in the world literature.

• • • **LOWER EXTREMITY REPLANTATION** • • •

○ **Although lower extremity replantation remains controversial, indications to proceed with replantation include?**

• Patient age (children do better with neurological regeneration)
• Overall condition (comorbidities and associated injuries)
• Ischemia time <6 hours
• Type and extent of injury (guillotine, single level)
• Bilateral amputations

○ **What are the contraindications to lower extremity replantation?**
- Poor baseline health
- Multilevel or crush injury
- Advanced age
- Severe polytrauma

○ **What can you do with the remaining amputated leg if replantation is not possible at a below-knee amputation site with significant soft-tissue loss?**
Foot fillet flap.

• • • PENIS REPLANTATION • • •

○ **Common cause of penile amputation?**
Self-mutilation.

○ **Vessels in penile replantation?**
Dorsal vein and deep arteries in corpora.

○ **What adjunctive therapy can be used to assist with ischemic tissues after replantation?**
Hyperbaric oxygen therapy.

• • • REFERENCES • • •

Agarwal JP, Trovato JM, Agarwal S, Hopkins PN, Brooks D, Buncke G. Selected outcomes of thumb replantation after isolated thumb amputation injury. *J Hand Surg Am.* 2010;35(9):1485–1490.

Allen DM, Levin LS. Digital replantation including postoperative care. *Tech Hand Up Extrem Surg.* 2002;6(4):171–177.

Alpert BS, Buncke HJ Jr, Mathes SJ. Surgical treatment of the totally avulsed scalp. *Clin Plast Surg.* 1982;9(2):145–159.

Bieber EJ, Wood MB, Cooney WP, Amadio PC. Thumb avulsion: results of replantation/revascularization. *J Hand Surg Am.* 1987;12(5 Pt 1): 786–790.

Buncke GM, Buncke HJ, Oliva A, Lineaweaver WC, Siko PP. Hand reconstruction with partial toe and multiple toe transplants. *Clin Plast Surg.* 1992;19:859–870.

Buncke HJ Jr. Microvascular hand surgery—transplants and replants—over the past 25 Years. *J Hand Surg Am.* 2000;25:415–428.

Buncke HJ. *Microsurgery: Transplantation, Replantation : An aAtlas Text.* Philadelphia, PA: Lea & Febiger; 1991.

Buncke HJ, Chang DW. History of microsurgery. *Sem Plast Surg.* 2003;17(1):5–16.

Buntic RF, Buncke HJ. Successful replantation of an amputated tongue. *Plast Reconstr Surg.* 1998;101:1604–1607.

de Chalain T, Jones G. Replantation of the avulsed pinna: 100% survival with a single arterial anastomosis and substitution of leeches for a venous anastomosis. *Plast Reconstr Surg.* 1995;95:1275–1279.

Classen DA. The indications and reliability of vein graft use in free flap transfer. *Can J Plast Surg.* 2004 Spring;12(1):27–29.

Conrad MH, Adams WP Jr. Pharmacologic optimization in microsurgery in the new millennium. *Plast Reconstr Surg.* 2001;108:2088–2096.

Converse JM. Reconstruction of the auricle. I. *Plast Reconstr Surg Transplant Bull.* 1958;22:150–163.

Datiashvili RO. Simultaneous replantation of both lower legs in a child: 23 years later. *J Reconstr Microsurg.* 2009;25(5):323–329.

Friedrich JB, Vedder NB. Thumb reconstruction. *Clin Plast Surg.* 2011;38(4):697–712.

Greenberg BM, May JW Jr. Great toe-to-hand transfer: role of the preoperative lateral arteriogram of foot. *J Hand Surg Am.* 1988; 13(3):411–414.

Goldner RD, Urbaniak JR. Replantation. In: Wolfe SW, Hotchkiss RN, Pederson WC, et al., eds. *Green's Operative Hand Surgery.* 6th ed. Philadelphia, PA: Churchill Livingstone; 2011:1585–1601.

Hanel DP, Chin SH. Wrist level and proximal-upper extremity replantation. *Hand Clin.* 2007;23(1):13–21.

Hammond DC, Bouwense CL, Hankins WT, Maxwell-Davis GS, Furdyna J, Capraro PA. Microsurgical replantation of the amputated nose. *Plast Reconstr Surg.* 2000;105:2133–2136.

Hierner R, Betz AM, Comtet JJ, Berger AC. Decision making and results in subtotal and total lower leg amputations: reconstruction versus amputation. *Microsurgery.* 1995;16(12):830–839.

Kay S, Werntz J, Wolff TW. Ring avulsion injuries: classification and prognosis. *J Hand Surg Am.* 1989;14:204–213.

Landström JT, Schuyler RW, Macris GP. Microsurgical penile replantation facilitated by postoperative HBO treatment. *Microsurgery.* 2004;24(1):49–55.

Mackenzie D, Seyfer AE. Reconstructive surgery: lower extremity coverage. In: Mathes SJ, Hentz VR, eds. *Plastic Surgery.* 2nd ed. Philadelphia, PA: WB Saunders; 2006:1369.

May JW Jr, Chait LA, O'Brien BM, Hurley JV. The no-reflow phenomenon in experimental free flaps. *Plast Reconstr Surg.* 1978;61(2): 256–267.

Mladick RA. Salvage of the ear in acute trauma. *Clin Plast Surg.* 1978;5:427–435.

O'Brien BM. Replantation surgery. *Clin Plast Surg.* 1974;1(3):405–426.

Pederson WC. Replantation. *Plast Reconstr Surg.* 2001;107:823–841.

Sud V, Freeland AE. Skeletal fixation in digital replantation. *Microsurgery.* 2002;22(4):165–171.

Walton RL, Beahm EK, Brown RE, et al. Microsurgical replantation of the lip: a multi-institutional experience. *Plast Reconstr Surg.* 1998;102:358–368.

Wei FC. Free style free flaps. *Plast Reconstr Surg.* 2001;114:910–916.

CHAPTER 44 Toe-to-Hand Transfer

Christopher G. Wallace, MD, MS, FRCS (Plast) and Fu-Chan Wei, MD, FACS

○ **What was Nicoladoni's contribution to thumb reconstruction?**

Carl Nicoladoni (1847–1902), a pioneering Austrian surgeon, was the first to perform the pedicled second toe-to-hand transfer for amputated thumb reconstruction. His description was published in 1900.

○ **On whose experimental work was the first human microvascular great toe-to-hand transfer based?**

Buncke. In 1966, Buncke et al. published their account of successful toe-to-hand microvascular transfer in rhesus monkeys. This work itself was inspired by Nicoladoni's concept of toe-to-hand transfer first performed at the end of the 19th century.

○ **Who performed the first microvascular second toe-to-hand transfer in humans?**

Yang Dongyue of Shanghai First Medical University in China performed the world's first successful microvascular toe-to-hand transfer, utilizing the second toe, in 1967.

○ **When were toe transplantations first used for reconstruction of congenital hand differences?**

In the late 1970s, when O'Brien and colleagues pioneered thumb reconstruction in children with congenital hand differences using microsurgical technique. These applications were popularized by Gilbert and others in the 1980s.

○ **Which two arterial pedicles may supply great toe or second toe transfers?**

The first dorsal metatarsal artery (FDMA) and the first plantar metatarsal artery (FPMA). The FDMA is dominant in 70% of cases, FPMA in 20%, and both are of equal caliber in 10% cases.

○ **Where in the foot is the FDMA located?**

The FDMA lies between the first and second metatarsals, at varying depths from superficial to the interosseous muscle to intramuscular to a position plantar to the interosseous muscle. The FDMA passes dorsal to the deep transverse metatarsal ligament, which connects the plantar plates of the metatarsophalangeal (MTP) joints.

○ **Is there a classification system to describe the various positions of the FDMA?**

There are at least three classification systems but it is not necessary to learn them. By commencing the dissection of the toe's vascular pedicle in the web space (instead of on the dorsum of the foot), the pedicle can be revealed retrograde and its pathway followed along whatever direction it takes.

○ **Are the dorsal metatarsal and plantar metatarsal arterial systems connected?**

Yes: first, by the communicating vessels, which pass between the first and second metatarsals; second, the two systems converge at the first web space.

○ **Which digital artery of the toe is more important, the dorsal or plantar system?**

The plantar digital artery. The dorsal digital artery is only rarely present.

○ **What venous system should be used to drain a great toe or second toe transfer?**

The intermediate level veins, which give rise to the greater saphenous vein.

○ **Which nerve supplies sensation to the first web space?**

The deep peroneal nerve.

○ **Which nerves are the most important for sensation of the transferred toe?**

The medial and lateral proper plantar digital nerves, which are terminal branches of the medial plantar nerve. The digital nerves are located plantar to the plantar digital arteries.

○ **Which tendon is cut when dissecting the FDMA on the foot dorsum?**

Extensor hallucis brevis.

○ **In which types of congenital hand conditions should a toe-to-hand transfer be considered?**

Constriction band syndrome, hands with no fingers but an adequate thumb, and thumb absence with a complex hand malformation. The latter two situations often have absent or anomalous recipient structures. A well-thought-out operative plan with alternative recipient vessels, nerves, and tendons must be devised. Pollicization should be considered for isolated thumb aplasia/significant hypoplasia and can offer better outcomes. For all these patients a thorough cardiorespiratory/anesthetic workup is mandatory as coexisting systems anomalies are not uncommon.

○ **How do outcomes differ between index finger pollicization and microsurgical second toe transfer for hypoplastic thumb reconstruction in children with radial deficiency?**

Tan and Tu compared a total of 30 children reconstructed with one of these two methods. They reported that patients who had undergone pollicization had earlier motor and sensory recovery and better range of motion. Patients who received toe transfers had higher parental satisfaction and performed better in some activities of daily living.

○ **In patients who may be future candidates for toe-to-hand transfer, which structures should be preserved during the initial emergent treatment? Why?**

Skin: Toe transfers have a paucity of skin; local flaps further injure and ultimately scar the hand, making recipient-site preparation more difficult; free flaps for skin coverage use all-important recipient vessels.

Joints: Intact proximal interphalangeal or metacarpophalangeal (MCP) joints will enhance mobility and function following transfer; preservation of only the proximal articular surface of the MCP joint is better than saving no articular surface because a composite joint reconstruction is possible.

Bone: Adequate bony length allows restoration of digital length with toe transfer, which improves appearance and function; the great toe should not be harvested proximal to the MTP joint, necessitating a staged reconstruction or second toe transfer if the thumb is excessively shortened.

Tendons: Maintaining flexor tendon length ensures preservation of the flexor pulley system; the complex extensor mechanism should be saved as it is difficult to reconstruct; less donor-site morbidity is incurred if tendons are preserved in the hand.

Vessels: Damage to recipient vessels either precludes transfer or necessitates riskier vein grafting.

Nerve: Preserving nerve length reduces donor-site dissection; a more distal nerve repair during transfer will speed up sensory recovery.

○ **How can closure of wounds in potential toe-to-hand candidates be achieved?**

Pedicled distant flaps (such as the pedicled groin flap) can import liberal fresh uninjured tissues and do not sacrifice local tissues or vessels.

○ **Should arteriography of the foot be performed prior to surgery?**

Preoperative arteriography is not required unless the donor foot has been injured or is congenitally anomalous or if the patient has significant peripheral vascular disease. The vascular pedicle is dissected in a retrograde manner, thus it is not necessary to know its proximal course.

○ **How does one increase pedicle length when harvesting a first plantar metatarsal artery dominant toe?**

The first plantar metatarsal artery is dominant in approximately 20% of patients. Its dissection is reasonably straightforward until the deep perforator is reached, which communicates between the plantar and dorsal systems. While it is feasible to trace the pedicle retrograde between the metatarsals, it is actually safer and more expedient to terminate the dissection at this point and extend the pedicle with vein grafts as necessary.

○ **Which pedicle should be chosen when neither the first plantar nor the first dorsal metatarsal artery is dominant in the web space?**

When the plantar and dorsal systems are codominant (which is the case in approximately 10% of cases), one should choose the dorsal system because it is easier to dissect and provides a lengthier pedicle.

○ **How should one extend the incision on the plantar and the dorsal feet when harvesting a toe?**

For a plantar system–dominant harvest, the incision should be extended in a straight line away from the weight-bearing surfaces. For a dorsal system–dominant harvest, the incision should be extended as a lazy-S incision.

○ **What risk factors predispose to vascular compromise requiring re-exploration of single-toe transplants?**

Multivariate analyses revealed that postoperative wound infection, metacarpal hand injuries, and preceding flap coverage were independently associated with re-exploration for vascular compromise.

○ **What are the most common causes of vascular compromise found at re-exploration of single-toe transplants?**

The most common causes for vascular compromise in single-toe transplants necessitating re-exploration are: arterial spasm (61%), arterial thrombosis (42%), and venous thrombosis (25%); more than one factor can be found at any one re-exploration.

○ **What type of secondary procedures might be necessary for patients who undergo toe-to-hand transfer?**

Approximately 14% of patients require surgical revisions to improve function including: flexor tendon tenolysis (7%), arthrodesis (2%), web space deepening (2%), osteotomy for malunion (2%), or bone grafting for nonunion. Some patients also request aesthetic improvement.

○ **What techniques are available to improve the cosmetic outcome of toe transplantation?**

Pulp plasty improves the appearance of the toe transplant but also may be indicated if the distal pulp is too bulky or needs improved stability. In addition, patients who have had trimmed toe or modified wraparound transfer may request osteotomy of the remaining tubercle (on the side of the skeleton that was not trimmed at the primary transfer) to remove the "swelling" on the fibular side of the interphalangeal joint of the neo-digit. Recently, Ju and Hou described a pulp transposition flap that simultaneously reduces pulp bulk whilst augmenting the waist of the second toe at time of transplantation to smoothen the contour of the reconstructed digit. Procedures to improve nail cosmesis are addressed in the following question.

○ **Describe a method to reduce the toenail (of the neo-thumb) to match that of the opposite normal thumb nail.**

Narrowing the toenail by excluding a portion of its tibial half from the transfer is probably the simplest and most widely practiced technique of improving nail symmetry compared to the unoperated contralateral thumb. However, this method risks nail growth and damages the specialized paronychial and eponychial contours to create an unnaturally straight edge to the nail plate. A method to create a near-normal and symmetric nail on the neo-thumb is perhaps the most significant remaining obstacle to a truly aesthetic thumb reconstruction.

○ **How many motor units power the thumb?**

Nine: four extrinsic muscles and five intrinsic muscles.

○ **In which important way does the motion of the great-toe MTP joint differ from the thumb MCP joint?**

The MTP range is one of hyperextension rather than flexion.

○ **What is the two-point discrimination of the great-toe in situ? Following transplantation and rehabilitation, is the sensation in the transplanted toe better or worse than before transfer?**

The great toe in situ has an average static two-point discrimination of 10 mm (2× standard deviation = ± 6 mm). Following transfer sensation varies considerably. Mean static two-point discrimination of 6.5 mm may be achieved in patients with optimal nerve coaptation and adequate sensory reeducation.

○ **What proportion of hand function does the thumb represent?**

40% to 50% of global hand function.

○ **What types of thumb to finger pinches are commonly discussed when analyzing prehensile function?**

Pulp-to-pulp, lateral (key), and chuck three-point (tripod) pinch. In addition the thumb assists the hand in power (cylinder) grasp. Hook grip requires only fingers. Without any digits present the hand may function as a bat.

○ **Any preoperative planning methods to decide the optimal position of the toe transplant for thumb reconstruction?**

Use of a prosthetic thumb by the patient can help determine the exact position of the future transplanted toe and for planning additional procedures, such as opponensplasties. Otherwise, careful preoperative discussion and analysis with the patient regarding prehension types and requirements, including at work, are important to this decision.

○ **What are the most common etiologies of a thumb absence/dysfunction that require reconstruction?**

Traumatic amputation, postoncologic resection, and certain types of congenital thumb differences.

○ **What is the best surgical procedure to treat an acutely amputated thumb?**

Replantation.

○ **If replantation is not possible, is primary toe-to-hand transfer possible?**

Yes. Advantages include decreased time in hospital and earlier return to work. There are no statistically significant differences in the rate of early postoperative complications between the primary and secondary transfers. However, subjectively, patients with primary reconstructions are less satisfied with the function and appearance of the reconstructed digit than patients who have lived for some time with the amputation. Primary toe-to-hand transfer must therefore be carefully and thoroughly discussed so that the patient has a realistic expectation of outcome; secondary reconstruction should be strongly considered if there is any doubt in the level of the patient's expectations.

○ **In assessing thumb amputations through the metacarpal, injury to which structures will most negatively influence the outcome of thumb reconstruction?**

Injury to the thenar muscles will dramatically affect thumb strength, stability, and mobility. When reconstructing a metacarpal hand injury with thumb involvement, inadequate thenar function will immediately downgrade the functional expectation and hence upgrade the classification of the metacarpal hand to IIC, no matter what the level of thumb amputation is.

○ **What main options are available to position the neo-thumb for opposable tripod pinch in thumb amputations proximal to the metacarpophalangeal joint with loss of thenar musculature function?**

Pronation osteosynthesis involves fixing the transplanted toe in a static opposable position at the time of toe transplant. Dynamic opponensplasty can additionally be performed, primarily or at a second stage, using the flexor digitorum superficialis tendon from the index or middle finger (or the palmaris longus tendon) and has been shown to improve acquisition of stable tripod pinch for these proximal reconstructions.

○ **How can circumduction be restored if the thumb basal joint is destroyed?**

Basal joint mobility for improved circumduction can be achieved with an interpositional suspension arthroplasty, usually using a strip of extensor carpi radialis longus or similar.

○ **What are the elements of an ideal thumb reconstruction?**

There are three main components: (1) functional reconstruction, requiring adequate motor power/excursion, at least protective sensation, correct thumb length and position, stability, and absence of pain; (2) cosmetically acceptable; (3) minimal donor-site morbidity.

○ **What is the minimum critical length of the thumb in an otherwise normal hand?**

The interphalangeal joint level. A reconstructed thumb may be made to this length if necessary or an amputation at this level may be tolerated.

○ **What structure differentiates between a proximal and a distal digital amputation?**

The insertion of the flexor digitorum superficialis into the middle phalanx.

○ **What factors determine the "correct" thumb length?**

A normal thumb reaches the middle of the proximal phalanx of the index finger when the thumb is adducted. The correct thumb length is determined by the thenar muscle function and the length and mobility of the remaining fingers. If the thumb will have minimal mobility, slightly shorter length is preferable. A shorter thumb may be tolerated if the fingers are normal or may be required in a metacarpal hand.

○ **What methods, other than toe-to-hand transfer, are available for thumb reconstruction?**

Pollicization of an injured digit, pollicization of an uninjured digit, osteoplastic thumb reconstruction, and distraction osteogenesis. For soft-tissue coverage of the distal tip, local and regional flaps may be used. For example, palmar advancement flaps and pedicled neurovascular island flaps.

○ **Is it necessary to use the ipsilateral great toe for thumb reconstruction? Why or why not?**

No. The left great toe is the first choice because the right foot is generally used for driving. However, either foot can be chosen according to the preference of the patient without detriment to the reconstruction.

○ **How do the great toe and thumb differ in appearance?**

The widest diameter of the great toe is 60% greater than that of the thumb. The great toe has a wider nail and larger bones.

○ **Where on the thumb should the web space attach to avoid an arachnodactylous appearance?**

The web space should meet at the MCP joint of the thumb.

○ **When might a second toe be considered for thumb reconstruction?**

A second toe may be preferred in the following circumstances: the patient refuses/cannot tolerate great toe loss; proximal metacarpal or transcarpometacarpal joint-level injuries; when the second toe and thumb are similar in size; in children; suboptimal reconstruction acceptable to the patient (such as on the nondominant hand).

○ **What are the advantages of the great toe over the second toe for thumb reconstruction?**

The great toe provides a broader, stronger, more stable reconstruction. The second toe is prone to develop a flexed posture, has a small nail and two interphalangeal joints, which leads to less stability.

○ **How can the flexed posture of the second toe be minimized?**

By releasing the extensor digitorum longus attachment from the MTP joint, suturing the extensor digitorum brevis to the extensor hood or interosseous tendon, tight extensor repair, pinning the interphalangeal joints in extension for 6 weeks, and nighttime extension splinting for at least 1 year.

○ **What are the main advantages of the second toe in thumb reconstruction?**

It may be harvested with a long segment of the second metatarsal, allowing for proximal thumb injury reconstructions. Donor-site morbidity is less than that of the great toe.

○ **What options are available for thumb reconstruction if the great toe is too big to give an acceptable aesthetic result?**

The great toe wraparound, the trimmed great toe or the twisted toe technique. The second toe generally gives a poorer aesthetic outcome.

○ **What are the advantages of using the wraparound great toe flap?**

Preservation of great toe skeleton/tendons; aesthetic thumb reconstruction; provision of glabrous skin, nail, and pulp with fibrous septa and sensibility.

○ **What are the disadvantages of the great toe wraparound for total thumb reconstruction?**

At least two secondary donor sites are required: iliac crest for thumb skeleton and a skin graft and/or regional flap to cover the remaining great toe. The reconstructed thumb has no interphalangeal joint. There is a risk of bone-graft resorption and fracture.

○ **How can pulp stability be improved when performing a wraparound toe transfer?**

The original description of the wraparound great toe transfer involved leaving the entire great toe skeleton at the donor site. The soft tissue of the great toe was then wrapped around an iliac crest bone graft. Unfortunately, patients found that the soft tissues of the great toe swiveled around the bone graft and this diminished prehensile stability. By simply harvesting a portion of the distal phalanx of the toe within the transfer, however, pulp stability could be dramatically improved as the fibrous septae that anchor the pulp in position are preserved.

○ **What are the advantages of the trimmed toe transfer?**

The trimmed toe provides a more aesthetic reconstruction than a total great toe transplantation and preserves skin for donor-site closure. It also preserves interphalangeal joint function. There is, however, a reduction in interphalangeal joint range of motion to around 18 degrees.

○ **What structures are reduced during a trimmed great toe transfer?**

For trimmed great toe transfer, the great toe skeleton and its soft tissues are reduced to match the uninjured thumb as closely as possible. The skin/fat is reduced according to circumferential measurements from the uninjured thumb taken at three levels: the eponychium, the widest girth of the interphalangeal joint, and the middle of the proximal phalanx (the remaining skin is left at the foot to aid wound closure). The skeleton is trimmed axially with an oscillating saw on the medial side of the toe. This axial osteotomy begins at the distal phalanx, through the joint and down the proximal phalanx, which removes approximately 4 to 6 mm of the medial joint prominence and 2 to 4 mm of the phalangeal shafts. It is also possible to reduce the anteroposterior dimensions of the skeleton with burring. Critical, however, is that the lateral (fibular) side of the toe is not trimmed so that the pedicle is not risked.

○ **Do patients who undergo toe-to-hand transfer for thumb amputation do better than those who don't?**

Yes. Patients who undergo toe transfer have a statistically significant better hand function, aesthetics, and satisfaction than those who do not. The strength and dexterity of the hand with the toe transfer are comparable to the opposite normal hands.

○ **What should one do if there is no flexor tendon in the amputated digit to flex the transferred toe?**

Utilize a neighboring flexor digitorum superficialis tendon instead.

○ **What are possible donor-site complications specific to the great toe transfer?**

Early complications include delayed wound healing and skin necrosis. Late complications include altered gait, change in weight bearing, and pain and cold intolerance.

○ **How can great toe donor-site complications best be avoided?**

Preservation of as much foot and web space skin as possible is important to allow direct closure without tension and critically without skin grafts. The first metatarsal head should not be sacrificed and 1 cm of proximal phalanx should be preserved to maintain adequate push-off when walking and foot span.

○ **If the great toe is harvested proximal to the MTP joint, how does gait change?**

There is a small but statistically significant decrease in stride length.

○ **List the flaps available for microvascular transfer from the forefoot for hand reconstruction.**

Great toe, wraparound great toe, trimmed great toe, pulp, hemi-pulp, onychocutaneous, first web space, second toe, wraparound second toe, vascularized second toe PIP joint, vascularized second toe MTP joint, combined second and third toe, combined third and fourth toe, third toe and twisted toe technique.

○ **List the unique physical characteristics of the fingertip that can be replaced only by tissue transplanted from a digit (toe or finger).**

Glabrous skin, fibrous septa, and the presence of a nail.

○ **What is glabrous skin?**

Glabrous skin, in distinction to hirsute skin, is thicker and hairless. Functionally important features of glabrous skin include friction ridges, increased mechanical strength, dense clustering of specialized sensory end organs, and numerous sweat glands. Hair interferes with sensation and is therefore absent from glabrous skin.

○ **Why are fibrous septa and nails important for manipulation?**

Fibrous septa between the fat of the pulp prevent excessive shearing, but still allow the pulp to conform to the object being held. The nail provides dorsal support and counterpressure to the pulp.

○ **What are indications for toe-to-hand transfer in a hand with only a single finger amputated?**

To improve hand aesthetics and function and to treat painful finger tip/neuroma.

○ **A patient has an index finger amputation at the middle of the proximal phalanx. Is she a good candidate for a second toe-to-index finger transfer?**

No. At this level the reconstructed finger will be noticeably shorter than the rest of the intact fingers. In hands with single finger loss the best reconstructive outcome is obtained when the amputation level is from the middle of the middle phalanx to the base of the distal phalanx.

○ **When using the second toe to reconstruct a distal finger, how is unnecessary bulkiness of the reconstructed digit avoided?**

Careful skeletonization of the vessels prevents bulky soft-tissue marring the aesthetic result and precludes unsightly skin grafting. Removal of the thick plantar subcutaneous fat at the MTP joint level will not only improve the appearance, but will also allow greater range of motion for the transferred digit.

○ **What is a "cobra deformity" and how can it be avoided?**

This term is used to describe an objectionable bulbous soft-tissue junction between a transferred toe and the amputation stump because it resembles the head and flare of a threatened cobra. It can be avoided by creating four equal triangular flaps through a cruciate incision at the amputation stump tip, undermining them so that they can freely move over the underlying skeleton of the stump and transferred toe, and by carefully interdigitating them with the flaps of the transferred toe.

○ **What are indications for toe-to-hand transfer in a mutilated hand?**

To improve or provide pulp-to-pulp, chuck, lateral pinch and hook grip and therefore overall hand function.

○ **What is a metacarpal hand?**

A hand that is unable to achieve any type of pinch or grip (no prehensile capacity) owing to amputation of all fingers. The thumb may or may not be preserved.

○ **How should a metacarpal hand be reconstructed?**

The variety and complexity of the metacarpal hand injuries demand careful planning to ensure proper use of limited donor tissues and to correctly address the most important deficiencies. Classification of the metacarpal hand helps determine the most appropriate reconstructive method, which may include two second toe transfers, combined second and third toe transfer, and great toe transfer.

○ **What should one do if positioning of the toe transfers is found to be erroneous immediately following metacarpal hand reconstruction with poor prehensile positioning?**

Prehensile positioning should be set as accurately as possible for any toe transfer, whether multiple (as in metacarpal hand reconstruction) or singleton (as in thumb reconstruction). However, slight adjustments are often required during the early stages of rehabilitation to perfect positioning. If rigid fixation is used, this may not be possible without an additional general anesthetic. Instead, if parallel intraosseous wiring is used for bony fixation at the osteotomy site, slight rotational and angular adjustments are feasible at the bedside within at least the first 2 weeks postoperatively without jeopardizing toe vascularity. This can be further optimized after 2 weeks by serial splinting.

○ **Classify the metacarpal hand.**

Type I: thumb preserved, all fingers amputated below the middle of the proximal phalanx. The level of finger amputation may be used to further subdivide patients into subtypes A, B, or C.

Type I metacarpal hand

Subtype	Level of Finger Amputation	Recommendations
I A	Proximal to middle of proximal phalanx	Two second toes or combined second/third
I B	Through MCP joint (intact proximal articular surface)	Combined second/third as composite joint transfer
I C	Proximal to MCP	Combined second/third

Type II: metacarpal hands have all fingers amputated proximal to the middle of the proximal phalanx plus a thumb amputation. Subtypes A, B, C, and D depend on the level of thumb amputation and status of two important structures: the thenar muscles and carpometacarpal (CMC) joint. Reconstruction of the fingers may be carried out concurrently or separately from the thumb reconstruction depending on the subtype.

Type II metacarpal hand

Subtype	Level of Thumb Amputation	Recommendations
II A	Distal to metacarpal neck	Great toe transfer
II B	Proximal to metacarpal neck, adequate thenar function	Preliminary procedure to lengthen thumb followed by great toe transfer or second toe transfer Concurrent transfer of combined second/third toe or two second toes
II C	Inadequate thenar function	Two-stage reconstruction Opponensplasty
II D	CMC joint damage	Thumb reconstructed as an immobile post

○ **What is the vascular supply for a combined second and third toe transfer?**

The FDMA and/or a plantar digital metatarsal artery provide the vascular pedicle. There is no difference in early outcome between using one versus two arterial pedicles.

○ **What are the advantages of providing a hand with two adjacent digits?**

This construct allows useful tripod (chuck) pinch, enhances lateral stability, provides a stronger hook grip, and allows a wider span for grasping larger objects.

○ **Is a combined second/third toe transplant appropriate to reconstruct the fingers for a type I A metacarpal hand with a preserved web space? Why or why not?**

No, two second toes should be used when the amputation is distal to the web space to avoid a long palm–short finger appearance.

○ **How many veins are required to drain the transferred toe(s) adequately?**

Even though all single- and double-toe transfers can be adequately drained by a single venous anastomosis, it is safe practice to harvest at least two good-sized dorsal veins at the foot (preferably draining separately). The preferred venous anastomosis should be allowed to drain the toe first; if inadequate (which is unusual) then the second vein can still be used to augment drainage.

○ **List the late donor-site complications specific to combined second/third toe transfer.**

Pain with ambulation and scissor deformity (migration of the fourth toe toward the great toe).

○ **What range of motion can be obtained using a vascularized joint for finger arthroplasty?**

Generally less than 40 degrees, often due to significant extensor lag of the transferred toe joint. If the extensor lag is improved, however, average range of motion can be increased to approximately 54 degrees.

○ **How can the extensor lag of vascularized joint transfer for proximal interphalangeal joint reconstruction be minimized?**

Two arrangements of the toe central slip have recently been described: type I is an attenuated central slip and type II is a distinct central slip. For a type I toe with sufficient recipient lateral bands, a centralization procedure is recommended and this should be repaired to the donor extensor tendon. If the lateral bands are insufficient, a modified Stack procedure is recommended (this involves passing one distally based slip of flexor digitorum superficialis through to the dorsal side via a drilled tunnel in the base of the toe middle phalanx, and repair to the recipient extensor tendon). In type II toe joints, a tight repair of the corresponding extensor tendons is recommended.

○ **What are the indications for vascularized joint transfer?**

A painful joint with posttraumatic arthritis, instability and/or deformity. Patients must be highly motivated, young, and have functioning flexor/extensor tendons.

○ **What advantages do vascularized joints have over other arthroplasty methods?**

Vascularized joint transfers utilize autologous tissue; growth potential in children; allow reconstruction of compound defects involving joint, bone, skin, and tendon in a single procedure.

○ **Describe a motor rehabilitation program for a neo-thumb reconstructed by toe transfer.**

Rehabilitation begins on the first postoperative day (Protective Stage) with planning and psychological support to the patient. By day 4, the vascularity of the transplanted toe can withstand gentle passive joint movements of 15 degrees (Early Mobilization Stage). This is gradually increased until full range of motion is achieved at the joint immediately distal to the osteotomy; the wrist should be kept in neutral. Near-full range of motion can be achieved between weeks 3 and 4 at joints proximal to the osteotomy. Active mobilization exercises commence after week 4 (Active Mobilization Stage), with blocking flexion/extension once tendons have healed. By week 7, rehabilitation can start to be tailored toward the precise requirements of the patient's dexterous needs to improve strength and joint motion (Activities of Daily Living Stage). From week 8, the final stage of rehabilitation commences (Prevocational Training), which is aimed at improving coordination and maximizing power according to vocational needs.

○ **Can toe transplantation be useful in a patient with hand amputation at wrist level?**

Yes. The concept of toe transfer to the wrist for prehension has existed for nearly a century. Oehlecker, inspired by Nicoladoni's work, successfully performed a distal forearm stump plasty using a pedicled great toe transfer in 1919. Nowadays, selected, highly motivated patients requiring key-grip to assist the other hand who do not want hand transplantation, and have not achieved satisfactory benefit from a prosthetic alternative, may be candidates for three-jointed second toe with great toe pulp flap transplantation to the antebrachial stump. Often termed the Vilkki procedure after the surgeon who described it, this involves osteoplastic moulding of the distal radius stump, osteosynthesis of the second toe metatarsal to the radius, insetting of the adjoined sensate great toe pulp flap to the distal radius stump, careful prehensile alignment of toe with pulp flap, and microvascular anastomoses.

○ **How should one instruct the patient to take care of the donor foot following toe harvest?**

The patient should only start taking steps on the hind foot from 2 weeks postoperatively; transfer of weight to the anterior foot is forbidden. The patient should then slowly begin to shift a little weight to the lateral and then the anterior foot as the next 2 weeks progress. Only once the foot has completed wound healing, after about 4 weeks, should the patient progress toward a more normal gait. It is critical that wound breakdown is avoided at the foot, as infection and subsequent dehiscence of the wound may ensue. Normal footwear can be used after approximately 6 weeks.

• • • REFERENCES • • •

Bannister LH. Integumental system: skin and breasts. In: Williams PL, ed. *Gray's Anatomy*. 38th ed. Toronto, Ontario, Canada: Churchill Livingstone; 1999:375–424.

Berry MM, Standring SM, Bannister LH. Nervous system. In: Williams PL, ed. *Gray's Anatomy*. 38th ed. Toronto, Ontario, Canada: Churchill Livingstone; 1999: 901–1398.

Buncke HJ Jr, Buncke CM, Schulz WP. Immediate Nicoladoni procedure in the Rhesus monkey, or hallux to-hand transplantation, utilising microminiature vascular anastomoses. *Br J Plast Surg*. 1966;19:332–337.

Cheng MH, Wei FC, Santamaria E, Cheng SL, Lin CH, Chen SH. Single versus double arterial anastomoses in combined second- and third-toe transplantation. *Plast Reconstr Surg*. 1998;108:2408–2412.

Chung KC, Wei FC. An outcome study of thumb reconstruction using microvascular toe transfer. *J Hand Surg*. 2000;25:651–658.

Dongyue Y, Yudong G. Thumb reconstruction utilizing second toe transplantation by microvascular anastomosis: report of 78 cases. *Chin Med J Engl*. 1979;92:295–309.

Eaton CJ, Lister GD. Toe transfer for congenital hand defects. *Microsurgery*. 1991;12:186–195.

Foucher G, Binhammer P. Free vascularized toe transfer. In: Foucher G, ed. *Reconstructive Surgery in Hand Mutilation*. London, UK: Mosby; 1997:57–66.

Frykman GK, O'Brien BM, Morrison WA, MacLeod AM. Functional evaluation of the hand and foot after one-stage toe-to-hand transfer. *J Hand Surg*. 1986;11:9–17.

Gilbert A. Congenital absence of the thumb and digits. *J Hand Surg Br*. 1989;14:6–17.

Gilbert A. Toe transfers for congenital hand defects. *J Hand Surg Am*. 1982;7:118–124.

Gilbert A. Vascular anatomy of the first web space of the foot. In: Landi A, ed. *Reconstruction of the Thumb*. London, UK: Chapman and Hall; 1989:199–204.

Gordon L. Toe-to-thumb transplantation. In: Green DP, Hotchkiss RN, Pederson WC, eds. *Green's Operative Hand Surgery*. 4th ed. Philadelphia, PA: Churchill Livingstone; 1999:1299–1326.

Ju JH, Hou RX. One-stage cosmetic finger reconstruction using a second toe island flap containing terminal branches of the toe artery. *Orthop Traumatol Surg Res*. 2015;101(3):345–351.

Kato H, Ogino T, Minami A, Usai M. Restoration of sensibility in fingers repaired with free sensory flaps from the toe. *J Hand Surg Am*. 1989;14:49–54.

Kleinman WB, Strickland JW. Thumb reconstruction. In: Green DP, Hotchkiss RN, Pederson WC, eds. *Green's Operative Hand Surgery*. 4th ed. Philadelphia, PA: Churchill Livingstone; 1999: 2068–2170.

Lam WL, Waughlock N, Hsu CC, Lin YT, Wei FC. Improving the extensor lag and range of motion following free vascularized joint transfer to the proximal interphalangeal joint: Part 2—A clinical series. *Plast Reconstr Surg*. 2013;132:271e–280e.

Leung PC. Sensory recovery in transplanted toes. *Microsurgery*. 1989;10:242–244.

Leung PC. Thumb reconstruction using the second toe. In: Landi A, ed. *Reconstruction of the Thumb*. London, UK: Chapman and Hall; 1989: 205–212.

Leung PC, Wong WL. The vessels of the first metatarsal web space. An operative and radiographic study. *J Bone Joint Surg Am*. 1983;65:235–239.

Lin CH, Lo S, Lin CH, Lin YT. Opponensplasty provides predictable opposable tripod pinch in toe transfer for proximal thumb ray defect reconstruction. *Plast Reconstr Surg*. 2012;130:810e–818e.

Lin YT, Su ST, Lo S, Hu CH, Lin CH, Wei FC. Risk factors for reexploration in toe-to-hand transfer: a multivariate analysis of 363 cases. *Plast Reconstr Surg*. 2015;135:501–506.

Lipton HA, May JW, Simon SR. Preoperative and postoperative gait analyses of patients undergoing great toe-to-thumb transfer. *J Hand Surg*. 1987;12:66–69.

Lister GD, Kalisman M, Tsai TM. Reconstruction of the hand with free microneurovascular toe-to-hand transfer: experience with 54 toe transfers. *Plast Reconstr Surg*. 1983;71:372–386.

Ma HS, el-Gammal T, Wei FC. Current concepts of toe-to-hand transfer: surgery and rehabilitation. *J Hand Ther*. 1996;9:41–46.

Mathes SJ. Great toe (hallux) flap. In: Mathes SJ, Nahai F, eds. *Reconstructive Surgery: Principles, Anatomy, and Technique*. New York, NY: Churchill Livingstone; 1997:891–925.

May JW. Microvascular great toe to hand transfer for reconstruction of the amputated thumb. In: McCarthy JG, May JW, Littler JW, eds. *Plastic Surgery*. Philadelphia, PA: WB Saunders; 1990:5183–5185.

May JW Jr, Chait LA, Cohen BE, O'Brien BM. Free neurovascular flap from the first web of the foot in hand reconstruction. *J Hand Surg Am*. 1977;2:387–393.

Morrison WA. The great toe wrap-around flap. In: Serafin D, ed. *Atlas of Microsurgical Composite Tissue Transplantation*. Philadelphia, PA: WB Saunders; 1996:131–135.

Nicoladoni C. Daumenplastik und organischer Ersatz des Fingerspitze (Anticheiroplastik und Daktyloplastik). *Archiv für klinische Chirurgie*. 1900; 61:606–628. [This article has been reprinted in translated form as follows: "The classic—plastic surgery of the thumb and organic substitution of the fingertip (anticheiroplastic surgery and finger plastic surgery)". By Carl Nicoladoni, 1900 (Translated in English by Arthur Lietze). *Clin Orthop Relat Res*. 1985;195:3–6.]

O'Brien B, Brennen MD, MacLeod AM. Microvascular free toe transfer. *Clin Plast Surg*. 1978;5:223–237.

Salmins S. In: Williams PL, ed. *Gray's Anatomy*. 38th ed. Toronto, Ontario, Canada: Churchill Livingstone; 1999:375–424.

Tan JS, Tu YK. Comparative study of outcomes between pollicization and microsurgical second toe-metatarsal bone transfer for congenital radial deficiency with hypoplastic thumb. *J Reconstr Microsurg*. 2013;29:587–592.

Tsai TM, Wang WZ. Vascularized joint transfers. *Hand Clin*. 1992;8:525–536.

Vilkki SK, Kotkansalo T. Present technique and long-term results of toe-to-antebrachial stump transplantation. *J Plast Reconstr Aesth Surg*. 2007;60:835–848.

Wallace CG, Wei FC. Further aesthetic refinement for great toe transfers. *J Plast Reconstr Aesthet Surg*. 2010;63:e109–110.

Wei FC. Tissue preservation in hand injury: the first step to toe-to-hand transplantation. *Plast Reconstr Surg*. 1998;102:2497–2501.

Wei FC, Chen HC, Chuang CC, Chen SH. Microsurgical thumb reconstruction with toe transfer: selection of various techniques. *Plast Reconstr Surg*. 1994;93:345–357; discussion 352–357.

Wei FC, Chen HC, Chuang CC, Noordhoff MS. Reconstruction of the thumb with a trimmed-toe transfer. *Plast Reconstr Surg*. 1988;82:506–513.

Wei FC, Colony LH. Microsurgical reconstruction if opposable digits in mutilating hand injuries. *Clin Plast Surg*. 1989;16:491–504.

Wei FC, Colony LH, Chen HC, Chuang CC, Noordhoff MS. Combined second and third toe transfer. *Plast Reconstr Surg*. 1989; 86:651–661.

Wei FC, El-Gammal TA. Toe-to-hand transfer. *Clin Plast Surg*. 1996;23:103–116.

Wei FC, El-Gammal TA, Lin CH, Chung CC, Chen HC, Chen SH. Metacarpal hand: classification and guidelines for microsurgical reconstruction with toe transfers. *Plast Reconstr Surg*. 1997;99:122–128.

Wei FC, Ma HS. Delayed sensory reeducation after toe-to-hand transfer. *Microsurgery*. 1995;16:583–585.

Wei FC, Santamaria E. Toe-to-finger reconstruction. In: Green DP, Hotchkiss RN, Pederson WC, eds. *Green's Operative Hand Surgery*. 4th ed. Philadelphia, PA: Churchill Livingstone; 1999:1327–1353.

Wei FC, Silverman RT, Hsu WM. Retrograde dissection of the vascular pedicle in toe harvest. *Plast Reconstr Surg*. 1995;96:1211–1214.

Wei FC, Yim KK. Pulp plasty after toe-to-hand transplantation. *Plast Reconstr Surg*. 1995;96:661–666.

Woo SH, Kim JS, Seul JH. Immediate toe-to-hand transfer in acute hand injuries: overall results, compared with results for elective cases. *Plast Reconstr Surg*. 2004;113:882–892.

Yim KK, Wei FC. Secondary procedures to improve function after toe-to-hand transfers. *Br J Plast Surg*. 1995;48:487–491.

Yim KK, Wei FC, Lin CH. A comparison between primary and secondary toe-to-hand transplantation. *Plast Reconstr Surg*. 2004;114: 107–112.

CHAPTER 45 Nerve Injury/Repair

Pieter G.L. Koolen, MD,
John B. Hijjawi, MD, FACS, and
Samuel J. Lin, MD, MBA, FACS

• • • ANATOMY OF PERIPHERAL NERVES • • •

○ **What are the basic elements of the peripheral nerves?**

Internal epineurium

External epineurium

Perineurium

Endoneurium

○ **What are the functions of the internal and external epineurium?**

The external epineurium surrounds the entire nerve and the internal epineurium surrounds groups of fascicles.

○ **Which layer is an extension of the blood–brain barrier?**

The perineurium. This layer has closely packed cells and surrounds individual fascicle that functions to block the spread of infection and to maintain a positive intrafascicular pressure.

○ **The layer that surrounds individual axons is termed?**

The endoneurium.

○ **What is a fascicular plexus?**

A region of interconnections between fascicles.

○ **Name three blood supply sources for peripheral nerves.**

1. Arteriae nervosum (vaso nervosus) (epineurium)

2. Extrinsic blood vessels (perineurium)

3. Capillary plexus (endoneurium)

○ **How is the nerve potential propagated down the nerve?**

Depolarizing current achieving the threshold membrane potential leads to activation of voltage-gated sodium channels.

○ **What is a node of Ranvier?**

A gap that represents a space between adjacent Schwann cells along the length of the axon.

○ **What is saltatory conduction?**

Propagation of the action potential via depolarization at the nodes of Ranvier (myelinated fibers 3–150 m/s).

○ **What is Wallerian degeneration?**

A process by which axoplasm and myelin are degraded and removed by phagocytosis.

○ **What are the key features of Wallerian degeneration?**

1. Granular disintegration of axoplasmic microtubules and neurofilaments.
2. Disappearance of myelin sheath and axons distal to a nerve lesion.
3. Loss of neural conductance within 48 to 96 hours.
4. Axonotmesis (Sunderland second degree).

○ **After laceration or injury to the nerve, Wallerian degeneration occurs in which segment?**

Distal segment.

○ **What are the bands of Büngner?**

Collapsed columns of Schwann cells in the distal segment of a complete nerve injury.

○ **What is neurotrophism?**

The ability of appropriate distal receptors to enhance the maturation of nerve fibers, which includes the production of a gradient of diffusible substances that direct axonal growth during regeneration.

● ● ● NERVE REPAIR CLASSIFICATION AND ASSESSMENT ● ● ●

○ **How are nerve injuries classified (Sunderland based)?**

First-degree or Neuropraxia	*Segmental Demyelination*
Second-degree or axonotmesis	Axonal injury
Third-degree combined with fibrosis of the endoneurium	Wallerian degeneration
Fourth-degree	Complete scar block
Fifth-degree or neurotmesis	Transection
Sixth-degree	Combination of IV injuries

○ **How is fibrosis resulting from nerve injuries classified (Millesi)?**

Type I: fibrosis of the epineurium

Type II: interfascicular fibrosis

Type III: intrafascicular fibrosis

○ **Which types of injuries can be expected to have complete recovery?**

Neuropraxia and axonotmesis.

○ **Nerve fiber regeneration occurs at what rate?**

1 mm/day or 1 in/month.

○ **What are clinical measurements of motor nerve injury?**

Weakness, loss of function, and atrophy.

○ **What are clinical measurements of sensory nerve injury?**

Moving and static two-point discrimination for <u>innervation density</u> and number of fibers.

Semmes–Weinstein monofilaments and vibration instruments as <u>threshold tests</u> for performance levels.

○ **Describe and classify the six levels of motor recovery following motor nerve injury.**

M0: no contraction

M1: contraction in proximal muscles

M2: contraction in distal muscles

M3: contraction sufficient to resist gravity

M4: contraction against strong resistance

M5: return to full muscle strength

○ **Describe and classify the six levels of sensory recovery following sensory nerve injury.**

S0: absence of sensibility

S1: deep-pain sensibility

S2: superficial sensibility

S3: full recovery of pain and touch (moving 2PD >15 mm)

S3+: localization of stimulus (moving and static 2PD 7–15 mm)

S4: complete recovery (2PD 3–6 mm)

○ **What does an "advancing Tinel sign" after nerve injury signify?**

Effect of triggered electric-current–like pain represents <u>outgrowing axon sprout ends.</u>

○ **What is the most sensitive test for eliciting nerve compression syndromes with demyelination?**

Nerve conduction velocity (NCV) tests.

○ **What is the most helpful test for eliciting a denervation with axonal loss?**
Electromyography (EMG)

○ **What is the earliest that EM studies will be helpful to evaluate a patient for a suspected peripheral nerve injury?**
3 weeks.

○ **Which imaging study is helpful in diagnosing injuries to peripheral nerves?**
Magnetic resonance imaging (MRI) neurograms.

○ **Which test is useful in helping to distinguish proximal and distal injuries?**
Somatosensory evoked potentials (SSEP).

○ **What are the normal values for static and moving two-point discrimination?**
1. Static 2PD: up to 6 mm
2. Moving 2PD: 2 to 3 mm

○ **Clinical tests for nerve function**

Function	Radial Nerve	Median Nerve	Ulnar Nerve
Extrinsic motor	Wrist extension	Profundus index finger	Profundus small finger
Intrinsic motor	None	Abductor pollicis brevis	First dorsal interosseous
Sensory	Dorsal first web space	Pulp of index finger	Pulp of small finger

● ● ● **TREATMENT OF NERVE INJURIES** ● ● ●

○ **What repair method is used when a nerve is partially transected and landmarks are preserved?**
Epineural repair.

○ **What repair method is generally used when a nerve injury includes a crushing component?**
Group fascicular repair.

○ **What repair method is generally used when there is a delayed repair requiring trimming of the nerve ends?**
Group fascicular repair.

○ **In an acute crush injury setting with evidence of transection and contusion of a peripheral nerve, what is the recommended treatment?**
Tagging the proximal and distal nerve endings followed by delayed repair after 3 weeks or until the wound permits.

○ **What is the advantage of early secondary nerve repair?**

Allows for terminated scar reaction along the nerve which the surgeon can estimate and graft.

○ **Have clinical studies demonstrated that fascicular repair is superior to epineural repair?**

No.

○ **Nerve elongation in secondary nerve repairs can provide how much additional length?**

Approximately 10%.

○ **How fast do nerves regenerate?**

Nerve advance in general at a rate of 1 mm/day or 1 in/month. Many clinical studies have reported nerve repair rates of 2 mm/day.

○ **Name six different types of nerve grafts.**

1. Trunk graft
2. Cable graft
3. Pedicle nerve graft
4. Interfascicular nerve graft
5. Fascicular nerve graft
6. Free vascularized nerve graft

○ **What is the best way to treat segmental peripheral nerve injuries?**

Autogenous nerve grafts.

○ **Sural nerve grafts can be harvested up to how many centimeters?**

35 to 40 cm.

○ **Harvest of the sural nerve results in a sensory deficit in which region?**

Lateral aspect of dorsum of foot.

○ **Reverse vein autograft <u>conduits</u> can be used for defects less than how many centimeters in the forearm?**

Up to 3 cm.

○ **Name four commonly harvested donor nerves for nerve grafting.**

1. Sural nerve
2. Lateral antebrachial cutaneous nerve
3. Medial antebrachial cutaneous nerve
4. Posterior interosseous nerve

○ **What is a nonsuture method used in nerve coaptation?**

Fibrin glue.

○ **Collagen conduits can be used for defects less than how many centimeters in the forearm?**
2 cm.

○ **Synthetic grafts that incorporate combinations of synthetic hydrogels, biologic materials, extracellular matrix components, and neurotrophic factors are also termed?**
Axonal guidance channels.

○ **Failure of the nerve growth cone to reach its peripheral targets causes which conditions?**
Terminal neuroma or neuroma in situ.

○ **The major treatment methods for treating neuromas include?**
• Excision and repair
• Embedding in muscle
• Proximal ligation

○ **The overall success rate for burying neuromas is?**
Approximately 75%.

○ **What is a nerve transfer?**
Transfer of the proximal portion of an intact donor nerve to reinnervate the distal portion of a more important injured nerve.

• • • PERIPHERAL NERVE ENTRAPMENT SYNDROMES • • •

○ **What does the surgical treatment of entrapment syndromes consist of?**
Decompression and/or neurolysis.

○ **What is the term given to compression of structure at the thoracic outlet?**
Thoracic outlet syndrome.

○ **The interscalene triangle borders consist of which structures?**
• Anterior scalene muscle anteriorly
• Middle scalene muscle posteriorly
• Medial surface of the first rib inferiorly

○ **The most common brachial plexus trunks involved in thoracic outlet syndrome?**
C8 and T1.

○ **Clinical maneuvers to diagnose thoracic outlet syndrome include?**
- Adson or Scalene test
- Costoclavicular or Military test
- Hyperabduction test
- Roos test

○ **The supraclavicular approach for surgical treatment of thoracic outlet syndrome endangers which nerve?**
The phrenic nerve.

○ **The transaxillary approach for surgical treatment of thoracic outlet syndrome endangers which nerve?**
The C8 or T1 nerve root.

○ **Suprascapular nerve entrapment may cause pain, weakness, and even atrophy of which muscles?**
Supraspinatus and infraspinatus.

○ **What is the most common anatomic site for suprascapular nerve entrapment?**
Suprascapular notch.

○ **The surgical treatment of suprascapular nerve entrapment consists of the release of which structure?**
Transverse scapular ligament.

○ **The two most common sites of ulnar nerve entrapment are located where?**
1. Cubital tunnel proximal to the elbow
2. Guyon canal in the wrist

○ **Inability to adduct the thumb without flexing the tip of the thumb is termed?**
Froment sign.

○ **Inability to adduct the little finger secondary to hypothenar and interossei atrophy is termed?**
Wartenberg sign.

○ **Hypothenar atrophy is secondary to compression or palsy of which nerve?**
Ulnar nerve.

○ **Surgical options for release of ulnar nerve compression at the elbow include?**
- Simple decompression
- Medial epicondylectomy
- Anterior transposition (subcutaneous *vs.* intramuscular *vs.* submuscular)
- Endoscopic decompression
- Combinations of the above

○ **As the ulnar nerve travels down the forearm, where is it positioned?**
Between the FDS and the FDP muscle bellies.

○ **The motor fascicular group of the ulnar nerve at the wrist is located in which position?**
Ulnar and dorsal.
Just remember that the <u>motor branch of the ulnar nerve</u> is the deep branch; so deep = more dorsal.

○ **Fractures from which bone can impinge on the ulnar nerve at Guyon canal?**
Hamate via fracture of the hook segment (hamulus).

○ **Laceration of the ulnar nerve in the distal forearm will result in the loss of which muscle groups?**
• Interossei
• Ulnar two lumbricals
• Hypothenar muscles
• Thumb adductor
• Half of the thumb flexor brevis

○ **Clawing of the hand is found with which types of ulnar nerve injuries?**
Low (distal) ulnar nerve injuries.

○ **Why does the hand claw with low ulnar nerve injuries?**
Unopposed FDP flexion of the IP joints and unopposed extension of the MP joints.

○ **What finding distinguishes a neuropathy of the ulnar nerve at the elbow from that at the wrist?**
Decreased sensation in the dorso-ulnar hand.

○ **What is the anatomic basis for the decreased sensation on the dorso-ulnar hand?**
The <u>dorsal sensory branch of the ulnar nerve</u> branches at approximately 8 cm proximal to the pisiform. Thus, it is unaffected by compression at the wrist but its fascicles are still with the main ulnar nerve at the elbow.

○ **What are sites of compression of the median nerve that cause pronator syndrome?**
• Ligament of Struthers
• Lacertus fibrosus (bicipital aponeurosis)
• Pronator teres (musculofascial band or compression between two muscular heads)
• FDS proximal arch

○ **What are the anatomic borders of the carpal tunnel?**
• Carpal bones (floor)
• Transverse carpal ligament (roof)
• Scaphoid and trapezium radially
• Pisiform and hook of the hamate ulnarly

○ **The motor fascicular group of the median nerve at the wrist is located in which position?**

Radial and volar. Just remember that the recurrent motor (muscular) branch branches off radially toward the thenar muscle group.

○ **Thenar atrophy is secondary to compression or palsy of which nerve?**

Median nerve.

○ **What is an important symptom to help distinguish the pronator syndrome from the carpal tunnel syndrome?**

Pain in the proximal palm. Patients will have abnormal sensibility over the thenar eminence in pronator syndrome.

○ **What is the anatomic basis for the above difference?**

The palmar cutaneous branch of the median nerve branches proximal to the wrist and is thus spared compression by the transverse carpal ligament.

○ **A splint to minimize pressure within the carpal canal would be designed with how much wrist and finger extension/flexion?**

Wrist neutral and fingers in extension.

○ **A characteristic symptom of anterior interosseous syndrome is?**

Inability to form a circle by pinching the thumb and index finger (O sign).

○ **What is the anatomic basis for the above finding?**

The AIN provides motor innervation to the FPL (thumb IP flexion) and the index and ling FDP (index DIP flexion). You cannot make an "O" without thumb IP and index DIP flexion. Incidentally, AIN also innervates the PQ.

○ **Does the anterior interosseous syndrome have any sensory component?**

No, motor only.

○ **What is Gantzer muscle?**

Accessory head of the FPL.

○ **What is innervation through a Martin-Gruber anastomosis?**

Median to ulnar nerve in the forearm. Remember FMG or **F**oreign **M**edical **G**raduate (**F**orearm-**M**artin-**G**ruber).

○ **What is innervation through a Riche–Cannieu anastomosis?**

Median to ulnar nerve in the hand.

○ **The radial nerve is derived from which cord of the brachial plexus?**

Posterior cord.

○ **The most common site of compression of the radial nerve occurs at?**

The arcade of Frohse, proximal fibrous edge of the supinator muscle. Remember the RAF of **R**oyal **A**ir **F**orce (**R**adial Nerve-**A**rcade of **F**rohse).

○ **Other sites of compression of the radial nerve include?**

• Fibrous fascia over the radiocapitellar joint.

• Vascular leash of Henry (radial recurrent artery). Remember RVH or **R**ight **V**entricular **H**ypertrophy (**R**adial Nerve-**V**ascular leash of **H**enry).

• Medial border of ECRB.

• Distal border of the supinator.

○ **Pain and tenderness in the dorsal lateral forearm is most consistently associated with which compression syndrome?**

Radial tunnel syndrome.

○ **What are symptoms commonly associated with posterior interosseous nerve syndrome?**

• Pain in the upper extensor forearm

• Dysesthesias in a superficial radial nerve distribution

• Weakening of the extension of the fingers, thumb, or wrist

○ **Compression of the superficial radial nerve as it emerges from under the brachioradialis is termed?**

Wartenberg's syndrome.

○ **What structures pass through the tarsal tunnel?**

• Tendons of the flexor hallucis longus muscle

• Flexor digitorum longus muscle

• Tibialis posterior muscle

• Posterior tibial nerve

• Posterior tibial artery

○ **Release of which structure is performed to decompress the tarsal tunnel?**

Flexor retinaculum (which is the roof of the tunnel).

○ **Erectile dysfunction following radical prostatectomy is considered to be largely neurogenic in origin; what is the origin of the fibers of the cavernous nerves?**

Parasympathetic fibers from S2 to S4.

○ **What is the location of the cavernous nerves in relation to the prostate?**

Within the cavernous nerve bundles along the posterolateral surface of the prostate, which corresponds anatomically to the peripheral zone, the most common site of prostate carcinogenesis.

○ **What are common strategies to preserve erectile function after radical prostatectomy?**

1. Nerve-sparing radical prostatectomy

2. Cavernous nerve interposition grafting

3. Neurotrophic treatment

○ **What is the most common nerve graft used in cavernous nerve interposition grafting?**

Sural nerve.

○ **What is the reported efficacy, or return of erectile function, for unilateral cavernous interposition nerve grafting? For bilateral cavernous interposition nerve grafting?**

Unilateral: approximately 50%

Bilateral: approximately 25%

○ **Spontaneous erectile activity following cavernous nerve regeneration has been observed how many months following surgery?**

- 5 to 8 months for mild tumescence.

- 14 to 18 months for erectile activity.

○ **What is the estimated probability of being able to have intercourse at 16 months?**

25%.

○ **What is the most frequent and avoidable complication after peripheral nerve decompression?**

Carpal tunnel: neuroma of the palmar cutaneous branch

Cubital tunnel: neuroma of the medial antebrachial cutaneous nerve

Tarsal tunnel: neuroma of posterior branch of saphenous nerve

• • • **REFERENCES** • • •

Chang DW, Wood CG, Kroll SS, et al. Cavernous nerve reconstruction to preserve erectile function following nonnerve-sparing radical retropubic prostatectomy: a prospective study. *Plast Reconstr Surg.* 2003;111:1174–1181.

Mackinnon SE, Novak CB. Thoracic outlet syndrome. *Curr Probl Surg.* 2002;39:1070–1145.

Mackinnon SE. Pathophysiology of nerve compression. *Hand Clin.* 2002;18:231–241.

Penkert G, Fansa H. *Peripheral Nerve Lesions: Nerve Surgery and Secondary Reconstructive Repair.* 1st ed. New York, NY: Springer-Verlag; 2004.

Rummler LS, Gupta R. Peripheral nerve repair: a review. *Curr Opin Orthop.* 2004;15:215–219.

Szabo RM. Entrapment and compression neuropathies. In: Green DP, Hotchkiss RN, Pederson WC, eds. *Green's Operative Hand Surgery.* 4th ed. New York, NY: Churchill Livingstone; 1999.

Section IV

HEAD AND NECK

CHAPTER 46 Facial Trauma

Jonathan Black, MD and
John N. Jensen, MD

● ● ● **GENERAL** ● ● ●

○ **What are the bones of the orbit?**

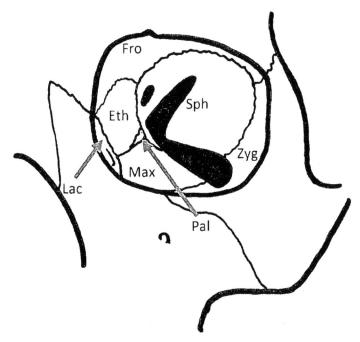

Fro, Frontal bone; Sph, Sphenoid; Zyg, Zygoma; Pal, Palatine bone; Max, Maxilla; Lac, Lacrimal bone; Eth, Ethmoid bone.

Roof: Frontal, lesser wing of sphenoid.

Medial wall: Ethmoid, lacrimal, frontal process of maxilla.

Lateral wall: Zygoma, greater wing of sphenoid.

Floor: Zygoma, maxilla.

○ **What are the buttresses of the facial skeleton?**

Vertical: Nasomaxillary (medial), zygomatico-maxillary/lateral orbit (lateral), mandibular ramus (posterior).
Horizontal: Fronto-orbital, inferior orbital rims, maxillary arch, mandibular arch, zygomatic arches.

○ **What is the most common facial fracture in children?**

A relatively recent study stratifies by age (0–6, 6–12, 12–18 years) and demonstrated a downward trend over time across age groups in skull and orbital fractures, and a concomitant upward trend in midface (maxillary, nasal, NOE, ZMC) fractures, mandible, and dentoalveolar fractures, as a percentage of total fractures remained stable from infancy through adolescence; in this study, orbital fractures were most common, followed by mandible or nasal, depending on the age.

○ **What is the current consensus of use of resorbable plates in facial fractures?**

Some studies show comparable results to titanium, but their use is not commonly employed, and remains controversial.

○ **What is the standard imaging for facial fractures?**

CT scan with axial and (reconstructed) coronal images are the minimum necessary; often sagittal and/or 3D reconstruction are critical to fully define the extent of injury.

○ **When is consideration made for tracheostomy in facial fractures?**

Unstable airway (bilateral mandible fractures and altered LOC); panfacial fractures with maxillary and mandibular fractures, especially with concomitant thoracic trauma and pulmonary contusion or brain injury.

○ **Is IMF an indication for gastrostomy?**

No. A liquid diet can be managed effectively per os (through a straw) in most cases.

○ **What finding should raise concerns with skull base fractures?**

Pulsatile proptosis, headache, visual loss, diplopia and periorbital and ocular erythema are signs of posttraumatic carotid-cavernous fistula. It may occur with fractures extending into the cranial fossa from either posterior or anterior cranial fossae. It is confirmed with angiography, and initially managed with VIR techniques.

○ **In facial nerve transection, how long before the distal segments lose the ability to be located with a nerve stimulator?**

24 to 48 hours.

○ **What general anatomic landmark may be used to determine the feasibility of facial nerve exploration and repair?**

Injuries medial to the lateral canthus are unlikely to be successfully repaired surgically.

○ **How often do patients with facial fractures from high-speed motor vehicle crashes sustain cervical spine injury?**

10%.

○ **How are parotid duct injuries managed acutely?**

Cannulation with a 5F pediatric feeding tube, with instillation of dye to locate laceration or transaction. Repair with fine suture (8-0 monofilament) acutely over the stent is advised.

○ **How effective is external carotid artery ligation in controlling facial hemorrhage following traumatic injury?**

Because of rich collateralization between internal and external carotid artery vascular territories, ligation is usually not very effective. Packing oral and nasal cavities is more likely to stem the hemorrhage and allow for coagulation and hemostasis.

○ **What is a "growing" skull fracture?**

Usually encountered in children under age 3 years, it occurs when a skull fracture is accompanied by an underlying dural tear that is untreated. Herniation of the underlying brain, sometimes referred to as a leptomeningeal cyst, prevents spontaneous bone healing, and the fracture appears to widen over time. It is managed with dural repair and cranioplasty.

○ **How does one approach the panfacial fracture?**

From stable to unstable; with concomitant maxillary and mandibular fractures, usually occlusion is established, followed by mandible, then maxilla ORIF.

○ **In cases of ORIF of the maxilla and/or mandible, what are the most likely causes of malocclusion after removal of intraoperative IMF?**

Inadequate reduction leading to inaccurate placement of miniplate fixation.

● ● ● FRONTAL SINUS ● ● ●

○ **How often do frontal sinus fractures present with CSF leak?**

About 20%

○ **What is the cause of a CSF leak in this setting?**

A dural tear (likely from a posterior table bone fragment or cribriform plate disruption) combined with a fracture pattern allowing the CSF to enter the paranasal sinuses.

○ **What are the conditions in frontal sinus fracture that warrant conservative management?**

Minimal displacement of fractures (anterior and posterior tables), even when CSF leak is present, are initially managed with observation. If CSF leak persists, a lumbar drain may be considered to reduce the flow across the dural tear, and allow for secondary healing.

○ **What are the features in frontal sinus fracture that determine which operative intervention is indicated?**

There are three: integrity of the barrier between the brain and frontal sinus, contour of the anterior table, and patency of nasofrontal ducts. The (colonized) sinus mucosa must be removed if there is communication with the dura/brain; therefore, cranialization is usually employed when there is a displaced posterior table fracture with or without CSF leak. ORIF of the anterior table addresses contour deformity, and outlet obstruction (assessed with instillation of dye in sinus, with patency confirmed with appearance of dye in nasal cavity) with intact posterior table is addressed by sinus obliteration or endoscopic sinus surgery.

○   **How is the frontal sinus cranialized?**

A coronal approach is generally employed, in the subpericranial plane. The fragments of the anterior table are marked for replacement, and additional osteotomy performed if necessary. The posterior table, usually comminuted, is removed, the dura repaired, the mucosa of the sinus thoroughly stripped, the sinus bony surface burred, and a pericranial flap raised from the frontal scalp, and placed in the base of the sinus to form a barrier between the intracranial space and frontonasal ducts. The anterior table is replaced with internal fixation, leaving a small gap above the brow to accommodate the pericranial flap.

○   **How is the frontal sinus obliterated?**

The anterior table fragments are recovered, the mucosa stripped and the bony cavity burred, the pericranial flap raised and inset, and the sinus cavity filled with fat, muscle, or bone. The anterior table is replaced with internal fixation.

○   **How is the mucosa properly stripped?**

All visible mucosa is manually removed. A fine burr is used over the entire bony surface of the sinus to remove the remaining mucosal invaginations (pits of Breschet).

○   **How do you test for CSF?**

Beta-2-transferrin is most specific; halo sign on filter paper is unreliable.

○   **What are the early complications of frontal sinus fracture?**

CSF leak, epistaxis, meningitis, intracranial bleed.

○   **What are the late complications of frontal sinus fracture?**

Osteomyelitis, mucocoele (from retained mucosa), intracranial abscess. These can occur years later; current recommendations are for annual surveillance imaging for 5 years, though there are many cases of mucocoele presenting more than 10 years post-injury.

● ● ● **NASAL** ● ● ●

○   **What is the sensory innervation of the nose?**

External branches of the anterior ethmoidal nerve (V1), infratrochlear nerve (V1) supply superior portion and tip; branches of infraorbital nerve (V2) supply inferior and lateral nasal skin.

○   **Why must a septal hematoma be drained?**

Failure to recognize and treat a septal hematoma may result in necrosis of the septal cartilage and perforation. It is most effectively accomplished with early intervention (at presentation) and apposition of mucosa to cartilage must be confirmed.

○   **What are the common features of a naso-orbital-ethmoid fracture?**

Telecanthus, epiphora, flattened nasal bridge, upturned nasal tip.

○ **What is the Markowitz–Manson classification schema for NOE fractures?**

Related to the fragment with the medial canthal insertion:

Type 1: large central fragment

Type 2: small fragment within comminuted segment

Type 3: extensive comminution/avulsion

○ **What is the key to minimizing postreduction nasal deformities requiring future septorhinoplasty?**

Addressing septal injury by primary reduction in a controlled setting with general anesthesia available.

● ● ● **ORBIT** ● ● ●

○ **What is the depth of the orbital floor?**

It varies according to size and age of patient, but generally about 40 to 45 mm in adults.

○ **Where is Whitnall's tubercle?**

The frontal process of the zygoma, about 5 to 10 mm deep to the lateral rim within the bony orbit. The lateral canthal ligament attaches here.

○ **Where does the medial canthal ligament attach?**

The frontal process of the maxilla; the thicker posterior portion inserts on the posterior lacrimal crest.

○ **What are the anatomic cues for fixation of the medial canthal ligament?**

The transnasal wire should be placed posterior and superior to the posterior lacrimal crest.

○ **What are the signs of orbital entrapment?**

Diplopia on upward gaze is the classic clinical finding, but may be present secondary to periorbital edema in the absence of entrapment following orbital fracture; CT scan has emerged as the most reliable sign in common practice, but a forced duction test remains a reliable tool as well.

○ **What is the Marcus–Gunn pupil and what is its significance?**

Also known as the afferent papillary defect (APD), it is an indication of optic nerve injury. It is present when there is no papillary constriction to direct light, but the consensual response is preserved, as the efferent (CN III parasympathetics) pathway remains intact. When a pupil remains dilated in response to direct light stimulation and the consensual response is absent, it is most likely a defect in the efferent pathway.

○ **What technical choices can be made to minimize the incidence of entropion following a transconjunctival approach to the inferior orbital rim?**

Avoid detachment of the lateral canthal tendon, which reduces the risk for misalignment/rotation of the lid margin when being reattached.

○ **What is the "trap door" pattern of orbital floor fracture?**

When the mechanism of injury is such that a defect in the orbital floor is transient, like a hinged trap door, and periorbita is entrapped, though in the absence of obvious orbital floor bony defect on imaging. In some cases it can induce the oculocardiac reflex.

○ **What is the Aschner phenomenon?**

Also known as the oculocardiac reflex, it occurs with traction of extraocular muscles (entrapment following blowout fracture) or compression of globe (during reconstruction of the orbital floor. Communications between V1 and the vagus nerve in the brainstem account for it, and can result in bradycardia, junctional rhythm, or asystole; it is a potentially life-threatening condition. When detected in the evaluation of a patient with facial injuries, it is an indication for immediate intervention.

○ **Which method of access to the orbital floor has the lowest risk of ectropion?**

It is widely reported that the transconjunctival approach has a lower incidence of postoperative ectropion, though probably it depends on the operator.

○ **How is ectropion initially treated?**

Conservatively with several weeks/months of scar massage.

○ **When is the lacrimal system explored?**

When there is visible sign of disruption of the duct, as with laceration.

○ **What is the proper plane of dissection in the transconjuctival approach to the orbital floor?**

Preseptal (between the orbicularis oculi and septum), following incision of the capsulopalpebral fascia.

○ **What are Jones I and II tests?**

They are used to detect obstruction of the lacrimal system. Jones I tests physiologic conditions and involves instillation of 2% fluorescein into the tear meniscus of the affected eye, insert a cotton swab under the anterior middle turbinate, wait 5 minutes, and check swab. If fluorescein is evident, there is no obstruction or only partial obstruction. If absent, it may mean obstruction at any point from the punctum to the nasal cavity. A Jones II test is then done by cannulating the punctum, and injecting saline (nonphysiologic conditions). It will overcome partial obstruction, or edema, or obstruction at the punctum. If reflux is encountered or no flow is evident, there is complete obstruction.

○ **What feature of orbital trauma is worrisome for optic nerve injury?**

Blunt force to superolateral aspect of orbit.

○ **What are the signs of retrobulbar hematoma?**

Eye pain, decreased visual acuity, proptosis, chemosis, intraocular hypertension, lid ecchymosis/hematoma, paralyzed extraocular muscles.

○ **What is the proper acute management of increased intraorbital pressure from a retrobulbar hematoma?**

Lateral canthotomy/cantholysis performed immediately (in ER); permanent visual loss can occur with delayed treatment.

○ **What are indications for ORIF of orbital floor fractures?**

Defect >2 cm (or >50% of orbital floor), entrapment of periorbital contents, enophthalmos.

○ **What are <u>not</u> indications for ORIF of orbital fractures?**

Diplopia, infraorbital nerve hypesthesia/anesthesia, and subconjunctival hemorrhage are common and often resolve without intervention.

○ **What is superior orbital fissure syndrome?**

Disruption of the four nerves passing through the superior orbital fissure: CN III, IV, VI and V1, giving extraocular muscle paralysis (ophthalmoplegia), ptosis, a fixed, dilated pupil with normal consensual response, and numbness of the forehead/brow/upper eyelid.

○ **What is orbital apex syndrome?**

Superior orbital fissure syndrome + optic nerve injury; presents with blindness.

○ **What are the surgical approaches to the orbit?**

Transconjunctival, subciliary, subtarsal, superior lid crease, brow, and transcaruncular.

○ **What is the mechanism of posttraumatic enophthalmos?**

Increased orbital volume is the predominant cause, possibly by inadequate floor reconstruction; posttraumatic fat atrophy, among other features, may contribute to a lesser degree.

● ● ● ZYGOMATICOMAXILLARY COMPLEX ● ● ●

○ **In the Gillies approach for zygomatic arch fracture reduction, what is the correct plane of dissection?**

Between the deep temporal fascia and temporalis muscle fibers; dissection in this plane allows safe placement of the instrument deep (medial) to the impacted fracture.

○ **Why is the lateral orbital wall a useful anatomic landmark to judge ZMC fracture reduction?**

In the standard fracture pattern with posterior and medial impaction of the zygomatic body, there usually is overlap of the fragments on the relatively flat surface of the lateral orbit (zygomaticosphenoid articulation), and alignment here is difficult to achieve without correction of the position of the zygomas. Reduction is still confirmed by visualization of anatomic alignment at the zygomaticofrontal suture, inferior orbital rim, and lateral buttress. However, use of these three areas alone can result in inadequate reduction as residual rotation is difficult to appreciate, especially if there is comminution of the lateral buttress.

○ **What are the four extensions alluded to in a "tetrapod" fracture?**

Inferior orbital rim, zygomatico-frontal suture (lateral orbit), zygomaticomaxillary buttress (lateral buttress), zygomatic arch.

○ **What are the indications for ORIF of a ZMC fracture?**

Unstable fractures. Complete fractures through the entire tetrapod, even if minimally displaced, have the potential to displace through the action of the masseter. Incomplete fractures that are displaced (usually medial and posteriorly) should be fixed. In nondisplaced incomplete fractures, infraorbital nerve anesthesia and malocclusion may resolve and may be observed. Comorbidity also plays a role in the decision to intervene.

○ **What are the additional indications for repairing a ZMC fracture?**

Malar flattening, enophthalmos.

○ **What are the indications to operatively repair an isolated zygomatic arch fracture?**

Trismus (inability to close the mandible) and aesthetic change from arch displacement.

○ **How does trismus occur in a ZMC fracture?**

Medial displacement of the arch portion impedes the coronoid process of the mandible from moving superiorly during elevation of the mandible.

○ **How can you prevent malar fat pad ptosis secondary to zygoma fracture reduction?**

It can be prevented by resuspension of overlying midface soft tissue after reduction of the fracture at the inferior orbital rim, or preservation of the periosteal attachments during dissection.

● ● ● **MAXILLARY FRACTURE** ● ● ●

○ **What are the classic midface fracture patterns, as described by Rene LeFort?**

LeFort 1: Horizontal fracture across both medial and lateral maxillary buttresses near base of piriform, and pterygoid plates.

LeFort 2: Pyramidal pattern across lateral buttresses but crosses medial buttresses more superiorly, and pterygoid plates.

LeFort 3: Craniofacial disjunction, with maintenance of lateral and medial buttresses, but fracture across zygomatic arches, orbital floors, nasofrontal junction, and pterygoid plates (Fig. 46-1).

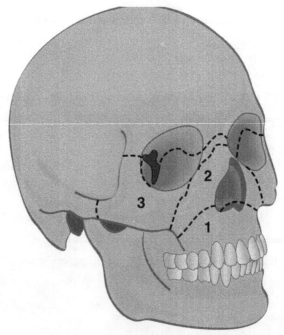

Figure 46-1 Classic midface fracture patterns (Le Fort fracture classification).

○ **In actual practice, how often are these patterns encountered?**

Commonly it is a combination of these patterns, usually with significant comminution, usually with high-energy blunt force trauma.

○ **In the surgical approach to maxillary fractures, what is the guiding principle?**

Reestablishment of a normal occlusive relationship; failure to do so is usually secondary to inadequate reduction of the fractures.

○ **How are palatal fractures managed?**

Because of the inelastic quality of the palatal mucoperiosteum, these fractures are usually stabilized with ORIF along the standard midface buttresses, as well as IMF, with suture repair of the mucoperiosteum assisting in stabilizing the fragments if necessary. Low-profile plates may be used on occasion, but often become exposed and necessitate removal. In severely comminuted cases, use of a custom-made splint should be considered.

● ● ● **MANDIBLE** ● ● ●

○ **What are the absolute indications for open reduction of a mandibular condylar neck fracture?**

Displacement of the condyle into the middle cranial fossa, bilateral injury with loss of posterior facial height, lateral displacement out of the glenoid fossa, and foreign body in the joint.

○ **What is an appropriate period of time to maintain a patient in intermaxillary fixation?**

Depends on the patient's age and comorbidity, and nature of the injury. If the injury extends into the joint, immobilization of more than 2 or 3 weeks is risky for ankylosis. Older patients are at greater risk as well. A standard of care is for IMF for 3 to 6 weeks, followed by several weeks of elastics if healing is incomplete.

○ **Is it true that most mandibular fractures are bilateral?**

No; about half are.

○ **What is the proper technique of placement of an Ivy loop?**

See Figure 46-2.

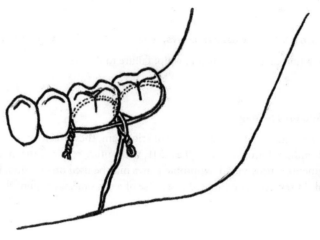

Figure 46-2 Ivy loop placement.

A 26-gauge wire is folded on itself, a few twists made at the bend, and the free ends passed from buccal to lingual at the site of the fracture. Each wire is brought around a tooth bordering the fracture, one end passed immediately inside the twists, and the ends twisted together to roughly bridal the border teeth. The central twisted segment is then further twisted to secure the circumdental fixation as a kind of weave. It is a good temporary fix to open, bleeding, displaced fractures in patients with life-threatening injuries precluding early operative intervention.

○ **What special considerations must be made for the pediatric population?**

Use of plate fixation requires periosteal stripping, and concomitant reduction of blood supply, which may adversely impact growth; additionally, in children in primary and mixed dentition, developing tooth follicles occupy much of the maxilla and mandible, and are at risk with ORIF. The unerupted permanent canine is traditionally thought to be at greatest risk.

○ **In children in primary and mixed dentition, how are mandible fractures managed?**

If the periosteal sleeve is essentially intact, mandible fractures often heal and remodel favorably in growing children. Subcondylar fractures are the most common in children, and are often treated conservatively with a soft diet. Immobilization (IMF) can afford comfort in some cases, and can be placed by crossing wire loops anteriorly anchored by piriform wires placed in an open manner, connected to circummandibular wires placed in a closed technique.

○ **In the classic case of unilateral subcondylar fracture with contralateral parasymphyseal fracture, what is the standard approach?**

ORIF of the parasymphyseal fracture with IMF.

○ **What are the two equivalent techniques for ORIF of noncomminuted mandibular angle fracture?**

Champy plate at the superior border with/without a short course of MMF OR two-plate fixation through an external approach.

○   **What is the Champy plate, and the principle behind it?**

It is a plate that wraps around the oblique line at the anterior junction of the ramus and body, placed through an intraoral approach. The notion is that some mandibular angle fractures are "favorable," and are essentially stabilized against rotation by the action of the masseteric/medial pterygoid sling, and require minimal fixation to heal well. Mesial to canines, the risk for rotation requires the standard two-plate (fixation plate + tension band) approach.

○   **Why do condylar neck fractures usually displace medially?**

The lateral pterygoid muscle inserts into the condylar neck; it displaces the neck medially when acting unopposed.

○   **What is a Joe Hall Morris device?**

A device for external fixation used to align badly comminuted mandibular fractures with significant soft tissue disruption is present (like gunshot wounds). Its advantage is minimal subperiosteal dissection to preserve blood supply.

○   **How does one manage a mandible fracture in the edentulous patient?**

ORIF if possible; otherwise, intermaxillary fixation must be managed either with a splint or the patient's dentures, if intact.

○   **In the treatment of early postoperative infection following mandible ORIF, when is it appropriate to leave the hardware in place?**

Usually it is appropriate, unless there is clear evidence of osteomyelitis. Most early post-op infections are related to diseased dentition, and if the underlying source is removed and the abscess drained, the hardware may be left in place and the patient observed.

○   **When are teeth extracted in managing mandible fractures?**

When they interfere with reduction, are comminuted, or clearly devitalized or decayed.

○   **In dental fractures, what is the significance of hot and cold sensitivity?**

Exposure of dentin, and possibly pulp (vascular supply).

○   **When mental nerve anesthesia is detected, what is the usual fracture pattern?**

Mandibular body, with displacement, affecting the inferior alveolar nerve; fractures through the mental nerve foramen can also cause anesthesia.

● ● ● **REFERENCES** ● ● ●

Bite U, Jackson IT, Forbes GS, et al. Orbital volume measurements in enophthalmos using 3-D CT imaging. *Plast Reconstr Surg.* 1985;75:502–508.

Crawley WA, Sandel AJ. Fractures of the mandible. In: Ferraro JW, ed. *Fundamentals of Maxillofacial Surgery.* New York, NY: Springer-Verlag; 1997:192–202.

Dufresne CR, Manson PN. Pediatric facial trauma. In: McCarthy JG, ed. *Plastic Surgery.* Vol 2. Philadelphia, PA: WB Saunders; 1990:1142–1187.

Ellis E. A prospective study of 3 treatment methods for isolated fractures of the mandibular angle. *J Oral Maxillofac Surg.* 2010;68: 2743–2754.

Kelly KJ. Pediatric facial trauma. In: Achauer BM, Eriksson E, Guyuron B, et al., eds. *Plastic Surgery: Indications, Operations, and Outcomes.* Vol 2. St Louis, MO: Mosby D Year Book; 2000:941–969.

Lettieri S. Facial trauma. In: Achauer BM, Eriksson E, Guyuron B, et al., eds. *Plastic Surgery: Indications, Operations, and Outcomes.* Vol 2. St Louis, MO: Mosby D Year Book; 2000:923–940.

Manson PN. Facial fractures. In: Aston SJ, Beasley RW, Thorne CH, eds. *Grabb & Smith's Plastic Surgery.* 5th ed. Philadelphia, PA: Lippincott-Raven; 1997:383–412.

Markowitz BL, Manson PN, Sargent L, et al. Management of the medial canthal tendon in nasoethmoid orbital fractures: the importance of the central fragment in classification and treatment. *Plast Reconstr Surg.* 1991;87:843–853.

McGuirt WF, Salisbury PL III. Mandibular fractures: their effect on growth and dentition. *Arch Otolaryngol Head Neck Surg.* 1987; 113:257–261.

Pollock RA. Nasal trauma: pathomechanics and surgical management of acute injuries. *Clin Plast Surg Am.* 1992;19:133–147.

Rohrich RJ, Adams WP. Nasal fracture management: Minimizing secondary nasal deformities. *Plast Reconstr Surg.* 2000;106:266–273.

Rohrich RJ, Hollier LH. Management of frontal sinus fractures: changing concepts. *Clin Plast Surg Am.* 1992;19:219–232.

Rohrich RJ, Hollier LH, Watamull D. Optimizing the management of orbitozygomatic fractures. *Clin Plast Surg Am.* 1992;19:149–165.

Rohrich RJ, Shewmake KB. Evolving concepts of craniomaxillofacial fracture management. *Clin Plast Surg Am.* 1992;19:1–10.

Schendel SA. Vertical maxillary defects. In: Ferraro JW, ed. *Fundamentals of Maxillofacial Surgery.* New York, NY: Springer-Verlag; 1997:284–286.

Smith ML, Williams JK, Gruss JS. Management of orbital fractures. *Oper Tech Plast Reconstr Surg.* 1998;5:312–324.

Wolfe SA, Johnson P. Frontal sinus injuries: primary care and management of late complications. *Plast Reconstr Surg.* 1988;82:781–791.

Wexler A. Anatomy of the head and neck. In: Ferraro JW, ed. *Fundamentals of Maxillofacial Surgery.* New York, NY: Springer-Verlag; 1997:53–113.

Yaremchuk MJ. Fractures of the maxilla. In: Cohen M, ed. *Mastery of Plastic and Reconstructive Surgery.* Vol 2. Boston, MA: Little Brown & Co; 1994:1156–1164.

Zide BM. The temporomandibular joint. In: McCarthy JG, ed. *Plastic Surgery.* Vol 2. Philadelphia, PA: WB Saunders; 1990:1474–1513.

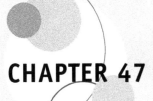

CHAPTER 47
Facial Nerve Anatomy and Paralysis

Douglas M. Sidle, MD, FACS and
Rakesh K. Chandra, MD

● ● ● **EMBRYOLOGY AND ANATOMY** ● ● ●

○ **What branchial arch does the facial nerve innervate?**

The second (hyoid) arch.

○ **What cartilage is associated with the second branchial arch?**

Reichert's cartilage.

○ **How many muscles does the facial nerve innervate?**

23 muscles per side:

- Occipitofrontalis
- Procerus
- Nasalis muscle
- Depressor septi nasi
- Orbicularis oculi
- Corrugator supercilii
- Depressor supercilii
- Auricular muscles (anterior, superior, posterior)
- Orbicularis oris
- Depressor anguli oris

- Risorius
- Zygomaticus major
- Zygomaticus minor
- Levator labii superioris
- Levator labii superioris alaeque nasi
- Depressor labii inferioris
- Levator anguli oris
- Buccinator
- Mentalis

The platysma in the neck is innervated by the facial nerve.

The stylohyoid muscle, stapedius and posterior belly of the digastric muscle are also innervated by the facial nerve, but are not considered muscles of facial expression.

○ **Through which foramen does the facial nerve exit the skull?**

Stylomastoid.

○ **What term is used to describe the network of anastomoses of the extratemporal facial nerve?**

The pes anserinus, and arborization.

○ **What does *pes anserinus* mean?**

The foot of a goose.

○ **What are the three major landmarks used to identify the facial nerve as it exits the stylomastoid foramen?**

1. The tympanomastoid fissure: 6 to 8 mm inferior to the drop-off of the fissure.

2. The tragal pointer: 1 cm anterior and 1 cm inferior to the point.

3. Retrograde dissection of the posterior belly of the digastric muscle.

The facial nerve is almost invariably found at a point where the tip of the mastoid, cartilaginous process of the auditory canal, and superior border of the posterior belly of the digastrics muscle meet.

○ **Where does the posterior belly of the digastric muscle insert on the skull?**

The medial aspect of the mastoid portion of the temporal bone.

○ **What are the extratemporal branches of the facial nerve?**

Temporal, Zygomatic, Buccal, Marginal Mandibular, Cervical (Mnemonic: *To Zanzibar By Motor Car*). Some patients have a branch to the postauricular musculature, but this is considered vestigial.

○ **What functional fiber types comprise the facial nerve?**

SVA: taste from anterior two-thirds of tongue via chorda tympani to the nucleus solitarius.

SVE: motor branches to muscles of facial expression, digastric, stapedius, and stylohyoid from the motor nucleus in the pons.

GSA: sensation from the conchal bowl and part of the external auditory canal. Possibly some V3 contribution to middle ear.

GVE: parasympathetic stimulation of lacrimal, submandibular, sublingual gland, and minor salivary glands (all glands in the head but the parotid).

○ **What is the blood supply to the facial nerve?**

Stylomastoid artery branch of posterior auricular artery. Greater superficial petrosal artery from the middle meningeal artery.

○ **What is SMAS?**

SMAS is an abbreviation for the submuscular aponeurotic system. The SMAS is a layer of tissue which covers the deeper structures of the cheek area and is linked to the superficial muscle covering the lower face and neck, called the platysma. Some techniques for facelift surgery, lift and reposition the SMAS along with the skin. In doing so, the jowls are lifted, the neck is tightened, and the cheeks are elevated.

Also known as the superficial musculo aponeurotic system, it is an inelastic fibrous tissue immediately below the skin and subcutaneous fat of the face into which the facial muscles insert. It is contiguous with the platysma inferiorly and the superficial temporal fascia and the galea superiorly.

○ **Where does the facial nerve course in the parotid region?**

Through the substance of the gland deep to the parotid fascia and SMAS.

○ **Where do the nerve branches exit the parotid fascia to course superficially?**

Branches exit at the anterior limit of the parotid gland, continuing deep to the SMAS.

○ **What is the most commonly permanently injured branch of the facial nerve during rhytidectomy?**

The temporal branch at the zygomatic arch.

○ **Where does the temporal branch cross the zygomatic arch?**

Halfway between the lateral canthus and the root of the auricular helix. Near McGregor's patch (zygomatic ligaments anchoring cheek).

○ **What is Pitanguy's line?**

It is a theoretical line reflecting the course of the temporal branch of the facial nerve. It is drawn from a point 0.5 cm below the tragus to a point 1.5 cm lateral to the superior orbital rim.

○ **Between which fascial layers does the temporal branch of the nerve course as it crosses the zygomatic arch?**

The branch courses deep to the SMAS and immediately superficial to the superficial layer of deep temporal fascia.

○ **A stroke patient may maintain function of the frontalis muscle even though all of the other facial muscles on the ipsilateral side are paralyzed. Why?**

Because the nerve fibers that project to the part of the facial nucleus in the pons that innervates the forehead project bilaterally, but those that project to the part of the nucleus that innervates the remaining facial muscles project only contralaterally.

○ **What fascial layer does the marginal mandibular nerve lay deep to as it crosses the mandible?**

The nerve lies immediately beneath the superficial layer of the deep cervical fascia.

○ **What branch of the facial nerve innervates the buccinator muscle?**

Buccal branch of the facial nerve.

○   **At what site is the primary action of botulinum toxin?**

Botulinum toxins block acetylcholine release at the presynaptic cell surface, causing a chemical denervation. The light chain, which has zinc metalloprotease activity, cleaves SNAP-25, which is involved in vesicle fusion and release of acetylcholine.

○   **What are the botulinum toxin subtypes?**

There are seven serologically distinct subtypes of botulinum toxin A through G. Only botulinum toxin type A is FDA approved for cosmetic use.

● ● ● FACIAL NERVE PATHOLOGY ● ● ●

○   **Why does a lesion proximal to the motor nucleus of VII produce paralysis of only the lower face, whereas a lesion below the motor nucleus produce complete facial paralysis?**

The lower face receives input from motor tract fibers that have crossed only once in the pons, while the upper face receives input from crossed and uncrossed fibers from the motor tract.

○   **What is the House–Brackmann grading system?**

A standard system to evaluate the degree of recovery of facial nerve function from 1 (normal) to 6 (complete paralysis). See Figure 47-1.

Grade	Description	Characteristics
I	Normal	Normal facial function in all areas
II	Mild dysfunction	Slight weakness noticeable on close inspection; may have very slight synkinesis
III	Moderate dysfunction	Obvious, but not disfiguring, difference between 2 sides; noticeable, but not severe, synkinesis, contracture, or hemifacial spasm; complete eye closure with effort
IV	Moderately severe dysfunction	Obvious weakness or disfiguring asymmetry; normal symmetry and tone at rest; incomplete eye closure
V	Severe dysfunction	Only barely perceptible motion; asymmetry at rest
VI	Total paralysis	No movement

Figure 47-1 The House–Brackmann grading system.

○   **What is the most common form of idiopathic facial paralysis?**

Bell's palsy, 15 to 40 per 100,000.

○   **What percentage of Bell palsy is recurrent?**

10% to 14%.

○   **What is Bell palsy?**

A diagnosis of exclusion, it is idiopathic facial paralysis with sudden onset and spontaneous resolution.

○ **What percentage of Bell palsy presents with complete paralysis?**

66%.

○ **Over what time period do the majority of Bell palsies resolve?**

4 to 6 months.

○ **What proportion of Bell palsy presenting with House–Brackmann grade 6 resolve completely?**

70%. More than 90% presenting with incomplete paralysis resolve.

○ **What other symptoms do patients with Bell palsy often present with?**

Viral prodrome, numbness of the ear, face, neck, dysgeusia, hyperacusis, and decreased tearing.

○ **If a Bell palsy patient is seen in the first few days, what medications can be prescribed?**

A prednisolone taper has been shown to improve outcomes. Less evidence supports antivirals, such as acyclovir, but they are commonly prescribed in conjunction with the prednisolone taper.

○ **What is Bell phenomenon?**

Upward/outward rotation of the eye with attempted eye closure. This is an unconscious movement to protect the cornea. It is a positive prognostic sign in regard to corneal protection. See Figure 47-2.

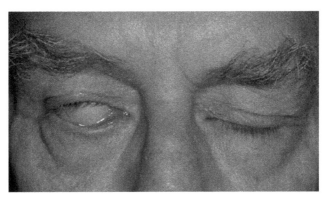

Figure 47-2 The Bell phenomenon.

○ **What percentage of patients with Lyme disease develop facial paralysis?**

10%. Paralysis may be bilateral. All resolve with appropriate Lyme disease treatment.

○ **What is the most common cause of bilateral facial paralysis?**

Guillain–Barrè syndrome.

○ **What is Melkersson–Rosenthal syndrome?**

Syndrome of unknown etiology characterized by recurrent facial nerve paralysis, woody facial edema, and a deeply fissured tongue.

○ **What is neuropraxia?**

Compression of a nerve resulting in decreased transmission without disruption of axons.

○ **What is axonotmesis?**

Disruption of axons resulting in Wallerian degeneration distal to the lesion with preservation of the neural sheaths (complete recovery expected).

○ **What is neurotmesis?**

Disruption of axons and support cells leading to Wallerian degeneration and uncertain return to function.

○ **What is synkinesis?**

Synkinesis is abnormal synchronization of movement, occurring with voluntary and reflex activity of muscles that normally do not contract together. This phenomenon occurs from faulty remyelination of regenerating nerve fibers.

○ **What is Bogorad syndrome?**

Nerves originally destined for the submandibular gland innervate the lacrimal gland leading to tearing during gustation. Also known as "crocodile tears."

○ **Where is the site of lesion leading to "crocodile tears"?**

The site of lesion must be at or proximal to the geniculate ganglion as the greater petrosal nerve segregates from the facial nerve at that point.

○ **What is Frey syndrome?**

Gustatory sweating is secondary to autonomic branches meant to drive parotid secretion cross-innervating sweat glands and blood vessels in the cheek.

○ **What are the most common causes of facial paralysis in children?**

Bell palsy (37%). Trauma (20%).

○ **What is the most common cause of facial paralysis in neonates?**

Birth trauma.

○ **What are the most common causes of facial nerve disorders in adults?**

Bell palsy (51%). Trauma (23%). Tumor (5%).

○ **The facial nerve should be electrically monitored when dissecting and extirpating which branchial cleft abnormality?**

Branchial cleft type I.

• • • **FACIAL NERVE EVALUATION AND REHABILITATION** • • •

○ **In the recovery suite immediately after a facelift, one side of the face is paralyzed. What should you do?**

Reassess the patient in 2 to 3 hours. Local anesthesia may still be affecting the nerve. Then consider steroids and nerve testing, since complete facial nerve injury after rhytidectomy is extremely rare.

○ **What is an EMG?**

EMG stands for ElectroMyoGraphy. It is a tool to measure voluntary nerve and muscle function. Probes are placed into the test muscles (in this case, facial muscles) and the patient volitionally tries to contract those muscles.

○ **What is the significance of fibrillation potentials on EMG?**

Fibrillation potentials are spontaneous muscle action potentials that occur 1 to 2 weeks after injury and signify denervation of the muscle. This signifies a poor prognosis. Thus, practitioners often wait 2 to 3 weeks to get an EMG.

○ **What is the significance of polyphasic potentials on EMG?**

Polyphasic potentials are recorded from nearby nerve fibers and signify reinnervation of the muscle. They are the earliest sign of nerve regeneration. This reveals good prognosis.

○ **What is ENoG (or EEMG)?**

In ElectroNeuroGraphy (or Evoked ElectroMyoGraphy), the nerve is electrically stimulated by a probe. This measures and compares the amplitude of summation potentials of the paralyzed face to the normal side.

○ **Where is the likely site of a facial nerve lesion in a newborn baby with a normal examination, no evidence of birth trauma, and unilateral facial paralysis?**

Likely temporal bone abnormalities. This is evaluated with a CT scan of the head and temporal bones. Likewise, serial electrical testing is performed. No activity on EMG and >90% reduction on ENoG (EEMG) suggest congenital cause, not birth trauma.

○ **What is the primary concern when initially managing a patient with facial paralysis?**

Protection of the eye from ophthalmologic sequelae including exposure keratitis, corneal ulcer, and potential blindness.

○ **What time constraints should you consider when facial nerve reinnervation techniques such as end-to-end anastomosis, hypoglossal crossover, or cable grafting (facial nerve grafting procedures) are being considered?**

Best performed in the first 12 to 18 months before muscle atrophy and loss of the motor end plates.

○ **What nonsurgical treatments exist for eye protection in facial paralysis?**

Hydrating drops, ointment, moisture chamber, lid taping at night, external eyelid weights, and physical therapy (using surface electromyography or mirror feedback).

○   **What surgical procedures are available for eye protection?**

Lateral canthoplasty, sling procedures, lower-lid shortening, tarsorrhaphy, and lid loading with gold or platinum weight placement, rarely medial canthoplasty.

○   **Where is an upper eyelid weight placed?**

It is placed superficial to the upper tarsal plate and the levator aponeurosis with the inferior edge a few millimeters above the lash line. It is generally placed centered over the junction of the central and medial one-third of the eyelid, generally over the medial limbus.

○   **What is the next alternative for eyelid weight placement in patients with contact allergy to gold?**

Platinum weight.

○   **What dynamic reanimation procedures may be accomplished?**

Temporalis transposition, free muscle transfer with microneuronal and microvascular anastomoses, masseteric nerve to facial nerve anastomosis, XII–VII crossover.

○   **What is a static sling procedure?**

Suspension of the affected musculature with Gore-Tex, fascia lata, or allograft dermal tissue.

○   **What procedures are used to restore neural input to the facial muscles?**

Primary repair of the nerve or neurorrhaphy, cable grafting, cross-face grafting, XII–VII crossover, XI–VII crossover, jump grafts, masseteric nerve to VII crossover.

○   **What proximal nerve can be used to provide a cable graft of 10 cm or less?**

Great auricular nerve.

○   **What nerve is used for cable grafts requiring >10 cm?**

Sural nerve (up to 35 cm).

○   **What is the technique of neurorrhaphy?**

Interrupted sutures of 9-0 nylon placed in the epineurium. A tension-free closure is essential.

○   **In the case of a severed nerve, what type of nerve repair generally produces the best outcomes?**

Generally, a primary repair of the nerve will produce better outcomes than a repair with an interposition, or jump graft.

○   **When evaluating a deep facial laceration, what landmark can be used to help determine if a primary nerve repair is warranted?**

A traumatically lacerated facial nerve is generally not repaired if it is torn distal to a line drawn vertically from the lateral canthus. This is in part due to the size of the distal nerve stumps and in part due to the arborization of distal nerve endings at that point.

○ **When a surgeon provides preoperative counseling to a patient who undergoing a nerve graft, how long should the patient told to wait for the procedure to achieve its best outcome postoperatively?**

Between 3 months and 2 years.

○ **When counseling your patient, what is the best results you can achieve with a nerve grafting procedure?**

House–Brackmann Grade III.

○ **In what situation should a XII–VII crossover be considered to reanimate a paralyzed face that is caused by a facial nerve disruption?**

When the proximal facial nerve stump is not available and the peripheral system is viable (less than 2 years from the time of the trauma).

○ **What is a XII–VII crossover with jump graft?**

The hypoglossal nerve is isolated and one-third to half of the nerve is incised. A great auricular nerve graft is sutured to the proximal cut segment of the hypoglossal nerve and is anastomosed to the cut facial nerve. This procedure shows comparable outcomes to the direct XII–VII crossover, provided it is performed in the first 30 days following nerve injury.

○ **What unique morbidity can result from a XII–VII crossover or XII–VII jump graft procedure?**

Disruption of the hypoglossal nerve can result in difficulties with mastication and articulation. To mitigate this complication, only one-third of the hypoglossal nerve is incised and a jump graft can be used.

○ **What is cross-facial nerve grafting?**

A nerve graft is anastamosed with contralateral buccal branches and tunneled to the opposite side of the face where it is anastamosed with the cut branches of the paralyzed side. This technique as primary therapy has largely fallen out of favor and is generally reserved for powering a free muscle graft.

○ **How long after paralysis may reinnervation techniques prove useful?**

Within 2 years of the onset of paralysis; after this point progressive muscle atrophy and fibrosis of the neuromuscular junctions precludes the use of reinnervation techniques.

○ **Describe the two-stage technique of microvascular free tissue transfer.**

Sural nerve graft is tunneled from an anastomosis with contralateral buccal branches to the involved side of the face and is tagged. Approximately 9 to 12 months later, free tissue transfer of gracilis muscle and neurovascular pedicle is performed, and the cross-facial nerve is anastamosed with the pedicle.

○ **What orientation is the sural nerve grafted?**

Reverse or rotated. However, newer evidence suggests directionality of the graft does not impact results.

○ **Describe the single-stage technique.**

Free muscle transfer is performed with cross-facial tunneling of the nerve pedicle to the contralateral buccal nerve branches. Likewise, nerve anastomosis can be made to the ipsilateral masseteric nerve.

○ **What is the advantage of single-stage repair?**

The axons need only traverse a single anastomotic line to reach the destination muscle. Less morbidity and quicker recovery is thus hypothesized.

○ **What are common muscles used in free tissue transfer facial reanimation procedures?**

Gracilis, pectoralis minor, and serratus anterior.

○ **What dynamic reanimation technique can be used to reanimate the paralyzed face in one-stage and provide immediate results?**

Temporalis transfer. Both the transfer of the temporalis tendon and transfer of the muscle are described.

• • • REFERENCES • • •

Bailey BJ. *Head and Neck Surgery: Otolaryngology*. 3rd ed. Philadelphia, PA: Lippincott Williams & Wilkins; 2001.

Gantz BJ, Rubinstein JT, Gidley P, Woodworth GG. Surgical management of Bell's palsy. *Laryngoscope*. 1999;109:1177–1188.

House JW, Brackmann DE. Facial nerve grading system. *Arch Otolaryngol Head Neck Surg*. 1985;93:146–147.

Lee KJ. *Essential Otolaryngology: Head and Neck Surgery*. 8th ed. New York, NY: McGraw-Hill; 2003.

May M. *The Facial Nerve*. 1st ed. New York, NY: Thieme; 1986.

McCabe BF. Autoimmune sensorineural hearing loss. *Ann Otol Rhinol Laryngol*. 1979;88(5):585–589.

Papel ID, Frodel JL, Holt GR, et al. *Facial Plastic and Reconstructive Surgery*. 2nd ed. New York, NY: Thieme; 2002.

Sullivan FM, Swan IR, Donnan PT, et al. Early treatment with prednisolone or acyclovir in Bell's palsy. *N Eng J Med*. 2007;357(16): 1598–1607.

Sidle DM, Fishman AJ. Modification of the orthodromic temporalis tendon transfer technique for reanimation of the paralyzed face. *Otolaryngol Head Neck Surg*. 2011;145(1):18–23.

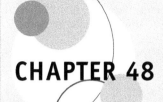

CHAPTER 48
Facial Paralysis: Static and Dynamic Treatment

Michael J.A. Klebuc, MD and Bradley Eisemann, MD

• • • ANATOMIC ESSENTIALS • • •

○ **What are the four functional components of the facial nerve?**

1. Somatic motor efferent—muscles of facial expression, auricular muscles, occipitalis, posterior belly digastric, stylohyoid and stapedius.

2. Special sensory afferent—(chorda tympani nerve running with lingual nerve) taste anterior 2/3 tongue, hard and soft palate.

3. General sensory somatic afferent—(posterior auricular nerve) sensation to skin of concha, small area behind ear, posterior ear canal. Arnold's nerve (CN X)—major contributor to external ear canal sensation.

4. Visceral motor efferent—(greater petrosal nerve) autonomic parasympathetic to mucus glands nose, hard palate, soft palate and lacrimal gland (chorda tympani nerve) submandibular, sublingual, and minor salivary glands.

○ **What landmarks are commonly utilized to identify the main trunk of the facial nerve?**

The nerve lies approximately 1 cm deep to the tragal pointer and medial to the posterior belly of the digastric muscle.

○ **What landmarks describe the course of the frontal branch of the facial nerve?**

Pitanguy's line: A line extending 0.5 cm below the tragus to 1.5 cm above the lateral brow with the nerve running on the undersurface of the temporoparietal fascia.

○ **What structures can facilitate identification and protection of the marginal mandibular nerve branches?**

The branches consistently lie on top of the facial artery and vein 1 to 3 cm below the mandibular border.

○ **Which facial muscles are innervated on their superficial surface?**

Most muscles of facial expression are innervated on their deep surface with the exception of the levator anguli oris, buccinator, and mentalis.

○ **Why does the anterior belly of the digastric muscle remain functional with facial nerve injury?**

The anterior belly is innervated by the mylohyoid branch of the inferior alveolar nerve (Trigeminal).

465

○ **Hyperacusis suggests injury at what level of the facial nerve?**

Injury of the facial nerve proximal to the branch of the stapedius muscle (middle ear) often produces increased perception of sound intensity.

• • • FACIAL PARALYSIS ETIOLOGY • • •

○ **A patient presents with the onset of mild flu-like symptoms and pain behind the right ear followed hours later by a complete unilateral hemi-facial paralysis. After neurologic evaluation to rule out a cerebrovascular accident what medical treatment is frequently prescribed?**

This is a classic presentation of Bell's palsy that is believed to represent a herpes simplex virus (HSV) type 1 infection of the facial nerve. A course of oral steroids should be prescribed within 72 hours of the onset of the paralysis. Antiviral medications (i.e., Acyclovir) are also frequently utilized, however, their benefit is less clear. Facial paralysis and painful vesicles involving the ear are associated with varicella zoster infection (VZV) known as Ramsay Hunt syndrome. The treatment for both is the same, however, more limited recoveries are frequently encountered with Ramsay Hunt syndrome when compared to Bell's palsy.

○ **A patient is referred by their primary care physician for surgical correction of Bell's palsy. The patient reports a slowly progressive, unilateral weakness of the midface and impaired ability to smile. What is the next step in this patient's treatment?**

Slow onset of facial weakness is highly suspicious for extratemporal causes of facial paralysis such as tumors of the parotid gland. A thorough head and neck examination followed by imaging (CT, MRI) should be undertaken prior to surgery.

○ **A patient presents with unilateral facial paralysis and reports a "bull's eye" rash, fatigue and fever after a hiking trip. What is the suspected diagnosis?**

Lyme disease is a spirochete (Borrelia burgdorferi) infection disseminated by tick bites. The diagnosis is confirmed with serologic testing and optimal treatment with antibiotics (ceftriaxone, doxycycline, azithromycin).

○ **Postoperative radiation therapy is planned following radical parotidectomy with segmental resection of the facial nerve. Should nerve graft reconstruction be delayed?**

There is no functional advantage to delaying nerve graft reconstruction until radiation therapy is completed. In addition, more accurate identification of the transected nerve branches will be possible during the initial surgical procedure.

○ **A child with bilateral facial paralysis presents for evaluation. What is the second most common cranial nerve effected by this syndrome?**

Moebius syndrome is a rare disorder effecting 1 in 50,000 births. It has a genetic component, however, most cases are sporadic and multifactorial. The facial nerve is involved in all cases. The abducens nerve (CN VI) is the second most frequently involved cranial nerve (approximately 75%) producing a lateral gaze palsy. The hypoglossal nerve (CN XII) is affected in approximately 25% of cases and is associated with a hypoplastic tongue. Cranial nerves VIII, III, and IV are usually spared. Other associated anomalies include club foot (approximately 30%), hand and upper limb deformities, Poland's anomaly (approximately 15%) and high-arched palate. Intelligence is usually normal, however, the autistic behavior spectrum is present in approximately 30% of cases.

○ **What is the optimal time for exploration of the facial nerve following sharp laceration?**

Exploration should take place within 72 hours. The transected distal nerve branches continue to conduct during this period allowing for more straightforward operative identification.

○ **Do facial nerve lacerations immediately adjacent to the nasolabial fold require repair?**

Reasonable recovery can be expected with cheek lacerations medial to the lateral canthus without direct nerve repair due to the extensive arborization of the buccal and zygomatic branches. However, all transected branches should be repaired if identified.

○ **What clinical presentation of a temporal bone fracture favors operative intervention?**

Immediate onset of facial paralysis often requires surgical exploration, while delayed paralysis is commonly managed with steroids and observation.

○ **Which facial nerve branch is most frequently injured during rhytidectomy?**

The buccal branches. The clinical sequelae of injury to the buccal branch is less than that seen with injury to the marginal and frontal branches. This is due to the extensive arborization of the marginal and frontal branches.

● ● ● SURGICAL REHABILITATION OF THE PARALYZED FACE ● ● ●

Treatment Goals

○ **What are the cosmetic goals of treating the paralyzed face?**

Restore static and dynamic facial symmetry.

○ **What are the functional goals of treating the paralyzed brow and periorbital region?**

Correct visual obstruction (brow ptosis) and avoid exposure keratitis (corneal protection and restoration of protective blink).

○ **What are the functional goals of treating the paralyzed midface and perioral region?**

Regain oral competence, facilitate speech (plosive and bilabial sounds), restore nonverbal communication (smile) and maintain a patent nasal airway.

○ **What are the functional goals of treating the paralyzed lower face?**

Restore lower lip symmetry and motion.

○ **What principle factors influence surgical planning and technique selection?**
1. Duration of paralysis (irreversible muscle atrophy after 18–24 months).
2. Availability of the proximal facial nerve trunk.
3. Viability of distal facial nerve branches.
4. Condition of muscles and soft tissue (trauma or radiation injury).
5. Advanced age and medical comorbidities.
6. Presence of additional cranial nerve injuries.

Regional Approaches

○ **What are the most common surgical treatments for the paralyzed brow?**

1. Direct browlift (hairline or via midbrow rhytid)

2. Pretrichial subcutaneous brow lift

3. Open coronal browlift

4. Endoscopic browlift

○ **What surgical procedures are most commonly used to treat acute paralysis (less than 18 months) of the upper eyelid with lagophthalmos?**

1. Nerve repair with or without interposition grafts

2. Cross-face nerve grafts

3. Insertion of upper eyelid weight (potentially temporary)

4. Lateral tarsorrhaphy (potentially temporary)

○ **What surgical procedures can be utilized to treat chronic paralysis (more than 18 months) of the upper eyelid with lagophthalmos?**

1. Insertion of upper eyelid weight (gold, platinum chain)

2. Palpebral spring

3. Temporalis transfer (a slip can be elevated from its origin and rerouted around the lateral orbital rim to the medial canthal ligament)

4. Free muscle flap (after cross-face nerve grafting)

○ **What are the most common surgical treatments for the paralyzed lower eyelid with ectropion?**

1. Lateral canthoplasty

2. Sling suspension

3. Horizontal lid shortening

4. Cartilage grafting

○ **What are the most common surgical treatments for the paralyzed nasal aperture?**

1. Static sling suspension

2. Alar base elevation

○ **What are the most common surgical treatments for dynamic reconstruction of acute (less than 18 months) paralysis of the midface and perioral region?**

1. Microsurgical nerve repair with or without interposition nerve grafts.

2. Nerve transfers (masseter-to-facial nerve, hypoglossal-to-facial nerve, cross-face nerve grafts)

3. "Baby sitter"- XII–VII or V–VII transfer combined with cross-face nerve grafts

○ **What are the most common surgical techniques for dynamic reconstruction of chronic (greater than 18 months) paralysis of the midface and perioral region?**

1. Free functional muscle flaps (gracilis, pectoralis minor, latissimus dorsi)

2. Regional muscle transfers (temporalis, masseter)

○ **What are the most common static techniques employed in the midface and perioral region?**

1. Static sling suspension (fascia lata graft, tendon graft, suture, Gortex/ADM)
2. Midface lift
3. Cervicofacial rhytidectomy

○ **What surgical treatments have been described to enhance motion and or symmetry in the chronically paralyzed lower lip?**

1. Myectomy of contralateral lower lip depressors (after initial trial of chemodenervation)
2. Transfer of anterior belly of digastric muscle (with or without neurotization from cross-face nerve graft)
3. Wedge excision (with or without obicularis oris muscle advancement flap)
4. Platysma flap
5. Fascia lata grafts

○ **What surgical treatments have been described to enhance motion and/or symmetry in acute (less than 18 months) lower lip paralysis?**

1. Microsurgical nerve repair with or without interposition grafts
2. Cross-face nerve graft
3. Mini-hypoglossal transfer
4. Direct muscle neurotization

Brow Paralysis

○ **What structure should be preserved during direct browlift through forehead excision?**

The supraorbital nerve should be preserved to preserve sensation to the forehead and scalp. This nerve runs just deep to the frontalis muscle at the lower forehead.

○ **Is there a role for weakening or paralyzing a *normal* hemi-forehead?**

Yes, particularly in younger patients. Improved upper facial symmetry and forehead tone may be obtained with botulinum toxin or frontal branch resection on a normal hemi-brow, at the variable expense of emotive upper facial expression. Care must be utilized in the older patient to avoid the production of excessive ptosis and visual obstruction.

Eyelid Closure and Lower Lid Support

○ **Upper eyelid treatments are aimed at balancing the unopposed action of which facial muscle?**

Levator palpebrae superioris (cranial nerve III).

○ **What are the most popular implant alloys for upper lid loading?**

Gold and platinum, both of which are highly immunoinert. Platinum allows for lower-profile implants and platinum chains may produce less visual disturbance and improved cosmesis.

○ **How are lid weights sized?**

Preoperatively in an awake patient, 0.8 to 1.8 g sizers are adhered to the upper lid with two-sided tape. The device that produces complete or near complete closure without ptosis is selected.

○ **Where are weights placed in the upper lid?**

Deep to the obicularis oculi muscle and directly on top of the tarsal plate with the weight's inferior boarder approximately above the lash line. The weight should be biased slightly medial to center as lateral placement often produces inadequate medial closure (see Fig. 48-1).

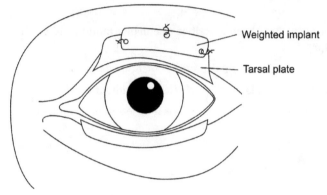

Weighted implant

Tarsal plate

Figure 48-1 Lid weight placement in the upper eyelid.

○ **What is the principal method for temporalis transfer to paralyzed upper lid?**

An inferiorly based strip of temporalis muscle is elevated from its origin in the temporal fossa and elongated with a strip of temporal fascia. This is then rerouted subcutaneously around the lateral orbital rim, across the tarsal plate, and inserted into the medial canthal tendon. With temporalis contraction the upper lid is pulled down.

○ **How do you perform a lateral tarsorrhaphy?**

Suture apposition of deepithelialized segments of the lateral upper and lower lids.

○ **What is an advantage of the lateral tarsorrhaphy for corneal protection?**

Reliable patient-independent improvement in corneal protection. This may be particularly useful in mentally debilitated or demented patients, in cases of involving an anesthetic cornea, or in cases with severe corneal exposure. Trade-offs include lateral visual obstruction and aesthetic asymmetries.

○ **Over time, with decreased midfacial tone and a paretic orbicularis oculi, a lower lid ectropion with scleral show can develop. How can this be treated?**

Static support of the lower lid (i.e., tendon or tensor fascia latae [TFL] sling, cartilage graft), lateral canthoplasty (e.g., dermal pennant or tarsal strip), horizontal lid shortening (e.g., Kuhnt–Szymanowski procedure), and/or cheek elevation procedures.

Midface and Perioral Restoration

○ **How does nasal airway obstruction develop?**

External nasal valve collapse due to external compression arising from a drooping midface as well as loss of dynamic compensation due to paralysis of the nasalis and levator alaeque nasi musculature. This is frequently treated with tendon or fascia sling to open the external nasal valve.

○ **When are cranial nerve transfers used to reanimate the midface and perioral region?**

Nerve transfers are employed when the proximal trunk of the facial nerve is not available (intracranial/intratemporal injury), there are identifiable distal nerve branches, and there are viable muscles of facial expression (not irreversibly atrophied or injured).

○ **What characteristics make the masseter-to-facial nerve transfer an effective technique for smile restoration?**

The descending branch of the masseter nerve can be transferred to selected zygomatic and buccal branches of the facial nerve without interposition grafts. The descending branch has a dense population of myelinated motor fibers (approximately 1,500) producing strong motion. Cerebral adaptation over time produces an effortless smile in the majority of young patients. There is limited donor-site morbidity because of functional overlap between the masseter and temporalis muscles.

○ **Where can the masseteric branch of the trigeminal nerve be found?**

The main trunk of the masseter nerve can be identified at a point 3 cm in front of the tragus and 1 cm below the zygomatic arch (cutaneous landmarks). The masseter muscle has three lobes. The nerve lies deep within the substance of the muscle on the superficial surface of the deep lobe (approximately 1.5 cm below the SMAS).

○ **What modification of the hypoglossal-to-facial nerve transfer has been made to decrease donor-site morbidity?**

Complete transection of the hypoglossal nerve produces hemi-tongue atrophy, mass facial motion, and impairment of speech and eating in a significant number of patients. These morbidities are greatly improved by partial transection of the nerve (approximately one-third) and the use of an interposition jump graft (usually greater auricular nerve).

○ **What is a "babysitter" procedure?**

Part of a staged strategy to restore spontaneous facial animation. Acutely deinnervated mimetic muscles are initially reinnervated by a local motor nerve (i.e., masseteric or hypoglossal nerve). This procedure minimizes mimetic muscular atrophy while a banked cross-facial nerve graft is allowed to mature.

○ **How can the temporalis muscle be utilized for smile restoration?**

Three variations of the temporalis transfer have been employed for creation of a smile.

1. Turning the central portion (approximately 4 cm wide) over the zygomatic arch and using an extension of the deep temporal fascia to reach the commissure (Gillies technique).

2. Releasing the temporalis insertion from the coronoid process and utilizing an interposition TFL graft to reach the corner of the mouth (McLaughlin technique, Fig. 48-2).

3. Releasing the coronoid insertion and mobilizing the entire muscle in the temporal fossa to reach the commissure without fascial grafts (lengthening temporalis myoplasty—Labbe technique).

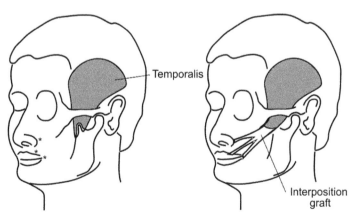

Figure 48-2 McLaughlin technique for smile restoration.

○ **What is the nerve supply to the temporalis muscle?**

The mandibular division of the trigeminal nerve (CN V). The temporal nerve splits into three branches innervating the anterior, middle, and posterior belly of the muscle. The nerve courses deep in the temporal fossa and enters the muscle at the junction of the lower and middle third. The primary arterial blood supply is the anterior and posterior temporal arteries arising from the maxillary artery.

○ **What muscles have been utilized for free functional muscle transplantation?**

Gracilis, pectoralis minor, latissimus dorsi, serratus anterior, rectus abdominis, extensor carpi radialis brevis, abductor hallucis, extensor digitorum brevis.

○ **What major benefit do free functional muscle flaps innervated by the contralateral facial nerve (cross-face nerve graft) have in contrast to other donor nerves?**

They consistently demonstrate spontaneous, synchronous facial motion.

○ **What are the potential benefits of free functional muscle flaps innervated by the masseter nerve?**

The reconstruction can be performed in a single stage. The dense population of motor axons facilitates the use of small muscle flaps and limits cheek fullness.

○ **If neither an ipsilateral nor contralateral facial nerve is available as a donor for spontaneous facial reanimation (i.e., Moebius syndrome), what alternatives are available?**

The masseteric nerve is most commonly utilized. The use of the spinal accessory (XI) and hypoglossal (XII) nerves has also been reported, however, nuclear agenesis of XII can occur in Moebius syndrome.

○ **What is a common donor nerve for cross-facial nerve grafting?**

Sural nerve.

○ **What deficit is produced by harvesting the sural nerve?**

Sensory deficit of the posterolateral leg, lateral ankle, lateral foot and cuboid joint.

○ **Why are cross-facial nerve grafts reversed?**

To maximize the number of regenerating axons that reaches the end of the nerve graft. Since the connective tissue of the nerve graft guides nerve regeneration, an anterograde graft would divert some regenerating axons to side branches occurring along the length of the nerve.

○ **How is the donor facial nerve branch selected for smile restoration with cross-face nerve grafts and free functional muscle flaps?**

A point approximately half way between the root of the helix and commissure (Zuker's point) describes the general location of the facial nerve branches best suited for smile restoration. Electrical stimulation is utilized to further select the branch that produces isolated activation of the zygomatic major muscle.

Lower Lip

○ **What is the effect of marginal mandibular palsy?**

Inability to depress, evert, and lateralize the ipsilateral lower lip. The deformity is most evident when talking or smiling as an asymmetric ability to show the lower teeth.

○ **Like the frontalis for upper brow paralysis, it is cosmetically and functionally acceptable to paralyze which normal perioral muscle for improved lower lip symmetry?**

The depressor labii inferioris. This can be accomplished with botulinum toxin (temporary) or with partial myectomy (permanent).

○ **Describe the digastric transfer for treatment of marginal mandibular palsy.**

The technique involves preserving the mental attachment and tunneling the anterior belly and intermediate tendon of the digastric through a subcutaneous tunnel to the lower lip. The intermediate tendon is split and attached to the mucocutaneous junction of the middle and lateral lower lip. Activation is not spontaneous unless modified through a cross-facial nerve graft. The anterior belly receives its motor innervation from the nerve to mylohyoid, which arises from the mandibular branch of the trigeminal nerve (V3) (see Fig. 48-3).

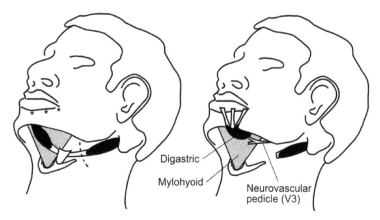

Figure 48-3 Digastric transfer for treatment of marginal mandibular palsy.

• • • REFERENCES • • •

Borschel GH, Kawamura DH, Kasukurthi R, Hunter DA, Zuker RM, Woo AS. The motor nerve to the masseter muscle: An anatomic and histomorphometric study to facilitate its use in facial reanimation. *J Plast Reconstr Aesthet Surg.* 2012;65:363–366.

Chan JY, Byrne PJ. Management of facial paralysis in the 21st century. *Facial Plast Surg.* 2011;27:346–357.

Chang CY, Cass SP. Management of facial nerve injury due to temporal bone trauma. *Am J Otol.* 1999;20:96–114.

Cocker NJ. Management of traumatic injuries to the facial nerve. *Otolaryngol Clin North Am.* 1991:24:215–227.

Dingman RO, Grabb WC. Surgical anatomy of the mandibular ramus of the facial nerve based on the dissection of 100 facial halves. *Plast Reconstr Surg Transplant Bull.* 1962;29:266–272.

Dorafshar AH, Borsuk DE, Bojovic B, et al. Surface anatomy of the middle division of the facial nerve: Zuker's point. *Plast Reconstr Surg.* 2013;131:253–257.

Evans GR, Brandt K, Ang K, et al. Peripheral nerve regeneration: the effects of postoperative irradiation. *Plast Reconstr Surg.* 1997: 100:375–380.

Fattah A, Borschel GH, Manktelow RT, Bezuhly M, Zuker RM. Facial palsy and reconstruction. *Plast Reconstr Surg.* 2012;129:340e–352e.

Hadlock TA, Greenfield LJ, Wernick-Robinson M, Cheney ML. Multimodality approach to management of the paralyzed face. *Laryngoscope.* 2006;116:1385–1389.

Kesser B. Anatomy of the facial nerve and associated structures. In: Slattery WH, Azizzadeh B, eds. *The Facial Nerve.* New York, NY: Thieme; 2014:1–22.

Klebuc MJ. Facial reanimation using the masseter-to-facial nerve transfer. *Plast Reconstr Surg.* 2011;127:1909–1915.

Kumar D. Moebius syndrome. *J Med Genet.* 1990:27:122–126.

Labbé D, Huault M. Lengthening temporalis myoplasty and lip reanimation. *Plast Reconstr Surg.* 2000;105:1289–1297; discussion 1298.

Levine RE, Shapiro JP. Reanimation of the paralyzed eyelid with the enhanced palpebral spring or the gold weight: modern replacements for tarsorrhaphy. *Facial Plast Surg.* 2000;16(4):325–336.

Manktelow RT. Use of the gold weight for lagophthalmos. *Operat Tech Plast Reconstr Surg.* 1999;6:157–158.

Manktelow RT, Tomat LR, Zuker RM, Chang M. Smile reconstruction in adults with free muscle transfers innervated by the masseter motor nerve: Effectiveness of cerebral adaptation. *Plast Reconstr Surg.* 2006;118:885–899.

Maurizio B. Differential diagnosis of acute facial paralysis. In: Slattery WH, Azizzadeh B, eds. *The Facial Nerve.* New York, NY: Thieme; 2014:57–62.

May M. Trauma to the facial nerve. *Otolaryngol Clin North Am.* 1983:16:661–670.

May M, Sobol SM, Mester SJ. Hypoglossal-facial nerve interpositional-jump graft for facial reanimation without tongue atrophy. *Otolaryngol Head Neck Surg.* 1991;104:818–825.

McLaughlin CR. Surgical support in permanent facial paralysis. *Plast Reconstr Surg (1946).* 1953;11:302–314.

Meltzer NE, Alam DS. Facial paralysis rehabilitation: state of the art. *Curr Opin Otolaryngol Head Neck Surg.* 2010;18:232–237.

Peitersen E. The natural history of Bell's palsy. *Am J Otol.* 1982;4:107–111.

Pitanguy I, Ramos AS. The frontal branch of the facial nerve: the importance of its variations in face lifting. *Plast Reconstr Surg.*1966;38:352–356.

Rubin LR, Lee GW, Simpson RL. Reanimation of the long-standing partial facial paralysis. *Plast Reconstr Surg.* 1986;77:41–49.

Seckel BR. Facial danger zone 2. In: Seckel BR, ed. *Facial Danger Zones Avoiding Nerve Injuries in Plastic Surgery.* St. Louis, MO:Quality Medical Publishing;1994;12–17.

Tan ST. Anterior belly of digastric muscle transfer: a useful technique in head and neck surgery. *Head Neck.* 2002;24:947–954.

Terzis JK. "Babysitters." An exciting new concept in facial reanimation. In: *Proceedings of the 6th International Symposium on the Facial Nerve.* Rio de Janeiro, Brazil: Kugler and Ghendini Publications; 1990.

Terzis JK, Kalantarian B. Microsurgical strategies in 74 patients for restoration of dynamic depressor muscle mechanism: a neglected target in facial reanimation. *Plast Reconstr Surg.* 2000;105:1917–1931.

Terzis JK, Karypidis D. The outcomes of dynamic procedures for blink restoration in pediatric facial paralysis. *Plast Reconstr Surg* 2010;125:629–644.

Terzis JK, Kyere SA. Minitendon graft transfer for suspension of the paralyzed lower eyelid: our experience. *Plast Reconstr Surg* 2008; 121:1206–1216.

Tucker H, May M. The facial nerve and extracranial surgery. In: May M, Schaitkin B, eds. *The Facial Nerve May's Second Edition.* 2nd ed. New York, NY: Thieme; 2000;491–503.

Yavuzer R, Jackson IT. Partial lip resection with orbicularis oris transposition for lower lip correction in unilateral facial paralysis. 2001;108:1874–1879.

Zuker RM, Manktelow RT, Hussain G. Facial paralysis. In: Mathes SJ, ed. *Plastic Surgery.* Vol 3. 2nd ed. Philadelphia, PA: Saunders; 2005:883–915.

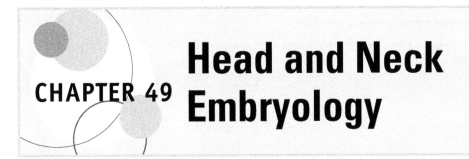

CHAPTER 49 Head and Neck Embryology

Priyesh Patel, MD and
Rakesh K. Chandra, MD

○ **Describe the anatomy of the branchial apparatus (see Fig. 49-1).**

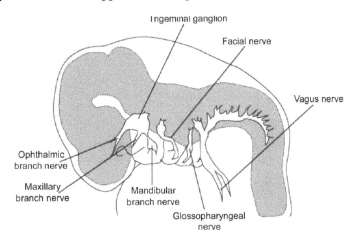

Figure 49-1 Branchial arches.

The branchial apparatus consists of five paired mesodermal arches that are separated by invaginations of ectoderm and endoderm known, respectively, as clefts and pouches. Each arch has a cartilage bar, an artery, and a nerve. The derivatives of the cartilage of each arch form the facial skeleton and laryngeal framework, while the artery and nerve supply and innervate the derivatives of the arch.

○ **What is derived from the ectoderm/branchial clefts?**

The ectoderm of the first cleft forms the major salivary glands, the mucosa of the oral cavity, and the lining of the anterior two-thirds of the tongue, while the ectoderm of the second, third, and fourth arches fuse to form a common cervical sinus (of His), which normally degenerates.

○ **What is derived from the endoderm/branchial pouches?**

The endoderm of the branchial pouches forms the middle ear, the glandular structures of the oropharynx, the parathyroid glands, and the thymus.

○ **What is the nerve of the first branchial arch?**

The trigeminal nerve.

○ **What is the artery of the first branchial arch?**

The artery of the first arch partly degenerates and partly remains as the maxillary artery.

○ **What are the derivatives of the cartilage of the first arch?**

Meckel's cartilage is the cartilage of the first arch and its derivatives are the mandible, the malleus (except for the manubrium), and the incus (except for the long process).

○ **What are the muscular derivatives of the first branchial arch?**

The muscular derivatives are the muscles of mastication (temporalis, masseter, medial and lateral pterygoids), the tensor tympani, the mylohyoid, anterior belly of the digastric, and the tensor veli palatini.

○ **What is the nerve of the second branchial arch?**

The facial nerve.

○ **What is the artery of the second branchial arch?**

The stapedial artery, which usually degenerates in normal development but occasionally persists in adulthood.

○ **What are the derivatives of the cartilage of the second arch?**

Reichert's cartilage is the cartilage of the second arch and its derivatives are the manubrium of the malleus, the long process of the incus, the stapes suprastructure, the styloid process, the stylohyoid ligament, and the body and lesser cornu of the hyoid bone.

○ **What are the muscular derivatives of the second branchial arch?**

The muscular derivatives of the second arch are the muscles of facial expression, the platysma, stylohyoid, posterior belly of the digastric, and the stapedius muscle.

○ **What is the nerve of the third branchial arch?**

The glossopharyngeal nerve.

○ **What is the artery of the third branchial arch?**

The internal carotid artery.

○ **What are the derivatives of the cartilage of the third arch?**

The body and greater cornu of the hyoid are the skeletal derivatives of the third arch.

○ **What are the muscular derivatives of the third branchial arch?**

The stylopharyngeus is the only muscle of the third arch.

○ **What is the nerve of the fourth branchial arch?**

The superior laryngeal nerve.

○ **What is the artery of the fourth branchial arch?**

The aortic arch is derived from the left arch, and the right subclavian artery is derived from the right arch. If the right fourth arch artery degenerates, the right subclavian artery will arise from the dorsal aorta and run posterior to the esophagus (retroesophageal subclavian).

○ **What are the derivatives of the cartilage of the fourth arch?**

The thyroid and cuneiform cartilage of the larynx.

○ **What are the mesodermal derivatives of the fourth branchial arch?**

The inferior pharyngeal constrictor, cricopharyngeal, and cricothyroid are the muscular derivatives of the fourth arch.

○ **What is derived from the fifth branchial arch?**

The fifth arch degenerates and has no derivatives in the human.

○ **What is the nerve of the sixth branchial arch?**

The recurrent laryngeal nerve.

○ **What is the artery of the sixth branchial arch?**

The pulmonary artery.

○ **What are the derivatives of the cartilage of the sixth arch?**

The skeletal derivatives are the cricoid, arytenoids, and corniculate cartilage.

○ **What are the muscular derivatives of the sixth branchial arch?**

The intrinsic muscles of the larynx.

○ **What are branchial cleft anomalies?**

Branchial cleft anomalies occur as cystic masses in the anterior triangle of the neck that arise from the failure of their respective branchial cleft remnants to obliterate during development. The etiology of the masses is not known, but the most common theory is that they are the result of entrapped remnants of the cervical sinus of His.

○ **How are the types of branchial cleft anomalies?**

Branchial cleft anomalies may occur as cysts, sinuses (with a blind-ended connection to either the pharynx or the skin), or as fistulas (with a connection between the pharynx and the skin). Branchial cleft anomalies are lined with squamous and respiratory epithelia.

○ **How do branchial cleft cysts present?**

Branchial cleft cysts most commonly present as fluctuant, nontender masses of the anterior cervical triangle. They may intermittently become infected during upper respiratory infections, and can present as a neck abscess. If a cutaneous connection via a sinus or fistula is present, mucoid discharge can often be expressed from the opening, and the opening may have increased or purulent drainage during an upper respiratory tract infection.

○ **How do branchial cleft sinuses or fistulas present?**

A branchial cleft sinus or fistula with a connection to the pharynx may present as recurrent unilateral infections of the tonsil or pyriform sinuses.

○ **Describe the classification of branchial cleft anomalies.**

Branchial cleft cysts arise from the first, second, and third branchial clefts. Branchial cleft anomalies are classified by anatomical location. They occur between the derivatives of two branchial arches and are named for the arch whose structures they lie deep to. There are two types of first branchial cleft cysts (type I and type II).

○ **Describe the anatomical location of a type I first branchial cleft cyst.**

A type I first branchial cleft cyst is a duplication of the external auditory canal and exists as a fistulous tract lying in close association with the lower portion of the parotid gland. They often have tracts that terminate in the external auditory canal, or the middle ear.

○ **Describe the anatomical location of a type II first branchial cleft cyst.**

A type II first branchial cleft cyst is typically located in the anterior triangle of the neck just inferior to the angle of the mandible. The tract of a type II first branchial cleft cysts extends superiorly through the substance of the parotid gland, over the angle of the mandible to the bony cartilaginous junction of the external auditory canal. Type II cysts are intimately related to the facial nerve, putting it at risk for injury during excision.

○ **Describe the anatomical location of second branchial cleft cyst.**

Second branchial cleft cysts are located deep to the structures of the second arch (the platysma and facial nerve), and superficial to the structures of the third arch (the internal carotid artery and the glossopharyngeal nerve). The tract of the second branchial cleft cyst ascends between the internal and external carotid arteries and opens into the pharynx at the tonsillar fossae.

○ **Describe the anatomical location of a third branchial cleft cyst.**

Third branchial cleft cysts are located in the anterior triangle of the neck deep to the structures of the third arch (glossopharyngeal nerve and the internal carotid artery), and superficial to the structures of the fourth arch (superior laryngeal nerves). The cyst enters the pharynx in the region of the thyrohyoid membrane or piriform sinus.

○ **What are the embryologic components of the midface (see Fig. 49-2)?**

The maxillary prominence, the lateral nasal prominence, and the medial nasal prominence are paired embryologic structures that fuse in the midline along with the frontonasal prominence to form the nose and upper lip. These prominences are made of neural crest–derived mesenchymal cells of the first branchial arch.

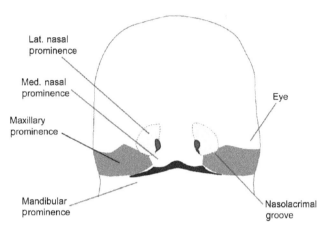

Figure 49-2 Seven-week embryo.

○ **Describe the embryogenesis of the nose and upper lip (see Fig. 49-2).**

Nasal placodes invaginate to form nasal pits during the fifth week of development. Medial and lateral nasal prominences are created on either side of the nasal pits. During the next 2 weeks, the maxillary prominences continue to grow in a medial direction and push the nasal prominences toward the midline. The medial nasal prominences fuse in the midline to form the tip of the nose and the philtrum of the upper lip. The lateral nasal prominences form the ala of the nose, and fuse with the maxillary prominence that forms the cheeks and lateral portions of the upper lip. The frontonasal prominence, which is located superiorly, fuses with the medial and lateral nasal prominences and forms the remaining portion of the nasal dorsum.

○ **Discuss the differential diagnosis of the congenital midline nasal mass.**

The differential diagnosis of the congenital midline nasal mass includes nasal dermoid cysts, nasal gliomas, and nasal encephaloceles.

○ **How do dermoid cysts present?**

Dermoid sinus cysts present as a mass on the dorsum of the nose or intranasally, with a pit or sinus tract opening on the nasal dorsum, hair around the external opening, and discharge of pus or sebaceous material.

○ **How do gliomas present?**

Nasal gliomas are firm masses that are nonpulsatile, present on the nasal dorsum and/or arise from the lateral nasal wall, have telangiectasias of the overlying skin, and do not enlarge with bilateral compression of the internal jugular veins (Furstenberg test).

○ **How do encephaloceles present?**

Encephaloceles may present as nasal broadening and/or as a blue, pulsatile, compressible mass near the nasal bridge or as an intranasal mass arising at the cribriform plate. Encephaloceles may be observed to transilluminate, or enlarge with crying or bilateral compression of the internal jugular veins.

○ **Where do congenital nasal masses arise from?**

During formation of the skull base and nose, the mesenchymal structures are formed from several neural crest–derived centers that will eventually fuse and ossify. Before their fusion there are recognized spaces including the fonticulus frontalis, the prenasal space, and the foramen cecum from which congenital nasal masses are thought to arise. The fonticulus frontalis is the space between the frontal and nasal bones. The prenasal space is between the nasal bones and the nasal capsule—the precursor of the septum and nasal cartilages. The foramen cecum is a midline opening present in the developing skull base in the basal frontal region.

○ **What is the primary palate?**

The primary palate is formed by the fusion of the medial nasal prominence. The primary palate is located anterior to the incisive foramen, and contains the four central incisors.

○ **What is the secondary palate?**

Development of the secondary palate begins after development of the primary palate is complete. The secondary palate is formed from laterally based palatal shelves of the maxillary prominences.

○ **Describe the embryogenesis of the palate.**

Both the primary and secondary palates are initially directed obliquely downward on either side of the developing tongue. As the maxillary prominences move medially, and as the developing tongue descends, the palatal shelves achieve their correct orientation in a horizontal plane. The palatal shelves then fuse from anterior (incisive foramen) to posterior (uvula).

○ **Describe the embryogenesis of the auricle.**

The external ear begins as six proliferations of mesenchymal tissue (known as Hillocks of His) located on either side of the dorsal end of the first branchial cleft. The first three hillocks are located on the first branchial arch and the last three hillocks are located on the second brachial arch.

○ **What arises from the first three Hillocks of His?**

The first three Hillocks of His form the tragus (1) and the helix (2, 3).

○ **What arises from the last three Hillocks of His?**

The last three Hillocks of His form the descending helix, antihelix (4, 5), and the antitragus (6).

○ **Describe the embryogenesis of the tongue.**

The anterior two-thirds of the tongue is derived from components of the first pharyngeal arch, which includes two paired lateral lingual swellings, and one medial swelling known as the tuberculum impar. The posterior one-third of the tongue is formed by the second, third, and fourth arches. The third arch component overgrows the second arch and the fourth arch component forms the most posterior portion of the tongue and the epiglottis.

○ **How does embryology explain tongue sensory innervation?**

The embryologic origin and development of the tongue explain why the anterior two-thirds is innervated by the lingual nerve (branch of trigeminal, nerve to first arch) and the posterior one-third is innervated by the glossopharyngeal nerve (nerve to the third arch).

○ **How do thyroglossal duct cysts present?**

Thyroglossal duct cysts typically present as asymptomatic midline neck mass. They are located near the level of the hyoid bone and elevate and descend with swallowing. Thyroglossal duct cysts are managed with excision of the cyst and the central portion of the hyoid bone (Sistrunk procedure).

○ **What do the paranasal sinuses develop from?**

The maxillary, ethmoid, and frontal sinuses are derived from evaginations of the lateral nasal wall. The sphenoid sinus originates as a posterior evagination of the nasal capsule.

○ **Which sinuses are present at birth?**

The ethmoid and maxillary sinuses are the only sinuses present at birth.

○ **Describe the development of the maxillary sinus?**

The maxillary sinus is the first sinus to develop, beginning as an outpouching of the lateral nasal wall in the 10th week. This outpouching is superior to the inferior turbinate and posterior to the developing uncinate. Maxillary sinus growth in its later stages involves invasion into the alveolar process after the eruption of permanent dentition. The sinus grows and matures at age 3, with another period of growth between ages 7 and 18.

○ **Describe the development of the ethmoid sinus?**

The ethmoid sinus develops in the 12th week and at birth there are three to four ethmoid air cells present. These cells pneumatize further between ages 3 and 12.

○ **Describe the development of the frontal sinus?**

Fontal sinus development involves upward extension of the nasal capsule and invasion of the frontal bone. The frontal sinus is not present at birth and does not appear until 5 to 6 years old. It reaches adult size by age 12 to 20.

○ **Describe the development of the sphenoid sinus?**

The sphenoid sinus remains largely undeveloped until middle childhood, with a rapid period of pneumatization and development occurring after age 7 until age 12 to 15.

• • • **REFERENCES** • • •

Chandler JR, Mitchell B. Branchial cleft cyst, sinuses, and fistulas. *Otolaryngol Clin North Am*. 1981;14:175–186.

Friedman O, Wang TD, Miluzuk HA. Cleft lip and palate. In: Cummings CW, Flint PW, Harker LA et al., eds. *Otolaryngology-Head and Neck Surgery*. 4th ed. Philadelphia, PA: Elsevier Mosby; 2005:4052–4085.

Goding GS, Eisele DW. Embryology of the face, head and neck. In: Papel ID, ed. *Facial Plastic and Reconstructive Surgery*. 2nd ed. New York, NY: Thieme; 2002:785–794.

Graney DO, Sie KC. Developmental anatomy. In: Cummings CW, Flint PW, Harker LA, et al., eds. *Otolaryngology-Head and Neck Surgery*. 4th ed. Philadelphia, PA: Elsevier Mosby; 2005:3938–3951.

Kubal WS. Sinonasal anatomy. *Neuroimaging Clin N Am*. 1998;8:143–156.

Sadler TW. Ear. In: Gruenwald P, ed. *Langman's Medical Embryology*. 7th ed. Baltimore, MD: Williams & Wilkins; 1995:347–357.

Sadler TW. Head and neck. In: Gruenwald P, ed. *Langman's Medical Embryology*. 7th ed. Baltimore, MD: Williams & Wilkins; 1995:312–346.

CHAPTER 50 Head and Neck Cancer

Ryan Gobble, MD and
Samuel J. Lin, MD, MBA, FACS

○ **A patient presents with numbness of left lower lip and a mass in floor of mouth. Examination demonstrates 2.5-cm biopsy-proven squamous cell carcinoma (SCC) of the floor of mouth with invasion of the mandible on CT scan and no lymph node involvement or distant metastases. According to the TNM classification, how would you stage this patient?**

T4aN0M0 (stage IVA). Based upon size this would be a T2 tumor, however, invasion of the mental nerve (numbness) and through mandibular cortex makes this a T4 tumor.

○ **Which surgical procedures are available for treating the mandible of the patient in Question 1?**

Segmental mandibulectomy. Marginal mandibulectomy can be used when the tumor abuts the mandibular cortex but does not directly invade it.

○ **How would you treat the neck of the patient in Question 1?**

The options are surgery +/− radiotherapy versus radiotherapy alone. Traditionally for midline T4 tumors, bilateral neck dissections with postoperative radiotherapy to the both primary and bilateral necks.

○ **What are the risk factors for increased risk of lymph node metastases?**

High-grade histology, large lesions (T4), spread involving the nonkeratinized (wet) mucosa of the lip or buccal mucosa in patients with recurrent disease, and invasion of the orbicularis oris muscle. These patients all need elective lymph node radiation or neck dissection.

○ **How would you treat the surgical defect if a segmental mandibulectomy were required for tumor clearance?**

Free fibula flap for bone reconstruction taken with a cutaneous skin paddle to reconstruct the floor of mouth defect.

○ **How would you treat the surgical defect if a rim/marginal resection only were required for tumor clearance?**

A free radial forearm flap or anterolateral thigh flap for intraoral lining.

○ **A 50-year-old patient presents with 1.5-cm tumor of the anterior tonsillar pillar with biopsy-proven SCC. The patient has no clinically palpable nodes or evidence of metastasis on work-up. How would you stage this tumor?**

T1N0M0 (stage I).

○ **What will be your treatment strategy?**

Radiation or surgical resection is equally effective in stage I and II oropharyngeal cancers. Elective cervical lymph node dissection should be considered in anterior tonsillar pillar, tonsil and base of tongue lesions as the incidence of lymph node metastases is up to 70%.

○ **What level of lymph nodes is the first to be involved?**

Level 2 (jugulodigastric nodes) followed sequentially by levels III, IV, and V.

○ **A 50-year-old patient presents with a 2-cm nonpulsatile mass in the level III of the neck. What is your management plan?**

FNA biopsy and CT scan of head and neck.

○ **If both CT and FNA are negative in the patient above, what is your plan?**

Open biopsy with frozen sectioning and progression to neck dissection if diagnosis of SCC is obtained. Pan endoscopies of naso/oro/hypo-pharynx, larynx, esophagus, stomach. If all look normal, multiple biopsies are performed including tonsils, base of tongue, nasopharynx, and piriform fossa. Treatment of the primary depends on the results of these biopsies.

○ **A patient presents with a 1-cm biopsy-proven tongue SCC and a palpable node in level II with no distant metastases. According to the TNM classification, how would you stage this patient clinically?**

T1N1M0.

○ **Following surgical excision pathological evaluation the tumor margins in the above patient were clear and the patient was staged as pT1N1M0. Would you perform radiotherapy to either the primary or the neck?**

No, unless there is presence of extracapsular spread.

○ **What are the indications for postoperative radiotherapy to the neck?**

More than one neck node involved or evidence of extracapsular nodal disease.

○ **What type of head and neck cancer is associated with Epstein–Barr viral infection?**

Nasopharynx. Most commonly with a nonkeratinizing undifferentiated carcinoma. These tumors are rare in the United States but endemic in East Asia and Africa. Treatment is usually with chemotherapy and radiation with surgery reserved for recurrent cancer.

○ **An 18-year-old male presents with progressive bilateral nasal obstruction and recurrent epistaxis. Anterior rhinoscopy demonstrates a soft, compressible purplish mass filling bilateral nasal cavities. What is the diagnosis?**

Nasopharyngeal angiofibroma occurs most commonly in adolescent males with unilateral or bilateral nasal obstruction and recurrent epistaxis. Advanced lesions can deform the nose, face, and orbits and may even erode into the cranial cavity causing diplopia from pressure on the optic chiasm.

○ **What is the treatment?**

Preoperative embolization and estrogen hormonal therapy to limit intraoperative blood loss followed by surgical resection. Postoperative radiation is usually given in cases with intracranial extension. These should never be biopsied in the office due to risk of bleeding.

○ **A patient requires segmental bony reconstruction of the mandible. This can be achieved by which methods?**

Reconstructive plate with no bone, reconstruction with nonvascularized bone, and reconstruction with vascularized bone (free flap or pedicle flap).

○ **When would you use a reconstruction plate?**

For patients in whom no other reconstruction is possible, where good soft tissue exists, and/or when radiotherapy has not been performed and is not planned.

○ **What types of vascularized bone on a pedicle flap exist?**

Clavicle on the sternocleidomastoid flap, rib on the pectoralis major muscle, and scapula on the trapezius muscle.

○ **What types of vascularized bone as a free flap would you consider?**

Deep circumflex iliac artery (iliac crest) flap, radial forearm flap, free fibula flap, and free scapula flap.

○ **Which free vascularized bone flap is most anatomically similar to a hemimandible?**

Deep circumflex iliac artery (iliac crest) flap. Typically used for defects less than 5 cm.

○ **Which free vascularized bone flap could you place osseointegrated implants into?**

Fibula flap and deep circumflex iliac artery flap. Survival rate for osseointegrated dental implants in a nonirradiated free fibular flap is 95%.

○ **Which free vascularized bone flap provides the longest length of bone?**

Fibula flap. This is important if you are performing more than one osteotomy. Multiple osteotomies may be easily performed without disrupting the blood supply to the fibula given its segmental distribution.

○ **A patient presents with a 2-cm mass in the parotid gland. Is the mass likely to be benign or malignant?**

Benign. 80% of salivary tumors originate in the parotid, and 80% of parotid tumors are benign.

○ **What factors from the history in a patient with a parotid mass suggest malignancy?**

Pain, obstruction, facial nerve involvement, invasion of other structures, and rapid progression.

○ **What are the most common benign tumors of the parotid?**

Pleomorphic adenoma (#1) and Warthin tumor (papillary cystadenoma lymphomatosum). Warthin tumors occur primarily in males and are bilateral in 10%.

○ **What are the most common malignant tumors of the parotid?**

Mucoepidermoid (#1), adenoid cystic carcinoma, and malignant transformation of pleomorphic adenoma. Also can have metastatic lesion from squamous cell cancer or melanoma.

○   **Which surgical methods are available to remove parotid tumors?**

Lumpectomy, superficial parotidectomy, and total parotidectomy. Superficial parotidectomy for benign lesion and total parotidectomy for malignant lesions. Facial nerve should be taken in cases of nerve invasion.

○   **A 45-year-old patient with parotid mass undergoes biopsy followed by total parotidectomy with facial nerve preservation. The final pathology demonstrates a cribriform ("Swiss cheese") pattern of cells with perineural invasion and residual microscopic disease at the deep margin. What is the type of cancer?**

Adenoid cystic carcinoma has three subtypes: cribriform ("Swiss cheese"), tubular, and solid. This is the second most common malignant tumor of salivary glands and most common malignant tumor of sublingual, submandibular, and minor salivary glands.

○   **What is the treatment plan?**

The patient should be treated with adjuvant radiation therapy for this stage III tumor (T3N0M0). Surgical reexcision of the margin should only be performed for gross disease either on postop physical examination or imaging. There is no role for chemotherapy except in palliative cases.

○   **What is Frey syndrome? How is it diagnosed? What is the treatment?**

Gustatory sweating. Auriculotemporal secretomotor nerve fibers disrupted during surgery reinnervate sweat glands following parotid surgery. Subsequent eating induces sweating in the distribution of the auriculotemporal nerve. Frey syndrome can be diagnosed via the Minor's starch iodine test. Treatment typically involves the injection of botulinum toxin A (Botox). Prevention can be accomplished by placing barrier (e.g., Alloderm, superficial temporal artery facial flap) between the deep parotid lobe and the skin at time of surgery.

○   **A patient has a biopsy-proven T1 oropharyngeal SCC. Which types of surgical access are possible?**

Transorally or through pharyngotomy. Mandibulotomy/mandibular swings are used for larger tumors.

○   **Which regions of the oropharynx are accessible transorally?**

Tonsil, soft palate, and superior pharyngeal wall.

○   **Which histological factors in the pathological report would influence your decision in performing postoperative radiotherapy to the primary?**

Close or positive margins, perineural or perivascular invasion, >5 mm tumor depth, presence of a noncohesive front, degree of differentiation, invasion of adjacent soft tissues, and subglottic extension.

○   **A patient presents with a 3-week hoarseness of voice with a normal clinical examination. What is your management?**

CT scan, laryngoscopy/biopsy.

○   **How are laryngeal tumors classified anatomically?**

Supraglottic, glottic, and subglottic.

○   **What is the rate of nodal metastasis for a T1–2 glottic tumor?**

Less than 10%; hence neck dissection rarely performed.

○   **What is the rate of nodal metastasis for a T1–2 supraglottic tumor?**

Approximately 50%; hence bilateral neck dissections frequently performed.

○   **For advanced laryngeal tumors what are the treatment options?**

Surgical excision, radiotherapy, chemotherapy, or a combination of all three. Organ preservation with chemoradiotherapy has shown comparable local control rates to traditional surgery.

○   **A 73-year-old man presents with recurrent laryngeal tumor 3 years after chemoradiation. He undergoes total laryngopharyngectomy with the resultant defect being from the base of the tongue to 2 cm proximal to the manubrium. What is the best single stage reconstructive option?**

Tubularized free anterolateral thigh free flap (skin forms the lining of the reconstructed GI tract). Restoration of swallowing can be achieved in most patients.

○   **A patient presents with mandibular pain and trismus. He has previously had an excision of a T2N0M0 floor of mouth SCC with close margins and postoperative radiotherapy 1 year ago. What is your differential diagnosis?**

Osteoradionecrosis, recurrence/another primary. Dental problems.

○   **Biopsy in the patient above suggests osteoradionecrosis. What is your initial management?**

Conservative—oral hygiene, antibiotics, analgesia.

○   **When would you consider surgery for osteoradionecrosis?**

Intractable pain, persistent bone exposure, fistulas, pathological fractures.

○   **Is there a role for hyperbaric oxygen in the management of osteoradionecrosis?**

Yes.

○   **Frequently, the involved mandible needs to be resected. How would you reconstruct the defect?**

With a free vascularized bone flap.

○   **A patient presents with postnasal drip, pain around the upper first and second molar, and cheek numbness on the left side. A CT scan shows a mass within the maxillary antrum and a biopsy confirms SCCa. Standard maxillectomy is planned. What access skin incision is traditionally used?**

Weber–Ferguson.

○   **Does a neck dissection need to be performed in the above patient?**

No. The risk of metastasis from maxillary tumors is rare.

○   **After resection of the tumor the resultant defect includes the left orbital floor, hemipalate, maxillary sinus, and nasal lining. How is the orbital floor reconstructed?**

Usually with nonvascularized bone graft, that is, rib or iliac crest.

○ **How is the maxillary defect reconstructed?**

A rectus abdominus free flap is the best treatment of the above defect. The skin from the abdomen can be used to reline the maxillary sinus and repair the palatal defect. Furthermore, the vascularized tissue obliterates the dead space and provides a barrier from the orbital floor reconstruction and the maxillary sinus or nasal cavity.

○ **A patient presents with a 3-cm nodal mass in the posterior triangle following radiotherapy to a nasopharyngeal tumor 2 years previously. An FNA biopsy confirms SCCa. What type of neck dissection would you perform, comprehensive or selective?**

Traditionally a comprehensive neck dissection.

○ **What is the difference between a selective and a comprehensive neck dissection?**

A selective neck dissection only removes the nodal levels most likely to harbor metastases. A comprehensive neck dissection removes lymph nodes from all levels.

○ **What different types of comprehensive neck dissections exist?**

Radical and modified radical neck dissections (MRNDs).

○ **How many types of modified MRND are there?**

Three.

○ **How do they differ?**

MRND type 1 preserves only the accessory nerve, MRND type 2 preserves both accessory and the internal jugular, and MRND type 3 preserves accessory, internal jugular, and sternocleidomastoid.

○ **A patient presents with a 2.4-mm malignant melanoma of the scalp clinically node negative. What is your management plan?**

For local control, a surgical excision of the malignant melanoma with a 2-cm margin. For staging of the clinically, N0 neck sentinel node biopsy is recommended.

○ **The sentinel node biopsy shows metastases of 2 mm in level 2 in the neck. What is your management plan?**

A staging CT scan to determine any other disease—if negative, an MRND is recommended.

○ **What if the sentinel node showed a micrometastases of 0.1 mm?**

A staging CT scan and, if negative, one should consider other pathological characteristics including whether the micrometastases were confined to the subcapsular sinus. For disease more than 0.1 mm, a completion lymphadenectomy is recommended. Patients with disease under 0.1 mm have a long-term prognosis similar to node-negative patients and can be spared completion lymphadenectomy.

○ **The neck dissection is clear of any further disease. Does the patient require radiotherapy?**

One should consult with an oncologist. Radiotherapy is usually unnecessary if only one node is involved with micrometastasis without extracapsular spread. For more than one node or extracapsular spread, radiotherapy should be considered.

○ **What about chemotherapy?**

Yes, all stage 3 patients should be offered chemotherapy in the context of a clinical trial.

○ **A patient presents with a clinically apparent 2-cm morphoeic BCC on the tip of the nose. What are the management options?**

The options are surgical and nonsurgical. For morphoeic BCCs, surgery would offer a better chance of local control. In such a cosmetically sensitive position, Mohs surgery would be the ideal management option followed by reconstruction.

○ **What option would you use if the defect included the nasal tip and dorsal sub units?**

Forehead flap.

○ **What if the nasal lining were involved, how would this be reconstructed?**

One would place a skin graft on the inner surface of the forehead flap and use the skin graft as lining. If cartilage was required, a second stage could be performed to insert the cartilage and thin the flap. A third stage would then be used to inset the flap and divide the pedicle.

○ **What if the donor site on the forehead does not close? How would you reconstruct?**

Secondary intention healing on the forehead leaves a reasonable cosmetic result and can be superior to skin grafting. It is important to make sure that during flap harvest the periosteal layer is left attached to the scalp. A few centimeters above the orbital rim, one can dissect under periosteum to protect the pedicle supply without compromising closure.

○ **An 85-year-old lady presents with a biopsy-proven radiorecurrent SCC of the temple. What is your management?**

CT staging scan and, if negative, surgical excision.

○ **What is your excision margin?**

1 cm with frozen-section analysis.

○ **The patient develops local recurrence 18 months later and CT scan shows involvement of temporalis but no other disease, what is your management?**

Excision of the mass and previous reconstruction with a 1-cm margin including temporalis. Reconstruction would require a large scalp rotation flap or free flap.

○ **A 45-year-old male presents with a slowly growing mass of the mandible that is causing significant distortion. Radiographically it is characterized as a multilocular mass with a "soap bubble" or "honeycomb" appearance. What type of mass is this?**

Ameloblastoma is derived from odontogenic epithelium. Treatment is typically with surgical resection and immediate repair with vascularized bone (e.g., free fibula flap). These are not usually cancerous so wide margins are not necessary, though rare cases of metastatic ameloblastic carcinoma have been reported, in which case the patient should receive adjuvant radiation.

○   **A 3-year-old female presents with a painless, slowly growing mass of the maxilla. An incisional biopsy is performed that demonstrates sinonasal myxoma. Postoperative MRI demonstrates residual tumor. What is the best course of treatment?**

Resection of the mass until negative margins. Tumors are not often encapsulated so a rim of normal tissue should be removed at the same time. Sinonasal myxoma most often present as slow growing masses in the maxilla or mandible.

● ● ● REFERENCES ● ● ●

Chrysomali E, Leventis M, Titsinedes S, Kyriakopoulos V, Sklavounou A. Odontogenic tumors. *J Craniofac Surg*. 2013;24:1521–1522.

Cordeiro PG, Chen CM. A 15-year review of midface reconstruction after total and subtotal maxillectomy: part I. Algorithm and outcomes. *Plast Reconstr Surg*. 2012;129:124–136.

Ettl T, Schwarz-Furlan S, Gosau M, Reichert TE. Salivary gland carcinomas. *Oral Maxillofac Surg*. 2012;16:267–283.

Futran ND, Parvathaneni U, Martins RG, et al. Malignant salivary gland tumors: part A: general principals and management. In: Harrison LB, Sessions RB, Hong WK, eds. *Head and Neck Cancer: A Multidisciplinary Approach*. 3rd ed. Philadelphia, PA: Lippincott Williams & Wilkins;2009:589–610.

Haddadin KJ, Soutar DS, Oliver RJ, Webster MH, Robertson AG, MacDonald DG. Improved survival for patients with clinically T1/ T2, N0 tongue tumors undergoing a prophylactic neck dissection. *Head Neck*. 1999;21:517–525.

Leemans CR, Tiwari R, Nauta JJ, van der Waal I, Snow GB. Regional lymph node involvement and its significance in the development of distant metastases in head and neck carcinoma. *Cancer*. 1993;71:452–456.

Leemans CR, Tiwari R, van der Waal I, Karim AB, Nauta JJ, Snow GB. The efficacy of comprehensive neck dissection with or without postoperative radiotherapy in nodal metastases of squamous cell carcinoma of the upper respiratory and digestive tracts. *Laryngoscope*. 1990;100:1194–1198.

Li C, Yang X, Pan J, Shi Z, Li L. Graft for prevention of Frey syndrome after parotidectomy: a systematic review and meta-analysis of randomized controlled trials. *J Oral Maxillofac Surg*. 2013;71:419–427.

Mann WJ, Jecker P, Amedee RG. Juvenile angiofibromas: changing surgical concept over the last 20 years. *Laryngoscope*. 2004;114: 291–293.

Neligan PC. Head and neck reconstruction. *Plast Reconstr Surg*. 2013;131:260e–269e.

Pillsbury HC 3rd, Clark M. A rationale for therapy of the N0 neck. *Laryngoscope*. 1997;107:1294–1315.

Robbins KT. Classification of neck dissection: current concepts and future considerations. *Otolaryngol Clin North Am*. 1998;31: 639–655.

Rotenberg BW, Daniel SJ, Nisha IA, Ngan BY, Forte V. Myxomatous lesions of the maxilla in children: a case series and review of management. *Int J Pediatr Otorhinolaryngol*. 2004;68:1251–1256.

Shah JP. Patterns of cervical lymph node metastasis from squamous carcinomas of the upper aerodigestive tract. *Am J Surg*. 1990;160: 405–409.

Spyropoulou GA, Lin PY, Chien CY, Kuo YR, Jeng SF. . Reconstruction of the hypopharynx with anterolateral thigh flap: defect classification, method, tips, and outcomes. *Plast Reconstr Surg*. 2011;127:161–172.

Van Akkooi AC, Nowecki ZI, Voit C, et al. Sentinel node tumor burden according to the Rotterdam criteria is the most important prognostic factor for survival in melanoma patients: a multicenter study in 388 patients with positive sentinel nodes. *Ann Surg*. 2008;248:949–955.

CHAPTER 51 Salivary Gland Tumors

Alex Senchenkov, MD, FCAS

○ **What are the histological features of salivary glands and how are they related to oncogenesis?**

The parenchyma of the salivary glands is formed from the acini that lead to the sequence of ducts. While origin of the salivary tumors is poorly understood, there may be a correlation between the salivary neoplasms and the cells forming salivary units. This unit consists of acinus, intercalated, striated, and excretory ducts. Table 51-1 illustrates the correlation between normal structure and tumor cells.

Table 51-1 Histogenic Scheme of Salivary Gland Neoplasms

Normal Structure	Cell of Origin	Neoplasm
Excretory duct	Excretory duct reserve cells	Squamous cell Ca Mucoepidermoid Ca
Acinus	Intercalated duct reserve cells	Acinic cell carcinoma Mixed tumor Monomorphic adenoma Myoepithelioma
Intercalated duct		Adenoid cystic Ca
Myoepithelium		Adenocarcinoma
Striated duct		Oncocytic tumors

Data from Regezi JA, Batsakis, JG. Histogenesis of salivary gland neoplasms. *Otol Clin N Am.* 1977;10:298.

○ **Which salivary gland is the most common site for salivary tumors?**

Parotid gland harbors 70% to 85% of all salivary tumors.

○ **What is the incidence of malignancy in different salivary glands?**

	Benign (%)	*Malignant (%)*
Parotid	80	20
Submandibular	50	50
Minor salivary	20	80

○ **Tumors of which salivary gland are most frequently malignant?**

Sublingual gland.

Starting with lowest to the highest chance of malignancy the sequence is as follows:

Parotid < submandibular < minor salivary < sublingual gland

○ **Overall, what salivary gland harbors the most of the malignant tumors?**

Parotid gland. Although about 80% of parotid tumors are benign, the remaining 20% are malignant, and since tumors in the parotid are much more frequent than in all other salivary glands combined, the majority of malignant salivary glands tumors occur in the parotid gland.

○ **What is the most common benign salivary neoplasm for all salivary glands?**

Pleomorphic adenoma (benign mixed tumor) is both the most common benign parotid neoplasm and the most common benign salivary neoplasm overall, comprising about 60% of all salivary tumors and about 80% of benign tumors. Mixed tumor is derived from dual epithelial (granular cells) and myoepithelial (mesenchymal) origin. The latter connective tissue (stromal) component often exhibits myxofibroid and cartilaginous differentiation. It has histologic appearance of stellate and spindle cells with a myxoid background. Pleomorphic adenoma has a potential for malignant transformation.

○ **The patient who was diagnosed with pleomorphic adenoma of the parotid (mixed parotid tumor) has another tumor in the same parotid gland. What is histology of the second primary parotid tumor most likely to be?**

Warthin's tumor (papillary cystadenoma lymphomatosum) has a reputation of the most common second primary parotid tumor. The tumor histologically characterized by papillary cysts with mucoid fluid and the presence of lymphoid tissue (Think of intercalated parotid lymph nodes); Warthin's is highly unusual outside the parotid gland and periparotid lymph nodes.

○ **Do any of the parotid tumors have propensity to be bilateral?**

Warthin's tumors are bilateral in 10% of patients.

○ **A patient who has a symptomatic Warthin's tumor in the parotid gland is found to have an occult contralateral parotid tumor on the CT scan. What would you do about it?**

In the patients with bilateral Warthin's tumors, the symptomatic side should be treated operatively, whereas you may observe an asymptomatic contralateral tumor. When it becomes symptomatic, you would remove it. Warthin's tumor is known for being bilateral and multicentric (Fig. 51-1).

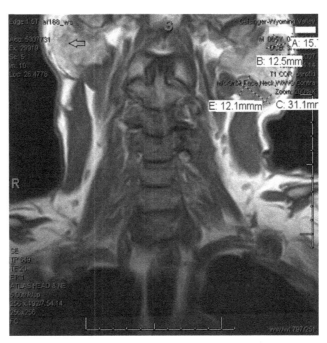

Figure 51-1 MRI of a bilateral and multicentric recurrence of Warthin's tumor after incomplete superficial parotidectomy.

○ **Why are oncocytomas frequently found on the Tc-99 scans and what do you do with them?**

Their origin is thought to correlate with striated ducts. This striation is related to the presence of large number of mitochondria. Tc-99 is preferentially picked up by tissues rich in mitochondria (gastric mucosa in the Meckel's diverticulum lights up on Tc-99 Meckel's scan). When oncocytoma is found on the scan and is not symptomatic, it may be observed initially.

○ **What is the most common malignant tumor of the parotid gland?**

Mucoepidermoid carcinoma is the most common malignancy of the parotid. Histologically, it contains two major components of mucin-producing cells and epidermoid epithelial cells hence its name. Low-grade tumor is more common and greater mucin-secreting component. High-grade, poorly differentiated variant is largely solid with paucity of mucin-producing elements with the loss of differentiation.

○ **What is the most common malignant tumor of the salivary gland outside the parotid?**

Adenoid cystic carcinoma (cylindroma) is the most common submandibular, sublingual, and minor salivary gland malignancy. There are three histologic types: the cribriform ("Swiss cheese" appearance), the tubular (resembles glandular architecture), and solid or basaloid pattern (solid sheets of cells without luminal or glandular appearance).

○   **What is the most common malignant tumor of the salivary glands overall?**

Mucoepidermoid carcinoma. Low-grade variant is more common and is predominantly cystic, whereas high-grade tumors are solid with small amount of mucin.

○   **How do salivary malignancies spread?**

Lymphatic, hematogenous, direct invasion of the surrounding structures, as well as perineurally.

○   **Which head and neck malignancies are notorious for perineural spread?**

Adenoid cystic carcinoma is a classic example. Malignant mixed tumor, melanoma, and squamous cell carcinoma also demonstrate perineural invasion.

○   **What are peculiar features of adenoid cystic carcinomas?**

Lack a tumor capsule, direct invasion of the surrounding tissues, and very high propensity for *perineural invasion*. These three features make it very challenging to achieve negative resection margins. This tumor has *hematogenous* route of spread, which leads to the lung, liver, and bone metastases. It has excellent 5-year survival (75%), but poor 10-year survival, and even worse 20-year survival (13%); it tends to recur late.

○   **What are the important clinical features of acinic carcinoma?**

While the majority of the acinic carcinomas are curable, about 10% can manifest very aggressively and be tenacious with a tendency to recur.

○   **What is an important consideration in planning the removal of malignant mixed tumors?**

Malignant mixed tumors (*or* carcinoma-ex-pleomorphic adenoma) are locally destructive and require wide resection and frequently, microvascular flap reconstruction.

○   **What is the most common parotid tumor of young children?**

Hemangioma.

○   **What are other common pediatric parotid tumors?**

Most common benign epithelial tumor is pleomorphic adenoma. Most common malignant tumor is mucoepidermoid carcinoma, similarly for adults.

○   **Does the ratio 80:20 between benign and malignant parotid tumors apply to children?**

No. Pediatric parotid tumors are much more likely to be malignant. In fact, an older child with a parotid mass has 50% chance of harboring malignancy.

○   **What is the most common presentation of parotid tumors?**

It is a mass below the angle of the mandible and not in front of the ear. The clinician needs to be aware that most parotid tumor present as *upper cervical masses*.

○ **Do you always feel parotid tumor on palpation?**

No. Sometimes the presentation is subtle. If the tumor is in the deep lobe, only diffuse enlargement of the gland can be appreciated, and you have to rely on imaging to demonstrate the tumor.

○ **What about the size of the tumor? If the tumor is large, is it more likely to be malignant?**

Not necessarily. You can have a large pleomorphic adenoma that has grown over past 20 years to be very large, yet still benign.

○ **A patient presents to you with a parotid mass, when should you think about malignancy?**

Start with history and physical examination. Patient's age, history of head and neck radiation, and history of previous malignancies and symptoms are important. Tumors in children and older individuals are more likely to be malignant. Pain and rapid growth are very suspicious for malignancy as are tumors that are adherent to surrounding structures on physical examination and have regional adenopathy. Facial nerve paralysis and eruption through the skin are rare even in advanced malignancy and are grave prognostic signs.

○ **A mass with facial nerve paralysis is a bad prognostic sign. What would be a benign condition that could have a similar presentation?**

Sarcoidosis is the most common cause for nonneoplastic parotid mass with facial nerve paralysis.

○ **What is importance of cystic parotid mass in an HIV patient?**

A benign lymphoepithelial cyst is a cystic degeneration of salivary gland inclusions within intercalated lymph nodes. The cyst is lined with lymphocytes. It is manifestation of progression to AIDS. Treatment is repeat aspiration and careful use of a sclerosing agent.

○   **The patient presents with xerostomia dry eyes and history of long-standing periodic cheek swelling. On physical examination the patient has a unilateral ill-defined parotid mass. What clinical entity should be considered?**

Clinical presentation of keratoconjunctivitis sicca and xerostomia is typical for Sjögren's syndrome, a chronic progressive autoimmune disorder resulting from lymphocyte-mediated destruction of lacrimal and salivary glands. As the disease progresses, a sizable parotid mass may develop (Fig. 51-2). It may manifest as an isolated (primary) or associated with other autoimmune disorders (secondary) forms. A biopsy of a minor salivary gland, usually form the lower lip under local anesthetic in the office is a valuable diagnostic tool. Representative serologies, such as rheumatoid factor, ANA, SS-A, and SS-B are also frequently obtained. The risk of primary non-Hodgkin's lymphoma of the parotid is increased.

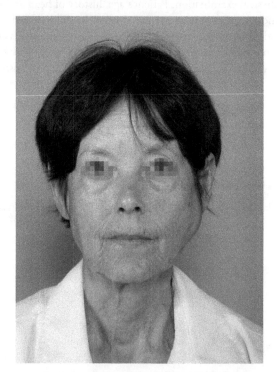

Figure 51-2 Left parotid mass in a patient with a long-standing Sjögren's syndrome. See Color insert.

The treatment is medical. Parotidectomy plays a very limited role in the case of Sjögren's syndrome patients and is reserved for parotitis refractory to medical management, gross disfigurement, and diagnostic concerns of parotid lymphoma.

○ **How do you workup a parotid mass?**

After thorough history and physical examination (Fig. 51-3A), MRI is the best study; however, a good quality head and neck CT is acceptable (Fig. 51-3B). These will evaluate local and regional extent of the disease. CT imaging of the tumors of deep lobes and parapharyngeal space is undermined by scattering from petrous pyramids and MRI is the study of choice for those locations.

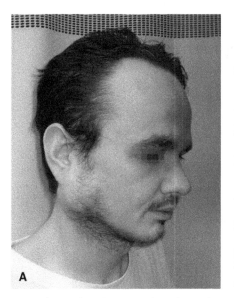
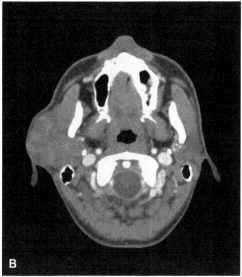

Figure 51-3 Large pleomorphic adenoma involving deep and superficial lobes of the right parotid. See Color insert.

Ultrasound is a versatile and important tool in the hands of an experienced practitioner. Some head and neck surgeons may choose to perform parotid and neck office ultrasound and an ultrasound-guided fine-needle aspiration (FNA) biopsy of the parotid mass and suspicions lymph nodes as the only preoperative imaging study and a biopsy (Fig. 51-4). If the tumor does not extend outside the parotid on ultrasound and FNA cytology is benign, MRI or CT may be avoided and the patient may proceed to the operative treatment.

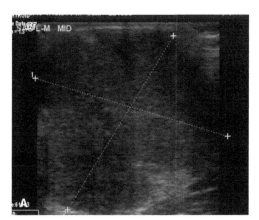
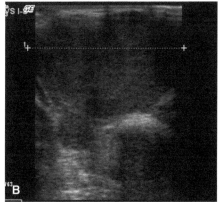

Figure 51-4 Surgeon-performed diagnostic ultrasound of the parotid tumor. AP and lateral images demonstrate the size of the tumor.

○ **How good is FNA for salivary tumors?**

It accurately diagnoses more than 95% of pleomorphic adenomas. It is very good in diagnosing malignancy, but may not tell you the type.

○   **How do you best perform FNA of a parotid mass?**

Routine use of ultrasound allows precise needle placement. Usually 21- to 25-gauge needle is used. Keeping the bevel of the needle up facilitates continuous sonographic visualization of the needle tip (Figure 51-5). One places the needle into the mass and performs several passes back and forth with continuous aspiration. It is very helpful to have a cytology technician on stand by to confirm that the first aspirate is sufficient. This may obviate the need for performing multiple aspirates. It is a common practice to irrigate the syringe with saline or CytoLyt® solution and send it for cell block preparation.

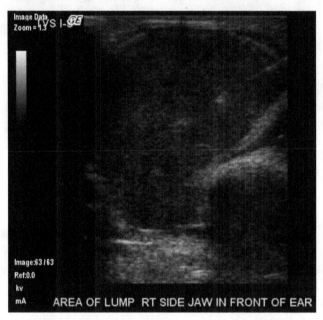

Figure 51-5 Surgeon-performed ultrasound guided FNA of the parotid mass. Note: bright echogenic reflection of the needle tip and the ultrasound waves reflected of the bevel of the needle turned upward.

○   **What about core needle biopsy used for breast masses? It gives histological, not cytological diagnosis. Would it help to establish the type of parotid malignancy preoperatively?**

Core needle biopsy for breast masses is performed with 14- and 11-gauge needles. Its use is contraindicated for the parotid masses because of the danger of transection of the facial nerve branch.

○   **You have a young patient with a small mobile mass that is very superficial in the parotid lobe. You performed an FNA and it is a pleomorphic adenoma. You explained to her that although it is a benign tumor it needs to be removed. She is asking if you can do "minimally invasive surgery" and just take out the lump.**

Enucleation or local excision of the adenoma is not a good option. The minimal operation for the parotid tumor is a superficial parotidectomy. Partial parotid resection have high rate of complications and should not be done.

○   **Some surgeons advocate not doing FNA, but just taking the patient with a parotid mass to the OR, performing superficial parotidectomy with frozen section, and having that be the biopsy. Why is it important to know whether the tumor is malignant preoperatively?**

This approach is also valid. However, knowing preoperatively that the patient has a malignant parotid tumor will allow better planning of the operation. While treatment of benign tumors is straightforward, a malignancy may require radical parotidectomy with resection of the mandible, neck dissection, facial nerve grafting, microvascular mandibular, and soft-tissue reconstruction and postoperative XRT. The patient and the family will have better understanding of what these all entail to make an informed consent.

○ **What are the clinical implications of perineural spread?**

Perineural spread is an important pathologic factor described in the majority of head and neck tumors. This process is a major cause of local failure and ultimately tumor-related mortality. High level of suspicion should be maintained in diagnostic and treatment efforts. Most of the time, it is clinically silent, but as the process becomes more advanced, the patient may present with *formication* (feeing of ants crawling) and eventual with loss of nerve function (numbness for the sensory or paralysis of the motor nerve). Thickening of the named nerves on MRI and changes in the skull foramina on CT is found in late cases. Certain tumor histologies (adenoid cystic carcinoma), suggestive locations of the tumors (areas of major nerves), perineural invasion identified on the diagnostic biopsies or excised tumor specimens are all factored into a complex clinical decision to sacrifice a named nerve for histologic evaluation. Ideally, negative margins on the involved nerves should be attained. These efforts are frequently limited by the advanced nature of the process (adenoid cystic carcinoma) and highly debilitating nature of these resections (Fig. 51-6).

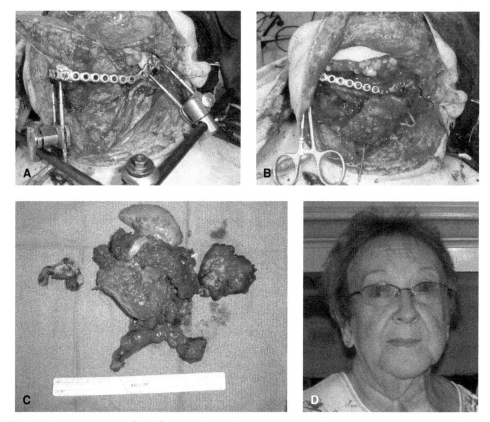

Figure 51-6 Adenoid cystic carcinoma of the left submandibular gland (size 2 cm physical examination) treated with composite resection, total parotidectomy with resection of lower division of the left facial nerve, free fibula (**A** and **B**), specimen (**C**) static sling, and postoperative radiation. Appearance of the patient without evidence of disease at 6 years (**D**). See Color insert.

○ **How do you stage parotid malignancies?**

TNM staging. T (primary tumor): T1: <2 cm, T2: 2 to 4 cm, T3: 4 to 6 cm, T4: >6 cm; a—no local extension, b—local extension

- **Stage I:** T1a or T2a/N0;
- **Stage II:** T1b, T2b, T3a/N0;
- **Stage III:** T3b, T4a or any T (except T4b) with N1,
- **Stage IV:** T4bN0 or Any T with N2–3 or M1

○ **The patient presents to you with pleural malignant effusion and multiple bilateral lung metastases. He had a 1.5-cm high-grade mucoepidermoid carcinoma of the parotid removed 2.5 years ago. He did not have neck dissection at that time because the neck was clinically negative and distant workup did not show metastasis. What is his stage now?**

Stage 1(T1N0M0)

A cancer patient is staged only once around the time his initial diagnosis and treatment based on anatomic extent of the tumor. This staging can be clinical *c*TNM or histologic *p*TNM, and this stage remains unchanged. Stage is predictor of prognosis drawn from retrospective analysis of outcomes. One cannot "restage" or "downstage" the cancer patient when he presents with a recurrence. In the setting of neoadjuvant chemotherapy or radiation therapy and *prior* to surgical resection, the change in the tumor extent is indicated by prefix *y*, for example, *yc*TNM or *yp*TNM.

○ **What is the surgical treatment for parotid tumors?**

Enucleation or lumpectomy is not an adequate treatment of the parotid tumors. Wide local excision with negative margins in conjunction with appropriate surgical treatment of the neck and durable reconstruction that would allow timely delivery of adjuvant radiation therapy if clinically indicated.

Benign tumor of the superficial lobe:	Superficial parotidectomy with facial nerve preservation
Benign tumor of the deep lobe:	Total parotidectomy with facial nerve preservation
Malignant parotid tumor:	
Without nerve involvement:	Total parotidectomy with facial nerve preservation
With nerve involvement:	Radical parotidectomy (involved branch, division, or trunk of the facial nerve is sacrificed)

○ **What is the difference between total and radical parotidectomy?**

In total parotidectomy, the facial nerve is preserved. The operation starts with superficial parotidectomy, then the facial nerve is dissected free off the deep lobe and the deep lobe is removed from underneath the nerve. In radical parotidectomy, the involved trunk of the facial nerve is removed *en bloc* with both lobes of parotid.

○ **How do you decide whether to perform total or radical parotidectomy?**

Direct invasion of the nerve is what determines the choice of the operation. If the patient's facial nerve is paralyzed preoperatively, radical parotidectomy is performed. If the nerve is not paralyzed, operation starts with superficial parotidectomy. If dissection plane between the tumor and the nerve branch cannot be established, that nerve or branch is resected with frozen-section evaluation. If the facial nerve cannot be dissected free, the branch, division, or trunk is sacrificed accordingly.

○ **You have mentioned superficial and deep lobes of the parotid. Could you define these terms?**

Division between the lobes of parotid is purely artificial. The parotid is one gland; however, during embryologic development facial nerve was trapped in the gland and the plane of the facial nerve branches defines the border between the lobes. Superficial lobe is much larger and encompasses approximately 80% to 90% of parotid parenchyma.

○ **Describe the steps of parotidectomy.**

After induction of general anesthesia with a short-acting paralysis, the patient is positioned with a shoulder roll and "donut" head rest with operated half of the face prepped in the field. The skin is injected with lidocaine with epinephrine, and a modified Blair or facelift incision is used (Fig. 51-7). SMAS is adherent for parotomasseteric fascia (parotid capsule) in the preauricular region; therefore, the sub-SMAS plane needs to be entered sharply. If oncologically safe, the dissection is performed between the SMAS and parotomasseteric fascia. With the index finger in the external auditory canal and double-prone skin hook placed in the canal's cartilage, subperichondrial dissection to the level of the tragal pointer if performed. Next, the plane between the sternocleidomastoid muscle and the tail of parotid is developed and the posterior belly of the digastric muscle is visualized. The tissue between this level and dissection and the tragal pointer is safely divided as the facial nerve is quite deep in this location (Fig. 51-8A). Once that is done, the trunk of the nerve is found under the thin layer of the fascia and fat just deep to the superior border of the posterior belly of the digastric (Fig. 51-8B). A split of the parotid tissue is created to visualize the upper and lower divisions, and only then, either superior or inferior mobilization of the gland can be safely performed without the risk of mistaking the facial nerve trunk for a division and risking the injury. The branches of the nerve then sequentially dissected (Fig. 51-8C). In the case of total parotidectomy, the facial nerve is dissected and elevated and the deep lobe is removed (Fig. 51-8D).

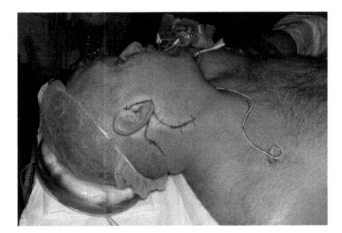

Figure 51-7 Positioning of parotidectomy patient on a shoulder roll and donut head rest. NIM facial nerve monitor for at least zygomatic (blue) and marginal mandibular (red) branches of the facial nerve as well as grounding electrodes (white and green) are placed. Both modified Blair and facelift incisions are outlined and lidocaine with epinephrine is injected prior to the prep. See Color insert.

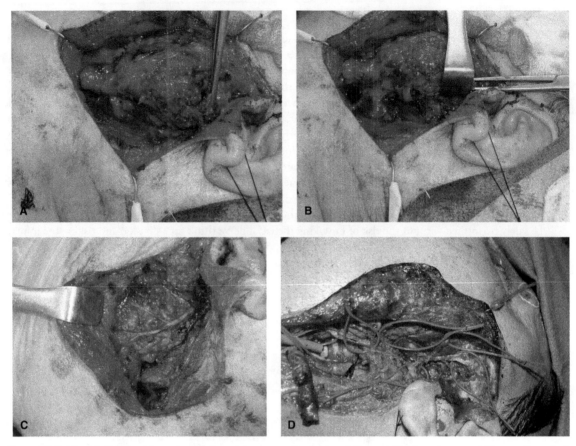

Figure 51-8 After sub-SMAS and external auditory canal dissection and separation of the parotid tail from the sternocleidomastoid muscle the deep points of dissection are connected by dividing the tissue between these points (**A**). The nerve trunk (**B**) and divisions are identified and the branches are sequentially dissected (**C**). In the case of total parotidectomy the nerve is dissected off the deep lobe, which is then removed (**D**). See Color insert.

○ **What recent technological advances that may improve efficiency of parotidectomy?**

Harmonic Focus® scalpel (Ethicon, Cincinnati, OH) utilizes ultrasound technology to achieve effective seal of the blood vessels and lymphatics. It was designed to optimize ergonomics of head and neck procedures (thyroidectomy, parotidectomy, and neck dissections). It has enhanced precision and decreased heat dissipation in the tissues, which makes it exceedingly effective in working around the cranial nerves.

Intraoperative facial nerve monitoring (Fig. 51-7) utilizes EMG technology. It assists in identifying facial nerve, recording intraoperative injurious potential, and confirming intact electrophysiologic function of the facial nerve. Although clear evidence of reduction of facial nerve injuries during parotidectomy is still not available, the technique does provide additional assurance, and is particularly useful in the cases with excessive facial nerve manipulation, for example, malignant tumors, deep lobe tumors, and parapharyngeal space procedures.

○ **The most critical part of the parotidectomy is finding of the facial nerve. How do you do that?**

(1) **Tragal pointer** is the medial end of the tragal cartilage. The dissection is carried out in the subperichondrial plane to expose the tragal pointer. The facial nerve trunk is 0.5 to 1 cm deep and inferior to the pointer. (2) The **Posterior belly of digastric muscle** is identified and followed superiorly to the digastric groove. The facial nerve is deep to cephalad border of the muscle. It is surrounded with small amount of fat that is incased in thin fascial envelope. (3) **Tympanomastoid suture** is the most constant landmark that can be palpated. The facial nerve is 6 to 8 mm deep to the inferior end of the suture line. (4) As a last resort, alternative method is **retrograde dissection** of the branches of the facial nerve.

○ **You have been called by your senior partner to give him a hand in the OR with a parotidectomy that he started 3 hours ago. He does not believe in preoperative FNA. The patient has a tumor of the superficial lobe of the parotid that was close to the nerve, but does not directly involve it. The pathologist is having a difficult time to determine the nature of the tumor on frozen section. How would you handle this situation?**

Some of the salivary malignancies are difficult to call on frozen section. In this case, sample upper cervical nodes (level 2) even they are not enlarged and send them for frozen section. If tumor is present in the nodes, perform total parotidectomy with neck dissection. If there is no tumor present in the nodes, *perform total parotidectomy* if suspicious for malignancy. In the worst case, add postoperative radiation if the tumor is malignant on permanent section. It is very important to avoid going back for completion parotidectomy in the previously operated field. Reoperative parotid surgery adds next level of complexity and risk to the facial nerve that can be avoided by performing initial total parotidectomy.

○ **How do you reconstruct total or radical parotidectomy defect?**

Unreconstructed total parotidectomy defect results in significant facial asymmetry. This problem is difficult to correct secondarily if there is a functional facial nerve present. These operations can be particularly difficult following adjuvant radiation therapy. Therefore, such reconstruction is best performed in the immediate setting. If the skin overlying the parotid has not been removed, the face and neck is delaminated in the manner similar to facelift technique. The most distal portion of this *cervicofacial flap* is tucked in, marked, and deepithelialized. The flap is secured with a mastoid stitch and sutured in place. The deepithelialized end of the flap usually provides sufficient volume to make the deformity less pronounced (Fig. 51-9).

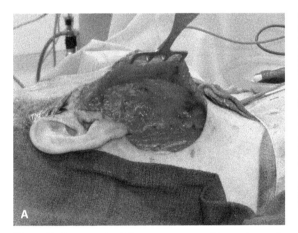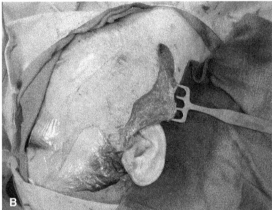

Figure 51-9 Cervicofacial flap reconstruction of the total parotidectomy defect. See Color insert.

Microvascular tissue transfer should be considered if the skin overlying the parotid is missing or the soft-tissue deficit is too great. Anterolateral thigh flap (ALT) has three advantages: (1) the fascia lata in the flap that will protect the facial nerve or facial nerve grafts during the future debulking procedures (Fig. 51-10); (2) the fascial lata from the ALT donor site is readily accessible for the construction of the static sling; (3) brunches of the femoral nerve can be used as facial nerve grafts (Fig. 51-11).

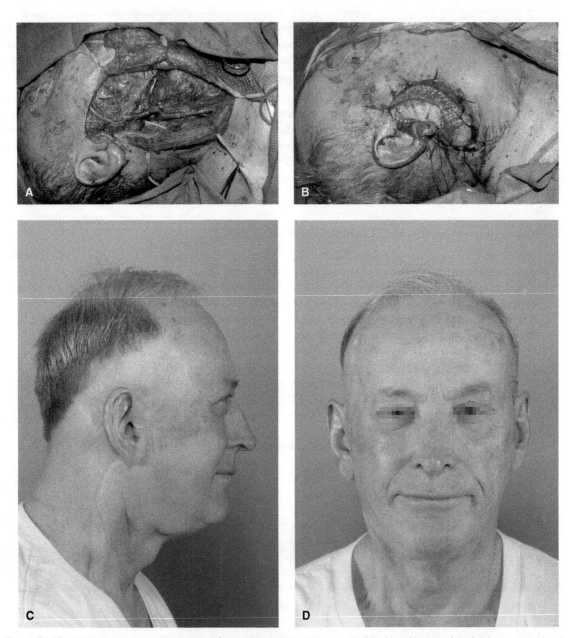

Figure 51-10 Metastatic squamous cell carcinoma of the temporal region with removal of the frontal branch of the facial nerve treated with total parotidectomy, neck dissection, and free ALT flap, followed by radiation, staged debulking, endoscopic browlift and upper blepharoplasty. See Color insert.

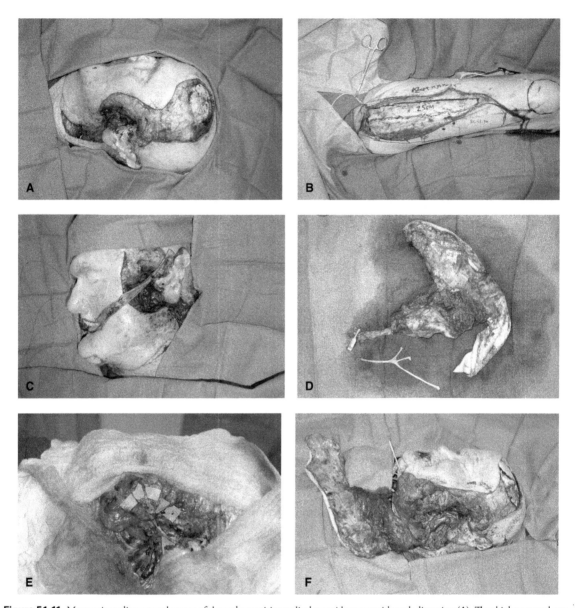

Figure 51-11 Metastatic malignant melanoma of the scalp requiring radical parotidectomy with neck dissection (**A**). The thigh was used as a donor site for ALT free flap, fascia lata graft (**B**) for static sling (**C**), and femoral nerve grafts (**D**). Both facial nerve graft reconstruction (**E**) and static sling (**C** and **F**) were performed in addition to ALT free flap (**F**). See Color insert.

○ **When do you perform neck dissection for the parotid tumors?**

Therapeutic neck dissection should be performed for all patients with clinically positive neck (N+). The patients with high-grade, high-stage, or requiring entrance of the neck for a free flap should undergo an elective (prophylactic) neck dissection with is usually selective, which implies removal of less than five lymph node levels.

○ **When is postoperative radiation therapy indicated?**

Grossly positive margins are treated with surgical resection when possible. Adjuvant radiation therapy is a treatment modality that aims to treat known or unknown local and regional microscopic disease that the surgeon left behind and thus enhance local and regional control of the tumor.

Tumors with close or microscopically positive margins that cannot be effectively re-resected; tumors in proximity to the facial nerve and the deep lobe, where margins are notoriously close and difficult to re-excise; tumors with presence or propensity for perineural spread; and tumors with lymphovascular invasion and cervical metastases should be considered for adjuvant radiation therapy.

○ **Is there any benign tumor that may benefit from postoperative radiation therapy?**

Recurrent pleomorphic adenoma.

○ **When fast neutron radiation can be considered?**

Adenoid cystic carcinoma and recurrent acinic carcinoma.

○ **You mentioned earlier that history of previous malignancies is important. Can you explain why?**

Parotid is a common site for metastases, both regional and distal.

○ **Why is the parotid a common site of regional metastases?**

Because of the embryologic delay of formation of the parotid capsule, lymph nodes became incorporated into the parotid. These *intercalated* nodes serve as regional lymph nodes for the area of skin between line over temporozygomatic arch to labial attachment of the nose inferiorly, sagittal line from the base of the nose to the vertex medially, and imaginary line from the vertex to the temporozygomatic arch posteriorly. In addition, it drains the external auditory canal, part of external ear including tragus, helical root, and superior helix, conjunctival sac, orbital content, posterior oral cavity, part of the pharynx, and the parotid gland itself.

○ **What is the most common metastatic tumor of the parotid?**

Malignant melanoma (40%) is the most common and squamous cell carcinoma is the next most common. In management of these tumors, the parotid is considered not as a gland, but rather as an additional cervical lymph node level; therefore, the decision to perform parotidectomy is guided by usual lymphadenectomy indications.
Sentinel node biopsy procedure allowed limiting elective parotidectomy and neck dissections in some low-risk patients.

○ **What tumors have propensity for hematogenous spread to the parotid?**

For the reasons that are not well understood, hematogenous metastases of the breast, lung, kidney, prostate, and gastrointestinal carcinomas have affinity for parotid tissues.

○ **What is gustatory sweating and how it relates to the parotid innervation?**

Postsynaptic sympathetic fibers arrive to the parotid in the adventitia of the branches of the external carotid artery. Preganglionic parasympathetic fibers travel within the glossopharyngeal nerve (cranial nerve IX) and then in tympanic branch (nerve of Jacobson) entering tympanic cavity, where it forms the tympanic plexus. The fibers leave the tympanic cavity through lesser superficial petrosal nerve entering middle cranial fossa. The nerve leaves the cranium via its own bony canal or the foramen ovale and terminates in the otic ganglion located on the medial surface of mandibular nerve (V_3). The postganglionic fibers join the auriculotemporal nerve (brunch of V_3), which in turn gives off the parotid branches to the gland.

Gustatory sweating or Frey's syndrome occurs following parotidectomy or rhytidectomy. It is caused by dysfunction of the auriculotemporal nerve. The pathways of this nerve are disrupted during the operation, and they regenerate incorrectly. Cross innervation of cholinergic postganglionic *parasympathetic* fibers from the otic ganglion and the cholinergic postganglionic *sympathetic* fibers innervating sweat glands of the skin. This results in parasympathetic innervation of the cholinergic postganglionic sympathetic fibers. Affected patients have facial sweating and flushing in response to gustatory stimulation.

○ **How do you manage it?**

Most patients with Frey's syndrome can be simply observed because the symptoms are usually mild. Injection of botulinum toxin (Botox) and operative placement of AlloDerm, dermis, or fascia graft under the affected skin to prevent improper nerve regeneration.

○ **What is the parapharyngeal space?**

It is an upside-down pyramid: superior border is skull base; inferior is lesser horn of the hyoid; medial is superior constrictor, tonsil, and eustachian tube; and lateral is ramus of the mandible. It is important that the lateral wall structures are rigid and the medial wall structures are pliable; tumors of the parapharyngeal space will present as a bulging tonsil.

○ **What does the parapharyngeal space have to do with salivary tumors?**

Tumors of parapharyngeal space are frequently of salivary gland origin. They can be tumors extending from the deep lobe of the parotid or tumors of accessory salivary gland rest.

○ **You have suspected that the patient has a parapharyngeal tumor, how do you work it up?**

Do not biopsy—some of the parapharyngeal tumors can be highly vascular and orientation of the tumor and the carotid artery cannot be determined on physical examination. Workup is largely based on imaging—get a CT scan with contrast.

○ **What in particular you look for on the CT scan?**

Axial cuts of the CT will show relation of the tumor to the styloid.
Prestyloid tumors are salivary in origin with the rare exception of connective tissue neoplasms.
Poststyloid tumors are neurogenic (CN IX, X, XI, and sympathetic chain), vascular (paragangliomas), or lymph node (metastases) in origin.

○ **Overall, what is the most common tumor of the parapharyngeal space?**

Metastatic lesions are the most common. The most common primary tumor is pleomorphic adenoma (50%).

○ **What are the lymph nodes in the parapharyngeal space?**

Nodes of Rouviere drain the nasopharynx.

○ **What is Vernet syndrome?**

Enlargement of the nodes extending to the jugular foramen that causes compression of CN IX, X, XI, and paralysis of their motor components.

○ **Does radical surgery for parotid tumors and radiation therapy significantly affect long-term survival?**

No. They do improve local and regional control, but do not change long-term survival. Unfortunately, outcome of parotid malignancies is largely predetermined by the histology of the tumor.

● ● ● **REFERENCES** ● ● ●

AJCC Cancer Staging Manual, 7th ed. New York, NY: Springer; 2010.

Batsakis JG. Tumors of the head and neck: clinical and pathological considerations. 2nd ed. Baltimore, MD: Williams Wilkins; 1979.

Close LG, Larson DL, Shah JP. Essentials of head and neck oncology. 1st ed. New York, NY: Thieme Medical Publishers, Inc.; 1998.

Janfaza P, Nadol JB, Galla RJ, Fabian RL, Montgomery WW. *Surgical Anatomy of the Head and Neck.* 1st ed. Philadelphia, PA: Lippincott Williams & Wilkins; 2001.

Medina JE. *Clinical Practice Guidelines for the Diagnosis and Management of Cancer of the Head and Neck.* American Head and Neck Society; 2002.

Regezi JA, Batsakis JG. Histogenesis of salivary gland neoplasms. *Otol Clin N Am.* 1977;10:297–307.

*Salivary Gland Tumors, NCCN Clinical Practice Guidelines in Oncology (NCCN Guidelines®), Version 2.*2014, National Comprehensive Cancer Network®; 2015.

Shah JP. *Head and neck surgery.* 2nd ed. London: Mosby-Wolfe; 1996.

Spiro RH. Salivary neoplasms: overview of a 35-year experience with 2,807 patients. *Head Neck Surg.* 1986;8(3):177–184.

Woods JE. Parotidectomy versus limited resection for benign parotid masses. *Am J Surg.* 1985;149(6):749–750.

CHAPTER 52

Head and Neck Reconstruction

Pieter G.L. Koolen, MD,
John B. Hijjawi, MD, FACS, and
Samuel J. Lin, MD, MBA, FACS

○ **Which muscles close the mouth?**

- Masseter
- Temporalis
- Medial pterygoid

○ **Which muscles open the mouth?**

- Digastric muscles
- Mylohyoid muscles
- Geniohyoid muscles
- Genioglossus muscles

○ **Which muscles protract the mandible?**

- Lateral pterygoid muscles
- Digastric muscles
- Mylohyoid muscles

○ **What are the goals of mandible reconstruction?**

- Restore shape of the lower third of the face.
- Preserve occlusion (if dentition).
- Allow for potential dental implants.
- Heal in a timely fashion—do not delay adjuvant therapy.

○ **When can nonvascularized bone grafts be used in mandible reconstruction?**

  • Isolated small defects in favorable locations for soft-tissue coverage (ramus, body).

  • No radiation history or plan for radiation therapy.

○ **In the medically compromised patient, what can be done to reconstruct a segmental defect at the time of mandibular resection?**

  • Reconstruction plate and regional tissue (pectoralis major, latissimus dorsi).

  • Avoid plate reconstruction with anterior defects.

○ **What are the disadvantages of plate reconstruction?**

  • Plate fatigue and fracture

  • Screw loosening

  • Plate exposure—beware with anterior defects and/or radiation therapy

  • Osteoradionecrosis

○ **What common microvascular flaps are available for mandible reconstruction?**

  • Fibula flap

  • Iliac crest flap

  • Scapula flap

  • Radial forearm osseous flap

○ **What is the blood supply to the iliac crest free flap?**

  Deep circumflex iliac artery.

○ **What are the advantages of the iliac crest free flap?**

  • Good length of bone.

  • Tall bone stock—good for implants. Abundant soft tissue—good for large-volume defects.

○ **What are the disadvantages of the iliac crest free flap?**

  • Short pedicle, small vessels.

  • Poor skin paddle mobility.

  • Protracted gait pain, risk of abdominal hernia.

  • Potential for meralgia paresthetica (lateral femoral cutaneous nerve injury/entrapment).

○ **What are the advantages of the fibula free flap?**

  • Reliable skin paddle for closure/monitoring.

  • Long, sturdy bone.

  • Long pedicle, large caliber vessels.

  • Supports osseointegrated implants.

  • Allows for simultaneous dissection while tumor is being resected.

  • Can make two skin islands based on separate perforators and include a portion of soleus muscle.

○ **What are the disadvantages of the fibula free flap?**

- Contraindicated with severe peripheral vascular disease.
- Donor-site healing can be difficult and prolonged in some patients.

○ **What options exist for reconstruction of the mandibular condyle?**

- Reinsert condylar process as a nonvascularized bone graft if disease free—viability may be unpredictable, especially with radiation therapy.
- Neocondyle—rounding off of the fibula flap transfer.
- Prosthetic reconstruction—not recommended if postoperative radiotherapy is planned.
- No reconstruction—mandible will rotate obliquely with opening.

○ **What is the typical dose to a tumor bed after resection of an oral cavity tumor?**

Typical dose is between 60 and 80 Gy.

○ **What effect does radiation therapy have on normal tissue?**

- Acute: dermatitis, mucositis, dysphagia, odynophagia, xerostomia, altered taste, fatigue.
- Late: xerostomia, hyperpigmentation, dental decay, osteoradionecrosis, dysphagia, strictures, cataracts, sensorineural hearing loss, soft-tissue fibrosis, neck lymphedema.

○ **What are the implications of xerostomia on oral function?**

- Accelerated tooth decay.
- Chewing, swallowing difficulties.
- Speech problems.

○ **Why is the mandible vulnerable to osteoradionecrosis?**

- Radiation therapy–induced obliteration of inferior alveolar artery without adequate redundant blood supply is believed to contribute.
- Histologically, scarcity of osteoblasts leads to fragile bone, susceptible to minimal injury.

○ **When does osteoradionecrosis manifest?**

- 1 to 3 years after radiation therapy, with an overall risk of 3% with current radiation techniques.
- Risk is present for the patient's entire life.

○ **How does radiation therapy complicate dental extractions?**

- The incidence of osteoradionecrosis increases significantly if dental extraction is performed *after* radiotherapy. Therefore, it should be done before radiotherapy.
- Should wait 10 to 14 days between extractions and radiation therapy.
- Atraumatic extraction with minimal mucoperiosteal flap undermining should be practiced if extraction is unavoidable.
- Hyperbaric oxygen and empiric antibiotic therapy have to be employed to minimize risk.

○ **What common reconstructive options are available for buccal defects?**

Any option employed should avoid intraoral contractures and avoid bulky flaps.

- Primary closure.
- Split-thickness skin graft—contracts 50% to 75%.
- FAMM flap—ensure facial artery patency, no more than 2 cm wide.
- Radial forearm flap—workhorse.
- Anterolateral thigh flap—may be too thick in some patients. Good option for large and through-and-through defects.
- Lateral arm flap—may be too thick in some patients.

○ **How do you minimize the risk of a fistula with oral cavity reconstruction?**

With an incidence of 5% to 15%, this can progress to microvascular failure.

- Ensure proper closure with nice mucosa–skin edge eversion. Avoid tight running or tight horizontal mattress sutures that may compromise the mucosal/skin edge blood supply.
- Obliterate dead space—this is the single most important measure. Include an appropriate amount of muscle to fill the submandibular dead space. With a good muscle filling, you really do not have to have watertight closure that is impossible in most cases. Tight closure should actually be avoided since it may cause ischemia of flap/ mucosa edges.
- Proper postoperative oral care.

○ **What are the tenets of flap choice and design for tongue and floor of mouth reconstruction?**

- Sealed communication between oral cavity and dissected neck. Some muscle filling is desirable.
- Overcorrect volume for total or subtotal glossectomy reconstruction, especially if XRT is planned so that the neotongue can touch the palate for better speech reproduction. It will also create a trough or gutter to route secretions posteriorly to minimize the risk of aspiration.
- For isolated floor of mouth or partial glossectomy defects, the flap should be thin to preserve the mobility of the remaining tongue.
- Design the flap to optimize protrusion of the residual tongue tip by recreating the ventral sulcus.
- A sensate flap may achieve better patient satisfaction and possibly better swallowing function.

○ **What are the common flap options for tongue and floor of mouth reconstruction after hemiglossectomy or total glossectomy?**

- Thin anterolateral thigh flap: good for FOM and hemiglossectomy reconstruction.
- Thick anterolateral thigh flap: good for total or subtotal glossectomy reconstruction.
- Radial forearm flap: good for FOM and hemiglossectomy reconstruction but not enough bulk for total glossectomy.
- Rectus abdominis/DIEP flap: good for total or subtotal glossectomy reconstruction, way too thick for hemiglossectomy or FOM reconstruction.
- Latissimus flap: good for total or subtotal glossectomy reconstruction.

○ **What is an "in-continuity" neck dissection?**

Removal of the lymphatic drainage pathways between the primary tumor and adjacent nodes that lie in proximity to the primary. This does present the possibility of fistula formation in floor of mouth/tongue tumors due to the potential communication between the oral defect and the neck.

○ **Is it necessary to innervate a free flap for partial or total tongue reconstruction?**

  • Anastomosis of a sensory nerve of the transferred flap is advantageous.

  • The preferred recipient sensory nerve is the lingual nerve.

  • Sensory recovery can be nearly complete.

  • Motor reinnervation of a muscle flap by anastomosing the motor nerve to the hypoglossal nerve is poor at best.

○ **What defects may exist after resection of an oral cancer of the tongue?**

  • Wedge resection.

  • Hemiglossectomy—may extend to floor of mouth and tonsillar pillar.

  • Near-total glossectomy—entire tip of tongue and up to half of the tongue base.

  • Total glossectomy—entire tip and tongue base. No functional residual tongue.

○ **What are the common complications of pharyngoesophageal reconstruction?**

  • Pharyngocutaneous fistula—1 to 4 weeks postoperation, manifests as a leakage of saliva or as a neck infection.

  • Anastomotic stricture—occurs months to years after reconstruction, usually at the distal anastomosis; minimized by converting a circumferential repair with a staggered anastomosis.

  • Neck infection—should rule out the possibility of anastomotic leakage.

  • Medical complications—usually respiratory or cardiac.

○ **Which free flap is least tolerant of ischemia and therefore microanastomosis should precede insetting?**
Jejunum flap.

○ **What are the common flaps used for partial or total pharyngoesophageal defects?**

  • Anterolateral thigh flap

  • Radial forearm flap

  • Jejunum flap

  • Pectoralis major flap

○ **What are the options for speech rehabilitation after pharyngolaryngectomy?**

  • Tracheoesophageal puncture (TEP) and insertion of voice prosthesis

  • Voice tube using transferred ileum, jejunum, or ileocecal valve

  • Electrolarynx

  • Esophageal speech

○ **What recipient vessels are commonly utilized for head and neck free flap reconstruction?**

  • Arteries: lingual artery, facial artery, superior thyroid artery, external carotid artery, superficial temporal artery.

  • Veins: common facial vein, internal jugular vein, superficial temporal vein, external jugular vein.

○ **Which recipient vessels can be considered in the radiated and previously operated neck?**

- Transverse cervical artery of the thyrocervical trunk

- Contralateral neck-vein grafts are usually needed

- Thoracoacromial artery

- Arteriovenous loop off the subclavian artery (cephalic vein ideal)

- Internal mammary vessels

○ **What is a "frozen neck"?**

Severe soft-tissue fibrosis of the neck as a result of neck dissection and radiation therapy. There is absence of surgical planes, as well as limitation of passive motion at the neck, making exposure potentially challenging.

○ **What are the problems associated with performing reconstruction in the frozen neck?**

- Risk of carotid artery rupture.

- Lack of recipient vessels for free tissue transfer.

- Neck skin deficit—may be significant.

○ **How does the surgeon avoid morbidity and mortality in reconstructing the pharyngoesophagus in the frozen neck?**

- Avoid dissection of the great vessels.

- Use alternative recipient vessels: transverse cervical vessels, internal mammary vessels, thoracoacromial trunk.

- Provide abundant skin coverage with flap transfer.

○ **When is a pectoralis flap used for pharyngoesophageal reconstruction?**

- Partial defects, male patients

- High-risk patients

- Failed free flap

○ **What happens if the patient has flap loss or is too fragile for reconstruction after pharyngectomy?**

- Create spit fistula at upper neck.

- Use pectoralis major flap or latissimus dorsi flap to protect neck vessels and divert saliva away from tracheostomy.

○ **If a patient has a hemipalatectomy or maxillectomy defect with intact contralateral maxillary dentition, what is the reconstruction of choice?**

Palatal obturator with denture is an acceptable option. The maxillectomy wound or the maxillary sinus can be skin grafted and the obturator separates the oral cavity from the nasal cavity to prevent VPI and nasal regurgitation. This is a quick and simple option, particularly useful for high-risk patients who <u>are not free flap</u> candidates. Postoperative radiation may cause skin-graft loss and bone exposure. For most patients with planned radiotherapy or with previous radiation, a soft-tissue flap reconstruction is the most popular option. For younger and more functional patients, especially with benign diseases, vascularized bone reconstruction with osteointegrated dental implants provides the best possible aesthetic and functional outcomes when the maxillectomy defect extends beyond the anterior midline to the contralateral side, vascularized bone reconstruction becomes the preferred choice.

○ **What are common free flaps for midface reconstruction of bony and soft-tissue defects?**

Bone flaps

- Fibula osteocutaneous free flap
- Iliac crest osteocutaneous flap
- Scapula osteocutaneous free flap
- Soft-tissue free flap with bone grafts

Soft-tissue flaps

- Anterolateral thigh flap
- Radial forearm flap
- Rectus abdominis myocutaneous flap
- Latissimus dorsi with bone graft

○ **What general principles guide skull base reconstruction?**

- Seal the dura from the aerodigestive tract.
- Tight seal of violated dura to prevent cerebrospinal fluid leak—muscle is desirable to eliminate dead space.

○ **What is Jackson and Hyde's classification of skull base reconstruction?**

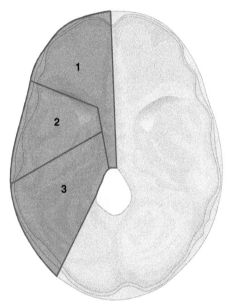

Figure 52-1 Regions of the skull base.

○ **What flaps are available for region 1 skull base defects?**

- Galea-frontalis flap (midline)
- Pericranial flap (midline)
- Temporalis flap (lateral defect)
- Temporoparietal fascial flap (lateral defects)

○ **What flaps are available for region 2 or region 3 skull base defects?**

- Temporalis flap
- Temporoparietal fascial flap
- Free flap (rectus abdominis or other muscle flap)

○ **What are the basic tenets to minimize flap pedicle and anastomotic problems besides meticulous anastomotic techniques?**

• Interrogate the recipient vessels for adequate inflow, venous outflow obstruction (valves, thrombus).

• Pedicle artery and vein should be parallel if possible. If this is not possible due to location of the respective recipient artery and vein, then the flap pedicle should be dissected and anastomosed so one should not compromise the other (long enough dissection to avoid kinking).

• Minimize redundancy—may cause kinking and twisting of pedicle.

• Minimize tension—vein grafts may be necessary.

• Avoid compression—especially an issue in the irradiated neck, never underestimate swelling at the end of the case or the need for a large flap skin paddle to close the defect. Flap insetting should not be tight. Some skin redundancy can be easily revised at a later stage. Trying to achieve the "best aesthetic result" by insetting the flap tight may cause pedicle (especially perforator) compression.

• Study and test the pedicle by moving the head back and forth. Before closing the neck incision, the head should return to a neutral position (from a turned away position) and the neck return from a hyperextended position. The pedicle position should then be carefully inspected again and any kinking or twisting should be corrected.

• The most common cause of venous occlusion (80%) is mechanical obstruction such as twisting, kinking, and compression. Therefore, great care should be taken to avoid these problems.

○ **What are the common free flaps for scalp reconstruction?**

• Latissimus dorsi muscle with skin grafting for large defects.

• Radial forearm or lateral arm flaps for smaller defects.

• Rectus abdominis muscle with or without skin components.

• Vastus lateralis muscle/anterolateral thigh flap.

• Scapular, parascapular flaps.

○ **What is the most common recipient vessel for scalp reconstruction and what are the potential problems with these vessels?**

The superficial temporal vessels are most commonly used as recipient vessels for scalp reconstruction due to their proximity to the defect. However, the superficial temporal vessels have a bad reputation of being prone to spasm and having higher failure rates. The key to avoid such problems is to use the very proximal part of the superficial temporal vessels near the zygomatic arch, to a point that they cannot be dissected any more. At this level, the diameter and flow are much greater and therefore most reliable. Only use the most proximal 1 cm of superficial temporal vessels for anastomosis.

• • • REFERENCES • • •

Coleman JJ. Reconstruction of the midface with vascularized bone and soft tissue. *Semin Plastic Surg*. 2003;17:291–303.

Cordeiro PG, Santamaria E. A classification system and algorithm for reconstruction of maxillectomy and midfacial defects. *Plast Reconstr Surg*. 2000;105:2347–2348.

Jackson IT, Hide TA. A systematic approach to tumors of the base of the skull. *J Maxillofac Surg*. 1982;10:92–98.

Neligan PC, Wei F-C, eds. *Microsurgical Reconstruction of the Head and Neck*. St Louis, MO: Quality Medical Publishing; 2010.

COLOR INSERT

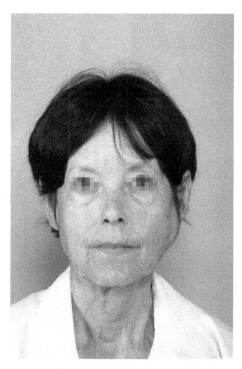

Figure 51-2 Left parotid mass in a patient with a long-standing Sjögren's syndrome.

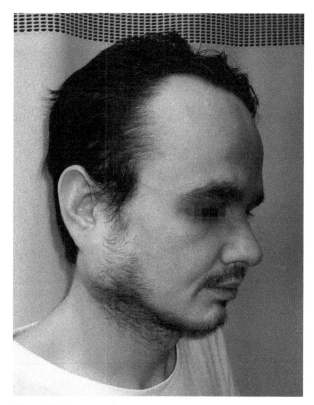

Figure 51-3 A: Large pleomorphic adenoma involving deep and superficial lobes of the right parotid.

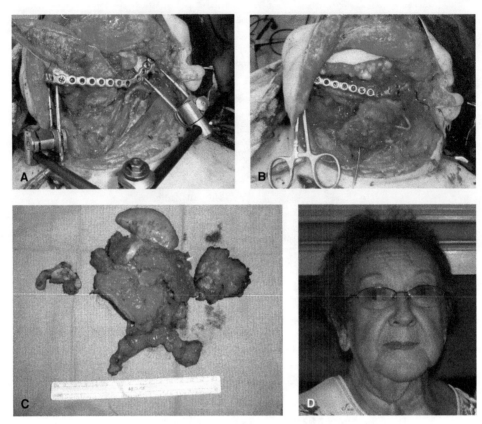

Figure 51-6 Adenoid cystic carcinoma of the left submandibular gland (size 2 cm physical examination) treated with composite resection, total parotidectomy with resection of lower division of the left facial nerve, free fibula (**A** and **B**), specimen (**C**) static sling, and postoperative radiation. Appearance of the patient without evidence of disease at 6 years (**D**).

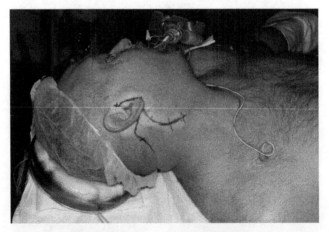

Figure 51-7 Positioning of parotidectomy patient on a shoulder roll and donut head rest. NIM facial nerve monitor for at least zygomatic (blue) and marginal mandibular (red) branches of the facial nerve as well as grounding electrodes (white and green) are placed. Both modified Blair and facelift incisions are outlined and lidocaine with epinephrine is injected prior to the prep.

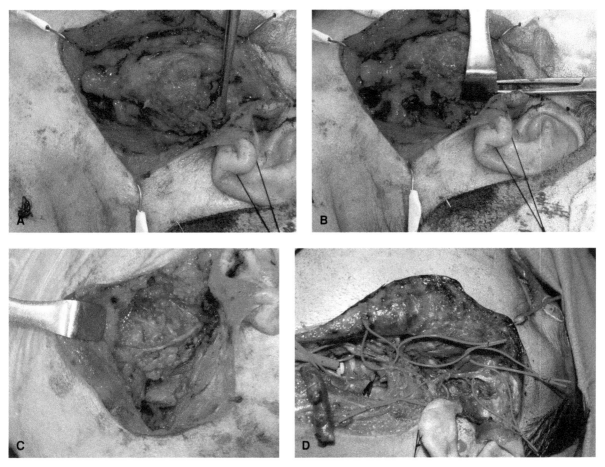

Figure 51-8 After sub-SMAS and external auditory canal dissection and separation of the parotid tail from the sternocleidomastoid muscle the deep points of dissection are connected by dividing the tissue between these points (**A**). The nerve trunk (**B**) and divisions are identified and the branches are sequentially dissected (**C**). In the case of total parotidectomy the nerve is dissected off the deep lobe, which is then removed (**D**).

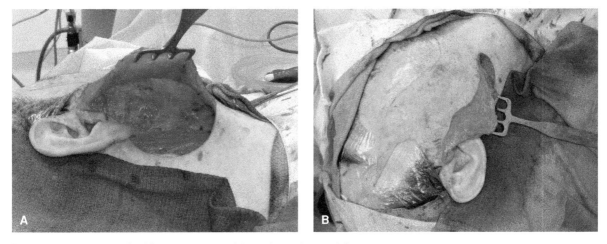

Figure 51-9 A, B: Cervicofacial flap reconstruction of the total parotidectomy defect.

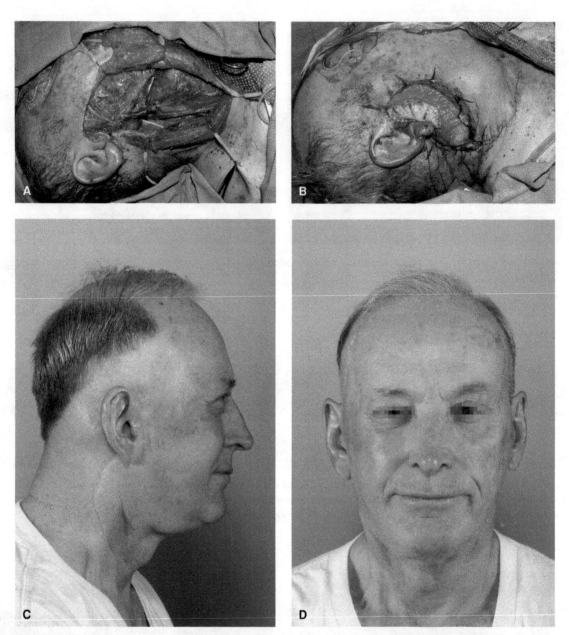

Figure 51-10 A–D: Metastatic squamous cell carcinoma of the temporal region with removal of the frontal branch of the facial nerve treated with total parotidectomy, neck dissection, and free ALT flap, followed by radiation, staged debulking, endoscopic browlift and upper blepharoplasty.

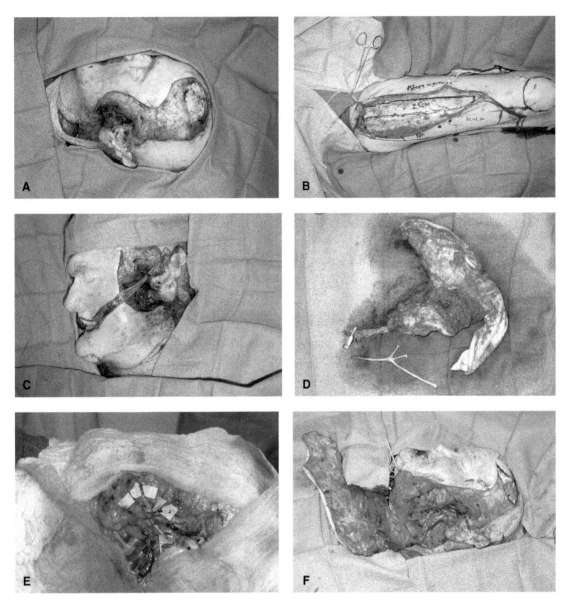

Figure 51-11 Metastatic malignant melanoma of the scalp requiring radical parotidectomy with neck dissection (**A**). The thigh was used as a donor site for ALT free flap, fascia lata graft (**B**) for static sling (**C**), and femoral nerve grafts (**D**). Both facial nerve graft reconstruction (**E**) and static sling (**C** and **F**) were performed in addition to ALT free flap (**F**).

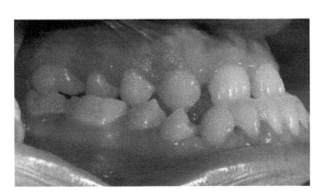

Figure 54-6 C: Dental crossbite.

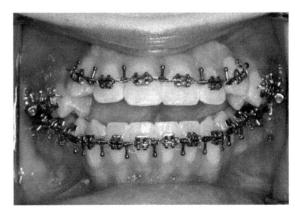

Figure 54-6 D: Anterior openbite.

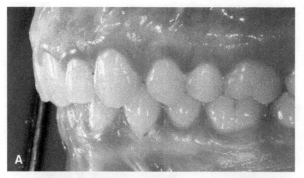

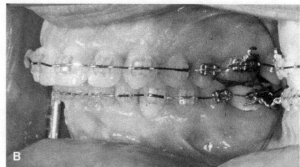

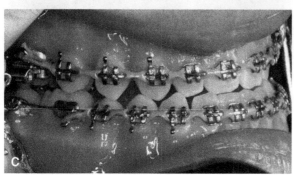

Figure 54-7 **A:** Angle class I molar relationship. **B:** Angle class II molar relationship—note the anterior overjet and maxillary canine anterior to the mandibular canine. **C:** Angle class III molar relationship—note the negative anterior overjet.

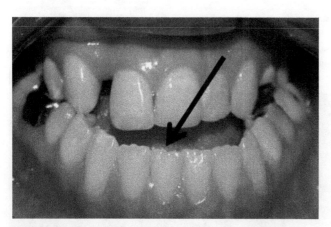

Figure 54-8 Mamelons in an anterior open bite.

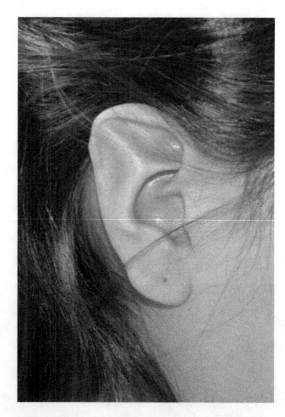

Figure 77-2 Example of a Stahl's ear.

Surgical Management of Migraine Headaches

CHAPTER 53

Aladdin H. Hassanein, MD, MMSc,
and William G. Austen, Jr., MD

○ **What is the difference between "headache" and a "migraine headache"?**

- A migraine is a specific type of headache which meets diagnostic criteria that is sub-categorized by the presence or absence of an aura (reversible neurological symptoms preceding the onset of migraine).

- Migraine without aura is defined as ≥5 attacks that (1) last 4 to 72 hours; (2) include ≥2 specific qualities (pulsating, unilateral location, moderate–severe intensity, aggravation by routine activities); and (3) associated with nausea/vomiting or photophobia.

- Migraine with aura is characterized by ≥2 episodes of headaches fulfilling "migraine without aura" criteria accompanied by aura ≤60 minutes in duration.

○ **How common are migraine headaches?**

- Affects 12% of the population

- Three times more common in women

○ **What is the pathophysiologic mechanism of migraine headaches?**

The exact etiology is unknown. The mechanism may involve activation of nociceptive sensory fibers of the trigeminal nerve which innervate meningeal vessels (trigeminovascular system). Altered cortical excitability and cortical spreading depression may affect the pathway. Peripheral nerve irritation/sensitization and myelin abnormalities recently have been implicated.

○ **What pharmacological therapies are available for migraines?**

- Acute analgesic—acetaminophen, nonsteroidal anti-inflammatory drugs, narcotics

- Acute abortive—triptans, ergotamine

- Prophylactic—beta-blockers, anticonvulsants, tricyclic antidepressants

○ **What nonpharmacological treatments are available for migraines?**

- Behavioral (e.g., avoidance of environmental triggers)
- Botulinum toxin (Botox)
- Surgical treatment

○ **How was a surgical option for migraine management discovered?**

Guyuron et al. observed improvement of headaches in patients that underwent aesthetic rejuvenation of the brow.

○ **Which patients may be considered candidates for surgical treatment of migraine?**

Patients with chronic, debilitating refractory migraine headaches that persist despite treatment by a neurologist with maximal medical therapy. Imaging is obtained to rule out intracranial or rhinogenic etiologies. History and physical examination should be consistent with a nerve trigger point. Response to Botox and/or nerve block can be correlative.

○ **What is the surgical goal of migraine treatment?**

Decompression/deactivation of peripheral nerve triggers that have been identified preoperatively as a likely migraine potentiator (synonymous to compressive neuropathies like carpal tunnel syndrome).

○ **What basic anatomical structures may compress/irritate involved peripheral nerves and trigger migraine?**

- Bone—compression through foramen/notch that nerve may exit (e.g., supraorbital foramen)
- Fascia—entrapment from fascial element (e.g., trapezius fascia)
- Muscle—compression from entry or exit into a muscle (e.g., corrugator muscle)
- Vascular—vessel crossing nerve (e.g., occipital artery)

○ **What are the migraine trigger points and which nerves are involved?**

Trigger Site	Nerves
Frontal	Supratrochlear (V_1), supraorbital (V_1)
Temporal	Zygomaticotemporal (V_2), auriculotemporal (V_3)
Occipital	Greater Occipital (C2), lesser Occipital (C2)

○ **What are nasoseptal triggers of migraine?**

- Aberrant intranasal mucosal contact points may trigger migraines by irritation of trigeminal nerve branches: anterior ethmoidal nerve (V_1) and sphenopalatine ganglion (V_2 contributions).
- Etiology includes deviated septum, spurs, turbinate hypertrophy, paradoxical turbinate curvature, concha bullosa (pneumatized turbinate), Haller cells (infraorbital ethmoid cells).

○ **How are nasoseptal causes of migraine surgically treated?**

Septoplasty and turbinate resection to relieve abnormal septal contact points.

○ **What are the three divisions of the trigeminal nerve (cranial nerve V) and the foramen that they exit?**
   • Ophthalmic division (V_1)—superior orbital fissure
   • Maxillary division (V_2)—foramen rotundum
   • Mandibular division (V_3)—foramen ovale

○ **What are the three branches of V_1?**
   • Frontal nerve
   • Lacrimal nerve
   • Nasociliary nerve

○ **What three nerves does the frontal branch of V_1 divide into?**
   • Supraorbital nerve
   • Supratrochlear nerve
   • Infratrochlear nerve

○ **Which nerves may be involved in frontal migraine headaches?**
   • Supraorbital nerve
   • Supratrochlear nerve

○ **Which muscles may compress the supratrochlear and supraorbital nerve?**
   Corrugator supercilii and depressor supercilii, which are resected during frontal migraine decompression.

○ **Does the supraorbital nerve more commonly exit through a notch or foramen?**
   Supraorbital notch is more common (83%). Either a foramen or notch (with fascial band) may cause compression.

○ **How is frontal migraine decompression surgically approached?**
   Either (1) endoscopically or (2) a transpalpebral (upper blepharoplasty) incision.

○ **Which nerves may be involved in temporal migraine headaches?**
   • Zygomaticotemporal nerve
   • Auriculotemporal nerve

○ **The zygomaticotemporal and auriculotemporal nerves are branches of which nerves?**
   • Zygomaticotemporal nerve: branch of the maxillary division of the trigeminal nerve (V_2)
   • Auriculotemporal nerve: branch of the mandibular division of the trigeminal nerve (V_3)

○ **Which muscle does the zygomaticotemporal nerve course through?**
   Temporalis muscle (50%).

○ **Which vessel travels closely with the auriculotemporal nerve?**

Superficial temporal artery and vein.

○ **Which nerves are implicated in occipital migraine headaches?**

- Greater occipital nerve (most common)
- Lesser occipital nerve
- Third occipital nerve—no longer considered a significant migraine trigger

○ **Are the nerves involved with occipital migraines branches from the trigeminal nerve? Which nerves do they arise from?**

- No, nerve triggers of occipital migraine triggers are from cervical spinal nerves not the trigeminal nerve.
- Greater and lesser occipital nerves are from the second cervicil spinal nerve (C2) and the third occipital nerve is from C3.

○ **Which structures can compress the greater occipital nerve**

- Capitis muscles (semispinalis, obliquus)
- Trapezius/trapezius fascia
- Occipital artery

○ **What is the success rate of surgical treatment of migraine in appropriately selected patients?**

- Up to 90% success rate (defined by reduction in symptoms by at least 50%).
- 50% experience total elimination of headaches.

○ **Is there any Level I evidence supporting a surgical migraine therapy?**

Yes, Guyuron et al. performed a placebo-controlled trial using a sham surgical group which demonstrated that operative treatment of migraines was effective.

● ● ● REFERENCES ● ● ●

Behin F, Behin B, Bigal ME, Lipton RB. Surgical treatment of patients with refractory migraine headaches and intranasal contact points. *Cephalalgia.* 2005;25:439–443.

Bernstein C, Burstein R. Sensitization of the trigeminovascular pathway: perspective and implications to migraine pathophysiology. *J Clin Neurol.* 2012;8:89–99.

Fallucco M, Janis JE, Hagan RR. The anatomical morphology of the supraorbital notch: clinical relevance to the surgical treatment of migraine headaches. *Plast Reconstr Surg.* 2012;130:1227–1233.

Gfrerer L, Maman DY, Tessler O, Austen WG Jr. Nonendoscopic deactivation of nerve triggers in migraine headache patients: surgical technique and outcomes. *Plast Reconstr Surg.* 2014;134:771–778.

Guyuron B. Rhinogenic migraine headaches. In: Guyuron B, ed. *Rhinoplasty.* 1st ed. China: Saunders; 2012:441–448.

Guyuron B, Kriegler JS, Davis J, Amini SB. Comprehensive surgical treatment of migraine headaches. *Plast Reconstr Surg.* 2005;115:1–9.

Guyuron B, Reed D, Kriegler JS, Davis J, Pashmini N, Amini S. A placebo-controlled surgical trial of the treatment of migraine headaches. *Plast Reconstr Surg.* 2009;124:461–468.

Guyuron B, Varghai A, Michelow BJ, Thomas T, Davis J. Corrugator supercilii muscle resection and migraine headaches. *Plast Reconstr Surg.* 2000;106:429–234.

Guyuron B, Yohannes E, Miller R, Chim H, Reed D, Chance MR. Electron microscopic and proteomic comparison of terminal branches of the trigeminal nerve in patients with and without migraine headaches. *Plast Reconstr Surg.* 2014;134:796e–805e.

International Headache Society (IHS). *IHS International Headache Classification II.* Available at: ihs-classification.org/en. Accessed March 30, 2015.

Janis JE, Barker JC, Javadi C, Ducic I, Hagan R, Guyuron B. A review of current evidence in the surgical treatment of migraine headaches. *Plast Reconstr Surg.* 2014;134:131S–41S.

Janis JE, Hatef DA, Ducic I, et al. The anatomy of the greater occipital nerve: Part II. Compression point topography. *Plast Reconstr Surg.* 2010;126:1563–1572.

Janis JE, Hatef DA, Hagan R, et al. Anatomy of the supratrochlear nerve: implications for the surgical treatment of migraine headaches. *Plast Reconstr Surg.* 2013;131:743–750.

Janis JE, Hatef DA, Thakar H, et al. The zygomaticotemporal branch of the trigeminal nerve: Part II. Anatomical variations. *Plast Reconstr Surg.* 2010;126:435–442.

Lee M, Lineberry K, Reed D, Guyuron B. The role of the third occipital nerve in surgical treatment of occipital migraine headaches. *J Plast Reconstr Aesthet Surg.* 2013;66:1335–1339.

Lipton RB, Bigal ME, Diamond M, Freitag F, Reed ML, Stewart WF; AMPP Advisory Group. Migraine prevalence, disease burden, and the need for preventive therapy. *Neurology.* 2007;68:343–349.

Olesen J, Burstein R, Ashina M, Tfelt-Hansen P. Origin of pain in migraine: evidence for peripheral sensitisation. *Lancet Neurol.* 2009; 8:679–690.

Pietrobon D, Striessnig J. Neurobiology of migraine. *Nat Rev Neurosci.* 2003;4:386–398.

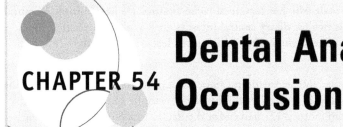

CHAPTER 54
Dental Anatomy and Occlusion

Anish Gupta, MD, DDS and
Ruba Khader, BDS

○ **What are the different types of teeth that are present in the adult dentition?**

1. Incisors—anterior teeth, single rooted, used for biting/incising

2. Canines—anterior teeth, cornerstones of the mouth, prominent cusp tips, single long roots

3. Premolars—aka bicuspids, posterior teeth, occlusal surface to chew, commonly single rooted in mandible and dual rooted in maxilla

4. Molars—posterior teeth used primarily for chewing, maxillary molars with three roots and mandibular molars with two roots

See Figure 54-1.

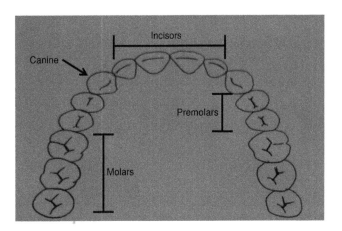

Figure 54-1 Types of teeth.

○ **You are called in to consult on a 27-year-old male who has sustained facial trauma. He has multiple intraoral and perioral lacerations and the crowns of his two maxillary central incisors are no longer present in his mouth. When calling the dental trauma consultant, which teeth will you tell her are fractured?**

Teeth 8 and 9.

The Universal Numbering System has been adopted by the American Dental Association. NUMBERS designate the 32 permanent (adult) teeth (1–32). Begin at the RIGHT maxillary third molar (#1) to the LEFT maxillary third molar (#16), down to the LEFT mandibular third molar (#17), and end at the RIGHT mandibular third molar (#32). Many individuals will have impacted third molars or have had their third molars extracted. Therefore, you will frequently begin counting at tooth #2.

LETTERS designate the 20 primary (deciduous) teeth (A–T). See Figure 54-2.

Other systems in use include the International Numbering System and the Palmer Notation Method.

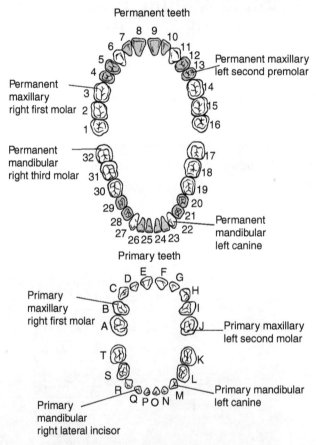

Figure 54-2 Universal numbering. Reproduced with permission from Tintinalli JE, Kelen GD, Stapczynski JS, et al. *Tintinalli's Emergency Medicine: A Comprehensive Study Guide.* 6th ed. New York, NY: McGraw-Hill; 2004. Fig. 242–2.

○ **What are the parts of the tooth and its housing?**

1. <u>Enamel</u>—hard outer highly mineralized covering of the tooth crown composed mainly of hydroxyapatite.

2. <u>Dentin</u>—less mineralized structure than enamel that also includes organic material and water containing microtubules. When exposed, teeth become sensitive.

3. <u>Cementum</u>—Located only on the root, it covers the dentin. It is less calcified than enamel or dentin and attaches to the periodontal ligament.

4. <u>Pulp</u>—neurovascular component of teeth also containing connective tissue and cells (odontoblasts). Pulpal inflammation or exposure causes significant pain.

5. <u>Periodontal ligament</u>—connective tissue that attaches cementum to bone, allowing for movement of the tooth in the socket as well as proprioception.

6. <u>Alveolar bone</u>—made of cortical and cancellous bone.

See Figure 54-3.

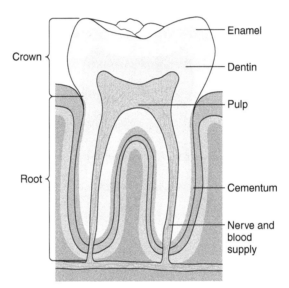

Figure 54-3 Anatomy of the tooth and surrounding structures. Reproduced from Stone CK, Humphries RL. *Current Diagnosis & Treatment: Emergency Medicine*, 2008. 6th ed. New York, NY: McGraw-Hill. Fig. 30–11.

○ **Describe the following anatomic terms used in describing surfaces of teeth:**

1. FACIAL: part of tooth that faces the lips or cheeks. Can be further subdivided into:

   a. LABIAL: facial surface of ANTERIOR teeth (incisors and canines).

   b. BUCCAL: facial surface of POSTERIOR teeth (premolars and molars).

2. PALATAL: surface of maxillary teeth that face the palate.

3. LINGUAL: describes both maxillary and mandibular surfaces that face the tongue.

4. MESIAL: TOWARD the dental midline.

5. DISTAL: AWAY from the dental midline.

6. OCCLUSAL: the chewing surface of the POSTERIOR teeth.

7. INCISAL: the biting surface of the ANTERIOR teeth.

See Figure 54-4.

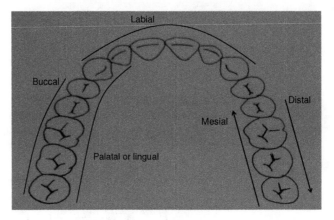

Figure 54-4 Surfaces of teeth.

○   **Describe the following dental terminology.**

CORONAL: refers to the crown of the tooth, which is the portion of the tooth which is visible in the mouth. "Coronal" can be used as a directional term. For example, the incisal edge of an incisor is coronal to the gingiva.

APICAL: the apex of the tooth is at the root end. The root is the portion of the tooth which is housed in the alveolar bone. The term "apical" can also be used as a directional term. For example, starting at the incisal edge and moving apically, one would reach the root of the tooth.

CINGULUM: the cingulum is a bulge on the lingual surface of anterior teeth.

HEIGHT OF CONTOUR: all teeth have heights of contour (crests of curvature) which refer to the location of greatest contour of the crown of the tooth.

See Figure 54-5.

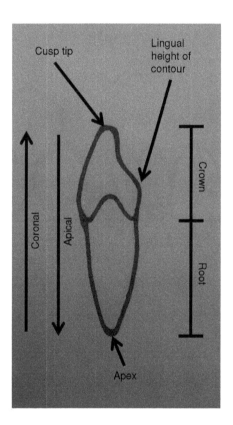

Figure 54-5 Tooth #24 profile view.

○ **Describe the following occlusal relationships.**

  1. Overbite: VERTICAL overlap between the maxillary and mandibular central incisal edges. See Figure 54-6A.

  2. Overjet: HORIZONTAL distance between the maxillary and mandibular central incisal edges. See Figure 54-6B.

  3. Crossbite: a NEGATIVE overJET relationship (mandibular teeth FACIAL to maxillary teeth). See Figure 54-6C.

  4. Openbite: a NEGATIVE overBITE relationship—a VERTICAL opening between maxillary and mandibular teeth incisal edges/occlusal surfaces. See Figure 54-6D.

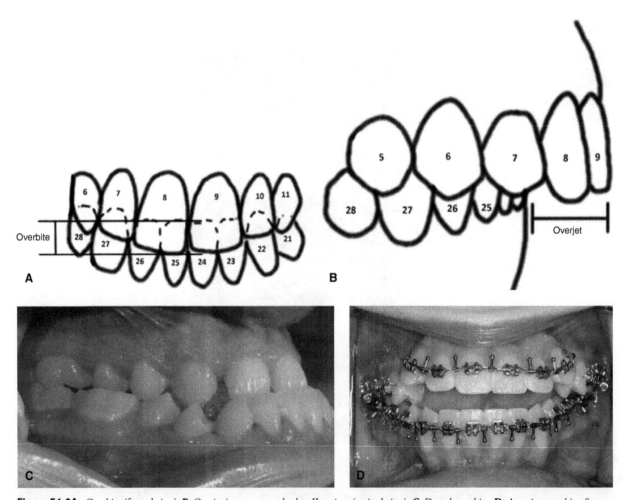

Figure 54-6A: Overbite (frontal view). **B:** Overjet in a severe angle class II patient (sagittal view). **C:** Dental crossbite. **D:** Anterior openbite. See Color insert.

○ **As part of your facial cosmetic treatment plan on a 42-year-old female patient, you have referred her to an orthodontist to correct her malposed teeth. The patient has a normal skeletal structure and an appropriate size and space for her full dentition. The orthodontist will place the patient in a normal overbite and overjet. What angle classification would you expect her final occlusal outcome to be?**

Class I. Angle classification provides a way to describe the patient's inter-arch occlusal relationship by defining inter-arch first molar relationship. A maxillary first molar has four cusp tips. The mesiobuccal cusp is the most anterior (mesial) and lateral (buccal) cusp. The mandibular molar has a buccal groove visible which appears to halve the lateral surface of the tooth. In class I molar occlusion, the mesiobuccal cusp tip of the maxillary first molar will lie on the buccal groove of the mandibular first molar when the patient is biting down and is completely in occlusion (maximum intercuspation). See Figure 54-7A.

In class II molar occlusion, the mesiobuccal cusp tip of the maxillary first molar will be **anterior** to the buccal groove of the mandibular first molar. In many cases, this can be interpreted as **anteriorly** placed maxillary teeth in relation to the mandibular teeth potentially leading to an increased overjet. Often, a class II occlusion is the result of **maxillary hyperplasia** or **mandibular hypoplasia.** See Figure 54-7B.

In class III molar occlusion, the mesiobuccal cusp tip of the maxillary tooth will be **posterior** to the buccal groove of the mandibular tooth. In many cases, this can be interpreted as **posteriorly** placed maxillary teeth in relation to the mandibular teeth potentially leading to a negative overjet (anterior crossbite). Often, a class III occlusion is the result of **maxillary hypoplasia** or **mandibular hyperplasia.** See Figure 54-7C.

More generally, a malocclusion is defined as any misalignment of the teeth or imperfect relationship between the two dental arches. Class II and class III angle classifications are specific types of malocclusion. Crowding and spacing within a single dental arch can also cause more localized malocclusions.

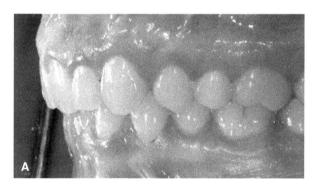
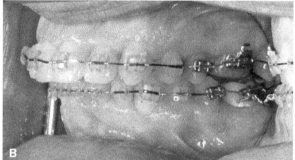
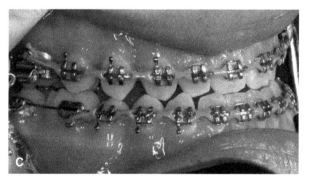

Figure 54-7 A: Angle class I molar relationship. **B:** Angle class II molar relationship—note the anterior overjet and maxillary canine anterior to the mandibular canine. **C:** Angle class III molar relationship—note the negative anterior overjet. See Color insert.

○ **Describe the difference between class II division 1 and class II division 2 malocclusion.**

Both have class II relationships. Division 1 patients have minimal crowding of maxillary teeth with a resultant large overjet of the incisors, while class II division 2 patients demonstrate incisors that crowd in such a way so as to diminish the overjet. The central incisors are lingually inclined ("shoveled") and the lateral incisors are facially malpositioned ("flared").

○ **Describe how the cingulum and height of contour contribute to the successful placement of Erich archbars.**

Tighten the wire while apical to the height of contour.

Think of the height of contour as the "waist" of the tooth. In anterior teeth, whose crowns appear triangular in shape when viewed in profile, the height of contour is at the neck of the tooth at the cingulum. It is critical to have the interdental wire apical to this cingulum.

○ **You are assessing a 32-year-old female patient who sustained a facial trauma. The patient had a helmeted motorcycle collision and fell off her vehicle after striking road debris at low speed. She didn't sustain any critical injuries, but was found to have an anterior openbite.**

○ **What signs in her occlusion would help you distinguish a preexisting openbite?**

Mamelons.

Mamelons are ridges on the incisal edges of teeth that are generally worn off of adult teeth due to occlusion and contact; however, they are often present in patients with open bites or severe class III malocclusions due to the lack of occlusal contact. If the patient above (adult) had mamelons, then it is safe to assume that she had a preexisting open bite. See Figure 54-8.

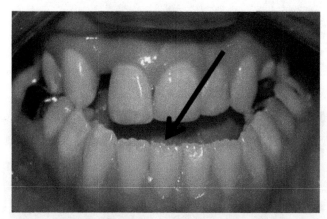

Figure 54-8 Mamelons in an anterior open bite. See Color insert.

In a trauma patient, the surfaces of the teeth will act as a guide to the pretraumatic occlusion. Other wear patterns or wear facets may also be helpful in identifying where the pretraumatic occlusion needs to be set. A patient's occlusion many times will resemble a jigsaw puzzle which needs to be snugly fit back together.

Causes of open bite:

1. Tongue thrust.
2. Foreign object placed chronically between teeth (i.e., thumb, pencil).
3. Trauma—often causing premature contacts on the posterior teeth.
4. Orthodontics—prior to orthognathic surgery.

○ **When assessing a patient's occlusion, you ask her to bite into maximum intercuspation. While gently holding this bite, you then ask her to slide her mandible to the right. On observation of this slide, you see that her posterior teeth are no longer in occlusion and that her canines are the only teeth touching. What do you call this phenomenon?**

Canine guidance.

Canine guidance is a characteristic of an ideal functional occlusion. In lateral excursions of the mandible, a patient with canine guidance will no longer occlude on the molars and premolars (immediate disclusion). In this lateral slide, the lower canine ramps against the upper canine and provides the opening of the bite.

Group function occurs when the premolars and molars continue to touch while the patient is performing the same lateral excursions. This has the potential to be traumatic and can cause wear on the posterior teeth.

Anterior guidance is an occlusal phenomenon which occurs when a patient protrudes his jaw while maintaining occlusal (or incisal) pressure. The anterior teeth (incisors and canines) ramp off each other and create posterior teeth disclusion.

○ **You are a local surgeon in a rural setting. A fight broke out at the local high school dance, and one of your patients in the ED received a punch to the face. Teeth 7, 8, 9, and 10 were avulsed and swallowed. You currently note that the buccal gingiva was also degloved on the buccal alveolus. When reapproximating the tissue, what structures will you suture together?**

The gingival papillae.

When adjacent teeth are in contact, healthy gingiva forms a scalloped margin between teeth. The collar of gingiva directly apical to the crown of the tooth is called the marginal gingiva.

The triangular gingival tissue between the crows of adjacent teeth is known at the gingival papilla or interdental papilla. Without the height of these papillae, unaesthetic "black triangles" form between the teeth. Care to reapproximate papilla in traumatic settings can prevent the formation of these empty spaces between the teeth.

See Figure 54-9.

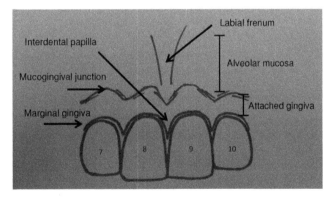

Figure 54-9 Gingival architecture.

○ **While doing an oral assessment on an intubated and sedated patient in the ICU you notice small quantities of blood in the oral cavity. The patient's RN states that there is bleeding after providing oral cares. You are unable to find any traumatic sources of bleeding, but you do note that multiple teeth are mobile and there is generalized erythema of the marginal gingiva. What is the likely source of the mobility and inflammation?**

Periodontal disease (gingivitis and periodontitis).

The two most common diseases involved with loss of teeth are caries and periodontal disease. With poor oral hygiene, bacterial load increases in the gingival sulcus around the teeth. This in turn starts an inflammatory process which ultimately leads to alveolar bone loss around the teeth and increases the depth of the gingival sulcus. Common findings include edematous rolled gingival borders, erythema, bleeding, and bone loss which shows the root surfaces of the teeth.

○   **A 12-year-old female patient with history of cleft palate was lost to follow up with your craniofacial practice. She also has not maintained follow ups with the remainder of the cleft lip and palate team. She returns for assessment with complaints of an oronasal fistula. She also has multiple malposed teeth with darkening and shadowing of the enamel surface at the points of crowding. What are these lesions?**

Carious lesions of the teeth.

Caries is a disease process attributed mainly to *Streptococcus mutans*, a normal oral inhabitant. Poor oral hygiene provides an opportunity for biofilm formation on the dentition. High-carbohydrate diet provides nutrients for the bacteria in the biofilm, and acid is created as a metabolic byproduct. This acid is what causes the erosion and destruction of the teeth. Carious lesions tend to start in locations where this biofilm is difficult to access, including at the contacts of teeth and otherwise crowded areas.

• • • **REFERENCES** • • •

Nelson SJ. *Wheeler's Dental Anatomy, Physiology, and Occlusion.* 10th ed. St. Louis, MO: Saunders; 2015.
Okeson JP. *Fundamentals of Occlusion and Temporomandibular Disorders.* 7th ed. St. Louis, MO: Mosby; 2012.

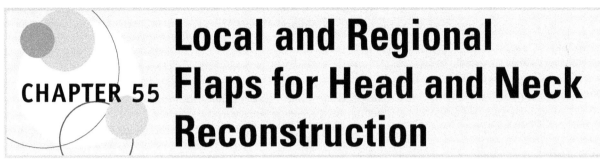

CHAPTER 55 Local and Regional Flaps for Head and Neck Reconstruction

Peter W. Henderson, MD, MBA and Evan Matros, MD, MMSc

● ● ● GENERAL RECONSTRUCTION PRINCIPLES ● ● ●

○ **What is the reconstructive ladder? What is the reconstructive elevator?**

The reconstructive ladder is the paradigm that dictates the traditional progression from least to most complex intervention for a given clinical scenario. The usual sequence moves from delayed wound healing to primary closure, to skin graft, to adjacent tissue transfer, to regional flap, and finally to free flap.

The "reconstructive elevator" is the concept that there are clinical scenarios which may benefit from performing a more complex procedure, "skipping" lower rungs on the ladder. Increasingly sophisticated microsurgical techniques can potentially allow for enhanced function with less donor site morbidity. For example, a superior outcome may be achieved with a free anterolateral thigh flap rather than combining a hemi-gastrocnemius and hemi-soleus for a large proximal and mid-tibial defect.

○ **What are the three basic modes of tissue movement of local flaps?**

Advancement, transposition, and rotation.

A rotation flap is a semicircular flap of skin and subcutaneous tissue that rotates about a pivot point into an immediately adjacent defect. A transposition flap is designed as a rectangle or square and crosses over areas of skin/subcutaneous tissue. In contrast, advancement flaps move directly forward without any rotation or lateral movement.

○ **What is difference between random pattern, axial pattern, and perforator pedicle flaps?**

A random pattern flap has no single dominant vascular supply, instead just random blood supply running through the various vascular plexuses (subepidermal, dermal, subdermal, subcutaneous, suprafascial, subfascial). Because of the limited blood supply, the length:width ratio is limited to 1–2:1.

An axial pattern flap contains a known vascular supply that is intentionally oriented longitudinally within a flap, thereby increasing the potential length:width ratio.

A perforator flap is based on one or more of the vessels that perforate either muscle or connective tissue in order to supply the skin and subcutaneous tissue used for the reconstruction. The axial vessel does not need to be sacrificed.

○ **What are Langer's lines? What are the relaxed skin tension lines? Are there any points at which they are in conflict?**

Langer's lines are defined by the direction that skin splits when pierced with a spike. It corresponds to the direction of collagen fibers in the dermis.

Relaxed skin tension lines (RSTL) run perpendicular to the direction of muscle contraction. It is thought that orienting incisions along RSTL results in improved cosmetic outcomes.

In most areas of the face, the Langer's lines and RSTL are in harmony; however, they are in conflict at the nasal supratip, the lateral canthi, and the glabella.

○ **Which anatomic landmarks of the head and neck do not tolerate asymmetry or distortion?**

Hairline, eyebrows, eyelids, medial and lateral canthi, nasal tip, nasal alae, earlobes, philtrum, vermillion, and oral commissures.

These landmarks do not tolerate distortion for a variety of reasons. In some instances, structures are paired, highlighting differences between the right and left side. In other cases, there are fixed proportions between two structures which cannot either exceed or be less than normal anthropometric proportions. For example, the nasolabial angle of the nasal tip rotation must be within a small range before abnormalities become obvious.

○ **What is a Burow triangle?**

Advancing a skin flap can result in excess bunching on either side of the flap's base. This excess, which lies in the skin immediately adjacent to the flap's base, results from a length discrepancy between the moving flap edge and the stationary adjacent skin. It can be excised as a triangle called a Burow triangle. A Burow triangle may also be excised along the outer edge of a rotational flap. Burow triangles often do not need to be excised in the scalp since they are often covered by hair and frequently become less prominent over time.

○ **What is a bilobed flap? Describe the key points of its design.**

The bilobed flap is a double transposition flap that fills a circular defect with a primary flap, and then transposes a secondary flap into the primary flap defect to recruit lax tissue from farther away than a single transposition flap would allow. The tension is distributed across both transpositions.

1. The primary flap should be the same size as the defect, and slightly longer because the flap will shorten as it is transposed.

2. Position the secondary flap in an area of laxity. For the nose, this is usually a vertically oriented pennant placed at the sidewall or dorsum. A horizontal secondary flap closure will elevate the nasal tip.

3. The secondary flap should be half the width of the primary flap.

See Figure 55-1.

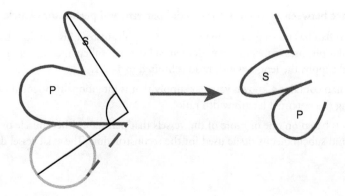

Figure 55-1 Bilobed flap.

○ **What is the maximum angle of transposition when using a bilobed flap?**

According to the Zitelli modification, the maximum angle of transposition is 90 to 100 degrees (45–50 degrees per lobe). The original bilobed flap described by Esser was rotated a total of 180 degrees, but resulted in excessive tension on the skin closure.

○ **What is a rhomboid flap? Describe the key points in its design.**

The rhomboid flap is a transposition flap that fills a rhomboidal defect with a matching adjacent rhomboidal flap. Circular defects can be made rhomboidal by excising a small amount of additional tissue.

1. The defect must be a rhomboid with 60- and 120-degree angles.
2. The sides of the defect should be equal in length and parallel. Flap dimensions should be the same size and shape as the defect.
3. Although four possible rhomboid flaps are available for any defect, the flap should be chosen based on location of laxity, scar direction, and vascularity.

See Figure 55-2.

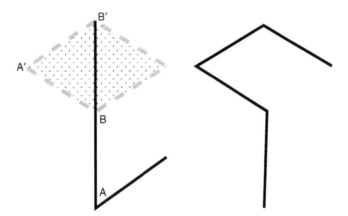

Figure 55-2 Rhomboid flap.

○ **How can a large circular defect be closed with rhomboid flaps?**

Conversion to a hexagon allows closure with three rhomboid flaps from the perimeter.

○ **How does the Dufourmentel flap differ from the Limberg rhomboid flap?**

The Dufourmentel flap uses a smaller degree of transposition and can thus be used for defects with angles up to 90 degrees. In Figure 55-3, C-F is oriented to bisect A-C-D, and E-F is parallel to D-B.

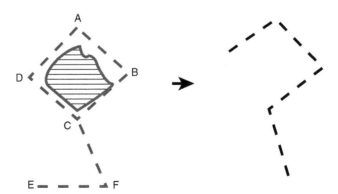

Figure 55-3 Dufourmentel flap.

○   **Describe the design of the V-Y advancement flap.**

The V-Y advancement flap is designed with the open side of the "V" adjacent to the defect. Flap length is approximately 1.5 to 2 times the defect length. After the flap is advanced into the defect, the resultant donor area is closed as a line which appears as a "Y."

○   **In addition to filling defects, how else can a V-Y advancement flap be used?**

A V-Y advancement flap can be used to lengthen structures such as the columella, and release tension in areas without a defect. The "V" incision is placed with the open side facing the direction of lengthening or excess tension. See Figure 55-4.

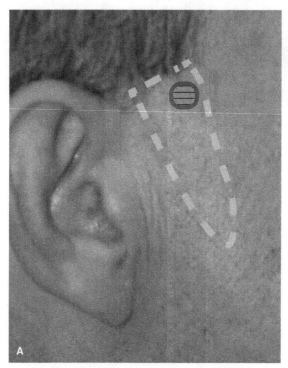 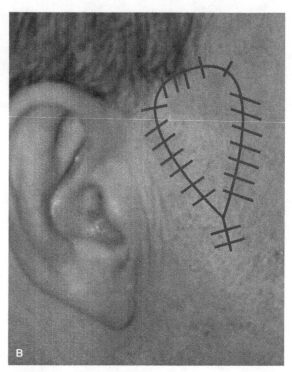

Figure 55-4 V-Y advancement flap.

○ **Describe the A-to-T or O-to-T flap.**

The A-to-T or O-to-T flap is a double advancement flap that can be used to close triangular or circular defects. The arms of the resultant "T" lie at the base of the triangular defect or tangent to the circular defect. See Figure 55-5.

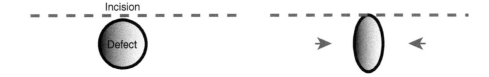

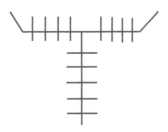

Figure 55-5 "A-to-T" or "O-to-T" flap.

○ **What is the total area that should be CPT-coded for a local rotational flap measuring 25 cm² to cover a cheek defect measuring 4 cm in diameter?**

For adjacent tissue transfers, the area to be coded is the sum of the primary defect and flap area. The primary defect in this case measures 13 cm² ($A = \pi r^2$), and the flap area measures 25 cm², for a total of 38 cm².

● ● ● **NASAL RECONSTRUCTION** ● ● ●

○ **What is the blood supply to the external nose?**

1. External carotid artery → facial artery → angular artery → **lateral nasal artery**

2. External carotid artery → facial artery → superior labial artery → **columellar branch**

3. External carotid artery → internal maxillary artery → **infraorbital artery**

4. Internal carotid artery → ophthalmic artery → anterior ethmoidal artery → **external nasal branch**

5. Internal carotid artery → ophthalmic artery → **dorsal nasal artery** (anastomoses with the lateral nasal artery)

○ **What is the innervation to the external nose? To the internal nose?**

External: Infratrochlear nerve (radix), infraorbital nerve (sidewalls), anterior ethmoid nerve—external branch (tip, alae)

Internal: Anterior ethmoid nerve—internal branch (septum, internal nasal walls), nasopalatine nerve (septum), lesser palatine nerve (nasal cavity)

○ **What are the two general contour classes into which the nasal subunits fall? And what is the ideal reconstructive element for each class?**

Convex (e.g., nasal tip and alae) and flat (e.g., sidewalls). Convexities are best replaced by flaps, which contract spherically, whereas flat areas can be replaced by full-thickness skin grafts, which contract in a linear manner.

○ **What are the three conceptual layers that must be considered when formulating a plan for nasal reconstruction?**

Lining (mucosa), support (cartilage), and coverage (skin).

○ **What are the differences in skin quality between the different nasal subunits?**

The skin of the dorsum and sidewalls tends to be thin and smooth, while the skin of the tip and alae is dense and sebaceous.

○ **How many aesthetic subunits compromise the external nose? How much of any given subunit must be lost in order to recommend removal of the entire subunit during reconstruction?**

Nine subunits (paired sidewall, paired alae, paired soft triangles, dorsum, tip, columella). Of note, some will include the nasal root as the tenth subunit.

If >50% of any given subunit is missing, some recommend removal of the entire subunit leads to be a better aesthetic result. See Figure 55-6.

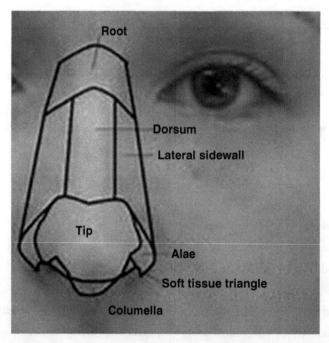

Figure 55-6 Aesthetic subunits of the nose.

○ **Is healing by secondary intention an appropriate option for management of nasal defects?**

Healing by secondary intention may be acceptable for smaller defects of the upper two-thirds of the nose, as well as neighboring areas, including the glabella and medial canthal region. It is generally unacceptable for defects of the lower nose, including the tip, ala, rim, and soft triangle, where contracture results in significant distortion and resultant skin quality is unsatisfactory.

○ **What are potential donor sites for full-thickness skin grafting of nasal defects?**

Preauricular, postauricular, and supraclavicular skin provide the best color and quality match for nasal skin.

○ **When may a superficial nasal defect be closed by a local flap?**

Defects of less than 1.5 cm can generally be filled with local flaps from the relatively mobile and pliable skin of the nasal sidewall.

○ **What are the indications for using a single-lobed flap such as a banner flap on the nose?**

Single-lobed flaps may be used in defects less than 1.5 cm in the upper two-thirds of the nose where the thin and pliable skin provides better aesthetic results than a skin graft. In the lower thirds of the nose, transposition of a single-lobed flap through a large arc can distort the ala or tip.

○ **What are the indications for using a bilobed flap in nasal reconstruction?**

Lower third nasal defects <1.5 cm in size. Typically a laterally based flap is used for nasal tip defects, whereas a medial-based flap is used for the ala.

○ **What layer should undermining for a bilobed flap in the nose be performed?**

Submuscular (superficial to the perichondrium and periosteum).

○ **Describe the nasolabial flap.**

The nasolabial flap is designed with its medial edge in the nasolabial crease to hide the resultant scar in the crease. It can be superiorly or inferiorly based and can be performed in one stage (island flap) or two stages (pedicled flap requiring delayed division).

○ **What is the blood supply of the nasolabial flap?**

Perforators from the facial artery and angular artery supply the inferiorly and superiorly based nasolabial flaps, respectively. It is considered to be a random flap.

○ **What are some indications for the superiorly and inferiorly based nasolabial flaps?**

Superiorly based flaps are well suited for large defects (1.5–2.5 cm) of the nasal ala, dorsum, and sidewall. Inferiorly based flaps are more suited for the reconstruction of the upper lip and oral cavity.

○ **What are some problems with using the nasolabial flap for nasal alar reconstruction?**

Potential mismatch between cheek and nasal skin color and texture. Loss of the concave border between the cheek and ala.

○ **When can the cheek be used for nasal reconstruction?**

Cheek advancement flaps can be used for nasal sidewall defects (~1.5 cm). However, doing so can lead to a loss of distinction between the cheek and nose (a "bowstring" appearance). These flaps should be divided at a later stage intentionally creating a scar at the junction between the aesthetic units.

○ **What is the dominant vascular supply to the frontonasal advancement flap?**

Otherwise known as a Rieger, dorsal nasal, or miter flap, the frontonasal advancement flap is supplied by the angular artery.

○   **What are the indications for use of the frontonasal flap?**

Transverse defects close to the midline in either the lower or middle third of the nose.

○   **What is a glabellar flap? What is the location of a defect best treated by a glabellar flap?**

The glabellar flap is essentially a vertically oriented banner (unilobe) flap harvested from the midline of the glabella. Glabellar flaps are good solutions for reconstructing defects of the medial canthi.

○   **The paramedian forehead flap is based on what vessel?**

The supratrochlear artery, with contributions from the rich anastomotic arcade comprised of the infratrochlear, dorsal nasal, and angular arteries.

○   **In which layers does the vascular pedicle to the paramedian forehead flap travel?**

The supraorbital and supratrochlear arteries travel just superficial to the periosteum initially, then emerge just deep to the dermis near the hairline. Therefore, the distal tip of the flap can be raised with just skin and a small amount of subcutaneous tissue, whereas near the orbital rims the dissection has to be carried deep to the frontalis, just above the periosteum.

○   **What are three ways to increase the length of a paramedian forehead flap?**

1. Extend the flap into hair-bearing scalp (requires secondary depilation procedure).
2. Extend the base of the flap up to 1.5 cm inferior to the superior orbital rim.
3. Score the frontalis muscle.

○   **What is the approach for dealing with the situation where an adequately sized paramedian forehead flap will leave too large a forehead defect for primary donor-site closure?**

Most paramedian forehead flap donor sites contract adequately with time and heal by secondary intention or can be easily camouflaged with a skin graft. Do not compromise the reconstruction of the recipient site for the sake of the donor site.

○   **What are some options for nasal lining replacement?**

1. Redundant skin folded over from the coverage flap.
2. Skin graft.
3. Mucoperichondrial flap from the septum.
4. Rotational or advancement flap from residual vestibular lining.
5. Facial artery musculomucosal (FAMM) flap.
6. Free flap from the radial forearm or anterolateral thigh.

○   **What are three common donor sites for reconstructing the cartilaginous framework of the nose?**

The nasal septum, auricular conchal cartilage, and rib cartilage.

○   **What is the ideal soft-tissue donor for the reconstruction of a small isolated alar margin defect?**

Composite auricular graft.

○ **What reconstructive option for small composite defects of the ala provides the best aesthetic results?**

Composite grafts including cartilage from the ear. Ear grafts provide excellent color, texture, and structural match. In addition, it provides both extranasal skin and intranasal skin for lining.

○ **The alar wings do not normally contain cartilage; why must they be supported by cartilage when reconstructed?**

To provide support for the thin soft-tissue contour that normally is not stressed, but after reconstruction is subject to the centripetal contractile forces of healing.

○ **How big a defect can a composite auricular graft reliably fill? What limits this size?**

Because an auricular composite graft for alar rim reconstruction contacts the wound bed along an edge, rather than a broad surface, neovascularization is significantly limited and in turn limits graft size to approximately 1.5 cm. No portion of the graft should be more than 5 to 8 mm away from the nourishing wound bed.

○ **What are some treatments that can potentially augment survival of auricular composite grafts?**

1. Cooling in the first few days after grafting can reduce the metabolic rate of the graft sufficiently while neovascularization is initiated. However, after the first week, this can be detrimental to graft survival due to vasoconstriction.

2. Hyperbaric oxygen.

○ **Describe the progression in physical appearance of an auricular composite graft from hours to months after grafting.**

1. 6 to 8 hours—pale

2. First day or two—pink tinged

3. First week—cyanotic due to venous congestion

4. Second–fourth weeks—pink, then red

5. 6 months—normalization of color

○ **What is the best option for reconstructing the columella?**

While more complex reconstructive options, such as ascending helical auricular free flaps, may be necessary for more extensive defects, auricular composite grafts are a good first choice in most situations.

○ **What is the presumed etiology of rhinophyma? What is the best treatment?**

The exact etiology of rhinophyma is unknown, but it is thought to be related to rosacea resulting in a bulbous, pustular nose. Historically, it was associated with alcohol consumption, but this relationship has been refuted.

The optimal treatment is tangential excision and skin grafting (though other modalities such as ablative laser and mechanical dermabrasion have been reported).

• • • LIP RECONSTRUCTION • • •

○ **What is the blood supply to the lip?**

The inferior and superior labial arteries from the facial artery.

○ **What is the location of the facial artery relative to the masseter muscle?**

Anterior and superficial.

○ **What nerve is at risk for injury when exposing the facial artery adjacent to the masseter?**

Marginal mandibular branch of facial nerve (cranial nerve VII).

○ **Where does the inferior labial artery branch from the facial artery?**

2.5 cm lateral and 1.5 cm inferior to the oral commissure.

○ **What does the facial artery continue as in the midface?**

It ascends as the angular artery, which contributes lateral nasal branches to the ala that anastomose with the dorsal nasal artery, a branch of the ophthalmic artery. The facial and labial arteries communicate with the subdermal plexus through a dense population of musculocutaneous perforators.

○ **What is the sensory innervation to the lip?**

Infraorbital nerve (central portion of upper lip), mental nerve (central portion of lower lip), and buccal branch of V3 (commissures).

○ **Which two nerves may become nonfunctional following hemi-mandible resection?**

Marginal mandibular branch of facial nerve (cranial nerve VII): particularly vulnerable when elevating the cheek to expose the mandible.

Inferior alveolar nerve: sacrificed during the bony resection (the nerve runs within the body of the mandible).

○ **What muscles of facial expression are innervated on their superficial surface?**

The mentalis, levator anguli oris, and buccinator ("MLB").

○ **What are the goals of lip reconstruction?**

1. Skin cover/oral lining.
2. Reestablishment of vermillion.
3. Adequate stomal diameter.
4. Sensation.
5. Oral competence (normal oral sphincter function).

○ **Do the upper and lower lips contribute equally to oral competence?**

No, the upper lip does not contribute significantly to oral competence.

○ **What are the limits of primary closure of the lower lip in terms of tissue loss? What about the upper lip?**

Lower lip defects up to 40% can be closed primarily whereas upper lips defects of only 25% can be closed primarily without significant anatomical distortion.

○ **What is the difference between direct primary closure of the upper lip as opposed to the lower lip?**

The unique anatomic landmarks of the upper lip (Cupid's bow, philtral columns) make the upper lip less flexible than its lower counterpart for direct primary closure.

○ **What options are available for replacement of vermilion tissue?**

1. Healing by secondary intention
2. Mucosal advancement flaps
3. Vermilion lip switch
4. Two-stage tongue flap
5. Buccal mucosal advancement
6. FAMM flap

○ **What layers are included in a FAMM flap?**

Mucosa, submucosa, buccinator, the deep layer of orbicularis oris, and the facial artery.

○ **How does the FAMM flap differ from buccal mucosal advancement flaps and musculomucosal V-Y advancement flaps in terms of blood supply?**

The FAMM flap provides tissue with an axial blood supply, whereas the latter flaps have only random pattern blood supplies.

○ **What is the key concern in using intraoral mucosa for the reconstruction of dry vermilion?**

Chronic dry lips.

○ **What general strategies are used in lip reconstruction?**

1. Rotation-advancement of the remaining uninvolved lip peripheral to the defect
2. Lip-switch flaps

○ **What is lip-switching?**

Using tissue from one lip to reconstruct the other, based on the dual blood supply to the lips from the facial artery. The two main procedures that employ a lip-switch technique are the Abbe and Estlander flaps.

○ **What is the blood supply to the Abbe flap?**

Typically, the Abbe flap is performed on the lower lip to reconstruct the upper lip, in which case it is based on the inferior labial artery. The artery runs deep to the orbicularis muscle. On sagittal sectioning it lies at the level of the white roll.

○ **What are the indications for using an Abbe flap?**

Closure of philtral or paramedian defects not involving the commissure.

○ **How large should an Abbe flap be?**

The flap should measure one-half the width of the upper lip defect. In reconstructing the philtrum, the flap should be no larger than 10 mm wide and 15 mm long; some surgeons advocate an even smaller flap.

○ **How does the Estlander flap differ from the Abbe flap? What artery is it based on, and what is it used for?**

Estlander's derivation of the Abbe flap involves a triangular flap based on the contralateral labial artery. It provides coverage for defects involving the commissure. While the flap typically is taken from the upper lip to reconstruct lower lip defects, it can also be reversed to cover upper lip defects with lower lip tissue. The Estlander flap is a usually a single stage procedure, whereas the Abbe flap requires a second procedure for pedicle division.

○   **What is the Gillies fan flap used for?**

As a rotational advancement flap, the Gillies fan flap donates upper lip and cheek tissue to close large central lower lip defects. Several modifications of this original concept have been established. McGregor (1983) initially described a rectangular musculocutaneous flap similar to Gillies, but with a more narrow base and thus without the distortion of the modiolus. The Gillies flap can also be used for the reconstruction of upper lip defects. The name is derived from the flap shape and direction of movement which resembles the opening of a fan.

○   **Describe the Karapandzic flap and its indications.**

The Karapandzic flap is an innervated orbicularis oris composite flap designed with a circumoral incision camouflaged in the nasolabial folds. It is used to repair midline and total upper and lower lip defects.

○   **What is unique about the Karapandzic flap compared to the Abbe and Estlander flaps?**

The Karapandzic flap is innervated (the buccal branch of the facial nerve, and the buccal trigeminal sensory branches).

○   **When local or regional flaps are not available, what is the next step in lip reconstruction? What are some problems with those options?**

The free tissue of choice in lower-lip reconstruction is the radial forearm free flap with palmaris tendon for oral competence. In general, however, this is far from ideal compared to local or regional flaps due to flap bulk, difficulty in restoring oral competence, and poor aesthetic match. Because the upper lip does not contribute significantly to oral competence, there is even less reason to use free tissue in upper lip reconstruction.

○   **For each flap (Abbe, Modified Bernard-Burow, Estlander, Gillies, Karapandzic) describe the advantages and disadvantages.**

Abbe flap:
- Advantages—ideal for central defects of the upper lip (philtral), color match, and rapid reinnervation
- Disadvantages—pedicled flap configuration requiring secondary division, minor secondary vermilion discrepancies

Estlander flap:
- Advantages—optimal for reconstruction of lateral commissure defects
- Disadvantages—microstomia, ablation of the natural shape of the commissure

Gillies fan flap:
- Advantages—suitable for large lower lip defects
- Disadvantages—may reduce the aperture of the mouth similar to the Estlander flap, disrupts and displaces the modiolus, and distortion of the lip and lack of neural supply can lead to severe aesthetic deformities and oral incompetence

Karapandzic flap:
- Advantages—neurovascular rotational flap provides reconstruction with a competent oral sphincter
- Disadvantages—similar to the Gillies and Estlander flaps, distortion and displacement of the modiolus occurs

Modified Bernard–Burow flap:
- Advantages—scars are camouflaged within natural creases along alar base and sill, can be used for defects up to 80% when the flap is raised bilaterally.
- Disadvantages—displacement of philtral columns, distortion of nasolabial fold

○ **How much of the oral circumference must be lost in order to develop microstomia? What trade-offs must be considered when deciding between local or free tissue transfer for the reconstruction of large lip defects?**

Resection of >50% of the total lip circumference often results in functional microstomia.

Utilizing a free flap (radial forearm, etc.) introduces additional tissue, thereby reducing the likelihood of microstomia. The trade-off is absent sensation and poor oral competence with chronic drooling.

○ **What is the "whistling deformity," and what causes it? How can it be treated?**

The "whistling deformity" is a deficiency in the vertical length of the lip that prevents complete closure. A whistling sound may be heard during normal respiration.

If it does occur, the most important element of reconstruction is repairing the orbicularis oris muscle. In addition, some sort of vermillion lengthening procedure can be performed (V-Y, z-plasty, etc.).

• • • CHEEK RECONSTRUCTION • • •

○ **What is the sensory and motor innervation to the cheek?**

Sensory: V2 and V3 branches of the trigeminal nerve (cranial nerve V).

Motor: Zygomatic, buccal, and marginal mandibular branches of the facial nerve (cranial nerve VII), and V3 branch of trigeminal nerve (cranial nerve V) which innervate the temporalis and masseter muscles.

○ **What are the aesthetic zones of the cheek?**

Suborbital, preauricular, and buccal mandibular.

○ **Which method creates the earliest postoperative smile restoration following facial nerve sacrifice: temporalis myoplasty, fascia lata sling, cross facial nerve graft, or V3 nerve transfer? Which creates the second-earliest?**

Earliest: Temporalis myoplasty.

Second-earliest: V3 nerve (nerve to masseter) transfer.

○ **What are the best options for reconstructing small, medium, and large cheek defects?**

1. Small: Local flaps (rhomboid, nasolabial, V-Y, banner/unilobed, bilobed flaps)
2. Medium: Cervicofacial flaps (Mustarde)
3. Large: Cervicopectoral flaps

○ **What are the indications for tissue expansion in cheek reconstruction?**

Because large skin grafts on the face result in poor color match and overall appearance, they are generally undesirable. A skin graft can be placed as a biologic dressing, followed by tissue expander placement, and finally a cervicofacial flap closure. Alternatively, for benign processes, such as AVM or congenital nevus, the tissue expander can be placed first, with immediate reconstruction at the time of tumor excision.

○ **Describe the submental flap.**

The submental flap is a musculocutaneous platysma flap based laterally on the submental artery. Blood supply is the submental branch of the facial artery that runs parallel to the anterior belly of the digastric muscle. It provides skin that is a good match for facial skin. In men, since this is typically hair-bearing skin, it can be advantageous for the reconstruction of hair-bearing areas.

○ **What are the indications for using the submental flap?**

1. Extraoral defects of the lower face, midface, and even inferior upper face.

2. Intraoral defects as far posteriorly as the base of the tongue and as far superiorly as the palate.

3. Combined intraoral and extraoral defects, by skin grafting the undersurface of the platysma muscle.

4. Since the flap comes from hair-bearing skin (in men), it can be used for the reconstruction of hair-bearing areas such as the upper lip.

○ **What is a contraindication to using the submental flap in head and neck tumor reconstruction?**

Ipsilateral neck dissection (excision of the submandibular gland usually results in ligation of the terminal branch of the facial artery).

○ **Describe the Juri cervicofacial flap.**

Juri's modification of the cervicofacial flap is a rotational flap, based inferomedially on the facial and submental arteries, used primarily to cover upper medial cheek defects. The incision extends laterally from the defect parallel to the zygomatic arch, turns inferiorly along the preauricular fold, then extends inferior to the ear before turning posteriorly along the retroauricular hairline. The flap is then rotated superomedially.

○ **What is the major advantage and disadvantage of using inferolaterally based cervicofacial flaps?**

Inferolaterally based flaps tend to exhibit less risk of necrosis. However, the incision is more anterior and medial in the face and neck. Where the incision crosses the mandibular border, a Z-plasty can serve to prevent later development of contracture.

○ **In what layer is the dissection of cervicofacial flaps carried out?**

Subcutaneous (staying superficial to superficial musculoaponeurotic system [SMAS] will reduce likelihood of facial nerve injury).

○ **Can the dissection be carried out in a different layer, and what is the advantage in doing so?**

Some authors advocate dissection of cervicofacial flaps in a sub-SMAS layer to improve the blood supply, especially in smokers and patients with poor skin quality (though this increases the risk of injury to the facial nerve).

○ **What complication can result from excessive tension at the malar eminence when using cervicofacial and cervicopectoral flaps?**

Lower lid ectropion can occur if downward tension is placed on the soft tissue of the malar eminence. To prevent this, anchor sutures can be placed in the periosteum of the zygomatic arch. In some instances, a lateral canthopexy can help as well.

○ **How can the frontal branch of the facial nerve be avoided when anchoring sutures to the periosteum of the zygomatic arch?**

The frontal branch does not cross the arch more than 3.5 cm anterior to the external auditory canal. By staying anterior to this, injury to the frontal branch can be avoided.

○ **Describe the cervicopectoral flap.**

The cervicopectoral flap is a myocutaneous flap based medially on anterior thoracic perforators off the internal mammary artery, used for defects of the lower lateral cheek. The incision extends from the defect posteriorly, passes inferior to the ear along the retroauricular hair line, travels inferiorly parallel to the anterior border of the trapezius, crosses the clavicle at the deltopectoral groove, and then can be extended a variable distance inferiorly. See Figure 55-7.

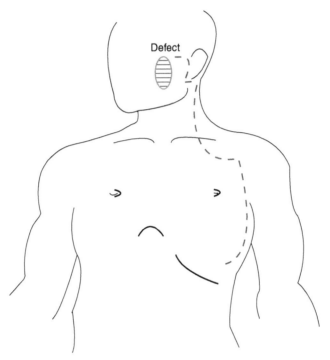

Figure 55-7 Cervicopectoral flap.

○ **In what layer is the dissection of cervicopectoral flaps carried out?**

Subcutaneously in the face, subplatysmal in the neck, and deep to the anterior pectoral fascia on the chest.

○ **What is the upper limit of defects that can be reliably covered by cervicopectoral flaps?**

Cervicopectoral flaps extending significantly above a line drawn between the tragus and oral commissure have increasing risk of necrosis. However, coverage of total cheek defects with extended cervicopectoral flaps has been described.

○ **What is the blood supply to the deltopectoral flap?**

Internal mammary artery and thoracoacromial artery (pectoral branch). Though not described as such when published by Bakamjian, the deltopectoral flap was one of the first axial (nonrandom) flaps.

○ **Describe the internal mammary artery perforator (IMAP) flap?**

The IMAP is an islandized variation on the deltopectoral flap based on only one internal mammary artery perforator. It provides thin, well-vascularized, and reliable tissue with a wide arc of rotation for coverage of cutaneous neck, pharyngeal, and tracheostomal defects.

○ **What is the blood supply to the temporalis muscle flap?**

The temporalis muscle is supplied by the anterior and posterior deep temporal branches of the internal maxillary artery, as well as the middle temporal artery—a branch of the superficial temporal artery. The temporalis muscle flap is based on the anterior and posterior deep temporal branches.

○ **What are some indications for the temporalis muscle flap in head and neck reconstruction?**

As a turnover flap, the temporalis can be used as intraoral lining for the posterior oral cavity or the nasopharynx, as well as coverage of the orbit, superior maxilla, and ear.

○ **What are two ways to increase the pedicle length of the temporalis muscle flap?**

   1. Temporary removal of the zygomatic arch.

   2. Disinsertion of the temporalis muscle from the coronoid process.

○ **What is the blood supply to the sternocleidomastoid muscle flap?**

The sternocleidomastoid (SCM) muscle is supplied by branches from the suprascapular, occipital, and superior thyroid arteries. The SCM flap can be based on either the occipital or suprascapular arteries, but it is relatively unfavorable for transposition because of its segmental blood supply (Mathes-Nahai Type IV, similar to the sartorius muscle).

○ **What is the blood supply to the platysma turnover flap?**

The platysma is a type II muscle supplied by the submental, superior thyroid, and transverse cervical arteries. The platysma musculocutaneous turnover flap is based on the submental artery.

○ **What are the indications for the platysma turnover flap?**

Intraoral lining, lip, and lower midface reconstruction.

○ **What is the vascular supply to the trapezius muscle?**

The trapezius has three portions: the upper, middle or transverse, and lower. The upper portion is supplied by the occipital artery. The middle or transverse portion is supplied by the superficial cervical artery, a branch of the transverse cervical artery. The lower portion is supplied by the deep branch of the transverse cervical artery (often referred to as the dorsal scapular artery) and intercostal vessels. The origin of the arteries supplying the trapezius muscle is highly variable, arising from different vascular trunks.

○ **What are the indications for a pedicled lower trapezius flap?**

The lower trapezius flap is typically used to reconstruct posterior cervical and occipital defects. When based on the superficial cervical artery, the large arc of rotation permits the flap to reach as far as the orbit, but requires division of the middle and upper trapezius. In contrast, when based on the deep branch of the transverse cervical artery the arc of rotation is more limited; however, the musculocutaneous island can be planned more distally on the back.

○ **Which free flaps are commonly used in cheek reconstruction? How could you make your own free flap for cheek coverage?**

Thin donor sites, such as radial forearm, scapular, parascapular, and anterolateral thigh are commonly used in cheek reconstruction. For very large recipients sites (e.g., total facial burn), a tissue-expanded free flap (with or without prefabrication) can be used.

• • • SCALP AND FOREHEAD RECONSTRUCTION • • •

○ **What are the layers of the scalp?**

Easy pneumonic is "SCALP": Skin, subcutaneous Connective tissue, Galea Aponeurotica, Loose areolar tissue, and Pericranium.

○ **What is the blood supply to the scalp?**

There are five paired arteries to the scalp:

1. Supraorbital artery from the internal carotid artery (ICA)
2. Supratrochlear artery from ICA
3. Superficial temporal artery from the external carotid artery (ECA)
4. Occipital artery from ECA
5. Posterior auricular artery from ECA

○ **How many vessels are necessary for scalp survival?**

Replantation with survival of the entire scalp has been performed based on a single vessel. This is more likely to be possible with the dominant vessels (superficial temporal and occipital) than the posterior auricular artery.

○ **In what layer does the frontal branch of the facial nerve run?**

The frontal branch runs within the superficial temporal fascia, into the frontalis muscle just above the orbital rim.

○ **What else is the galea aponeurotica continuous with, outside the scalp and forehead?**

The temporoparietal fascia or superficial temporal fascia laterally, and the SMAS in the face.

○ **Which anatomic layers are a continuation of the calvarial periosteum outside the scalp and forehead?**

The deep temporal fascia, which separates into superficial and deep layers at the temporal fusion line and envelops the superficial temporal fat pad.

○ **The forehead and scalp are often considered together in reconstruction due to their similarities. What are the two major differences?**

1. The scalp is hair bearing.
2. The frontalis muscle in the forehead is continuous with the galea and occipitalis muscle in the scalp.

○ **What size forehead defects can be effectively closed by local flaps?**

For defects up to 3 cm in diameter, options include direct closure or local flaps such as rhomboid, banner, bilobed, V-Y, A-T/O-T, and shutter flaps.

○ **How can additional length be gained in direct closure or local flaps of the forehead and scalp?**

Flap length can be extended a small amount by scoring the galea perpendicular to the axis of the flap at 5- to 10-mm intervals.

○ **What is the Orticochea scalp reconstruction technique?**

In the pre-free flap era, the Orticochea technique was the best option for very large scalp defects. Utilizing either 3 or 4 extensive flaps, Orticochea himself described it as "peeling a banana" and then reconfiguring such that the defect was closed.

○ **How should rotation-advancement scalp flaps be designed?**

Moderate-sized defects of the scalp up to 9 cm can be closed with adequately designed rotation-advancement flaps.

1. Attempt to design the flap so that both primary and secondary defects can be closed directly; this may not be possible with defects larger than 6 cm.
2. Incorporate at least one major vessel in the flap.
3. Keep the flap base as wide as possible.
4. Flap length should be at least five times the diameter of the defect.
5. Bevel the incision in the direction of hair follicles to prevent incisional alopecia.
6. Score galea as needed to gain additional length; make back cuts conservatively.

○ **What local flaps provide the best aesthetic results for small- and moderate-sized forehead defects?**

Bipedicled H flaps, A-to-T and O-to-T flaps, and V-to-Y flaps. Rotational-advancement flaps can be designed with incisions along the hairline and superior eyebrow border.

○ **What options are available for defects larger than 6 cm in which the rotation-advancement flap donor site likely cannot be closed directly?**

Skin grafting is possible for defects with intact pericranium, or when bone has been prepared with burring or removal of the outer table. Tissue expansion can also provide tissue for closure of moderate-sized defects. These options may not be viable in irradiated scalp tissue, in which case free tissue transfer may be necessary even for moderate-sized defects.

○ **Which free flap is most commonly used in scalp reconstruction and why?**

The most commonly used flap is a latissimus dorsi, raised either as a musculocutaneous flap or more commonly as a muscle flap with split-thickness skin graft coverage. This flap has a large surface area and is very thin; for men the skin graft can appear quite natural, and for women the thin flap facilitates wearing a wig.

○ **What is the Crane principle?**

Temporary coverage of a forehead defect with a scalp flap to regenerate adequate subcutaneous tissue for skin grafting. In a second stage, the flap is returned to its donor site, and a skin graft is placed on the new subcutaneous tissue of the original defect.

● ● ● **REFERENCES** ● ● ●

Austen WG Jr, Parrett BM, Taghinia A, Wolfort SF, Upton J. The subcutaneous cervicofacial flap revisited. *Ann Plast Surg.* 2009; 62(2):149–153.

Buncke HJ, Rose EH, Brownstein MJ, Chater NL. Successful replantation of two avulsed scalps by microvascular anastomoses. *Plast Reconstr Surg.* 1978;61(5):666–672.

Burget GC, Menick FJ. The subunit principle in nasal reconstruction. *Plast Reconst Surg.* 1985;76(2):239–247.

Crosby MA. Nasal reconstruction. In: Janis JE, ed. *Essentials of Plastic Surgery.* St Louis, MO: Quality Medical Publishing; 2007: 295–306.

Davies JC, Agur AM, Fatah AY. Anatomic landmarks for localization of the branches of the facial nerve. *Clin Anatomy.* 2013;1(4): 33–40.

Gosman, AA. Basics of flaps. In: Janis JE, ed. *Essentials of Plastic Surgery.* St Louis, MO: Quality Medical Publishing; 2007:20–38.

Gottlieb LJ, Krieger LM. From the reconstructive ladder to the reconstructive elevator. *Plast Reconstr Surg.* 1994;93(7):1503–1504.

Guo L, Pribaz JR, Pribaz JJ. Nasal reconstruction with local flaps: a simple algorithm for management of small defects. *Plast Reconstr Surg.* 2008;122(5):130e–139e.

Haas F, Weiglein A, Schwarzl F, Scharnagl E. The lower trapezius musculocutaneous flap from pedicled to free flap: anatomical basis and clinical applications based on the dorsal scapular artery. *Plast Reconstr Surg.* 2004;113(6):1580–1590.

Heniford BW, Bailin PL, Marsico RE Jr. Field guide to local flaps. *Dermatol Clin.* 1998;16(1):65–74.

Hong RW, Menick FJ. Nasal reconstruction. In: Weinzweig J, ed. *Plastic Surgery Secrets.* 2nd ed. Philadelphia, PA: Mosby-Elsevier; 2010:381–387.

Jackson IT. Local flaps for facial coverage. In: Mathes SJ, ed. *Plastic Surgery.* Vol 5. 2nd ed. Philadelphia, PA: Saunders-Elsevier; 2006:345–390.

Kierner AC, Aigner M, Zelenka I, Riedl G, Burian M. The blood supply of the sternocleidomastoid muscle and its clinical implications. *Arch Surg.* 1999;134(2):144–147.

Leedy JE. Scalp and calvarial reconstruction. In: Janis JE, ed. *Essentials of Plastic Surgery.* St Louis, MO: Quality Medical Publishing; 2007:279–286.

Lenert JJ, Evans GRD. Oral cavity reconstruction. In: Mathes SJ, ed. *Plastic Surgery.* 2nd ed. Philadelphia, PA: Saunders-Elsevier; 2006:917–955.

Lesavoy MA, Smith AD. Lower third face and lip reconstruction. In: Mathes SJ, ed. *Plastic Surgery.* Vol 1. 2nd ed. Philadelphia, PA: Saunders-Elsevier; 2006:799–857.

Mankani MH, Mathes SJ. Forehead reconstruction. In: Mathes SJ, ed. *Plastic Surgery.* Vol 1. 2nd ed. Philadelphia, PA: Saunders-Elsevier, 2006:699–731.

Mankani MH, Mathes SJ. Forehead reconstruction. In: Weinzweig J, ed. *Plastic Surgery Secrets.* 2nd ed. Philadelphia, PA: Mosby-Elsevier; 2010:373–380.

Mathes DW, Garcia CA. Cheek reconstruction. In: Janis JE, ed. *Essentials of Plastic Surgery.* St Louis, MO: Quality Medical Publishing; 2007:307–313.

Mathes SJ, Hansen SL. Flap classification and applications. In: Mathes SJ, ed. *Plastic Surgery.* 2nd ed. Philadelphia; PA: Saunders-Elsevier; 2006:365–481.

McConnell MP, Evans GRD. Local flaps of the head and neck. In: Weinzweig J, ed. *Plastic Surgery Secrets.* 2nd ed. Philadelphia, PA: Mosby-Elsevier; 2010:363–372.

Menick FJ. Reconstruction of the cheek. *Plast Reconstr Surg.* 2001;108(2):496–505.

Mosser SW. Lip reconstruction. In: Janis JE, ed. *Essentials of Plastic Surgery.* St Louis, MO: Quality Medical Publishing; 2007:324–336.

Orticochea M. Four flap scalp reconstruction technique. *Br J Plast Surg.* 1967;20:159–171.

Pribaz JJ, Chester CH, Barrall DT. The extended V-Y flap. *Plast Reconstr Surg.* 1992;90(2):275–280.

Pribaz JJ, Meara JG, Wright S, Smith JD, Stephens W, Breuing KH. Lip and vermilion reconstruction with the facial artery musculomucosal flap. *Plast Reconstr Surg.* 2000;105(3):864–872.

Sati S, Makki AS, Shashikant M, Ramasastry SS. Scalp reconstruction. In: Weinzweig J, ed. *Plastic Surgery Secrets.* 2nd ed. Philadelphia, PA: Mosby-Elsevier; 2010:422–426.

Seki JT. Lip reconstruction. In: Weinzweig J, ed. *Plastic Surgery Secrets.* 2nd ed. Philadelphia, PA: Mosby-Elsevier; 2010:401–408.

Shah AM, Jung H, Skirboll S. Materials used in cranioplasty: a history and analysis. *Neurosurg Focus.* 2014;36(4):E19.

Stevens CR, Tan L, Kassir R, Calhoun K. Biomechanics of A-to-T flap design. *Laryngoscope.* 1999;109(1):113–117.

Taghinia AH, Movassaghi K, Wang AX, Pribaz JJ. Reconstruction of the upper aerodigestive tract with the submental artery flap. *Plast Reconstr Surg.* 2009;123(2):562–570.

Weinzweig J, Weinzweig N. Techniques and geometry of wound repair. In: Weinzweig J, ed. *Plastic Surgery Secrets.* 2nd ed. Philadelphia, PA: Mosby-Elsevier; 2010:8–14.

Wells MD. Scalp reconstruction. In: Mathes SJ, ed. *Plastic Surgery.* Vol 1. 2nd ed. Philadelphia, PA: Saunders-Elsevier; 2006:607–631.

Wilhelmi BJ, Blackwell SJ, Phillips LG. Langer's lines: to use or not to use. *Plast Reconstr Surg.* 1999;104(1):208–214.

Wolfe SA, Rivas-Torres MT, Ozerdem O. Reconstruction of the periorbital adnexa. In: Mathes SJ, ed. *Plastic Surgery.* Vol 1. 2nd ed. Philadelphia, PA: Saunders-Elsevier; 2006:733–761.

Xue CY, Li L, Guo LL, Li JH, Xing X. The bilobed flap for reconstruction of distal nasal defect in Asians. *Aesthetic Plast Surg.* 2009; 33(4):600–604.

Younai SS, Seckel BR. Surgical anatomy of the facial nerve. In: Weinzweig J, ed. *Plastic Surgery Secrets.* 2nd ed. Philadelphia, PA: Mosby-Elsevier; 2010:427–430.

Yu P, Roblin P, Chevray P. Internal mammary artery perforator (IMAP) flap for tracheostoma reconstruction. *Head Neck.* 2006;28(8): 723–729.

Zavod MB, Zavod MB, Goldman GD. The dorsal nasal flap. *Dermatol Clin.* 2005;23(1):73–85, vi.

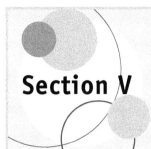

Section V INTEGUMENT

CHAPTER 56 Benign Skin Lesions

Marissa Heller, MD

• • • BENIGN MELANOCYTIC LESIONS • • •

○ **What is a nevus?**

A cutaneous hamartoma or benign proliferation of cells. Usually refers to a melanocytic nevus.

○ **What are the three histologic types of melanocytic nevi?**

Junctional, compound, and intradermal.

○ **True/False: Melanocytes develop from neural crest cells.**

True.

○ **During fetal development neural crest cells migrate to what eventual location?**

Epidermal side of the dermal–epidermal junction.

○ **What is a blue nevus?**

A deep dermal accumulation of melanocytic cells. Its deep dermal location gives a blue, gray, or black appearance.

○ **Can blue nevi become malignant?**

Yes, rarely.

○ **What is a Spitz nevus?**

A melanocytic nevus that occurs most commonly in children.

○ **Where does a Spitz nevus appear?**

Usually presents as a small pink nodule on the face or lower extremities. Histologically composed of pleomorphic and cytologically atypical cells, sometimes confused for a melanoma.

○ **Is the risk of malignancy within a congenital melanocytic nevus (CMN) related to size?**

Yes.

○ **When is the risk of malignant transformation of a CMN greatest in childhood?**

Usually before age 9.

○ **What is a Becker nevus?**

Area of hyperpigmentation and hypertrichosis, most commonly found on the upper back, shoulder, or chest in males. Usually presents at puberty.

○ **What is the recommended treatment for an atypical or dysplastic nevus?**

Excision with 2-mm margins.

○ **What is a nevus of Ota?**

It is a blue to gray hyperpigmentation of the skin, mucosa, or conjunctiva in the distribution of the trigeminal nerve.

○ **What is a nevus of Ito?**

Similar in appearance to a nevus of Ota but found on the neck or shoulder.

○ **What is a Mongolian spot?**

Congenital hyperpigmented spot found in the sacrococcygeal region. Usually disappears in the first 3 to 5 years of life.

○ **What is a nevus spilus?**

An irregularly shaped light brown macule with darkly pigmented macules or papules scattered randomly within the lesion.

○ **What is a labial lentigo?**

Hyperpigmented macule that develops on the lip, usually in young women.

○ **Which autosomal-dominant syndrome consists of multiple lentigines and gastrointestinal polyps?**

Peutz-Jeghers syndrome.

○ **What is a halo nevus?**

A melanocytic nevus with surrounding depigmentation. This is most frequent on the trunk of teenagers.

• • • BENIGN VASCULAR LESIONS • • •

○ **What is the most common vascular neoplasm of childhood?**

Hemangioma.

○ **What is a hemangioma?**

It is a benign tumor of vascular endothelium. Presents at age 4 to 8 weeks.

○ **What is the natural history of a hemangioma?**

The lesion proliferates for the first 6 months to a year, and then goes through involution (regression). Classically, 50% completely regress by age 5.

○ **What is the most common complication of hemangiomas?**

Ulceration.

○ **What are complications after regression of a hemangioma?**

Hypopigmentation, telangiectasia, excess skin, fibrofatty deposits, and scarring after ulceration.

○ **What is a port-wine stain?**

A capillary malformation presents at birth that grows proportionate to the patient and has normal endothelial turnover.

○ **What laser is used to treat a port-wine stain? Why?**

Pulsed dye. Wavelength (585 nm) specific for absorption of oxyhemoglobin with an extremely short duration (400 ms). The short duration limits heating of adjacent tissues.

○ **When a facial port-wine stain is seen with leptomeningeal angiomatosis, what is it called?**

Sturge–Weber syndrome.

○ **Where does the port-wine stain occur most commonly in Sturge–Weber syndrome?**

The cutaneous areas innervated by CN V1 and V2.

○ **Regular ophthalmologic examinations are important for which patients with port-wine stains?**

All patients with V1 facial distribution.

○ **What are blue-black hyperkeratotic vascular papules?**

Angiokeratomas.

○ **Who gets cherry angiomas?**

Middle-aged and elderly patients.

○ **What occurs in an extremity as a painful, purple nodule? (Hint: sometimes seen in the fingertip.)**

Glomus tumor.

○ **True/False: A condition with inherited multiple glomus tumors is transmitted in an autosomal-dominant manner.**

True.

○ **What syndrome has telangiectasias on the face, lips, tongue, ears, hands, feet, GI, GU, pulmonary, CNS, and liver?**

Osler–Weber–Rendu syndrome (Hereditary hemorrhagic telangiectasia).

○ **What are the common causes of facial telangiectasias?**

Chronic UV light, rosacea, connective tissue disease, abuse of potent topical steroids, and radiation.

○ **True/False: Pyogenic granulomas often develop as rapidly growing bleeding papules during pregnancy (see Fig. 56-1)?**

True.

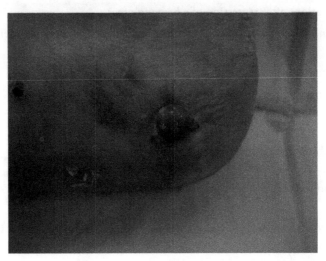

Figure 56-1 Pyogenic granuloma.

○ **What is PHACE syndrome?**

P (posterior fossa abnormalities), H (hemangiomas), A (arterial lesions), C (coarctation of the aorta/cardiac malformations), E (eye abnormalities).

○ **Which syndrome has a capillary malformation of the lower extremity associated with soft-tissue hypertrophy, lymphedema, and venous malformations?**

Klippel–Trenaunay syndrome (Angio-osteohypertrophy syndrome).

● ● ● BENIGN FIBROUS AND INFLAMMATORY LESIONS ● ● ●

○ **What is a solitary, firm, hyperkeratotic, sometimes pedunculated papule frequently found on the digits overlying an IP joint, but can be found anywhere on the hands or feet?**

Acquired digital fibrokeratoma.

○ **What is a lesion that is skin colored or red found on the lateral or dorsal surface of a digit on an infant or young child?**

Infantile digital fibromatosis.

○ **What are common pedunculated papules that are often found in intertriginous folds?**

Acrochordons (or skin tags, or fibroepithelial polyps).

○ **What is a flesh-colored, pedunculated papule that can be found anywhere on the body and what autosomal-dominant syndrome it is associated with?**

Neurofibromas are found in neurofibromatosis or Von Recklinghausen disease.

○ **What is a firm nodule or papule often found on the extremities (see Fig. 56-2)?**

Dermatofibroma.

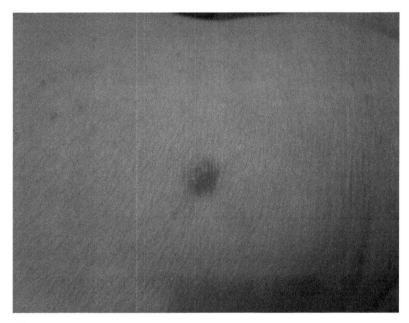

Figure 56-2 Dermatofibroma.

○ **What is a firm tender nodule that may have rolled borders and central ulceration and can mimic a malignant cutaneous neoplasm?**

Chondrodermatitis nodularis helicis.

○ **What is the most common treatment modality for keloids?**

Intralesional corticosteroid injections.

○ **What are the most common side effects of this treatment for keloids?**

Dermal atrophy and hypopigmentation.

○ **What is the most common malignant tumor that can arise in a nevus sebaceous?**

Basal cell carcinoma.

○ **Which reddish-brown lesion exhibits Darier's sign (urticates upon stroking)?**

Cutaneous mastocytoma.

• • • BENIGN PREMALIGNANT LESIONS • • •

○ **True/False: Seborrheic keratoses are premalignant lesions.**

False.

○ **Cutaneous horns are related to what premalignant skin lesion?**

Actinic keratoses.

○ **Name the acceptable treatment modalities for actinic keratoses.**

Excision, curettage, cryosurgery, dermabrasion, chemical peels, topical 5-FU, and laser ablation.

○ **What is an eczematous condition of the nipple and areola with or without an underlying mass?**

Paget disease.

○ **What is actinic cheilitis?**

A scaly, fissured, eroded lesion on the lower lip with is secondary to chronic ultraviolet light exposure. Squamous cell carcinoma can develop from this condition.

○ **Which human papillomavirus (HPV) subtypes, found in some condyloma acuminata, are considered high risk and are associated with cancer?**

HPV 16 and 18.

• • • BENIGN SUBCUTANEOUS LESIONS • • •

○ **What are the most common subcutaneous soft-tissue tumors?**

Lipomas.

○ **What are the two most common types of keratinous cysts?**

Epidermal inclusion cysts (often incorrectly termed "sebaceous cysts"), and pilar or trichilemmal cysts.

○ **Where are pilar cysts most commonly found?**

Scalp.

○ **What is the etiology of dermoid cysts?**

Improper embryonic epithelium growth at fusion sites during craniofacial development.

○ **What are angiolipomas?**

Painful subcutaneous nodules which are otherwise similar to lipomas.

○ **What are the cutaneous findings in Gardner syndrome?**

Epidermal inclusion cysts, osteomas, fibromas, lipomas, leiomyomas, desmoid tumors, and fibrosarcomas.

● ● ● REFERENCES ● ● ●

Giandoni MB. Fibrous tumors of the skin. In: Fitzpatrick JE, Aeling JL. *Dermatology Secrets*. 1st ed. Philadelphia, PA: Hanley & Belfus; 1996:278–283.

Grevelink SV, Mulliken JB. Vascular anomalies and tumors of skin and subcutaneous tissues. In: Freedberg IM, Eisen AZ, Wolff K, et al., eds. *Fitzpatrick's Dermatology in General Medicine*. 6th ed. New York, NY: McGraw-Hill; 2003:1002–1019.

Grichnik JM, Rhodes AR, Sober AJ. Benign hyperplasias and neoplasias of melanocytes. In: Freedberg IM, Eisen AZ, Wolff K, et al., eds. *Fitzpatrick's Dermatology in General Medicine*. 6th ed. New York, NY: McGraw-Hill; 2003:881–905.

Kint A, Baran R, De Keyser H. Acquired (digital) fibrokeratomas. *J Am Acad Dermatol*. 1985;12:816–821.

Morelli JG. Vascular neoplasms. In: Fitzpatrick JE, Aeling JL, eds. *Dermatology Secrets*. 1st ed. Philadelphia, PA: Hanley & Belfus; 1996: 275–277.

Morelli JG, Tan OT, Yohn JJ, Weston WL. Treatment of ulcerated hemangiomas in infancy. *Arch Pediatr Adoescl Med*. 1994;148: 1104–1105.

Netscher D, Spira M, Cohen V. Benign and premalignant skin conditions. In: Achauer BM, Eriksson E, Guyuron B, et al., eds. *Plastic Surgery Indications, Operations, and Outcomes*. 1st ed. St. Louis, MO: Mosby; 2000:293–314.

Skohler S. Muscle, adipose and cartilage neoplasms. In: Bolognia JL, Jorizzo JL, Rapini RP, eds. *Dermatology*. 2nd ed. St Louis, MO: Mosby; 2008:1831–1844.

Stone MS. Cysts. In: Bolognia JL, Jorizzo JL, Rapini RP, eds. *Dermatology*. 2nd ed. St Louis, MO: Mosby; 2008:1681–1691.

Tsao H, Sober AJ. Atypical melanocytic nevi. In: Freedberg IM, Eisen AZ, Wolff K, et al., eds. *Fitzpatrick's Dermatology in General Medicine*. 6th ed. New York, NY: McGraw-Hill; 2003:906–916.

Walsh P. Benign melanocytic tumors. In: Fitzpatrick JE, Aeling JL, eds. *Dermatology Secrets*. 1st ed. Philadelphia, PA: Hanley & Belfus; 1996:269–274.

Malignant Skin Lesions (Basal Cell and Squamous Cell Carcinoma)

CHAPTER 57

Kristina Liu, MD and Daihung Do, MD

○ **How common is skin cancer in the United States?**

There are currently approximately 3.5 million new cases of skin cancer in the United States annually making skin cancer the most common type of cancer. The incidence rate has increased dramatically over the past two decades. Sharply increased skin cancer rates have been reported worldwide.

○ **What are the two most common types of skin cancer?**

Basal cell carcinoma (BCC) is the most common type of skin cancer. It accounts for 75% to 80% of all skin cancers making BCC the most common type of cancer in humans. Squamous cell carcinoma (SCC) is the second most common type of skin cancer. Together, BCC and SCC account for 95% of all nonmelanoma skin cancers (NMSCs).

○ **How does skin pigmentation affect risk for skin cancer?**

Lightly pigmented patients are 70 times more likely to develop NMSC than patients with darkly pigmented skin. BCC is the most common type of skin cancer in Caucasians. In patients with a dark skin type, SCC is more common than BCC and tends to occur in non–sun-exposed sites. In contrast, BCC tends to occur in sun-exposed areas in dark-skinned patients with lighter complexions.

○ **How does ultraviolet radiation contribute to carcinogenicity?**

Ultraviolet (UV) light leads to the formation of pyrimidine dimers. UVB (315–290 nm) is regarded as the most carcinogenic ultraviolet radiation by causing direct damage to DNA and DNA repair mechanisms. UVA (400–315 nm) is now considered to be a co-carcinogen because it potentiates the effects of UVB.

• • • BASAL CELL CARCINOMA • • •

○ **What are the risk factors for developing BCC?**

The most common risk factor is UV light exposure. Patients with fair skin and little melanin are more likely to develop BCC. The incidence of BCC rises with decreasing latitude (closer to the equator). UV exposure from tanning beds and PUVA (therapeutic UV exposure) also predisposes to the development of BCC. Intermittent sun overexposure (sunburns) early in life (childhood and adolescence) is linked with the development of BCC. Other risk factors are less common such as ionizing radiation, arsenic exposure, topical nitrogen mustard use, and certain genetic syndromes.

○ **What inherited conditions predispose to basal cell carcinoma and other skin cancers?**

- Basal cell nevus syndrome
- Xeroderma pigmentosum
- Albinism

○ **Other than sun-exposed sites, what are the classic locations for the development of BCC?**

BCC has a predilection for developing in certain locations. They may develop in an old scar (e.g., vaccination scar), in thermal burns, or at the site of a nevus sebaceous.

○ **What are some of the *clinical* types of BCC?**

- **Superficial BCCs** present as a pink to red, slightly scaly plaque. There may be areas of skin atrophy and hypopigmentation present within the plaque. Occasionally, they may develop significant subclinical spread.

- **Nodular BCC** presents as a skin-colored to pink papule or plaque. It may be translucent in color leading to their classic description as "pearly." The border is often heaped and there are typically overlying telangiectases that may require magnification to visualize.

- **Ulcerative BCC** presents as an ulcer. It usually develops from a nodular BCC that over the course of time has become so invasive with central necrosis that an ulcer has formed. They are often long standing and have a heaped pearly rim with telangiectases. When an ulcerative BCC becomes extensive and invades deeply and widely, it may be referred to as a *rodent ulcer* because the tissue appears to have been gnawed by a rat.

- **Pigmented BCC** presents as a dark papule and more commonly as a dark plaque. The pigmentation may be uniform across the lesion or it may be focal. This type of BCC is often mistaken for a nevus, melanoma, or solar lentigo.

- **Morpheaform BCC** presents as a hypopigmented shiny plaque that resembles the lesions of morphea. Overlying telangiectases may be present. There is often extensive subclinical spread with a high risk of recurrence.

○ **What are the treatment options for BCC?**

Curettage and electrodessication, excision, cryotherapy, photodynamic therapy, imiquimod cream, 5-fluorouracil cream, and Vismodegib.

○ **What are the contraindications for curettage and electrodessication?**

- Aggressive histologic subtypes that curette poorly such as morpheaform BCC, sclerosing BCC, infiltrative BCC, recurrent BCC, and micronodular BCC.

- Anatomic areas rich in pilosebaceous units such as the nose and scalp. In these areas, BCC can hide between hair follicles.

- Deeply invasive tumors. Once the tumor has invaded through the dermis, it cannot be removed through curettage.

- Areas with soft skin texture such as the eyelid and lip. In these areas, curettage is more difficult to perform and normal skin is likely to be removed with curettage.

○ **What is Mohs surgery?**

Mohs surgery is a tissue-sparing microscopically controlled technique of excising skin cancers pioneered by Dr. Frederick Mohs. It is often contrasted with routine surgical excision or surgical excision with frozen-section analysis. In the latter technique, conventional histologic analysis of elliptical tissue specimens uses the "breadloaf" technique in which serial transverse sections are examined, which covers less than 0.1% of the true surgical margin. In Mohs surgery, saucer-shaped specimens are removed and processed with tangential sectioning that allows 100% of the true surgical margin to be assessed. Specimen orientation is meticulously tracked during this process so that residual tumor at the specimen margin can be mapped back to the patient for additional tissue removal. In this manner, tumors can be removed with a minimal margin of normal tissue. With its high technical precision, Mohs surgery has been shown to offer high cure rates for highly aggressive tumors in critical and sensitive anatomic locations while offering maximum tissue preservation.

○ **What are the indications for Mohs surgery?**

Mohs surgery is indicated when there is a high risk for local recurrence or when tissue conservation is highly desirable.

- Recurrent tumors.
- Tumor size >2 cm.
- Tumors in high-risk locations such as the H-zone of the face, hands/feet, and genitalia.
- Aggressive histologic subtypes such as infiltrative, morpheaform, micronodular, metatypical BCC.
- Indistinct tumor margins.

● ● ● SQUAMOUS CELL CARCINOMA ● ● ●

○ **What are the risk factors for developing SCC?**

- UV light exposure: fair skin, chronic cumulative UV exposure, geographic location closer to the equator, PUVA therapy
- Immunosuppression
- History of prior NMSC
- Genodermatoses
- Chronic scarring or inflammatory conditions
- Human papilloma virus infection
- Chemical carcinogens:
  - Polycyclic aromatic hydrocarbons such as soot, pitch, tar, shale oil, and mineral oil
  - Arsenic
  - Ionizing radiation

○ **What is the precursor to cutaneous SCC?**

Actinic keratoses (AK) are characterized by their rough texture ("gritty"), erythematous base, and ill-defined border. Hypertrophic actinic keratoses may be difficult to distinguish clinically from SCC.

○ **What is the treatment for actinic keratoses?**

Actinic keratoses are usually treated with cryosurgery. Field treatment for large numbers of actinic keratoses includes ingenol mebutate, imiquimod, topical 5-FU, and photodynamic therapy.

○   **What is a keratoacanthoma (KA)?**

A KA is a dome-shaped nodule with a central keratin crater that is characterized by rapid growth and a tendency for self-involution. It is controversial whether it should be considered a benign lesion or a truly malignant lesion.

○   **What is SCC in-situ (SCCis) or Bowen's disease?**

An SCCiS or Bowen's disease is an intraepidermal carcinoma that has the potential for transformation into an SCC. It usually appears as a pink to red scaly papule.

○   **What is the metastatic risk for SCC?**

The overall risk of metastasis is 2% to 6%. Primary tumors have a 5% metastatic risk while recurrent tumors have a 30% risk. Lesions with a size less than 2 cm have a 9% metastatic risk, and lesions greater than 2 cm in size have a 30% risk. Lesions that invade more than 4 mm have a metastatic risk of 45%.

○   **Where are the most common sites of SCC metastasis?**

The most common metastatic locations are regional lymph nodes, liver, and lung. SCCs of the scalp, forehead, ears, nose, and lips also carry a higher risk of metastasis. SCCs originating in the lip and pinna metastasize in 10% to 20% of cases. Five-year survival for metastatic SCC is 34%.

• • • **REFERENCES** • • •

Ad Hoc Task Force, Connolly SM, Baker DR, et al. AAD/ACMS/ASDSA/ASMS 2012 appropriate use criteria for Mohs micrographic surgery: A report of the American Academy of Dermatology, American College of Mohs Surgery, American Society for Dermatologic Surgery Association, and the American Society for Mohs Surgery. *J Am Acad Dermatol.* 2012;67(4):531–550.

Balch CM, Gershenwald JE, Soong SM, et al. Final version of 2009 AJCC melanoma staging and classification. *J Clin Oncol.* 2009;27(36):6199–6206.

Bolognia JL, Jorizzo JL, Rapini RP, et al. *Dermatology.* 2nd ed. Spain: Mosby; 2008.

Gilchrest BA, Eller MS, Geller AC, Yaar M. The pathogenesis of melanoma induced by ultraviolet radiation. *N Engl J Med.* 1999;340(17):1341–1348.

Goldenberg G, Perl M. Actinic keratosis: update on field therapy. *J Clin Aesthet Dermatol.* 2014;7(10):28–31.

Rigel DS, Friedman RJ, Dzubow LM, et al. *Cancer of the Skin.* 1st ed. New York, NY: Saunders; 2005.

Rogers HW, Weinstock MA, Harris AR, et al. Incidence estimate of nonmelanoma skin cancer in the United States, 2006. *Arch Dermatol.* 2010;146(3):283–287.

CHAPTER 58
Malignant Melanoma: Basis and Treatment

David Michael Miller, MD, PhD, FAAD and Lydia Anne Helliwell, MD

○ **Approximately how many new melanomas are diagnosed each year and roughly how many patients die from melanoma annually?**

There are approximately 75,000 new cases of melanoma diagnosed each year and between 9,000 and 10,000 patients die from melanoma annually.

○ **What are the ABCDEs of melanoma?**

A: Asymmetry

B: Border irregularity

C: Color variegation or change

D: Diameter greater than 6 mm

E: Evolutionary changes in color, symmetry, size, shape, or symptoms

○ **What are some of the common known risk factors for the development of melanoma?**

Environmental:

1. Exposure to ultraviolet radiation (UVR)

2. History of sunburns, particularly in childhood or sunburns that induce severe pain/blistering

Personal:

1. Red hair

2. Skin type

3. Sun sensitivity

4. Family history

5. Number of moles present (risk increases as number of moles increases)

6. Personal history of melanoma

7. Female sex

8. Immunosuppression

9. Diagnosis of xeroderma pigmentosum

10. History of dysplastic nevi

11. Inherited genetic mutations (e.g., mutations in CDKN2A, CDK4, and TERT)

○   **What is the most common type of melanoma?**

Superficial Spreading Melanoma (SSM)

Accounting for approximately 60% to 70% of all melanomas, SSM is the most common type. SSM is most frequently diagnosed in the fifth, sixth, and seventh decades of life and is most commonly found on the legs of females and the trunk of males. Nodular melanoma accounts for approximately 15% to 30% of all melanomas and is the second most common type of cutaneous melanoma in light-skinned individuals. Lentigo maligna melanoma makes up approximately 10% of all melanomas and is found most commonly on the face. Nevoid and Spitzoid melanomas are uncommon variants of melanoma.

○   **What are the recommended surgical margins for melanoma in situ (MIS)?**

NCCN guidelines for resection margins for MIS recommend a measured margin of 0.5 to 1 cm around the clinically visible lesion. They state that certain types of MIS, for example, lentigo maligna melanoma, may require resection margins beyond 5 mm. No definitive resection recommendations beyond the current recommendations of 5 mm have been given. Published recurrence rates for wide local excision (WLE) in the literature range from 8% to 20%. Despite this, WLE remains the gold standard treatment for MIS although a number of published stage excision protocols have shown recurrence rates ranging from 0% to 7.3%.

○   **What are the recommended surgical resection margins for a 2.1 mm thick primary cutaneous melanoma?**

2.0 cm.

The current recommended margins for surgical resection of primary melanoma:

Melanoma in situ	0.5–1.0 cm
Less than 1.0 mm thick	1.0 cm
1.0–2.0 mm thick	1.0–2.0 cm
Greater than 2.0 mm thick	2.0 cm

○   **What is the overall rate of local recurrence following surgical excision of melanoma with appropriate margins?**

The rate of local recurrence approaches 4%.

○   **What are the current recommended surgical resection margins for recurrent or in transit melanoma?**

True local scar recurrence, which most likely represents locally persistent disease after inadequate initial excision, is treated similarly to the primary tumor. Following confirmatory biopsy, re-excision to the appropriate margins based on Breslow thickness is recommended. In contrast, there are no definitive data to guide management at this time for local recurrences (defined as regrowth within 2 cm of the surgical scar after definitive excision) or disease in transit (any skin or subcutaneous metastases that are >2 cm from the primary lesion and distal to the regional nodal basin). These lesions (local recurrence and in transit disease) are thought to represent dermal lymphatic disease and impart a prognosis similar to regional nodal disease; whereas, there are no conclusive data that true local scar recurrence negatively affects outcome. National Cancer Comprehensive Network (NCCN) guidelines recommend complete surgical excision to clear margins if feasible.

○   **What are the indications for sentinel lymph node biopsy in melanoma patients?**

1. Patients with lesion thickness greater than 1.0 mm and no evidence of metastatic disease nor clinical lymph node involvement should be offered SLNB.

2. SLNB should be discussed and offered to patient's with lesions that are 0.76 to 1.0 mm thick with either ulceration or mitotic rate ≥ 1 per mm^2.

The 2015 NCCN guidelines state that in general, SLNB is not recommended for lesions 0.75 mm or less, regardless of other characteristics. It does state, however, that in the rare event that a high-risk feature is present (e.g., ulceration, high mitotic rate, and/or lymphovascular invasion), the decision to perform an SLNB should be left to the physician and patient.

3. Patient request. This is highly controversial due to the lack of definitive guidelines regarding the use of sentinel lymph node biopsy in melanoma. Patients must be aware of the complication rate of sentinel node biopsy (approximately 6%) in comparison to their chance of having a positive node (between 5% and 8% in patients with melanomas less than 1.0 mm thick).

○ **Assign the following primary melanoma lesions with the corresponding American Joint Committee on Cancer (AJCC) stage.**

1. 0.76 mm thick lesion, with evidence of ulceration, no clinical LAD

2. 2.2 mm thick lesion, no evidence of ulceration, no clinical LAD

3. 2.9 mm thick lesion, no ulceration, one clinically enlarged lymph node, that is confirmed positive on lymphadenectomy

4. 3.1 mm thick lesion, no ulceration, positive SLNB, positive metastasis in the liver

5. 0.56 mm thick lesion, no evidence of ulceration, no clinical LAD

The current AJCC staging system is set up such that stages 1 and 2 represent local disease, stage 3 is regional metastasis, and stage 4 is distant metastasis. Please see the chart below for the complete staging system.

Stage	Tumor (T)	Nodes (N)	Metastasis (M)
IA	≤1.0 mm without ulceration and mitosis <1/mm²	None	None
IB	≤1.0 mm with ulceration or mitosis ≥1/mm² 1.01–2.0 mm without ulceration	None	None
IIA	1.01–2.0 mm with ulceration 2.01–4.0 mm without ulceration	None	None
IIB	2.01–4.0 mm with ulceration >4.0 mm without ulceration	None	None
IIC	>4.0 mm with ulceration	None	None
IIIA	Any thickness without ulceration	1–3 micrometastatic	None
IIIB	1. Any thickness without ulceration 2. Any thickness with ulceration 3. Any thickness	1. 1–3 macrometastatic 2. 1–3 micrometastatic 3. 2–3 positive nodes	1. None 2. None 3. In transit/satellite metastasis
IIIC	1. Any thickness with ulceration 2. Any thickness	1. 1–3 macrometastatic 2. Four or more positive nodes or matted nodes	1. None 2. In transit/satellite metastasis
IV	Any thickness	Any nodes	Distant metastasis

Answers: (1) IB, (2) IIA, (3) IIIB, (4) IV, and (5) IA.

○ **What are the estimated 5- and 10-year survival rates associated with the various stages of melanoma?**

Stage	5-Year Survival Rate (%)	10-Year Survival Rate (%)
1A	97	95
1B	92	86
2A	81	67
2B	70	57
2C	53	40
3A	78	68
3B	59	43
3C	40	24
4[a]	15–20[a]	10–15[a]

[a]Survival is higher if metastasis is to distant parts of the skin or lymph nodes rather than internal organs or if the blood lactate dehydrogenase (LDH) is within normal limits.

The above survival rates are observed (non–disease-related) survival rates. They include patients who have been diagnosed with melanoma but may have died from causes other than melanoma. These statistics may slightly underestimate the percentage of people surviving melanoma.

○ **What are some of the prognostic factors associated with melanoma?**

BETTER PROGNOSIS WITH:

Age 65 years or younger

Female sex

Lesions on the extremity

Thickness less than 1.0 mm

Low mitotic rate

Presence of tumor-infiltrating lymphocytes*

Desmoplastic type*

Clark's level 1, 2, 3

WORSE PROGNOSIS WITH THE PRESENCE OF:

Ulceration

Tumor vascular invasion

Microsatellite lesions

Regression*

Poor performance status (stage 4 disease)

Disease in lymph node basin

Distant metastasis (particularly pleural, GI, and liver or multiple sites)

*Uncertain or disputed importance within the literature.

○ **What are the common sites of melanoma distant metastasis?**

Location	Estimated Rates of Metastasis (%)
Skin, lymph nodes, subcutaneous tissue	42–59
Lungs	18–36
Liver	14–20
Brain	12–20
Bone	11–17
Gastrointestinal	1–7

○ **What technique should be used to biopsy a lesion suspicious for cutaneous melanoma?**

Ideally, a patient with a lesion suspicious for melanoma should have a narrow excisional biopsy. This biopsy can be performed with a variety of techniques (e.g., elliptical excision, punch biopsy, or saucerization). Whichever technique is chosen, the goal is to achieve clinically negative lateral margins (usually 1- to 3-mm margins are necessary to remove the subclinical component) and a depth that ensures that the lesion is not transected. The orientation of the excisional biopsy should be planned with definitive treatment in mind (i.e., in a longitudinal axis on the extremities). Full-thickness excisional biopsy is often regarded as the procedure of choice, as it is generally accepted to produce the lowest transection rates. Nevertheless, punch biopsies and saucerization biopsies are performed routinely by experienced clinicians when they can produce full excision. In certain situations, an excisional biopsy may be inappropriate (e.g., lesions on the face, acral areas, or subungual lesions). In these cases, full-thickness incisional biopsy remains an acceptable option. Care must be taken when performing incisional biopsies to plan ahead for further excision and should involve the thickest portion of the lesion.

○ **What is the surgical management for metastatic melanoma to the lymph nodes identified clinically or on sentinel node biopsy?**

NCCN guidelines call for complete lymph node dissection in patients with positive sentinel lymph node biopsy and those patients with stage 3 clinical disease.

○ **What are the limits of a complete axillary node dissection?**

Complete axillary lymph node dissection consists of the removal of all lymph node bearing tissue (zones 1, 2, and 3) including tissue anterior, superior, posterior, and inferior to the axillary vessels.

The limits of the complete axillary dissection are as follows:

Superior: Subclavius muscle

Inferior: Insertion of the thoracodorsal nerve into the latissimus muscle

Medial: First rib medial to the edge of the pectoralis minor muscle and including the tissue above the pectoralis major and in between the pectoralis major and minor

Lateral: Edge of latissimus dorsi muscle

○ **What are the limits of a complete inguinal lymph node dissection?**

Complete inguinal lymph node dissection consists of the removal of the superficial lymph node basin with dissection and removal of the deep lymph node basin for metastasis of the Cloquet node or palpable deep node involvement.

The limits of the complete inguinal dissection are as follows:

Superior: 5 cm above the inguinal ligament

Inferior: The confluence of the sartorius and the adductor longus

Medial: The adductor longus muscle and the pubic tubercle

Inferior: The sartorius muscle and the anterior superior iliac spine

○ **How many lymph nodes does an axillary or inguinal lymph node dissection require in order to be complete?**

Recent NCCN guidelines state that there is an insufficient amount of data to determine the number of lymph nodes required to deem a dissection complete. Complete dissections should be determined by anatomic boundaries as listed above.

○ **What is the most significant determining factor of melanoma clinical behavior?**

Lesion thickness.

○ **Can a sentinel node biopsy be performed after wide local excision?**

Yes. Sentinel lymph node biopsy should be offered if inadequate initial margins of resection are present. WLE of the entire scar based on current recommended resection guidelines with a sentinel lymph node biopsy is the treatment of choice. Multiple studies have shown that even though lymphatic channels may have been damaged during the initial resection, SLN biopsy has equal predictive value compared to that having been done at the initial resection.

○ **What percentage of melanoma patients have no identifiable primary tumor?**

2% to 6% of melanoma patients will have no identifiable primary tumor. Five-year survival rate for these patients has been estimated to be 83% in patients with in-transit metastasis (cutaneous or subcutaneous), 50% in patients with metastasis in the lymph node basin, and 6% in patients with distant or disseminated disease.

○ **What is the recommended follow-up/surveillance for melanoma patients?**

Stage	History and Physical	Imaging	Laboratory Tests
0	Yearly	None	None
1	Every 6–12 months for 5 years, then annually as indicated	Routine radiologic imaging for asymptomatic individuals is not recommended	Routine blood tests are not recommended for asymptomatic individuals
2A	Every 6–12 months for 5 years, then annually as indicated	Routine radiologic imaging for asymptomatic individuals is not recommended	Routine blood tests are not recommended for asymptomatic individuals
2B/C	Every 3–6 months for 2 years, then 3–12 months for 3 years, then annually as indicated	Consider chest x-ray, CT, and/or PET/CT every 4 to 12 months, and annual brain MRI, for 5 years	Routine blood tests are not recommended for asymptomatic individuals
3	Every 3–6 months for 2 years, then 3–12 months for 3 years, then annually as indicated	Consider chest x-ray, CT, and/or PET/CT every 4 to 12 months, and annual brain MRI, for 5 years	Routine blood tests are not recommended for asymptomatic individuals
4	Individualized	Individualized	Individualized

○ **What is the differential diagnosis of a pigmented nailbed lesion?**

Subungual hematoma, onychomycosis, frictional melanonychia, Coumadin-associated melanonychia, melanonychia striata, junctional nevus, Addison's disease, and Peutz–Jegher's disease.

○ **What are concerning symptoms of a pigmented nailbed lesion that should raise concern for subungual melanoma?**

Irregular borders, ulceration, size increase, onycholysis, nail plate dystrophy, extension beyond nail bed into proximal nail fold (Hutchinson sign).

○ **How long should you observe a pigmented nailbed lesion without concerning symptoms before biopsy?**

3 to 4 weeks. If nail plate grows distally past pigmentation or concerning symptoms develop, perform a full-thickness nailbed biopsy.

○ **What are the current treatment recommendations for biopsy proven subungual melanoma?**

Historically, amputation at the distal phalangeal joint has been the widely accepted treatment for subungual melanoma. However, conclusive data to support this aggressive form of treatment is lacking. Wide local excision, especially for melanoma in situ, may be appropriate for some lesions. Further studies are needed.

○ **What is the most common form of malignant melanoma in black Americans?**

Acral lentiginous melanoma (ALM) is the most common form of malignant melanoma in black Americans. ALM occurs on non–hair-bearing surfaces of the body, often not exposed to sunlight. It is most commonly on the palms, soles, nailbeds, and oral mucosa. ALM is often misdiagnosed as a more benign process, and therefore African Americans often present with late-stage disease leading to decreased survival times.

○ **Where is the most common site for malignant melanoma in Asian populations?**

Plantar surface of the foot. Acral lentiginous melanoma is also more common in this patient population.

● ● ● **REFERENCES** ● ● ●

Agbai, ON, Buster K, Sanchez M, et al. Skin cancer and photoprotection in people of color: a review and recommendations for physicians and the public. *J Am Acad Dermatol.* 2014;70:748–762.

Australian Cancer Network Melanoma Guidelines Revision Working Party. Prognostic factors and survival outcomes in cutaneous melanoma. In: *Australian Cancer Network Melanoma Guidelines Revision Working Party. Clinical Practice Guidelines for the Management of Melanoma in Australia and New Zealand.* Wellington, NZ: The Cancer Council of Australia. Australian Cancer Network, Sydney and New Zealand Guidelines Group; 2008:157–162.

Balch CM, Gershenwald JE, Soong SJ, et al. Final version 2009 AJCC melanoma staging and classification. *J Clin Oncol.* 2009; 27(36):6199–6206.

Balch CM, Urist MM, Karakousis CP, et al. Efficacy of 2-cm surgical margins for intermediate-thickness melanomas (1 to 4 mm). Results of a multi-institutional randomized surgical trial. *Ann Surg.* 1993;218:262–267.

Bichakjian CK, Halpern AC, Johnson TM, et al. Guidelines of care for the management of primary cutaneous melanoma. *J Am Acad Dermatol.* 2011;65(5):1032–1047.

Bosbous MW, Dzwierzynski WW, Neuburg M. Lentigo maligna: diagnosis and treatment. *Clin Plast Surg.* 2010;37(1):35–46.

Cho YR, Chang MP. Epidemiology, staging (new system), and prognosis of cutaneous melanoma. *Clin Plast Surg.* 2010;37(1):47–53.

Cochran AM, Buchanan PJ, Bueno RA Jr, Neumeister MW. Subungual melanoma: a review of current treatment. *Plast Reconstr Surg.* 2014;134:259–273.

Coit DG, Thompson JA, Andtbacka R, et al. *NCCN Clinical Practice Guidelines in Oncology: Melanoma.* Version 3, 2015. Available at: http://www.nccn.org/professionals/physician_gls/pdf/melanoma.pdf. Accessed March 15, 2015.

Dzwierzynski WW. Complete lymph node dissection for regional nodal metastasis. *Clin Plast Surg.* 2010;37(1):113–125.

Farma JM, Kulkarni N, Hsu C. Surgical management of primary and recurrent melanoma. *Surg Oncol Clin N Am.* 2015;24(2):239–247.

Finley RK 3rd, Driscoll DL, Blumenson LE, Karakousis CP. Subungual melanoma: an eighteen-year review. *Surgery.* 1994;116:96–100.

Garbe C, Bauer J. Melanoma. In: Bolongnia JL, Jorrizo JL, Schaffer JV, eds. Vol 2. 3rd ed. *Dermatology.* Philadelphia, PA: Elsevier; 2012: 1885–1914.

Heaton KM, el-Naggar A, Ensign LG, Ross MI, Balch CM. Surgical management and prognostic factors in patients with subungual melanoma. *Ann Surg.* 1994;219:197–198.

Homsi J, Kashani-Sabet M, Messina JL, Daud A. Cutaneous melanoma: prognostic factors. *Cancer Control.* 2005;12(4):223–229.

Kelemen PR, Essner R, Foshag LJ, Morton DL. Lymphatic mapping and sentinel lymphadenectomy after wide local excision of primary melanoma. *J Am Coll Surg.* 1999;189:247–252.

Kozlow JH, Rees RS. Surgical management of primary disease. *Clin Plast Surg.* 2010;37(1):65–71.

Larson DL, Larson JD. Head and neck melanoma. *Clin Plast Surg.* 2010;37(1):73–77.

Leong SP, Thelmo MC, Kim RP, et al. Delayed harvesting of sentinel lymph nodes after previous wide local excision of extremity melanoma. *Ann Surg Oncol.* 2003;10(2):196–200.

Lifchez SD, Kelamis JA. Melanoma workup and surveillance. *Clin Plast Surg.* 2010;37(1):55–63.

Mir M, Chan CS, Khan F, Krishnan B, Orengo I, Rosen T. The rate of melanoma transection with various biopsy techniques and the influence of tumor transection on patient survival. *J Am Acad Dermatol.* 2013;68(3):452–458.

O'Leary JA, Berend KR, Johnson JL, Levin LS, Seigler HF. Subungual melanoma. *Clin Orthop Rel Res.* 2000;(378):206–212.

Patterson RH, Helwig EB. Subungual malignant melanoma: a clinical-pathological study. *Cancer.* 1980;46:2074–2087.

Saida T, Ohshima Y. Clinical and histopathologic characteristics of early lesions of subungual malignant melanoma. *Cancer.* 1989;63:556–560.

Schlagenhauff B, Stroebel W, Ellwanger U, et al. Metastatic melanoma of unknown primary origin shows prognostic similarities to regional metastatic melanoma recommendation for initial staging examinations. *Cancer.* 1997;80:60–65.

Standelmann WK. The role of lymphatic mapping and sentinel lymph node biopsy in the staging and treatment of melanoma. *Clin Plast Surg.* 2010;37(1):79–99.

Stubblefield J, Kelly B. Melanoma in non-caucasian populations. *Surg Clin N Am.* 2014;94:1115–1126.

Swetter SM, Boldrick JC, Jung SY, Egbert BM, Harvell JD. Increasing incidence of lentigo maligna melanoma subtypes: northern California and national trends 1990–2000. *J Invest Dermatol.* 2005;125:685–691.

Wells KE, Joseph E, Ross M, et al. Lymphatic mapping for melanoma before and after wide local excision: 4th World Conference on Melanoma. Sydney, Australia: Melanoma Research; 1997:S105.

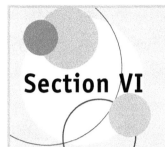

Section VI   PEDIATRICS

CHAPTER 59 Craniofacial Syndromes

Nicholas Do, MD and
John N. Jensen, MD

○ **In which gene is the mutation responsible for Saethre–Chotzen syndrome?**

TWIST (p21–p22).

○ **How many subtypes of Pfeiffer syndrome are documented?**

Three:

Type 1—craniosynostosis, broad thumb/toes, normal or near-normal intelligence (classic form)

Type 2—cloverleaf skull, severe CNS involvement, elbow synostosis, early death

Type 3—like type 2 without cloverleaf skull; poor prognosis

○ **What mutations are associated with Pfeiffer syndrome?**

FGFR1 (8p11.22–p12) and *FGFR2* (10q25–q26); *FGFR1* mutations associated with less severe extremity involvement.

○ **What mutation is associated with Apert syndrome?**

FGFR2 (10q25–q26).

○ **What mutation is associated with Crouzon syndrome?**

FGFR2 (10q25–q26).

○ **What is the mutation associated with the variant of Crouzon syndrome that includes acanthosis nigricans?**

Ala391Glu substitution of the *FGFR3* (4p) gene.

○ **What is the mutation associated with Muenke syndrome?**

Point mutation of *FGFR3* (4p) gene.

○ **Which of the craniosynostosis syndromes follows an autosomal recessive pattern of inheritance?**

Carpenter syndrome.

○ **Which of the craniosynostosis syndromes follows an X-linked pattern of inheritance?**
Craniofrontonasal dysplasia.

○ **What is the purported mechanism of FGF receptor mutations in craniosynostosis syndromes?**
Gain of function.

○ **What is Kleeblattschädel?**
Cloverleaf skull, or pancraniosynostosis (except squamosal).

○ **Which of the craniosynostosis syndromes is unique in that almost all mutations are one of the two specific substitution mutations on *FGFR2*?**
Apert syndrome.

○ **What is the Pierre Robin sequence?**
Retrognathia, glossoptosis, airway obstruction.

○ **What is the classic cleft morphology characteristic of the Robin sequence?**
Wide, U-shaped cleft.

○ **What are the most commonly associated anomalies in clefting syndromes?**
Clubfoot, cardiac anomalies.

○ **Which cleft-associated syndrome has as its hallmark feature lip pits?**
Van der Woude syndrome; hypodontia also a feature.

○ **What is the pattern of inheritance for van der Woude syndrome?**
Autosomal dominant but with variable penetrance.

○ **Which gene contains the mutation for van der Woude syndrome?**
Interferon regulatory factor 6 (IRF6) on chromosome 1.

○ **Which cleft-associated syndrome is associated with progressive blindness?**
Stickler syndrome.

○ **How many syndromes have been described to include cleft lip and/or palate?**
More than 300.

○ **What syndrome has malar hypoplasia and variable thumb and upper extremity hypoplasia?**
Nager syndrome.

○ **What is the inheritance pattern of Treacher–Collins syndrome?**
Autosomal dominant.

○ **What is the genetic mutation in Treacher–Collins syndrome?**
TCOF1 (5q31.3–32).

○ **Which nerves are involved in Moebius sequence?**
CN VI and VII.

○ **How is the genetic defect common to Velocardiofacial, DiGeorge, and Conotruncal Anomaly Face syndromes identified?**
FISH (fluorescent in situ hybridization) detection of the 22q11 deletion.

○ **What are the clinical findings associated with 22q11.2 deletion?**
Developmental disabilities, learning disabilities, or both; conotruncal cardiac anomalies, palatal defects, nasal regurgitation, and/or hypernasal speech; behavioral problems, psychiatric illness, or both; immunodeficiency; hypocalcemia; and characteristic elongated facial features.

○ **What electrolyte abnormality can complicate the post op course of a 22q11.2 deletion patient?**
Hypocalcemia can occur postoperatively and thus a serum calcium concentration should be checked in the first 6 hours after surgery.

○ **Is clefting the most common mechanism of velopharyngeal dysfunction in velocardiofacial syndrome?**
No, VPD occurs commonly without clefting in these patients.

○ **Which syndrome is most likely to be present in a patient with Pierre Robin sequence?**
Stickler syndrome.

○ **What does the OMENS classification system describe?**
Severity of craniofacial microsomia by anatomic divisions:
O—orbit
M—mandible
E—ear
N—nerve
S—soft tissue

○ **What features distinguish Goldenhar syndrome from craniofacial microsomia?**
Epibulbar dermoids and vertebral abnormalities.

○ **What is Virchow's principle?**
Cranial bone normally grows perpendicular to cranial sutures.

○ **Which of the craniofacial syndromes often demonstrate critical airway instability at birth?**
Robin sequence, Treacher–Collins, and bilateral craniofacial microsomia.

○ **What treatment modalities have been described for the newborn with Robin sequence and airway obstruction?**

Positioning, NP airway, tongue–lip adhesion, mandibular distraction, tracheostomy.

○ **What disease process has associated with the coup de sabre deformity?**

Romberg disease, or progressive hemifacial atrophy.

○ **When does Romberg disease usually present?**

First two decades.

○ **On a plain PA radiograph, what does the harlequin sign indicate?**

Superiorly displaced lesser wing of the sphenoid, usually associated with unicoronal synostosis.

○ **What tests are commonly used to assess airway obstruction in neonates with suspected airway obstruction?**

Laryngoscopy, bronchoscopy, and polysomnography (sleep study).

○ **What are the contraindications for tongue–lip adhesion or mandibular distraction in the Robin sequence?**

Subglottic obstruction.

○ **What is the rationale for avoiding distraction of the hypoplastic mandible in Robin sequence?**

"Catch up" growth eventually occurs.

○ **What is the presumed mechanism for neurocognitive maldevelopment in syndromic synostosis?**

Increased intracranial pressure; probably present in fewer than half of the affected patients.

○ **What methods are used to assess increased intracranial pressure?**

Direct pressure monitoring with invasive probe; CT findings and papilledema are less reliable/predictive.

○ **Aside from craniosynostosis, what considerations must be made for patients with Apert, Crouzon, and Pfeiffer syndromes?**

Airway, exposure keratopathy, occlusal relationship.

○ **How has management of midface hypoplasia in Apert, Crouzon, and Pfeiffer syndromes evolved?**

Le Fort III distraction in childhood, now standard in most centers.

○ **In velocardiofacial syndrome, what consideration is made prior to surgical correction of velopharyngeal dysfunction?**

The possibility of medially deviated internal carotid arteries; unlikely in the absence of clinical signs on nasoendoscopy and physical examination, but MRA is definitive test.

○ **In common usage, hemifacial microsomia refers to a spectrum of disorders; what other terms are used?**

Craniofacial microsomia, oculo-auriculo–vertebral spectrum, first and second branchial arch syndromes, and Goldenhar syndrome.

○ **What does the literature suggest about the efficacy of cranial expansion in craniosynostosis on neurocognitive development?**
Its benefit is questionable.

○ **After Tessier cleft 7 (macrostomia), what is the most common atypical facial cleft?**
Tessier 3/11.

○ **What are the commonly encountered diagnoses associated with hypertelorism?**
Encephalocoele, frontonasal dysplasia, atypical facial clefting, Crouzon syndrome, bilateral cleft lip/palate.

○ **How is hypertelorism classified?**
Intraocular distance (Tessier):
Type 1 (mild): 30–34 mm
Type 2 (moderate): 35–39 mm
Type 3 (severe): ≥40 mm

○ **Which of the cranial sutures is the only one normally to undergo fusion before the brain stops growing?**
Metopic suture.

○ **Match the skull morphology to corresponding sutural synostosis.**
Scaphocephaly—sagittal synostosis
Trigonocephaly—metopic synostosis
Plagiocephaly, anterior—unicoronal synostosis
Plagiocephaly, posterior—lambdoid synostosis
Brachycephaly—bicoronal synostosis

○ **What is the average cephalic index in normal adult Caucasians?**
0.78.

○ **How is the cephalic (or cranial) index defined?**
Eurion–eurion distance/glabella–opisthocranion distance × 100.

○ **In unicoronal synostosis, in which direction is the nasal root deviated?**
The affected side (toward fused suture).

○ **What are the anatomic features seen in lambdoid synostosis, but not in deformational plagiocephaly?**
Ipsilateral mastoid bulge, trapezoid shape.

○ **What is the pathognomonic finding in Binder syndrome?**
Absent anterior nasal spine.

○ **Some define the Treacher–Collins craniofacial deformity in terms of which of the atypical facial clefts?**

Tessier 6, 7, 8.

○ **What is PHACE syndrome?**

Posterior fossa, **H**emangioma, **A**rterial anomalies, **C**ardiac defects, **E**ye anomalies. This condition should be suspected when patients present with a large segmental hemangioma of the face.

○ **What study should be obtained when a patient presents with a large segmental hemangioma, especially of the face in the trigeminal nerve distribution?**

Magnetic resonance angiography (MRA) of the brain to rule out ipsilateral cerebral artery anomalies.

○ **What is CHARGE association?**

CHARGE (**C**oloboma of the eye, **H**eart defects, **A**tresia of the nasal choanae, **R**etardation of growth and/or development, **G**enital and/or urinary abnormalities, and **E**ar abnormalities and deafness) syndrome.

○ **What study should be conducted for a patient presenting with an ear anomaly associated with syndromic appearing facial features?**

Renal ultrasound should be ordered to rule out structural renal anomalies as there is a higher incidence in syndromes associated with ear deformities (CHARGE syndrome, Townes–Brocks syndrome, branchio-oto-renal syndrome, Nager syndrome, Miller syndrome, and diabetic embryopathy).

● ● ● **REFERENCES** ● ● ●

Bassett AS, McDonald-McGinn DM, Devriendt K, et al; International 22q11.2 Deletion Syndrome Consortium. Practical guidelines for managing patients with 22q11.2 deletion syndrome. *J Pediatr*. 2011;159(2):332–339.

Blake KD, Davenport SL, Hall BD, et al. CHARGE association: an update and review for the primary pediatrician. *Clin Pediatr (Phila)*. 1998;37(3):159–173.

Bradley JP, Hurwitz DJ, Carstens MH. Embryology, classifications, and descriptions of craniofacial clefts. In: Mathes SJ, ed. *Plastic Surgery*. 2nd ed. Philadelphia, PA: Saunders Elsevier; 2006.

Farkas LG, ed. *Anthropometry of the Head and Face*. 2nd ed. New York, NY: Raven; 1994.

Jones KL. *Smith's Recognizable Patterns of Human Malformation*. 6th ed. Philadelphia, PA: Elsevier Saunders; 2006.

Lam AK, David DJ, Townsend GC, Anderson PJ. Van der Woude syndrome: dentofacial features and implications for clinical practice. *Aust Dent J*. 2010;55(1):51–58.

McCarthy JG, Hopper RA, Grayson, BH. Craniofacial microsomia. In: Mathes SJ, ed. *Plastic Surgery*. 2nd ed. Philadelphia, PA: Saunders Elsevier; 2006.

Metry DW, Haggstrom AN, Drolet BA, et al. A prospective study of PHACE syndrome in infantile hemangiomas: demographic features, clinical findings, and complications. *Am J Med Genet A*. 2006;140(9):975–986.

Shen L, Gu H, Wang D, et al. Influence of chromosome 22q11.2 microdeletion on postoperative calcium level after cardiac-correction surgery. *Pediatr Cardiol*. 2011;32(7):904–909.

Stuppia L, Capogreco M, Marzo G, et al. Genetics of syndromic and nonsyndromic cleft lip and palate. *J Craniofac Surg*. 2011;22(5): 1722–1726.

Vander Kolk CA, Menezes J. Craniofacial syndromes. In: Mathes SJ, ed. *Plastic Surgery*. 2nd ed. Philadelphia, PA: Saunders Elsevier; 2006.

Wilkie AOM. Molecular genetics of craniosynostosis. In: Lin KY, Ogle RC, Jane JA, eds. *Craniofacial Surgery: Science & Surgical Technique*. Philadelphia, PA: WB Saunders; 2002.

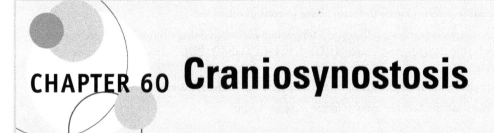

CHAPTER 60 Craniosynostosis

Pieter G.L. Koolen, MD and
Samuel J. Lin, MD, MBA, FACS

○ **What is the incidence of craniosynostosis?**

1 in 2,000 births.

○ **True/False: Facial sutures fuse before cranial sutures.**

False.

○ **When do the facial sutures fuse?**

Facial sutures (except for the midpalatal suture) fuse in the seventh decade. Suture—time of fusion: frontonasal—68 years, frontozygomatic—72 years.

○ **When do the cranial sutures fuse?**

Cranial sutures fuse earlier than the facial sutures.

Suture—Time of fusion: metopic—2 years (may persist throughout life in 10%), sagittal—22 years, coronal—24 years, lambdoid—26 years, palatal—30 to 35 years.

○ **What is the pattern of cranial suture fusion?**

Front to back, lateral to medial.

○ **What is the function of cranial and facial sutures?**

<u>Cranial:</u> Bone overlap during birth, principal site of skull expansion, and shock-absorbing function in childhood.

<u>Facial:</u> Shock-absorbing function related to mastication.

○ **What is Moss's functional matrix theory?**

Cranial bones enlarge as a result of growth and expansion of the underlying brain.

○ **What role may osteoblast-derived growth factors have in craniosynostosis?**

In vitro studies of craniosynostotic bone cells reveal a longer population doubling time, which suggests that suppression of osteoblastic-derived growth factors (IGF-I, IGF-II, TGF-b1, PDGF, and bFGF) may be a factor.

○ **What is the genetic abnormality of Crouzon, Apert, and Jackson–Weiss syndromes?**

Chromosome 10, mutation of fibroblast growth factor receptor 2 gene.

○ **What is the genetic abnormality of Pfeiffer syndrome?**

Chromosomes 8 and 10, mutation of the fibroblast growth factor receptor 1 or 2 gene.

○ **Which form of suture synostosis has an increased frequency of mutation in the genetic loci for fibroblast growth factor receptor 3 *(FGFR-3)*?**

Coronal.

○ **What is the genetic transmission of Saethre Chotzen, Crouzon, Apert, and Pfeiffer syndromes?**

Autosomal dominant.

○ **What is the genetic transmission of Carpenter and Baller–Gerhold syndromes?**

Autosomal recessive.

○ **What is the cause of contralateral frontal bone bossing and bilateral temporal bulges in coronal suture craniosynostosis?**

Bone growth occurs at the perimeter sutures with increased bone deposition directed away from the abnormally fused bone plate.

○ **True/False: Virchow (1851) noted that skull growth is inhibited parallel to the synostosed suture.**

False (inhibited perpendicular, compensatory expansion parallel).

○ **What are the three types of forehead plagiocephaly (asymmetry of the head)?**

Synostotic plagiocephaly, compensational plagiocephaly, deformational plagiocephaly.

○ **What is the incidence of synostotic forehead plagiocephaly?**

1 in 10,000 live births.

○ **True/False: 79% of synostotic forehead plagiocephaly occurs in females.**

True.

○ **What are the distinguishing features of synostotic forehead plagiocephaly?**

- Forehead flat on affected side.
- Eyebrow elevated on affected side.
- Ear on affected side rotated anterior-superiorly.
- Face C-shaped with nose and chin deviated to opposite side.
- Forehead prominence opposite side.
- Ipsilateral cheek forward.

○ **What is the cause of head tilting in uncorrected unilateral synostosis?**

Strabismus secondary to paresis of the ipsilateral superior oblique muscle.

○ **What are the radiographic features of synostotic forehead plagiocephaly?**

- Radiographs—perisutural sclerosis, absence of coronal suture, harlequin mask appearance of orbit.
- 3D CT scan—fused suture, extent of skull, and facial deformity.

○ **What percentage of patients with synostotic forehead plagiocephaly have torticollis?**

14%, usually contralateral side.

○ **What is the cause of compensational plagiocephaly?**

Premature fusion of the contralateral lambdoid suture. Uncommon condition, fused suture revealed on radiographs. Clinical distinguishing factor from deformational plagiocephaly, no improvement on follow-up.

○ **What are the causes of deformational plagiocephaly?**

Compressive forces in utero, by birth trauma and postnatal deformation by laying too much on one side.

○ **What is the incidence of deformational forehead plagiocephaly?**

1 in 300 live births.

○ **What are the distinguishing features of deformational plagiocephaly?**

- Superior orbital rim lower on the affected side.
- Eyebrow down.
- Ear rotated posterior-inferiorly on the flattened side.
- Malar eminence flattened ipsilaterally.
- Nose and chin rotated to affected side.
- Deformity not as severe as in synostosis.

○ **What are the radiographic findings?**

Patent sutures.

○ **True/False: Torticollis is most commonly ipsilateral in deformational forehead plagiocephaly.**
True.

○ **True/False: Unlike synostotic forehead plagiocephaly, 76% of patients are male in deformational forehead plagiocephaly.**
False.

○ **True/False: On follow-up examination, physical findings in deformational plagiocephaly do not improve.**
False.

○ **What is the cause of brachycephaly?**

Bilateral coronal suture craniosynostosis.

○ **What are the clinical features of brachycephaly?**

Reduced anterior–posterior distance, increased bitemporal distance.

○ **What is the normal ratio of anterior–posterior to bitemporal distance? What is the ratio in brachycephaly?**

3:2, 1:1.

○ **What are the radiographic findings of brachycephaly?**

• X-ray—bilateral fused coronal sutures and harlequin mask appearance.

• CT scan—fused sutures, abnormal shape of frontal bone.

• 3D CT scan—receding supraorbital borders, compensatory bulging of upper forehead.

○ **What is the cause of trigonocephaly?**

Metopic suture craniosynostosis.

○ **What are the clinical features of trigonocephaly?**

Triangular forehead with bilateral recession of lateral supraorbital borders and hypotelorism.

○ **What are the radiographic findings of trigonocephaly?**

• X-ray—hypotelorism.

• CT scan—triangular-shaped forehead.

• 3D CT scan—altered shape of forehead.

○ **Which form of synostosis is most frequently associated with abnormalities of the corpus callosum and increased incidence of developmental delay?**

Metopic synostosis, trigonocephaly.

○ **What is the cause of scaphocephaly?**

Sagittal suture craniosynostosis.

○ **True/False: Scaphocephaly is the most common form of craniosynostosis, more than 50% of cases.**

True.

○ **What are the clinical features of scaphocephaly?**

Dolichocephalic (scaphocephalic) cranial shape with biparietal narrowing and often frontal and/or occipital bossing. Palpable midline ridge. The cranial vault is long and narrow with a low posterior vault. Apex of the vault is anterior whereas under normal circumstances it is posterior.

○ **What percentage of patients also have lambdoid synostosis?**

5% to 10%.

Clinical findings—foreshortening of skull in occipital region with prominent frontal bossing.

○ **What is the incidence of lambdoid suture craniosynostosis?**

1% to 5% of all craniosynostosis cases. Much less common than deformational posterior plagiocephaly.

○ **What are the clinical features of lambdoid craniosynostosis?**

Flatness on one or both sides of the posterior skull, posterior rotation of ipsilateral ear, compensatory flatness on contralateral frontal area—brachycephaly.

○ **What are the radiographic findings?**

Extensive sclerosis along the suture line difficult to distinguish from the mild sclerosis of deformational plagiocephaly.

○ **What is Kleeblattschädel (cloverleaf skull)?**

It is the most severe form of craniosynostosis, fusion of the coronal, lambdoid, and metopic sutures. Anterior sagittal and squamosal sutures are open.

○ **What are the clinical features of Kleeblattschädel?**

• Bulging of frontal and temporal bones.

• Markedly receding supraorbital borders.

• Severe exorbitism.

• Skull circumference significantly reduced.

• Hydrocephalus usually present.

○ **What are some of the congenital anomalies that may be associated with Kleeblattschädel?**

• Choanal atresia

• High-arched palate

• Cleft palate

○ **What are the ocular complications seen in Kleeblattschädel?**

Because of retraction of the eyelids behind the globe, corneal opacity and perforations may occur if surgery is delayed.

○ **Which craniosynostosis syndrome is commonly associated with Kleeblattschädel?**

Pfeiffer syndrome.

○ **What is cranioscoliosis?**

Curvature of the midline of the craniofacial skeleton without fusion of sutures or torticollis or neck deformities. Diagnosis of exclusion.

○ **What are the features of Saethre–Chotzen syndrome (craniocephalosyndactyly)?**

- Bilateral coronal synostosis
- Brachycephaly
- Ptosis
- Maxillary hypoplasia
- Low hair line
- Prominent ear crus along concha
- Strabismus
- Cleft or high arched palate
- Syndactyly
- Brachydactyly or clinodactyly
- Vertebral anomalies
- Normal intelligence

○ **What are the features of Crouzon syndrome (craniofacial dysostosis)?**

Bilateral coronal synostosis

- Oxycephaly (high, wide forehead, bulging anterior fontanelle)
- Cranial base synostosis, hypertelorism
- Exophthalmos
- Maxillary hypoplasia
- Parrot beak nose
- Micrognathia
- No hand or feet abnormality

○ **What are the features of Apert syndrome (acrocephalosyndactyly)?**

- Skull: Bilateral coronal synostosis, brachycephaly.
- Maxillary hypoplasia: High-arched palate, cleft palate or submucosal cleft palate, crowding dental arch, anterior open bite.
- Orbit: Hypertelorism, exorbitism, oculomotor paralysis, ptosis, down-slanting palpebral fissure.
- Hands: Syndactyly all fingers (mitten hands), short humerus.
- Feet: Syndactyly all toes.
- Coarse skin and acne.
- Enlarged ear lobes.
- Mental retardation: Variable.

○ **What are the features of Carpenter syndrome (group of acrocephalosyndactyly)?**

- Craniosynostosis single or multiple sutures
- Deafness
- Mental retardation
- Brachydactyly (hands and feet)
- Syndactyly (hands and feet)
- Polydactyly (hands, preaxial)

○ **What is the incidence of Crouzon and Apert syndromes?**

1 in 60,000 and 16 per million births, respectively.

○ **What are the clinical features of Pfeiffer syndrome?**

- Craniosynostosis
- Wide thumbs and great toes
- Brachydactyly
- Partial syndactyly
- Maxillary hypoplasia
- Intelligence usually normal

○ **What is Jackson–Weiss syndrome?**

- Craniosynostosis
- Hypertelorism
- Midface hypoplasia
- Broad great toes
- Syndactyly toes (occasionally fingers)
- Medial deviation tarsal–metatarsal coalescence

○ **What is Baller–Gerhold syndrome?**

- Craniosynostosis
- Radial aplasia
- Anal anomalies
- Urologic defects
- Cardiac deformity
- CNS abnormalities
- Vertebral defects

○ **What is Antley–Bixler syndrome?**

- Craniosynostosis (brachycephaly, frontal bossing, large anterior fontanelle)
- Midfacial hypoplasia
- Depressed nasal bridge
- Proptosis
- Choanal stenosis and/or atresia
- Dysplastic ears
- Radiohumeral synostosis
- Joint contractures (upper and lower extremities)
- Arachnodactyly
- Renal defects
- High incidence of respiratory compromise

○ **What is the timing of surgery in Kleeblattschädel (cloverleaf deformity)?**

Kleeblattschädel: First few days of life, urgent decompression is needed to decrease intracranial pressure as well as fronto-orbital advancement and tarsorrhaphy for ocular protection.

○ **What is the general timing of surgical intervention for any form of single-suture craniosynostosis?**

Endoscopic approaches and strip craniectomies may be performed as early as 2 to 3 months of age and generally require helmeting for up to 1 year postoperation.

Fronto-orbital advancement and/or total vault reconstruction is generally undertaken at 6 months of age or later, but can be done as early as 3 months of age. Helmeting is only needed in ambulating patients for up to 1 to 2 months if required.

○ **What principles guide the timing of surgical correction for craniosynostosis?**

Osteogenetic potential of the dura is greatest under 18 months of age; gaps after reconstruction are well tolerated because the dura will fill them with new bone. This osteogenic potential of the dura is generally lost after 2 years of age.

The cranial bone is more malleable at an early age. It becomes substantially more brittle and more difficult to shape after the age of 18 months making good aesthetic outcomes more difficult to attain.

Surgical blood loss is much less in the younger age groups making surgery safer in patients younger than 18 months.

By operating early it is believed by some that the rapid brain growth will help to guide and maintain the head shape after surgery.

The best window for operation is between 3 and 12 months of age for decreased surgical morbidity and optimized surgical outcomes.

○ **What is the risk of increased intracranial pressure and adverse effect on mental development in synostosis of one suture?**

7% chance, risk increases with multiple sutures.

○ **True/False: Cosmetic appearance is the primary factor for operative intervention in craniosynostosis.**

False.

○ **What are the goals of therapy in craniosynostosis?**

- Release the synostosis and provide adequate skull volume for brain development.

- Create an aesthetically normal forehead and skull shape.

- It is still quite controversial whether surgical intervention improves developmental outcomes. Current literature seems to suggest that it does not, except in the case of symptomatic, increase intracranial pressure.

○ **What are the interventions for deformational plagiocephaly?**

- Sternomastoid stretching exercises for torticollis

- Tummy time

- Avoid extensive periods of time spent in car seats

- Increase amount of time spent carrying the child

- At feeding times baby encouraged to turn head toward breast or bottle

- Orthotic cranioplasty—helmet to mold skull as it grows

○ **At what age is orthotic cranioplasty effective and what is the time course of therapy?**

Molding can be begun as early as 4 months of age. It is not effective after 18 months of age. Helmet is worn 23 hours a day for 2 to 4 months. Inadequate response may require surgical intervention in severe cases. Outcomes are best with early application.

○ **What is the surgical management of unilateral coronal suture synostosis?**

Unilateral (mild deformity) or bilateral (severe deformity) fronto-orbital advancement.

○ **What is the determining factor in the surgical management of bilateral coronal suture synostosis?**

Presence of concomitant brachycephaly.

○ **What is the surgical management of bilateral coronal suture synostosis?**

Bilateral fronto-orbital advancement in patients without brachycephaly. Total calvarial reconstruction with barrel staving of occipital bones in patients with brachycephaly.

○ **What is the surgical management of metopic synostosis?**

Fronto-orbital advancement by removal of supraorbital bar, corticotomy, and correction of midline angle to 150 degrees with bone graft or miniplates. Correction of coronal synostosis. Examination of metopic suture and release. Hypotelorism corrects with growth.

○ **What is the primary determinant in the choice of operation for patients with sagittal synostosis?**

Patient age followed by previous intervention. Procedures are most effective and less extensive in younger patients less than 6 months. Ideal age is 2 to 4 months. More extensive procedures are needed at age 6 to 9 months. In children older than 1 year even more extensive procedures are needed and morbidity increases significantly due to increased blood loss.

○ **What are the standard surgical interventions for sagittal synostosis?**

The "pi" or "t" craniectomy techniques (or modifications thereof) that utilize strip craniectomies with partial wedge osteotomies. In selected cases with more severe deformity (frontal and occipital bossing), anterior and posterior parietal wedges or barrel-stave osteotomies to facilitate biparietal expansion. Total calvarial reconstruction may be used in children older than 1 year or reoperations, may require bone replacement.

Early strip craniectomy by open or endoscopic technique with helmeting.

○ **What is the Melbourne technique?**

This is a new surgical technique of total vault reconstruction generally applied to the complete correction of severe scaphocephaly. Tony Holmes of the Royal Children's Hospital (RCH) in Melbourne, Australia, developed this technique. It can also be used for cranial expansion. Fronto-orbital advancement can be easily added to the technique.

○ **What aspects of the scaphocephalic deformity are addressed by the Melbourne technique?**

The surgical goals of the Melbourne technique are the correction of frontal bossing, reduction of forehead height, correction of biparietal narrowing, anterior advancement of the occiput, elevation of posterior vault, and cranial expansion for increased intracranial volume. The Melbourne technique for total vault reconstruction developed at the RCH craniofacial unit addresses all of these reconstructive parameters.

○ **What is the major risk of surgical management of sagittal synostosis?**

Sagittal sinus injury with blood loss or venous infarction.

○ **What is the disadvantage of simple suture removal?**

Immediate correction of cranial shape is not achieved, many patients have residual deformity secondary to suture reclosure before adequate cranial remodeling.

○ **What is the advantage of early operation in sagittal synostosis?**

High potential for new bone growth, quicker operative options with less blood loss, continued brain growth for skull expansion, and increased skull flexibility for easier remodeling. Strip craniectomies are more effective if performed early, under 3 months of age, but require helmeting for continued molding.

○ **How long does it take for bone defects to fill in?**

Approximately 6 months.

○ **What is the rate of reoperation, what are the outcomes?**

Less than 5% reoperation. More than 90% excellent cosmetic results, the remaining good cosmetic results. This varies by type of craniosynostosis, severity of disease, and whether it is a syndromic or nonsyndromic case. Outcomes tend to be better in nonsyndromic (single suture) synostosis.

○ **What is the surgical management of lambdoidal synostosis?**

Under age 6 months excision of lambdoid suture. Over age 6 months posterior skull remodeling with occipital bandeau, barrel staving of bone below the bandeau, and bending with Tessier bone bender. Alternate method: spiral osteotomy.

○ **What is the preoperative management of Kleeblattschädel?**

- Management of more serious medical problems.

- Airway management.

- Eye protection—artificial tears, ophthalmic ointment.

- R/O cervical spine and craniovertebral anomalies.

- Radiologic workup 3D CT scans.

○ **What is the indication for emergent management Kleeblattschädel?**

- Management of hydrocephalus.

- VP shunt may be indicated at the same time or at a subsequent procedure.

- Ocular compromise.

○ **What is the operative management of Kleeblattschädel?**

Anterior calvariectomy with fronto-orbital advancement. Bone removal from constricting band of coronal, frontosphenoid, frontoethmoid, and lambdoid sutures. Total calvarial reconstruction may be indicated.

○ **Will further intervention be needed?**

In severe cases a second-stage posterior calvarial release is necessary at 1 to 2 months of age. A second anterior surgical release is often required at 6 to 12 months. A third correction of anterior and/or posterior skull deformities again before age 4.

○ **What are some of the potential operative and early postoperative complications of craniosynostosis cases?**

- Death

- Anesthetic complications

- Excessive blood loss

- Sagittal sinus tear with venous infarction

- Cerebral edema

- Increased ICP

- Subdural hematoma

- Periorbital injury

- Nerve injury (frontal branch VII, supraorbital nerve)

- Loss of vision

- Corneal abrasion

- CSF leak via dural tear

- Infection

- Skin necrosis

- SIADH

○ **What are some of the late postoperative complications of craniosynostosis operations?**

- Alopecia
- Hypertrophic scarring
- Palpable hardware
- Forehead defects and irregularities
- Deficient frontal bone advancement
- Temporal depression
- Pseudomeningoceles
- Metal plates
- Orbital deformities
- Asymmetry
- Recurrence
- Bone graft resorption
- Increased ICP
- Patient dissatisfaction

● ● ● **REFERENCES** ● ● ●

Anderson FM, Geiger L. Craniosynostosis: a survey of 204 cases. *J Neurosurg.* 1965;22:229–240.

Bruneteau RJ, Mulliken JB. Frontal plagiocephaly: synostotic, compensational, or deformational. *Plast Reconstr Surg.* 1992;89:21–31.

Cassileth LB, Bartlett SP, Glat PM, et al. Clinical characteristics of patients with unicoronal synostosis and mutations of fibroblast growth factor receptor 3: a preliminary report. *Plast Reconstr Surg.* 2001;108:1849–1854.

David DJ, Poswillo D, Simpson DA. *The Craniosynostosis; Causes, Natural History and Management.* New York, NY: Springer-Verlag; 1982.

Delashaw JB, Persing JA, Broaddus WC, Jane JA. Cranial vault growth in craniosynostosis. *J Neurosurg.* 1989;70:159–165.

Fearon JA, Munro IR. Cranioscoliosis. *Plast Reconstr Surg.* 1993;92:202–208.

Gosain AK, Steele MA, McCarthy JG, Thorne CH. A prospective study of the relationship between strabismus and head posture in patients with frontal plagiocephaly. *Plast Reconstr Surg.* 1996;97:881–891.

Greensmith AL, Holmes, AD, Lo, P, Maxiner W, Heggie A, Meara JG. Complete correction of severe scaphocephaly: the Melbourne method of total vault remodeling. *Plast Reconstr Surg.* 2008;121(4):1300–1310.

Hinton DR, Becker LE, Muakkessa KF, Hoffman HJ. Lambdoid synostosis. Part 1. The lambdoid suture: normal development and pathology of "synostosis." *J Neurosurg.* 1984;61:333–339.

Huang MH, Mouradian WE, Cohen SR, Gruss JS. The differential diagnosis of abnormal head shapes: separating craniosynostosis from positional deformities and normal variants. *Cleft Palate Craniofac J.* 1998;35(3):204–211.

Losken HW, Pollack IF. Craniosynostosis. In: Bentz ML, ed. *Pediatric Plastic Surgery.* 1st ed. Stamford: Appleton & Lange; 1998:129–157.

Sidoti EJ Jr, Marsh JL, Marty-Grames L, Noetzel MJ. Long-term studies of metopic synostosis: frequency of cognitive impairment and behavioral disturbances. *Plast Reconstr Surg.* 1996;97:276–281.

Speltz ML, Kapp-Simon K, Collett B, et al. Neurodevelopment of infants with single-suture craniosynostosis: presurgery comparisons with case-matched controls. *Plast Reconstr Surg.* 2007;119(6):1874–1881.

Watters EC, Hiles DA, Johnson BL. Cloverleaf skull syndrome. *Am J Ophthalmol.* 1973;76:716–720.

Whitaker LA, Bartlett SP, Schut L, Bruce D. Craniosynostosis: an analysis of the timing, treatment, and complications in 164 consecutive patients. *Plast Reconstr Surg.* 1987;80(2):195–212.

Zampino G, DiRocco C, Butera G, et al. Opitz C trigonocephaly syndrome and midline brain anomalies. *Am J Med Genet.* 1997;73:484–488.

CHAPTER 61 Cleft Lip and Palate

John N. Jensen, MD

○ **What anatomic feature divides the primary and secondary palates?**

The incisive foramen.

○ **Which muscles control the velum?**

Levator veli palatini, tensor veli palatini, palatopharyngeus, palatoglossus, and musculus uvulae.

○ **What are the anatomic features of a submucous cleft palate?**

Bifid uvula, zona pellucida (muscle diastasis), V-notch to posterior palatal edge.

○ **What is the probability of a patient with a submucous cleft having velopharyngeal dysfunction?**

Trick question; patients with a submucous cleft who are asymptomatic are unlikely to present to medical professionals; the probability may be estimated at less than 10%.

○ **What is the fundamental argument for surgical repair of the palate prior to 18 months of age?**

Preservation of speech.

○ **Which of the paired velar muscles is innervated by CN V, mandibular division?**

Tensor veli palatini.

○ **What is the reason to "stage" a palatal repair?**

Delay of elevation of hard palatal mucoperiosteum may preserve midface growth potential.

○ **What is the principal vascular supply to the palatal mucoperiosteal flap?**

Greater palatine artery and vein.

○ **What is the target of innervation of the greater and lesser palatine nerves?**

They contribute sensory innervation to the palatal mucosa.

○ **What is the motor innervation of the velar musculature except the tensor veli palatini?**
CN X (vagus) via the pharyngeal plexus.

○ **Which teeth usually originate in the premaxilla?**
Central and lateral incisors.

○ **Which tooth is most likely to be abnormal in cleft lip?**
Lateral incisor.

○ **What is the significance for lateral incisor agenesis in children with cleft patients?**
It is a predictor for the need for maxillary advancement.

○ **Where is the lesser palatine foramen?**
Posterior to the greater palatine foramen within the palatine bone.

○ **Which muscles of the palate control eustachian tube function?**
Tensor veli palatini, and to a lesser extent, levator veli palatini.

○ **What is the blood supply of the soft palate?**
Ascending palatine artery is the major source.

○ **What is the argument against gingivoperiosteoplasty in infancy?**
Restricted maxillary growth.

○ **What are the putative etiological factors in clefting?**
Advanced paternal age, genetic, prenatal exposure to drugs, other environmental agents (multifactorial).

○ **Which muscles form the anterior and posterior tonsillar pillars?**
Palatoglossus and palatopharyngeus, respectively.

○ **What is the main function of the levator veli palatini?**
To elevate the soft palate.

○ **Does the tensor veli palatini elevate the palate?**
No, it primarily controls eustachian tube function and possibly contributes to swallowing.

○ **What is the probability that a parent with nonsyndromic cleft lip/palate will have a child with a cleft?**
4% for the first child, and 17% for the second child if the first child has a cleft.

○ **What is the probability that parents without clefts who already have a child with a (nonsyndromic) cleft will have another child with a cleft?**
4%.

○ **What is the probability that a parent with Van Der Woude syndrome will have a child with a cleft?**

50% (autosomal dominant inheritance: roughly follows Mendelian pattern).

○ **What is a Simonart band?**

Soft tissue at the nasal sill on the affected side; it is a feature that commonly defines "incomplete" cleft lip, but it is abnormal tissue and variable in thickness.

○ **At what point in gestation is the error responsible for cleft lip and palate likely to occur?**

Weeks 5 to 6 (lip) and 7 to 8 (palate).

○ **In embryology, what are the five facial prominences that eventually form the face, and what is the error in cleft lip?**

The five facial prominences: Frontonasal process, paired maxillary prominences, paired mandibular prominences.

The frontonasal process derives medial and lateral nasal processes; failure of fusion of one or both of the medial nasal processes and corresponding maxillary processes results in cleft lip.

○ **What is the purpose of presurgical orthopedics?**

To narrow the cleft and align the alveolar segments, facilitating surgical repair by reducing tension.

○ **What is the rate of postoperative cleft palate fistula formation?**

It varies widely in reports: 2% to roughly 30%.

○ **What is the essential advantageous feature of the Furlow palatoplasty?**

It effectively lengthens the palate.

○ **What is a criticism of the Furlow palatoplasty?**

Ischemic flaps induce fibrosis and reduce mobility of the velum.

○ **What is the most pertinent outcome measure of success of palatoplasty?**

Speech intelligibility.

○ **Which cleft palate surgical technique is shown to give superior speech results?**

A recent review found a statistically significant reduction in secondary speech surgery in patients treated with Furlow double-opposing Z-plasty compared to straight line repair.

○ **What is the theoretical purpose of the intravelar veloplasty?**

To detach from the hard palate and correctly reorient the levator muscle and optimize its function.

○ **What governs the timing of alveolar bone grafting?**

Eruption of the permanent canine on the affected side (usually 8–10 years).

○   **In cleft patients with large negative overjets (>8–10 mm) and normal mandibular projection, what is the most appropriate treatment for correction of their malocclusion?**

Le Fort I distraction osteogenesis.

○   **At what age can Le Fort I distraction be considered?**

When the developing dentition has descended sufficiently to accommodate the osteotomy.

○   **How does nasoalveolar molding differ from standard presurgical orthopedics?**

It addresses the nasal deformity with passive stretching of the nasal vestibule and alar dome.

○   **Does presurgical nasoalveolar molding improve surgical outcomes in cleft lip/nose repair?**

In most studies, there is clear benefit, ranging from improved nasal symmetry to reduced need for secondary procedures.

○   **What is the difference between presurgical orthopedics and presurgical orthodontics?**

Orthopedics refers to the movement of bone, not teeth, and is applicable in the newborn cleft patient when referring to realignment of the alveolar segments.

○   **Is the prevalence of orofacial clefts on the rise in the United States?**

No.

○   **Do children with cleft lip/palate suffer from reduced oral health-related quality of life?**

Yes.

○   **What is the incidence of clefts?**

About 1 in 700: Asian > Caucasian > African.

○   **Why are left-sided clefts thought to occur about twice as commonly as those on the right?**

Fusion of the left embryonic processes occurs later, increasing the probability of exposure to mutagenic mechanisms.

○   **What is the principle that distinguishes the Veau–Wardill–Kilner technique of palatoplasty?**

The V-Y "pushback," which attempts to posteriorly displace the reconstructed soft palate.

○   **What is the Noordhoff flap?**

A triangular vermillion flap on the lateral segment that addresses the deficiency of dry vermillion on the medial segment, as well as contributing bulk to the vermillion.

○   **What is the function of myringotomy tubes?**

To ventilate the middle ear.

○ **What is the purpose of cleft feeding aids?**

To compensate for a lack of suction in the cleft palate baby, by allowing the manual delivery of formula or breast milk.

○ **How can speech development be impeded by a cleft lip/palate?**

Velopharyngeal dysfunction, conductive hearing loss, dental derangement.

○ **What is the theoretical advantage of the gingivoperiosteoplasty in infancy?**

It may preclude the necessity for alveolar bone grafting in mixed dentition.

○ **What is the expected rate of growth in cleft infants?**

0.5 to 1 ounce per day (normal growth).

○ **True or False: Children with unilateral cleft lip/palate exhibit normal growth from 2 to 10 years of age.**

True.

○ **Where is enamel hypoplasia of the permanent dentition most commonly seen in cleft patients?**

In the anterior dentition, at the site of the cleft.

○ **What reasons could explain poor weight gain in a patient with isolated cleft palate?**

Poor feeding technique, neuromotor dysfunction, occult airway obstruction.

○ **What disciplines are represented in the typical cleft team?**

Plastic surgery, otolaryngology, speech pathology, audiology, pediatric dentistry, orthodontics, prosthodontics, psychology, social work, genetics, nursing.

○ **What genes have been identified as involved in susceptibility to nonsyndromic cleft lip/palate?**

TGF A, TGFb3, MSX1, IRF6, TBX22, CYP1A1, GSTM1, NAT2, MTHFR, RARA, PVRL1.

○ **What is a Latham appliance?**

A presurgical orthopedic device that actively realigns alveolar segments.

○ **When does a middle ear effusion typically become apparent in a patient with cleft palate?**

Within about 8 weeks from birth.

○ **What is the essential feature of the von Langenbeck palatoplasty?**

Incomplete elevation of hard palatal mucoperiosteal flaps.

○ **What are the abnormal anatomic features in unilateral cleft lip?**

Overall deficiency of lip tissue on the cleft side, shortened columella on the cleft side, upwardly rotated Cupid's bow, disruption and aberrant insertion of the orbicularis muscle, often profound nasal asymmetry, anterior nasal spine deviated to noncleft side, sagittal retrusion of alveolus and piriform on cleft side.

○ **What anatomic features distinguish the bilateral cleft lip deformity from unilateral clefts?**

Wide nasal tip with splaying of lower lateral cartilages, greater severity in columellar deficiency, greater projection of the premaxilla, effaced sulcus on the prolabium, absent muscle in the prolabium, and deficient muscle in the lateral segments of the upper lip.

○ **What characterizes the nasal deformity in clefts of the lip/primary palate?**

Diminutive lower lateral cartilage, caudally rotated, resulting in a depressed alar dome with a widened base on the cleft side as well as (often severe) septal deviation.

○ **What are the essential features of the Millard technique of cleft lip repair?**

It levels the Cupid's bow by rotating a medial flap downward, and advancing the lateral segment into the defect, which also narrows the alar base and restores symmetry to the nose; its result is to place the scar along the philtral column, preserving the philtral dimple.

○ **What is the Randall–Tennison repair?**

This technique lengthens the columella by inserting a rotated triangular flap from the lateral lip, leaving a scar within the philtrum and flattening the philtral dimple.

○ **What is a "forme fruste" cleft lip?**

A better term is microform or minor cleft and refers to that end of the spectrum of severity of clefting with lesser but variable involvement of the vermillion, muscle, and alveolus.

○ **What percentage of cleft lips are incomplete?**

Estimates range from 10% to 30%.

○ **What is the ratio of left-sided clefts to right-sided clefts to bilateral clefts?**

6:3:1.

○ **What is the "M" flap in the Millard rotation-advancement technique of cleft lip repair?**

If the cleft is viewed as a geometric void, it is the medial boundary and may be elevated to add lining to the sulcus or add tissue to reconstruct the nasal floor.

○ **What is the "L" flap in the Millard rotation-advancement technique of cleft lip repair?**

The lateral extent of the void, or superior aspect of the abnormal vermillion on the cleft side; it may be elevated as a flap based on the nasal mucosa to reconstruct the nasal floor and expand the nasal vestibule on the cleft side.

○ **What is the "C" flap in the Millard rotation-advancement technique of cleft lip repair?**

The skin on the medial aspect of the cleft bounded by the medial vermillion as it extends into the cleft itself and the medial incision; it is used to reconstruct the columella.

○ **What is the Mohler modification of the Millard rotation-advancement?**

The medial incision is carried onto the columellar skin to add length to the medial lip and allows for downward rotation of the Cupid's bow while restricting the scar to the philtral column, columella, and nasolabial junction; in the classic Millard repair, severely rotated medial segments may require extended back cuts that can leave the scar positioned obliquely across the philtrum.

What is the forked flap?

In Millard bilateral cleft lip repair, the lateral segments of the prolabium are preserved and transposed to the nasal sill, to be reelevated and advanced to midline some years later to effect columellar lengthening.

When is lip adhesion employed?

It is the first of a staged repair, where a simple surgical repair joins the lip segments, without rotation or advancement, in a way that does not compromise the later, definitive repair. It is usually employed in wide clefts to have an orthopedic effect on the alveolar segments that serve to narrow the cleft for less tension for the definitive repair.

What is the significance of palatal cleft morphology?

Wide, U-shaped clefts are more often associated with the Pierre Robin sequence and may indicate underlying airway compromise.

When is the cleft nasal deformity addressed?

Usually at the time of cleft lip repair.

When is secondary cleft nasal surgery usually undertaken?

At age 5 to 6 years, but no firm rule is generally accepted.

What is the arterial supply of the upper lip?

Superior labial artery, branching from the facial artery.

What is the nerve supply of the upper lip?

Primarily branches of the infraorbital nerve (CN V_2).

When is the Abbe–Estlander flap employed in cleft surgery?

Often in bilateral cleft lip the disparity between upper and lower lip transverse dimension is so great that transfer of lower lip tissue is indicated to address the short, immobile upper lip that can result in bilateral repair.

• • • REFERENCES • • •

Cutting CB. Bilateral cleft lip repair. In: Mathes SJ, ed. *Plastic Surgery*. 2nd ed. Philadelphia, PA: Saunders Elsevier; 2006.

Grayson BH, Garfinkle JS. Early cleft management: the case for nasoalveolar molding. *Am J Orthodont Dentofacial Orthop*. 2014; 145(2):134–142.

Hoffman WY, Mount D. Cleft palate repair. In: Mathes SJ, ed. *Plastic Surgery*. 2nd ed. Philadelphia, PA: Saunders Elsevier; 2006.

Hollier L. Cleft palate and velopharyngeal incompetence. In: Barton FE, ed. *Selected Readings in Plastic Surgery*. Vol. 8. 23rd ed. Dallas, TX: UT-Southwestern Medical Center; 1997.

Jones KL. Smith DM. *Recognizable Patterns of Human Malformation*. 6th ed. Philadelphia, PA: Elsevier Saunders; 2006.

Lai LH, Hui BK, Nguyen PD, et al. Lateral incisor agenesis predicts maxillary hypoplasia and Le Fort I advancement surgery in cleft patients. *Plast Reconstr Surg*. 2015;135(1):142e–148e.

Losee JE, Kirschner RE, eds. *Comprehensive Cleft Care*. New York, NY: McGraw-Hill; 2009.

Margulis A, Bauer BS. Cleft palate deformities. In: Bentz ML, Bauer BS, Zucker RL, eds. *Principles & Practice of Pediatric Plastic Surgery*. St Louis, MO: Quality Medical Publishing; 2008.

Marques IL, Nackashi J, Borgo HC et al. Longitudinal study of growth of children with unilateral cleft lip and palate: 2 to 10 years of age. *Cleft Palate Craniofacial J.* 2015;52(2):192–197.

Noordhoff MS, Chen PKT. Unilateral cheiloplasty. In: Mathes SJ, ed. *Plastic Surgery.* 2nd ed. Philadelphia, PA: Saunders Elsevier; 2006.

Ruiz LA, Maya RR, D'Alpino PH, Atta MT, da Rocha Svizero N. Prevalence of enamel defects in permanent teeth of patients with complete cleft lip and palate. *Cleft Palate Craniofac J.* 2013;50(4).394–399.

Stuppia L, Capogreco M, Marzo G, et al. Genetics of syndromic and nonsyndromic cleft lip and palate. *J Craniofac Surg.* 2011;22(5): 1722–1726.

Timbang MR, Gharb BB, Rampazzo A, Papay F, Zins J, Doumit G. A systematic review comparing Furlow double-opposing Z-plasty and straight-line intravelar veloplasty methods of cleft palate repair. *Plast Reconstr Surg.* 2014;134(5):1014–1022.

Ward JA, Vig KW, Firestone AR, Mercado A, da Fonseca M, Johnston W. Oral health-related quality of life in children with orofacial clefts. *Cleft Palate Craniofac J.* 2013;50(2):174–181.

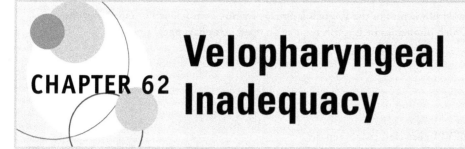

CHAPTER 62
Velopharyngeal Inadequacy

Jugpal S. Arneja, MD, MBA, FAAP, FACS, FRCSC and Arun K. Gosain, MD

○ **Describe what is meant by velopharyngeal incompetence (VPI)?**

1. The velopharyngeal structures cannot produce full closure of the velopharyngeal port.

2. The velopharyngeal system is structurally inadequate for production of good speech.

3. The structure of the velopharyngeal system or its neuromotor control is inadequate for production of good speech.

4. An individual's speech is perceived as showing characteristics associated with disorders of the velopharyngeal system.

○ **What terms are associated with VPI?**

Velopharyngeal incompetence, inadequacy, deficiency, or insufficiency.

○ **Is there a difference in the meaning of the relative terms associated with VPI?**

These terms are specific to different aspects of inadequacy of the velopharyngeal mechanism:

1. *Incompetence* refers to impaired motion of the velopharyngeal mechanism.

2. *Insufficiency* refers to tissue deficiency of the velum.

3. *Inadequacy* refers to a combination of incompetence and insufficiency, and is the more generic term. Therefore, velopharyngeal inadequacy is more properly referred to as VPI.

○ **What are the symptoms and signs of VPI?**

Speech: Hypernasality, compensatory misarticulations, airflow escape, facial grimacing.

Reflux: Oronasal regurgitation (fluids >> solids).

Hearing loss (conductive): Eustachian tube dysfunction.

○ **What is the hallmark characteristic of VPI on perceptual speech evaluation?**

Hypernasality.

○   **The majority of articulated phonemes in the English language require competency or closure of the velopharyngeal port. Which phonemes in English require an open velopharyngeal port?**

1. /m/

2. /n/

3. /ng/

○   **What is the incidence of VPI post-cleft palate repair?**

The incidence varies between 7% and 25% post-palate repair.

○   **What are the etiologies of VPI?**

1. Idiopathic insufficiency of palatal musculature.

2. Congenital palatal insufficiency.

3. Submucous cleft palate (SMCP).

4. Post-cleft palate repair.

5. Postpharyngeal flap or pharyngoplasty.

6. Postadenoidectomy or adenoid involution.

7. Enlarged tonsils.

8. Postmidface advancement.

9. Neurogenic causes.

10. Adynamic velopharyngeal sphincter.

11. Functional or hysterical hypernasality.

12. Palatopharyngeal disproportion.

○   **What is the most common cause of VPI?**

Post-cleft palate repair.

○   **What anatomically makes up the velopharyngeal space?**

Velum/soft palate (anterior border), posterior pharyngeal wall (posterior border), lateral pharyngeal walls (lateral borders).

○   **What muscles contribute to closure of the velopharynx?**

Levator veli palatini, superior pharyngeal constrictor, palatopharyngeus, tensor tympani, musculus uvulae.

○   **What is the most important muscle regarding closure of the velopharyngeal space for speech?**

Levator veli palatini muscle.

○   **Discuss functions during opening and closing of the velopharynx.**

Opening of the velopharynx: Facilitates breathing and normal speech production of nasal phoneme articulations.
Closure of the velopharynx: Allows normal speech production of oral consonants and prevents oronasal reflux.

○ **How does the velopharynx close?**

The velum moves posteriorly and superiorly, the posterior pharyngeal wall moves anteriorly, the lateral pharyngeal walls move medially, and the tonsils and adenoids may augment or interfere with the function of the walls during velopharyngeal closure.

○ **Who contributes to the evaluation of VPI?**

An interdisciplinary team consisting of:

1. Plastic surgeon

2. Speech/language pathologist

3. Otolaryngologist

4. Audiologist

5. Radiologist

6. Geneticist

○ **How should VPI be evaluated?**

The initial assessment of speech should be based on a perceptual assessment by a trained speech-language pathologist. Based on this assessment a patient is given a diagnosis of VPI. Whereas not all speech-language pathologists make this diagnosis based on a numeric scale, use of such scales is highly recommended for consistency and interrater reliability. Patients who are given a diagnosis of VPI can then undergo further testing.

Indirect methods: Mirror test, nasometry

Direct methods: Nasopharyngeal endoscopy, multiview videofluoroscopy

○ **What methodology employed by the speech-language pathologist has been the most consistent for intercenter auditing of cleft speech?**

The Cleft Audit Protocol for Speech—Augmented (CAPS-A).

○ **How has the CAPS-A methodology impacted speech assessment worldwide?**

CAPS-A now forms the basis for both the EuroCleft and the AmeriCleft protocols for speech evaluation.

○ **What are the parameters used for rating speech by the CAPS-A?**

The patient's speech is evaluated perceptually (auditory and visual input) by a trained speech pathologist. CAPS-A establishes a numeric scale by which to rate cleft speech based on the following parameters, each of which provides a relative score in which 0 is normal, and the higher the number, the more severe the inadequacy:

1. Intelligibility/Distinctiveness of speech (score: 0–4)

2. Voice characteristics (score: 0–1)

3. Resonance

    a. Hypernasality (score: 0–4)

    b. Hyponasaility (score: 0–2)

4. Nasal airflow

    a. Audible nasal emission (score: 0–2)

    b. Nasal turbulence (score: 0–2)

5. Grimace (score: 0–1)

○ **What modality has been recently studied that might have efficacy in the evaluation of VPI?**

Functional magnetic resonance imaging (fMRI).

○ **At what age should a perceptual speech assessment be performed?**

Although a baseline evaluation can be performed at approximately 1.5 years of age, an objective assessment of velopharyngeal function can rarely be obtained prior to 2.5 to 3 years of age as patients need to be cooperative for a thorough perceptual speech assessment.

○ **What are the closure patterns seen with nasopharyngeal endoscopy?**

Four types of closure patterns are found on nasopharyngeal endoscopy:

1. Coronal (most common, 55%)
2. Circular (20%)
3. Circular with Passavant's ridge (15–20%)
4. Sagittal (10–15%)

○ **What can a plastic surgeon fix?**

The goal of surgery is to prevent airflow escape through the nose during phonation; surgeons can fix fistula(e), lengthen the palate (Furlow or via addition of buccal flaps), augment the palate or posterior wall, create a passive obstruction (pharyngeal flap), or create a dynamic posterior sphincter (sphincter pharyngoplasty). The remainder of speech-related problems associated with VPI must be corrected with speech therapy.

○ **What nonsurgical treatments are available for VPI?**

Speech therapy, palatal lift, palatal prosthesis, velopharyngeal obturator.

○ **What surgical treatments are available for VPI?**

Palatal lengthening (Furlow palatoplasty or V-Y pushback palatoplasty), posterior wall augmentation (alloplastic or autogenous materials), sphincter pharyngoplasty, pharyngeal flap.

○ **What materials are available for posterior wall augmentation?**

Alloplastic: Teflon, silastic, silicone gel, proplast, hyaluronic acid derivatives Autogenous: Autologous cartilage, autologous fascia, fat.

○ **Is posterior wall augmentation used in practice today?**

Most centers have abandoned posterior wall augmentation because of unpredictable results and implant migration, extrusion, or exposure. However, recently some centers have found success using fat grafting for augmentation of the posterior wall or soft palate.

○ **What is a sphincter pharyngoplasty?**

A surgical procedure designed to tighten the central orifice and occlude the lateral aspects of the velopharyngeal sphincter.

○ **Which muscle forms the basis for a successful sphincter pharyngoplasty? How is it done?**

Palatopharyngeus; two (right and left) myomucosal (palatopharyngeus) flaps are elevated from the posterior tonsillar pillars and are sutured to each other and to the posterior pharyngeal wall.

○ **When should a sphincter pharyngoplasty be performed?**

There is no consensus in the literature, but historically sphincter pharyngoplasties have been performed for documented cases of sufficient palatal length and mobility, with poor lateral wall motion in the setting of hypernasality/airflow escape on perceptual speech evaluation.

○ **What are the complications of a sphincter pharyngoplasty?**

Flap dehiscence, sleep apnea, snoring, airway obstruction, persistent hypernasality.

○ **What is a pharyngeal flap?**

The creation of a midline subtotal obstruction of the oral and nasal cavities with two small lateral openings (ports) that remain patent during respiration and nasal consonant production and closed during oral consonant production.

○ **How is a pharyngeal flap done?**

A myomucosal flap based on the superior constrictor muscle is elevated from the posterior pharyngeal wall and is attached to the soft palate creating an incomplete midline obstruction; the donor site can be closed primarily or allowed to heal secondarily.

○ **Should a superiorly or inferiorly based pharyngeal flap be performed?**

Superiorly based flaps are most frequently used since inferiorly based flaps can tether the velopharyngeal port closure in an inferior direction, opposite to the necessary superior direction for correct velopharyngeal closure.

○ **When should a pharyngeal flap be performed?**

Again, there are no clear indications, but historically pharyngeal flaps are performed when there is sufficient lateral wall motion but a short soft palate or adynamic anteroposterior palate closure in the setting of hypernasality/airflow escape on perceptual speech evaluation.

○ **What are the complications of a pharyngeal flap?**

Flap dehiscence, sleep apnea, snoring, airway obstruction, hyponasality, persistent hypernasality.

○ **What is velocardiofacial (VCF) syndrome? What is the concern to a surgeon treating VPI in patients with VCF syndrome?**

VCF syndrome is an autosomal dominant condition associated with deletions on the long arm of chromosome 22.

Major clinical findings include cleft palate, congenital heart anomalies, cognitive impairment, and abnormal facies. The concern of a VPI surgeon is that patients with VCF may have medially displaced carotid arteries that make injury to the carotids a possibility during pharyngeal surgery.

○ **What test is essential prior to surgical correction of VPI in patients with VCF syndrome?**

Magnetic resonance angiography (MRA) or angiography.

○ **What is the recommended surgical treatment for VPI in VCF patients?**

This remains controversial, but some groups report high success rates using a high, wide pharyngeal flap.

○ **What is a submucous cleft palate (SMCP)?**

A SMCP is classically defined as patients having a bifid uvula, a zona pellucida (palatal muscle diastasis), and absence of the posterior nasal spine (identified as a bony notch in the posterior aspect of the hard palate in lieu of a posterior nasal spine).

○ **What is the incidence of VPI in patients with an SMCP?**

One in nine (11%).

○ **What should the treatment be of an SMCP?**

SMCP should be initially evaluated by perceptual speech evaluation; surgery should only be performed for documented cases of VPI following a thorough speech evaluation.

○ **What is the "black hole" in VPI?**

On nasoendoscopic evaluation of the velopharyngeal space, there is confirmation of both poor lateral wall motion and a large anterior–posterior velopharyngeal gap.

● ● ● **REFERENCES** ● ● ●

Arneja JS, Hettinger P, Gosain AK. Through and through dissection of the soft palate for pharyngeal flap inset. A new technique for velopharyngeal incompetence in velocardiofacial syndrome. *Plast Reconstr Surg.* 2008;122:845–852.

Bicknell S, McFadden LR, Curran JB. Frequency of pharyngoplasty after primary repair of cleft palate. *J Can Dent Assoc.* 2002;68: 688–692.

Boneti C, Ray PD, Macklem EB, Kohanzadeh S, de la Torre J, Grant JH. Effectiveness and Safety of autologous fat grafting to the soft palate alone. *Ann Plast Surg.* 2015;74:S190–S192.

Conley SF, Gosain AK, Marks SM, Larson DL. Identification and assessment of velopharyngeal inadequacy. *Am J Otolaryngol.* 1997; 18:38–46.

Croft CB, Shprintzen RJ, Rakoff SJ. Patterns of velopharyngeal valving in normal and cleft palate subjects: a multiview videofluoroscopic and nasendoscopic study. *Laryngoscope.* 1981;91:265–271.

David DJ, Bagnall AD. Velopharyngeal incompetence. In: McCarthy JG, ed. *Plastic Surgery.* 1st ed. Philadelphia, PA: WB Saunders, 1990:2903–2921.

Denny AD, Marks SM, Oliff-Carneol S. Correction of velopharyngeal insufficiency by pharyngeal augmentation using autologous cartilage: a preliminary report. *Cleft Palate Craniofac J.* 1993;30:46–54.

Dworkin JP, Marunick MT, Krouse JH. Velopharyngeal dysfunction: speech characteristics, variable etiologies, evaluation techniques, and differential treatments. *Lang Speech Hear Serv Sch.* 2004;35:333–352.

Folkins JW. Velopharyngeal nomenclature: incompetence, inadequacy, insufficiency, and dysfunction. *Cleft Palate J.* 1988;25:413–416.

Gart MS, Gosain AK. Surgical management of velopharyngeal insufficiency. *Clin Plast Surg.* 2014;41(2):253–270.

Gosain AK, Arneja JS. Management of the black hole in velopharyngeal incompetence: combined use of a Furlow palatoplasty and sphincter pharyngoplasty. *Plast Recon Surg.* 2007;119:1538–1545.

Gosain AK, Conley SF, Marks S, Larson DL. Submucous cleft palate: diagnostic methods and outcomes of surgical treatment. *Plast Reconstr Surg.* 1996;97:1497–1509.

John A, Sell D, Sweeney T, Harding-Bell A, Williams A. The Cleft Audit Protocol for Speech—Augmented: a validated and reliable measure for auditing cleft speech. *Cleft Palate Craniofac J.* 2006,43:272–288.

Marsh JL. Management of velopharyngeal dysfunction: differential diagnosis for differential management. *J Craniofac Surg.* 2003;14: 621–628.

Marsh JL. The evaluation and management of velopharyngeal dysfunction. *Clin Plastic Surg.* 2004;31:261–269.

Mitnick RJ, Bello JA, Golding-Kushner KJ, Argamaso RV, Shprintzen RJ. The use of magnetic resonance angiography prior to pharyngeal flap surgery in patients with velocardiofacial syndrome. *Plast Reconstr Surg.* 1996;97:908–919.

Schendel SA, Lorenz HP, Dagenais D, Hopkins E, Chang J. A single surgeon's experience with the Delaire palatoplasty. *Plast Reconstr Surg.* 1999;104:1993–1997.

Sirois M, Caouette-Laberge L, Spier S, Larocque Y, Egerszegi EP. Sleep apnea following a pharyngeal flap: a feared complication. *Plast Reconstr Surg.* 1994;93:943–947.

Sloan GM. Posterior pharyngeal flap and sphincter pharyngoplasty: the state of the art. *Cleft Palate Craniofac J.* 2000;37:112–122.

Tatum SA 3rd, Chang J, Havkin N, Shprintzen RJ. Pharyngeal flap and the internal carotid in velocardiofacial syndrome. *Arch Facial Plast Surg.* 2002;4:73–80.

Vedung S. Pharyngeal flaps after one- and two-stage repair of the cleft palate: a 25-year review of 520 patients. *Cleft Palate Craniofac J.* 1995;32:206–215.

Witt PD, D'Antonio LL. Velopharyngeal insufficiency and secondary palatal management. a new look at an old problem.. *Clin Plast Surg.* 1993;20:707–721.

Witt PD, Marsh JL, Muntz HR, Watchmaker GP. Acute obstructive sleep apnea as a complication of sphincter pharyngoplasty. *Cleft Palate Craniofac J.* 1996;33:183–189.

Witt PD. Velopharyngeal insufficiency. In: Achauer B, ed. *Plastic Surgery: Indications, Operations, and Outcomes.* 1st ed. St Louis, MO: CV Mosby, 2000:819–833.

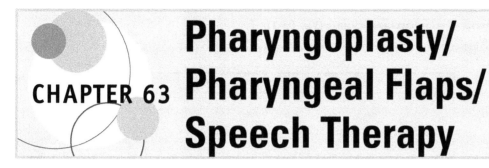

Pharyngoplasty/ Pharyngeal Flaps/ Speech Therapy

CHAPTER 63

Kristen A. Hudak, MD and
Arlen D. Denny, MD

○ **Name the six primary muscles of the velopharyngeal mechanism.**

Levator veli palatini, tensor veli palatini, musculus uvulae, palatoglossus, palatopharyngeus, superior constrictor.

○ **Which of these muscles is innervated by V3?**

Tensor veli palatini. (The others are all innervated by from the pharyngeal plexus—IX, X, XI)

○ **What is the primary function of tensor veli palatini?**

Opening of the eustachian tube.

○ **In what direction(s) does the soft palate move to close the velopharyngeal portal?**

Posteriorly and superiorly.

○ **What muscle is primarily responsible for this movement?**

Levator veli palatini.

○ **What muscle is primarily responsible for medial movement of the lateral pharyngeal walls during closure of the velopharyngeal portal?**

Levator veli palatini.

○ **Name the four patterns of velopharyngeal closure (Fig. 63-1).**

Coronal, sagittal, sphincteric, and sphincteric with Passavant's ridge.

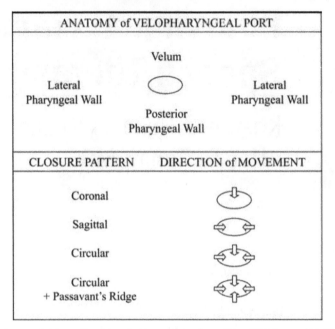

Figure 63-1 Pattern of velopharyngeal closure. (Reproduced with permission from, Fisher DM, Sommerlad BC. Cleft lip, cleft palate, and velopharyngeal insufficiency. *Plast Reconstr Surg*. 2011;128(4):342e–360e.)

○ **What is Passavant's ridge?**

Transversely oriented ridge on the posterior pharyngeal wall, due to bulging of the fibers of superior constrictor.

○ **Where does Passavant's ridge usually lie relative to the level of velopharyngeal closure?**

Approximately 1 cm inferior, often does not close the velopharyngeal gap.

○ **Which arteries supply the soft palate?**

Lesser palatine artery, ascending palatine branch of facial artery, palatine branches of ascending pharyngeal artery.

○ **What is the difference between velopharyngeal incompetence (VPI) and velopharyngeal insufficiency?**

VPI is the inability to adequately close the palate against the pharyngeal wall leading to nasal air escape.

Insufficiency refers to an anatomic or structural defect that can be congenital or due to surgery. Examples include: cleft palate, congenitally short palate/large pharynx, or after an adenoidectomy or an ablative surgery.

Incompetence refers to neuromuscular deficit. Examples include: myasthenia gravis, cerebral palsy, stroke, head injury, or upper/lower motor neuron lesions.

○ **What is rhinolalia aperta?**

Hypernasal speech due to inadequate closure of the velopharyngeal portal.

○ **Can hypernasality be quantified?**

Yes, with a nasometer. This device uses a nasal microphone, an oral microphone, and a computer to analyze the relative sound output from each source. It calculates the nasalance as a ratio of the nasal acoustic emission to the nasal and oral acoustic emission.

○ **What is a fricative?**

Consonant sound produced by the constriction of the air stream to create friction, as in f, v, s, z, th, or sh.

○ **What distinguishes the different fricatives?**

Position of the articulators (e.g., the tongue articulates with the teeth for th, and with the alveolar ridge for s or z).

○ **What is a pharyngeal fricative?**

Fricative produced by articulation of the tongue base against the posterior pharyngeal wall.

○ **Name an example of a pharyngeal fricative in normal English speech.**

There is none. A pharyngeal fricative is used by patients with VPI as a substitute for a normal oral fricative.

○ **What is a stop plosive?**

Consonant sound produced by the sudden release of intraoral pressure, as in p, b, t, d, k, or g.

○ **What is a glottal stop?**

Plosive sound made after the adducted vocal cords suddenly open. It is a common misarticulation by patients with VPI. The only example in normal English is "uh."

○ **What is a posterior nasal fricative?**

The back of the tongue articulates against the velum (attempt to close the posterior nasal aperture). This sounds like a nasal snort.

○ **What is an anterior nasal fricative?**

Nasal grimacing (attempt to close anterior nasal aperture).

○ **What is a diphthong?**

Single syllable with two vowel sounds (e.g., cow, toy, about). Diphthongs require significant velar elevation and mobility, and are thus difficult for patients with VPI.

○ **Besides hypernasality, what other category of speech disturbance is associated with VPI?**

Misarticulations.

○ **Besides VPI, what are other common reasons for misarticulation in the pediatric plastic surgery population?**

Congenital hearing loss, developmental delay, abnormal dentition (e.g., V-shaped maxillary dentition in Apert syndrome), malocclusion.

○ **Describe the Cul-de-sac test.**

Cul-de-sac resonance is when sound resonates in a cavity, however, cannot get out due to obstruction. To test you ask the patient to repeat a word like "bat" or "boot" twice, the second time with the patient's nose pinched. If the resonance is different, the oral and nasal cavities are coupled (i.e., there is inadequate velopharyngeal closure).

○ **What is pressure–flow instrumentation?**

Objective assessment of nasal airflow and differential oral–nasal air pressure.

○ **What are the two most common imaging modalities for the assessment of VPI?**

Videofluoroscopy and nasal endoscopy.

○ **What is the advantage of videofluoroscopy?**

Ability to define the level of velopharyngeal closure in the sagittal plane (i.e., with respect to Passavant's ridge). This test requires less cooperation than nasal endoscopy.

○ **What is the advantage of nasal endoscopy?**

Ability to directly visualize the entire velopharyngeal mechanism during speech. This allows characterization of the closure pattern.

○ **What are the indications for a palatal obturator?**

Extremely wide cleft with little or no velar movement (in whom surgery would be expected to have a poor outcome), neuromuscular deficit, poor surgical candidate, surgical failure.

○ **What is the orientation of the levator fibers within the normal soft palate and in the cleft palate?**

Transverse/horizontal in the normal palate.
Longitudinal with abnormal insertion at the posterior hard palate in the cleft palate patient.

○ **What is an intravelar veloplasty?**

Redirection of the aberrantly oriented levator muscles to the transverse plane, permitting functional mobility of the soft palate.

○ **What is the incidence of VPI after standard palatoplasty and intravelar veloplasty?**

Approximately 20%.

○ **What common palatoplasty technique has the lowest incidence of postoperative VPI?**

Furlow double-opposing Z-plasty.

○ **What is the incidence of VPI in individuals with submucous cleft palate?**

10% to 15%, first refer for speech therapy, if repair needed use double-opposing Z-palatoplasty

○ **What is pharyngeal augmentation?**

Placement of autologous tissue or alloplastic material in the retropharyngeal space with the goal of reducing the size of the velopharyngeal gap. Reported substances include bone, cartilage, fascia, mucosa, fat, and calcium hydroxyapatite. No study has demonstrated a safe, effective and reliable material for long-term reduction in velopharyngeal gap.

○ **The retropharyngeal space lies between what two fascial planes?**

Buccopharyngeal fascia and prevertebral fascia.

○ **What layers are included in the posterior pharyngeal flap (PPF)?**

A rectangular flap is designed either superiorly or inferiorly on the posterior pharyngeal wall including: mucosa, muscle (superior constrictor), buccopharyngeal fascia. This flap is elevated superficial to the prevertebral fascia and inset at the posterior soft palate (Fig. 63-2).

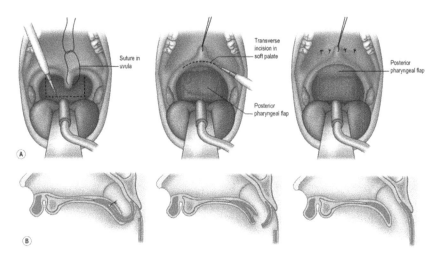

Figure 63-2 Posterior pharyngeal flap. (Reproduced with permission from, Kirschner RE, Baylis AL. Velopharyngeal dysfunction. In: Neligan PC. *Plastic Surgery*. New York, NY: Elsevier; 2013.)

○ **What important vascular structure lies 1 to 1.5 cm lateral to the PPF?**

Internal carotid artery.

○ **The internal carotid artery is often medially displaced in what common craniofacial syndrome?**

Velocardiofacial syndrome. A magnetic resonance angiography can be obtained to evaluate preoperatively.

○ **What can be done to prevent contracture and rolling of a PPF?**

Lining the raw surface with nasal mucosal flaps from the soft palate.

○ **What are the most serious complications of PPF surgery?**

Hemorrhage and sleep apnea.

○ **What are the risk factors for postoperative sleep apnea?**

Age <5 years, microretrognathia, upper respiratory tract infection, history of perinatal respiratory dysfunction, tonsillar or adenoid enlargement (some recommend tonsillectomy prior/during surgery).

○ **What is a sphincter pharyngoplasty (SP)?**

Wrapping of superiorly based lateral pharyngeal flaps along posterior pharyngeal wall to create a dynamic ridge (Fig. 63-3).

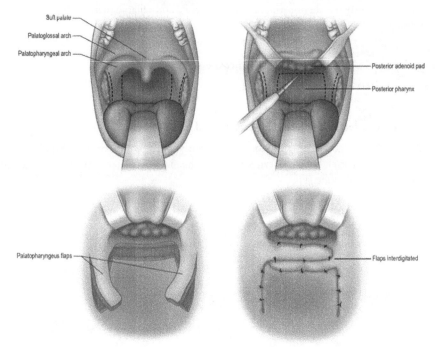

Figure 63-3 Sphincter pharyngoplasty. (Reproduced with permission from, Kirschner RE, Baylis AL. Velopharyngeal dysfunction. In: Neligan PC. *Plastic Surgery*. New York, NY: Elsevier; 2013.)

○ **What muscle is included in the sphincter pharyngoplasty flaps?**

Palatopharyngeus.

○ **What is the innervation of the muscle included in the sphincter pharyngoplasty?**

Cranial part of accessory nerve (XI) and pharyngeal branch of vagus (X) via pharyngeal plexus.

○ **What is the difference between the Hynes and Orticochea pharyngoplasties?**

Hynes pharyngoplasty: The palatopharyngeal flaps are inset within a transverse incision in the posterior pharyngeal wall.

Orticochea pharyngoplasty: The palatopharyngeal flaps are inset under an inferiorly based mucosal flap from the posterior pharyngeal wall. Jackson modified the Orticochea procedure by insetting the flaps under a superiorly based mucosal flap.

○ **At what level should the palatopharyngeal flaps be inset?**

At the level of velopharyngeal closure, as determined by videofluoroscopy. Usually this means insetting the flaps as high as possible, above Passavant's ridge and above the level of the arch of the atlas.

○ **In what fraction of SPs does the transferred palatopharyngeus muscle retain significant contractility?**

Approximately one-third.

○ **Is SP better than PFF?**

It is not clear. Two randomized trials found no difference between the two procedures in terms of speech improvement, operative complications, or incidence of sleep apnea. However, a meta-analysis showed possible improved outcomes with a pharyngeal flap. The velopharyngeal closure pattern may impact the relative efficacy of these procedures. SP is thought to be easier to perform than PPF, with no need to divide the soft palate. SP is also easily revisable, in that the flaps can be reelevated and made tighter (if hypernasality persists) or looser (if sleep apnea becomes a problem).

○ **For each of the following velopharyngeal closure patterns, what treatment is (theoretically) most appropriate?**

Coronal pattern, with little lateral wall movement	Sphincter pharyngoplasty
Sagittal pattern, with good lateral movement but poor velar movement	Pharyngeal flap
Sphincteric pattern, with small gap	Sphincter pharyngoplasty
Sphincteric pattern, with large gap	Pharyngeal flap
No closure (poor velar and lateral movement)	Large pharyngeal flap or obturator
Good velar movement, small gap, anteriorly directed velar muscles	Double-opposing Z-plasty (Furlow)

• • • REFERENCES • • •

Abyholm F, D'Antonio L, Davidson Ward SL, et al. Pharyngeal flap and sphincteroplasty for velopharyngeal insufficiency have equal outcome at 1 year postoperatively: results of a randomized trial. *Cleft Palate Craniofac J.* 2005;42(5):501–511.

Armour A, Fischbach S, Klaiman P, Fisher DM. Does velopharyngeal closure pattern affect the success of pharyngeal flap pharyngoplasty? *Plast Reconstr Surg.* 2005;115(1):45–52.

Collins J, Cheung K, Farrokhyar F, Strumas N. Pharyngeal flap versus sphincter pharyngoplasty for the treatment of velopharyngeal insufficiency: a meta-analysis. *J Plast Reconstr Aesthet Surg.* 2012;65(7):864–868.

Fisher DM, Sommerlad BC. Cleft lip, cleft palate, and velopharyngeal insufficiency. *Plast Reconstr Surg.* 2011;128(4):342e–360e.

Khosla RK, Mabry K, Castiglione CL. Clinical outcomes of the Furlow Z-Plasty for primary cleft palate repair. *Cleft Palate Craniofac J.* 2008;45(5):501–510.

Kirschner RE, Baylis AL. Velopharyngeal dysfunction. In: Neligan PC, ed. *Plastic Surgery.* New York, NY: Elsevier; 2013.

Sullivan SR, Vasudavan S, Marrinan EM, Mulliken JB. Submucous cleft palate and velopharyngeal insufficiency: comparison of speech outcomes using three operative techniques by one surgeon. *Cleft Palate Craniofac J. 2011;*48(5):561–570.

Ysunza A, Pamplona C, Ramírez E, Molina F, Mendoza M, Silva A. Velopharyngeal surgery: a prospective randomized study of pharyngeal flaps and sphincter pharyngoplasties. *Plast Reconstr Surg.* 2002;110(6):1401–1407.

CHAPTER 64 Distraction Osteogenesis

Pieter G.L. Koolen, MD and
Samuel J. Lin, MD, MBA, FACS

○ **When was the field of craniofacial surgery established?**

In 1967 after publication of Paul Tessier's work in the paper "Osteotomies totales de face, Syndrome de Crouzon, Syndrome D'Apert, Oxycephalies, Scaphocephalies, Turricephalies."

○ **What are the main insights that have helped to overcome the limitations in craniofacial surgery over the past 25 years?**

Understanding of the pathologic anatomy through better imaging (3D CT scan), extensive bone grafting of bony defects, rigid fixation of osteotomized segments, and most recently, the evolving applications of distraction osteogenesis.

○ **What is distraction osteogenesis?**

A concept of fixation that actively mobilizes osteotomy segments and promotes osteogenesis. Also known as callostasis (stretching of callus, as in a fracture).

○ **What is the concept of distraction osteogenesis?**

1. Distraction zone: location of the bone separation by osteotomy or corticotomy
2. Latency period: time allowed for reparative callus formation in the distraction zone
3. Activation period: gradual distraction forces applied to callus, elongation of callus under tension
4. Consolidation period: external fixation maintained after activation, allows consolidation of distraction generate.

○ **What are the advantages of distraction osteogenesis?**

Reduced risk of infection seen in nonvascularized bone grafts, eliminated need for a donor site hence no donor site morbidity or limitations, simple design, more predictable bone survival, potential for three-dimensional changes, reduced operative blood loss, reduced number of subsequent procedures, possibility of repeated applications, avoids in situ metal plates and screws or maxillomandibular fixation (MMF), early closure of tracheostomy in cases of micrognathia, ability to be used in irradiated bone, well tolerated, no known evidence of growth retardation, possibility of better aesthetic results.

○ **True/False: Distraction osteogenesis has a higher rate of morbidity and greater need for secondary midface procedures compared to bone grafting.**

False.

○ **True/False: Distraction osteogenesis actually causes enlargement of the overlying surrounding tissue via histiogenesis.**

True.

○ **What are the disadvantages of mandibular distraction osteogenesis?**

Hypertrophic scarring at pin site (most common disadvantage), pin tract infection (osteomyelitis not reported to date), pin extrusion or migration, facial nerve injury, sensory deficits of inferior alveolar nerve, intolerance or noncompliance (uncommon), dentigerous cyst formation, ankylosis, tooth bud injury in patients younger than 1 year, may still require secondary procedures.

○ **How is new bone formed during distraction osteogenesis?**

Intramembranous ossification.

○ **True/False: Distraction is a unique form of fracture healing that occurs in the craniofacial skeleton without a cartilaginous intermediate.**

True.

○ **What are the zones of distraction osteogenesis that result in mature bone formation?**

Zone of fibrous tissue (zone I): the fibrous interzone (FIZ) is composed of highly organized, longitudinally oriented, parallel strands of collagen with spindle-shaped fibroblasts and undifferentiated mesenchymal precursor cells through the matrix. Central region of the distraction gap.

Zone of extending bone formation (zone II): the primary mineralization front (PMF) found on both the edges of the FIZ composed of fibroblasts and undifferentiated mesenchymal precursor cells in direct continuity with osteoblasts on the surface of bone spicules (osteoblasts longitudinally oriented and parallel to direction of distraction). Spindle-shaped fibroblastic cells transform into bone-forming cells. Increased levels of alkaline phosphatase, pyruvic acid, and lactic acid. Also known as the transitional zone.

Zone of bone remodeling (zone III): advancing fields of bone resorption and apposition, increased number of osteoclasts.

Zone of mature bone (zone IV): early compact cortical bone located adjacent to mature bone in unexpanded areas. Bone spicules thicker, less longitudinal orientation.

○ **When are chondrocytes present during distraction osteogenesis?**

When there is excessive motion, fibrocartilage nonunion occurs.

○ **What growth factor is currently thought to play a key role in the process of distraction osteogenesis?**

Transforming growth factor-beta 1.

○ **True/False: The blood supply in the distraction zone is decreased compared to the normal side.**

False.

○ **How long does it take the bone in the distraction zone to achieve 90% of normal bony structure?**

Usually within 8 months.

○ **What are the clinical phases of distraction osteogenesis?**

<u>Latency phase:</u> 5 to 7 days after corticotomy or osteotomy, initial fracture healing bridges the cut bony surfaces before initiating distraction.

<u>Distraction phase:</u> 3- to 5-week period of active stretching of the FIZ at 1 mm/day.

<u>Mineralization phase:</u> The period of consolidation, a 7- to 9-week period after distraction when the PMF advances from each end toward the center, bridging the FIZ with bone.

○ **True/False: Failure of distraction osteogenesis has not been reported clinically in the craniofacial skeleton.**

True.

○ **Although failure of distraction osteogenesis has not been recorded in the craniofacial skeleton, what are some of the factors Aronson has suggested could contribute to failure?**

<u>Ischemic fibrogenesis:</u> inadequate local blood supply, fibrous tissue formation without bone formation.

<u>Cystic degeneration:</u> caused by blockage of venous outflow, distraction gap fills with cystic cavity.

<u>Fibrocartilage nonunion:</u> caused by unstable fixation, cartilage fills distraction gap.

<u>Buckling of regenerate bone:</u> fixation device destabilized or removed prematurely.

○ **At what age are bones potentially too soft to allow distraction?**

Before age 18 months distraction is used with caution. Distraction is primarily used in the mandible between 18 months and 22 years of age. Recent literature supports the use of mandibular distraction in neonates with tongue-based airway compromise as seen in Pierre Robin sequence.

○ **What is the only indication for distraction in patients younger than 2 years?**

Tongue-based airway compromise secondary to mandibular hypoplasia. Pulling the mandible forward pulls the tongue forward relieving the obstruction. Good outcomes have been seen in multiple institutions.

○ **What are the specific clinical indications for mandibular distraction in patients with Pierre Robin sequence?**

- Syndromic patients with poor mandibular growth.
- Beyond 9 months and continued airway compromise secondary to tongue base obstruction.
- Candidates for tracheostomy.
- Failure of nonsurgical management.
- Age 2 to 4 difficult time to distract.
- May also need adenoidectomy or tracheal reconstruction.

○ **True/False: Children younger than 2 years with hypoplasia or aplasia of the mandible without airway compromise should not undergo distraction osteogenesis of the mandible because of the risk for permanent dental injury.**

True.

○ **In which grades of mandibular hypoplasia is distraction osteogenesis indicated?**

Grades I, IIA, and IIB. In grade III, elongation is not possible because the ramus is absent.

○ **True/False: Distraction can be accomplished regardless of soft-tissue deficiency since the soft tissues are simultaneously expanded with bone distraction.**

True.

○ **What is included in the clinical assessment of patients for mandibular distraction?**

Anthropometric measurements, facial nerve function, dental occlusion, dental cast impressions, preoperative photos (full face, profile, three-fourth, basal views, biting tongue blade for occlusal slant), cephalometric radiographs (lateral, AP), Panorex and or 3D CT scans—most accurate measure of mandible size and deficiency.

○ **True/False: Bone grafting is preferred over distraction osteogenesis for advancements of more than 10 mm because a more stable result that is less prone to relapse can be attained.**

False.

○ **Why is distraction less prone to relapse than bone grafting in advancements larger than 10 mm?**

There is a more gradual stretching of the soft tissues, which makes relapse less likely.

○ **What are the principles of mandibular distraction?**

Preserve periosteum if possible, place osteotomy and pin sites with adequate bone stock away from tooth buds, corticotomy preferred to osteotomy (to avoid inferior alveolar nerve injury).

○ **What are the surgical approaches to the mandible?**

Extraoral approach (modified Risdon) or internal approach.

○ **What is the primary advantage of an external distraction device versus an internal distraction device?**

External distraction device can be removed in the office avoiding a second operative procedure. Better control of the distraction vector.

○ **What is a common protocol for mandibular distraction after device placement?**

Begin distraction on fifth to seventh postoperative day by rotating the screw 0.25 mm four times a day (better tolerated than 0.5 mm twice a day) or 1 mm of distraction a day. Distraction completed in 3 to 5 weeks, slight overcorrection useful to prevent postoperative relapse. Pins and device left in place 8 to 9 weeks longer or until radiographic evidence of new bone bridging seen.

○ **When should the distraction device be removed?**

Only when new bone has a radiodensity equivalent to the host bone surfaces and a macrostructure resembling host bone with equivalent cross-sectional area and formation of cortex and medullary canal.

○ **How is the posterior open bite achieved during distraction maintained?**

Bite block or similar orthodontic appliance until maxillary growth and tooth eruption fills the gap.

○ **What are the complications of mandibular distraction?**

Injury to the inferior alveolar nerve (direct injury or slow traction when distraction distance is significant)—usually temporary, pin tract infection, loosening of pins, relapse after device removal, injury to tooth buds, ankylosis of temporal mandibular joint (TMJ), facial nerve paresis, failure of distraction (not reported).

○ **True/False: Osteomyelitis of the mandible during distraction has not been reported.**

True.

○ **What patient population may benefit most from the clinical application of distraction osteogenesis of the midface?**

Cleft palate patients with maxillary hypoplasia. Maxillary advancement may cause speech problems; distraction may limit velopharyngeal compromise.

○ **What patient population may benefit from orbital expansion by distraction in the future?**

Patients with anophthalmos, congenital absence of ocular tissue. It is predicted to result in fewer surgical procedures, better fit of orbital prosthesis, and improved cosmetic outcome.

○ **What are the indications for palatal distraction?**

Anatomic or relative maxillary deficiency, nasal stenosis when conchae are compressed against the septum, all types of class III occlusion, mature cleft patient, anteroposterior maxillary deficiency, selected arch length problems.

● ● ● REFERENCES ● ● ●

Aronson J. Experimental and clinical experience with distraction osteogenesis. *Cleft Palate Craniofac J.* 1994;31:473–482.

Cruz MJ, Kerschner JE, Beste DJ, Conley SF. Pierre Robin sequence: secondary respiratory difficulties and intrinsic feeding abnormalities. *Laryngoscope.* 1999;109:1632–1636.

Denny AD, Talisman R, Hanson PR, Recinos RF. Mandibular distraction osteogenesis in very young patients to correct airway obstruction. *Plast Reconstr Surg.* 2001;108(2):302–311.

Gantous A, Phillips JH, Catton P, Holmberg D. Distraction osteogenesis in the irradiated canine mandible. *Plast Reconstr Surg.* 1994;93:164–168.

Glat PM, McCarthy JG. Distraction of the mandible: experimental studies. In: McCarthy JG, ed. *Distraction of the Craniofacial Skeleton.* New York, NY: Springer-Verlag; 1999:67–79.

Gosain AK; Plastic Surgery Educational Foundation DATA Committee. Distraction osteogenesis of the craniofacial skeleton. *Plast Reconstr Surg.* 2001;107:278–280.

Haas AJ. Long-term post treatment evaluation of rapid palatal expansion. *Angle Orthod.* 1980;50:189–217.

Ilizarov GA. The tension-stress effect on the genesis and growth of tissues. Part I. The influence of stability of fixation and soft-tissue preservation. *Clin Orthop Relat Res.* 1989;(238):249–281.

Ilizarov GA. The tension-stress effect on the genesis and growth of tissues. Part II. The influence of rate and frequency of distraction. *Clin Orthop Relat Res.* 1989;(239):263–285.

Karp IS, McCarthy JG, Schreiber JS, Sissons HA, Throne CH. Membranous bone lengthening a serial histological study. *Ann Plast Surg.* 1992;29:2–7.

McCarthy JG, Schrieber J, Karp N, Throne CH, Grayson BH. Lengthening the human mandible by gradual distraction. *Plast Reconstr Surg.* 1992;89:1–8.

McCarthy JG, Stelnicki EJ, Mehrara BJ, Longaker MT. Distraction osteogenesis of the craniofacial skeleton. *Plast Reconstr Surg.* 2001;107:1812–1827.

McCarthy JG. Principles of craniofacial distraction. In: Thorne CH, Beasley RW, Aston SJ, Bartlett SP, Gurtner GC, Spear SL, eds. *Grabb and Smith's Plastic Surgery.* 6th ed. Philadelphia, PA: Lippincott Williams & Wilkins; 2007:96–102.

Personal notes from Presymposia on Pierre Robin Sequence. *ACPA.* 2009.

Singhal VK, Losken HW, Patterson G. Craniofacial distraction. In: Benz ML, ed. *Pediatric Plastic Surgery.* 1st ed. Stamford, CT: Appleton & Lange; 1998:341–357.

CHAPTER 65 Orthognathic Surgery

Steven R. Sewall, DDS and Kyle Smith, DDS

○ **What is orthognathic surgery?**

Orthognathic surgery is the surgical correction of abnormalities of the mandible, maxilla, or both. The underlying abnormality may be present at birth or may become evident as the patient grows and develops or may be the result of traumatic injuries. The severity of these deformities precludes adequate treatment through dental treatment alone.

○ **What are the main osteotomies performed in orthognathic surgery?**

1. Maxilla:
    a. Le Fort I osteotomy
        i. One-piece
        ii. Segmented
2. Mandible:
    a. Sagittal split ramus osteotomy
    b. Transoral vertical ramus osteotomy
    c. Transcutaneous vertical ramus osteotomy

○ **What are the facial categorizations?**

Mesocephalic: equal vertical facial thirds

Brachycephalic: broader, shorter, square face

Dolichocephalic: ovoid and narrow face with an increased lower third

○   **What are the different classifications of skeletal relationships?**

See Figure 65-1.

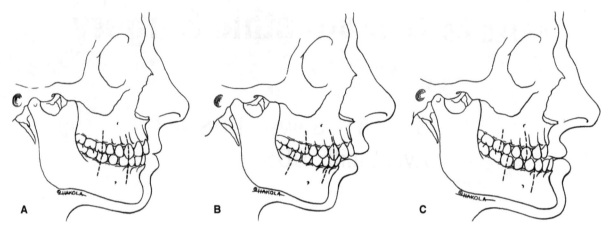

Figure 65-1 A: Class I orthognathic. **B:** Class II retrognathic. **C:** Class III prognathic. (Reproduced with permission from Ferraro JW. *Fundamentals of Maxillofacial Surgery*. New York, NY: Springer-Verlag Inc.; 1997.)

○   **How do you perform a dentofacial analysis?**

A dentofacial analysis is a clinical examination of soft and hard tissue of the dentofacial complex assessing vertical and transverse proportions in a thorough, systematic, and consistent approach. Direct measurement of the patient's resting and dynamic relationships is performed.

See Figure 65-2.

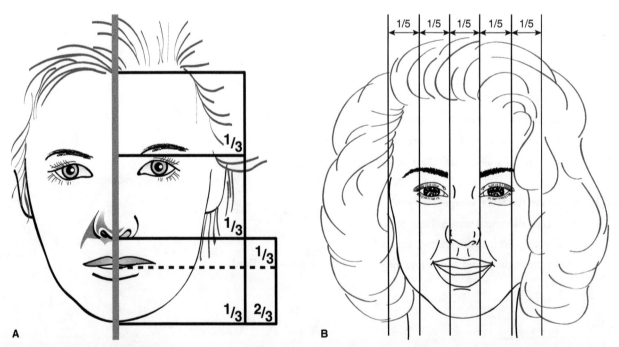

Figure 65-2 A: Reproduced with permission from Booth PW, Schendel SA, Hausamen JE. *Maxillofacial Surgery*. 2nd ed. Vol. 2. St Louis, MO: Churchill Livingstone; 2007. **B:** Reproduced with permission from Ferraro JW. *Fundamentals of Maxillofacial Surgery*. New York, NY: Springer-Verlag Inc.; 1997.

○ **What records are needed for treatment planning for orthognathic surgery?**

1. Photographs:

   a. Frontal view at rest

   b. Frontal view with smile

   c. Profile view at rest

   d. Dental occlusal relationship

2. Plaster study models mounted on an articulator utilizing a face-bow transfer

3. Centric relation record

4. Cephalometric prediction

5. Radiographs:

   a. Cephalometric radiographs

      i. Lateral

      ii. Posteroanterior

   b. Panorex

○ **What are the most pertinent points/angles that should be traced on a lateral cephalometric radiograph?**

1. Sella (S): Center of the pituitary fossa of the sphenoid bone.

2. Nasion (N): Intersection of the internasal suture with the nasofrontal suture in the midsagittal plane.

3. Glabella (G): Most anterior portion of the frontal bone.

4. Orbitale (Or): Lowest point of the roof of orbit; most inferior point of the external border of the orbital cavity.

5. Subnasale (Sn): Point where the nose connects to the center of upper lip.

6. Anterior nasal spine (ANS): The tip of the ANS.

7. A-point: Deepest point of the curve of the maxilla between the ANS and the dental alveolus.

8. B-point: Most posterior point in the concavity along the anterior border of the symphysis.

9. Stomion superius: Most inferior point on the curve of the upper lip.

10. Stomion inferius: Most superior point on the curve of the lower lip.

11. Pogonion (Pg): Most anterior point on the midsagittal symphysis.

12. Gnathion (Gn): Midpoint between the most anterior and the inferior point on the bony chin.

13. Menton (Me): Most inferior point of the symphysis.

14. Porion (Po): Highest point of the ear canal; most superior point of the external auditory meatus.

15. Condylion (Co): Most posterior superior aspect of the condyle.

16. Gonion (Go): Most convex point along the inferior border of the ramus.

17. SNA:

    a. Angle of sella, nasion, and A-point.

    b. Relationship of maxilla to the cranial base—mean is 82 ± 2 degrees.

18. SNB:

    a. Angle of sella, nasion, and B-point.

    b. Relationship of the mandible to the cranial base—mean is 80 ± 2 degrees.

19. ANB:

   a. Angle of A-point, nasion, to B-point.

   b. Relative position of maxilla/mandible to each other—mean is 2 ± 2 degrees.

   c. N-ANS (mm) and ANS-Me (mm): Hard tissue proportion of the middle facial height to the lower facial height—mean ratio is 7:8.

20. MP-FH: Divergence of the mandible from the horizontal plane—mean is 25 degrees.

21. G-Sn-Pg′: Soft-tissue angle relative to facial form—mean is 12 ± 4 degrees.

22. G-Sn/Sn-Me: Soft-tissue proportion of the middle facial height to the lower facial height—mean ratio is 1:1 (Fig. 65-3).

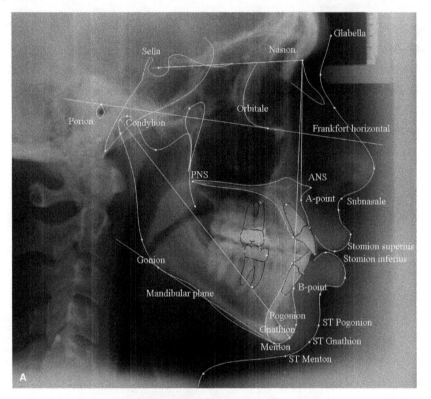

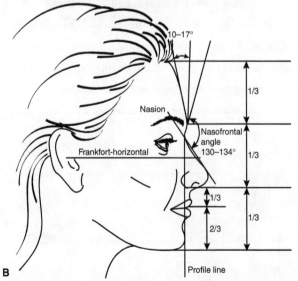

Figure 65-3 A: Lateral cephalometric radiograph. **B:** Profile of face demonstrating vertical and sagittal relationships. (**B:** Reproduced with permission from Ferraro JW. *Fundamentals of Maxillofacial Surgery.* New York, NY: Springer-Verlag Inc.; 1997.)

○ **What does a cephalometric prediction accomplish in treatment planning for orthognathic surgery?**

A cephalometric prediction anticipates hard and soft-tissue changes of the planned surgery that cannot be visualized on the plaster model surgery. The purpose is to develop an accurate surgical treatment plan that will achieve the best functional and aesthetic results.

○ **What are the key features and surgical correction of short face syndrome?**

The short face syndrome is characterized by a *reduced facial height secondary to vertical maxillary deficiency*. Examination notes a square-shaped face, a low mandibular plane angle, little or no show of the maxillary, anterior teeth with lips reposed, a deep labiomental fold, and an acute nasolabial angle. Dental analysis varies from an Angle Class I to an Angle Class II malocclusion. Surgical correction of the problem is with a Le Fort I osteotomy with bone grafting to position the maxilla inferiorly.

○ **What are the key features and surgical correction for long face syndrome?**

The long face syndrome is characterized by vertical maxillary excess resulting in a narrow nose, narrow alar bases, a prominent nasal dorsum, and depressed paranasal areas. Analysis of the lower third of the face usually reveals excessive exposure of the maxillary anterior teeth and gingiva on smiling, lip incompetence, long lower third facial height, a retropositioned chin, and a normal-to-obtuse nasolabial angle. Examination of the dentition notes a high, constricted palatal vault with a wide space between the root apices and the nasal floor, as well as a steep mandibular plane. An Angle Class II malocclusion is a frequent finding with or without the presence of an anterior open bite. Surgical correction of the long face syndrome decreases the anterior facial height with a Le Fort I maxillary impaction, autorotation of the mandible, and sagittal osteotomies of the mandible if necessary.

○ **What are the key characteristics and surgical correction of mandibular excess without midface deficiency?**

Mandibular excess is characterized by a prominent lower third of the face. Analysis of the data notes normal soft and hard tissue position of the midface; maxillary anterior teeth that are protrusive to the alveolus; the mandibular anterior teeth are upright to lingually inclined relative to the alveolus; bilateral, posterior crossbites are usually present; an Angle Class III molar and cuspid malocclusion, and cephalometric measurements greater than the mean for anteroposterior position of the mandible. Surgical correction is aimed at reducing the mandible and dentition with either transoral vertical or sagittal ramus osteotomies or transcutaneous vertical ramus osteotomies.

○ **What are key characteristics and surgical correction of anteroposterior maxillary deficiency without mandibular excess?**

Anteroposterior maxillary deficiency unrelated to one of the anomalous syndromes is characterized by a retrusive upper lip; flatness of the paranasal areas, a narrow nose, an obtuse nasolabial angle, nasal "prominence" in the anteroposterior plane, normal hard and soft-tissue position of the mandible, anterior and posterior crossbites, maxillary anterior teeth are protrusive to the alveolus, mandibular anterior teeth are upright to the alveolus, an Angle Class III malocclusion, and cephalometric data less than the mean for anteroposterior position of the maxilla. Surgical correction is with a Le Fort I maxillary advancement osteotomy.

○ **What are the key characteristics and surgical correction of mandibular deficiency?**

The soft-tissue characteristics are variable depending on the severity of the deficiency; however, a retruded position of the chin in profile view is a constant feature. Dental relationships are also variable depending on the severity of the deficiency; however, the Angle Class II malocclusion is a constant characteristic. Unusual inclinations of the cranial base are common for patients with mandibular deficiency and therefore the standard cranial base planes may not be satisfactory references. For patients with suspected mandibular deficiency, it is important to take cephalometric films in a natural head position and utilize the patient's physiologic horizontal reference, the visual axis, as a reference plane. Surgical correction is with transoral sagittal ramus osteotomies to advance the mandible.

○ **What are the key characteristics and surgical correction of an open bite deformity?**

Skeletal characteristics include long lower third of the face, narrow V-shaped maxilla, excessive exposure of maxillary anterior teeth show at rest, normal or short mandibular ramus, tipped palatal plane which is higher in front than in back, steep mandibular plane angle with the mandible rotated down and backward causing increased facial height.

Surgical correction is Le Fort I maxillary osteotomy with superior repositioning, when the extrusion is primarily a maxillary problem, possibly combined with mandibular advancement if there is an anteroposterior deficiency.

○ **What is the most important clinical measurement when treatment planning for vertical maxillary changes?**

The amount of maxillary incisor exposure with the lips in a relaxed position is the most important clinical measurement. Approximately 2 to 4 mm of incisor exposure is normal.

○ **What are the osteotomies needed to complete surgically assisted rapid palatal expansion?**

Horizontal osteotomy from pyriform rim to pterygomaxillary fissure, midline palatal osteotomy from ANS to posterior nasal spine then extending interdentally between the maxillary incisors, pterygoid, and nasal septal separation.

○ **A 17-year-old boy s/p cleft lip and palate repair presents to your office for management of malocclusion. Evaluation notes a significant deficiency of SNA, a normal SNB, and a negative 15-mm overjet. What surgical procedure is the most appropriate for the correction?**

1. A Le Fort I advancement by distraction osteogenesis.

2. Expanding the soft-tissue envelope is often the rate-limiting step in large maxillary advancements. Distraction osteogenesis should be considered for patients, with repaired cleft lip and palate, who require greater than 10 mm advancement.

○ **What are the phases of distraction osteogenesis in the craniofacial region?**

1. Latency period: 3 to 7 days depending on the surgical site.

2. Activation:

    • Distraction rate: 1.0 mm per day (0.5–2.0 mm)

    • Distraction rhythm: Continuous force application is best, but device activation two times a day allows for better patient compliance.

3. Consolidation: Until cortical outline can be seen radiographically across the distraction gap, usually 6 weeks.

○ **What is the blood supply of the maxilla following osteotomy?**

Ascending pharyngeal artery and the ascending palatine branch of the facial artery, and the descending palatine branch of the maxillary artery (Fig. 65-4).

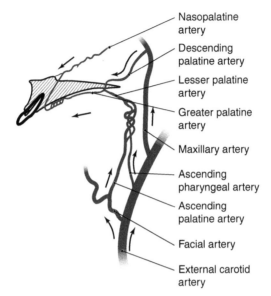

Nasopalatine artery

Descending palatine artery

Lesser palatine artery

Greater palatine artery

Maxillary artery

Ascending pharyngeal artery

Ascending palatine artery

Facial artery

External carotid artery

Figure 65-4 Reproduced with permission from Miloro M, Ghali GE, Larsen PE, Waite PD, et al. *Peterson's Principles of Oral and Maxillofacial Surgery.* 2nd ed. Vol. 2. Hamilton: BC Decker Inc.; 2004.

○ **A 22-year-old woman undergoes a downfracture of the maxilla during Le Fort I osteotomy. Profuse bleeding is noted in the posterior aspect of the lateral nasal wall. Which artery is most likely involved?**

Descending palatine artery, which is a branch of the maxillary artery, descends vertically within the perpendicular laminae of the palatine bone along the inferior lateral nasal wall.

○ **What are the potential complications when performing mandibular osteotomies?**

1. Ramus fractures of the proximal and distal segments of a sagittal osteotomy.

2. Nerve injuries:

   a. Inferior alveolar and lingual nerves with transoral osteotomies.

   b. Inferior alveolar and facial nerves with transcutaneous osteotomies.

3. Temporomandibular joint dysfunction.

4. Infection.

5. Necrosis of the proximal segment with a vertical ramus osteotomy.

6. Relapse secondary to malposition of the proximal segment.

○ **What are the complications of genioplasty?**

1. Dehiscence of the incision

2. Mental nerve paresthesia

3. Ptosis of mentalis muscle

4. Damage to root apices

5. Infection

○ **At what age is it appropriate to perform orthognathic surgery?**

Once skeletal maturity is reached. In females, this occurs at ages 14 to 16 years old. In males, this occurs at ages 16 to 18 years old. This can be verified with serial lateral cephalometric and wrist radiographs. The patient during this time will have undergone presurgical orthodontics, which includes alignment and positioning of the dentition over basal bone and decompensation of the dentition.

○ **What are the key features and surgical correction for a cleft lip and palate?**

Clefts are characterized by maxillary deficiency in the transverse, anteroposterior, and vertical dimensions. Examination reveals anterior and posterior dental crossbites, an Angle Class III malocclusion, midface sagittal deficiency, and vertical overclosure. The incidence of maxillary hypoplasia has been reported to be approximately 21%. This is an iatrogenic cause as a result from scar tissue formation after primary lip repair, followed by the palatoplasty. In cleft patients without repair, the skeletal and dental growth patterns are relatively normal.

Surgical correction is a Le Fort I maxillary advancement osteotomy.

○ **What is the surgical approach to the cleft maxilla for a Le Fort I osteotomy?**

In unilateral cleft palates and those without severe scarring, a traditional circumvestibular incision, at least 5 mm apical to the mucogingival junction and extending to the zygomaticomaxillary buttresses, can be performed.

For a bilateral cleft palate, severe palatal scarring, or a previous island palatal repair, an anterior buccal pedicle with a small vertical incision to allow for tunneling, should be left intact to allow for adequate perfusion of the premaxilla.

When performing the osteotomy and mobilizing the maxilla, the greatest point of resistance is usually in the vertical portion of the palatine bone near the descending palatine vessels.

○ **An 18-year-old female with mandibular hypoplasia undergoes a bilateral sagittal split osteotomy. An elevator is inserted along the inferior border of the mandible to elevate the masseteric sling, when all of a sudden, profuse bleeding occurs. Which artery is most likely involved?**

The facial artery, which courses along the submandibular gland and passes lateral and superior to mandible at the antegonial notch.

Other vessels that can be injured during a mandibular osteotomy are the masseteric, inferior alveolar, medial pterygoid, and retromandibular. Most injuries are due to indirect trauma from a retractor placement, an osteotome, or bur.

○ **A 17-year-old male undergoes a bilateral sagittal split osteotomy. Upon separation of the proximal and distal segments, a fracture occurred in the distal segment posterior to the last erupted tooth. What is the next step?**

The split must be completed through the planned osteotomy. The free segment can then be fixated with bicortical screws to the proximal segment, which is then fixated to the distal segment, usually with a plate.

Unfavorable mandibular fractures can occur 1.9% to 3.9% during bilateral sagittal split osteotomies. There is a slightly higher incidence when third molars are present, and it is recommended that third molars be removed at least 9 to 12 months prior to the osteotomy.

○ **What are nasal complications after a Le Fort I osteotomy?**

  a. Septal deviation

  b. Inadequate turbinate reduction

  c. Alar base widening

  d. Nasal tip over-rotation

  e. Dorsal deformities

○ **A 20-year-old male with vertical maxillary excess undergoes a Le Fort I maxillary impaction. After fixating the maxilla, and immediately following the release of maxillomandibular fixation, the patient developed an anterior open bite. What is the cause?**

There was inadequate reduction of the posterior maxilla, creating interferences that displaced the condyles from the fossa during fixation of the maxilla. Upon release of the maxillomandibular fixation, the condyles are repositioned correctly into the fossa, which causes the apertognathia.

○ **A 19-year-old female with mandibular hyperplasia, a Class III Angle molar and cuspid malocclusion, and bilateral TMJ arthralgia and anterior disc displacement. What is an appropriate surgical procedure?**

An intraoral vertical ramus osteotomy will allow for a mandibular setback to correct the malocclusion, and results in an anterior and inferior displacement of the condyle. This increases the joint space and can promote disc reduction.

○ **A 16-year-old female with the diagnosis of bilateral idiopathic condylar resorption presents to the office with severe retrognathia, a high mandibular plan angle, loss of chin projection, and an anterior open bite. What is an appropriate surgical procedure for correction of this patient's deformity?**

Bilateral total temporomandibular joint arthroplasties and a Le Fort I osteotomy with a counterclockwise rotation of the maxillomandibular complex. Idiopathic condylar resorption, rheumatoid arthritis, trauma, and condylar hypoplasia which can present as a shortened ramus height and steep mandibular plane angle. These can be corrected with an alloplastic TMJ replacement in conjunction with a Le Fort I osteotomy.

● ● ● REFERENCES ● ● ●

Bell WH, Proffit WR, White RP. *Surgical Correction of Dentofacial Deformities*. Vols. 1 & 2. Philadelphia, PA: WB Saunders; 1980.

Booth PW, Schendel SA, Hausamen JE. *Maxillofacial Surgery*. 2nd ed. Vol. 2. St Louis, MO: Churchill Livingstone; 2007.

Ferraro JW. *Fundamentals of Maxillofacial Surgery*. New York, NY: Springer-Verlag; 1997.

Fonseca RJ, Marciani R, Turvey T, et al. *Oral and Maxillofacial Surgery*. Vol. 3. 2nd ed. St Louis, MO: WB Saunders; 2009.

James JN, Costello BJ, Ruiz RL. Management of cleft lip and palate and cleft orthognathic considerations. *Oral and Maxillofacial Surgery Clinics*. 2014;26:4.

Miloro M, Ghali GE, Larsen PE, Waite, PD, et al. *Peterson's Principles of Oral and Maxillofacial Surgery*. Vol. 2. 2nd ed. Hamilton: BC Decker; 2004.

Nale JC. Orthognathic surgery and the temporomandibular joint patient. *Oral and Maxillofacial Surgery Clinics*. 2014;26:4.

Piecuch JF. *OMS Knowledge Update Self-Study Program*. Vol. 2. Rosemont: American Association of Oral and Maxillofacial Surgeons; 1998.

Proffit WR, Turvey TA, Phillips C. The hierarchy of stability and predictability in orthognathic surgery with rigid fixation: an update and extension. *Head Face Med*. 2007;3:21.

Robl MT, Farrell BB, Tucker MR. Complication in orthognathic surgery, a report of 1000 cases. *Oral and Maxillofacial Surgery Clinics*. 2014;26:4.

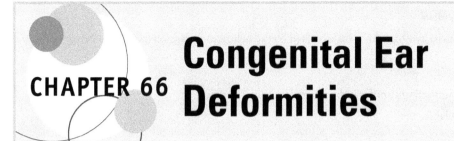

CHAPTER 66
Congenital Ear Deformities

Jonathan Bank, MD,
Donald B. Johnson, MD, and
Bruce S. Bauer, MD, FACS, FAAP

○ **What structures develop from the hillocks of the first branchial arch?**

The tragus, the helical crus, and helical root (lymphatic drainage to parotid nodes).

○ **What structures develop from the three hillocks of the second branchial arch?**

The helix, scapha, concha, antihelix, antitragus, and lobule (lymphatic drainage to posterior auricular nodes). The most common auricular sinus lies at the junction between the helical root and the superior helix (rises at the boundary between the first and second arch contributions).

○ **What embryologic structure gives rise to the external auditory meatus?**

The first branchial groove (lymphatic drainage to both parotid and posterior auricular nodes).

○ **What is the normal size of the ear?**

5.5 to 6.5 cm for the normal adult ear height and 3 to 4.5 cm for the normal adult ear width. The width varies from 66% of the height in children to 55% of the height in adults. For children 4 years of age, a subnormal ear height (i.e., <2 SD) is below 4.5 cm.

○ **Describe normal ear growth.**

85% of ear development occurs by 3 years of age with full development achieved between 6 and 15 years of age.

○ **What is the normal position of the ear?**

1. One ear length posterior to the lateral orbital rim.

2. Mean inclination from vertical of 20-degree posteriorly.

○ **What is the normal scalp-to-helix distance for each third of the ear? (Upper, middle, and lobule)**

1. Upper: 1.0 to 1.2 cm

2. Middle: 1.6 to 1.8 cm

3. Lobule: 2.0 to 2.2 cm

○ **How is the concha subdivided?**

The concha cavum and concha cymba, which are separated by the helical root (also referred to as the root of the helical crus).

○ **The superior crus of the antihelix is bordered by what structures?**

The scapha and the triangular fossa.

○ **The inferior crus of the antihelix is bordered by what structures?**

The triangular fossa and the concha cymba.

○ **What is the triangular fossa?**

The concave area between the superior crus and the inferior crus.

○ **Describe the arterial blood supply to the ear.**

Superficial temporal artery supplies the anterior surface. Posterior auricular artery supplies the posterior surface of the ear, lobule, and retroauricular skin. There are numerous perforating vessels interconnecting the two territories.

○ **Describe the venous drainage of the ear.**

Anterior ear is drained by the superficial temporal and retromandibular veins. Posterior ear is drained by posterior auricular veins draining into the external jugular vein.

○ **Describe the innervation of the ear (Fig. 66-1).**

Sensory supply of the anterior surface of the ear is via the auriculotemporal (V3) and great auricular (CN II–III) nerves. The posterior surface is innervated by the great auricular nerve, and the mastoid branches of the lesser occipital nerve. The region of the meatus (and medial concha) is supplied by the nerve of Arnold from the Vagus nerve (oropharyngeal cancer may present with referred pain to the ear via vagal nerve fibers common to the oropharynx and concha).

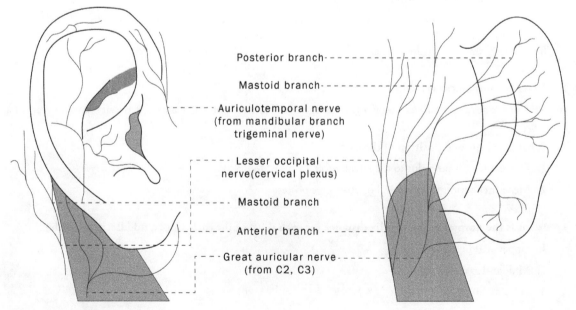

Figure 66-1 Innervation of the ear.

Illustrations by Matthew Gould.

○ **Microtia is seen in what syndromes (Fig. 66-2)?**

1. Hemifacial microsomia (first and second branchial arch syndrome).
2. Goldenhar syndrome (oculoauriculovertebral dysplasia; characteristically has bilateral ear deformities).
3. Treacher Collins syndrome (bilateral deformities).

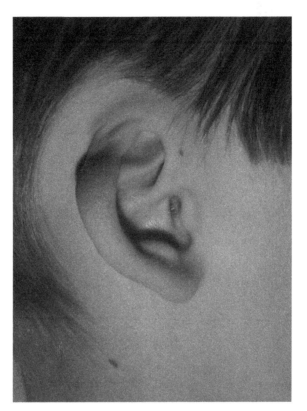

Figure 66-2 Microtia.

○ **What is the proposed pathogenesis of microtia?**

Obliteration of the stapedial artery. The bilateral deformity in Treacher Collins syndrome has been demonstrated to arise from a different event occurring early in gastrulation (Poswillo) and has also been associated with thalidomide.

○ **For the microtia patient, at what age is it usually recommended for the child to undergo total ear reconstruction?**

Traditional recommendations advocated reconstruction by age 6 or 7 before starting school. However, optimal reconstruction requires costal cartilage of sufficient size and shape to carve the key framework details and maintain the strength to display these details through the overlying skin envelope. Better results can be obtained at age 9 to 10 years or later, with a lower rate of revision. One must balance potential psychological issues of dealing with the deformity versus the benefits of delaying surgery.

○ **How many stages are usually required for total ear reconstruction?**

Two or three, depending on the particular technique.

○ **What is usually involved in the first stage?**

Harvest of a costal cartilage graft and creation of a cartilage framework, elevation of a flap for coverage of the framework and insertion of the framework in the pocket. The majority of surgeons today rotate the lobule in the first stage and design the framework to include the tragus.

○ **What is usually involved in the second and third stages?**

Elevation of the reconstructed ear, placement of a banked cartilage graft for additional framework elevation, and coverage with fascia flap and skin graft. In cases where lobule was not rotated in the first stage and the tragus not reconstructed, these procedures are performed in the second and third stages along with elevation of the ear.

○ **Which ribs are usually harvested for the cartilage framework?**

Portions of costal cartilages 6 through 9, ipsilateral or contralateral (surgeon preference).

○ **What morbidities are associated with the harvest of costal cartilage?**

Harvesting costal cartilage may lead to chest wall deformity, scarring, and substantial pain; of these, distortion of the chest wall is the greatest concern. Delaying reconstruction until 10 years of age, preserving the perichondrial margin during harvest, and reconstituting the donor-site defect with cartilage fragments may significantly reduce the potential for deformity.

○ **What regional flap can be utilized when the standard skin flaps are unsuitable for ear reconstruction?**

The most readily available is the temporoparietal fascia flap based on the superficial temporal artery with split thickness skin graft.

○ **What are the advantages/disadvantages of using polyethylene implants (Medpor®) in ear reconstruction?**

Porous polyethylene implants offer excellent definition and contralateral ear matching, reconstruction at a younger age, a shorter duration of treatment (typically 4 months), and are not associated with autologous reconstruction chest morbidities. Conversely, allopathic materials have a higher rate of infection and extrusion, and implant exposure commonly results in loss of the temporoparietal fascia used for implant coverage.

○ **In microtia patients, what must be present for canal and middle ear reconstruction?**

Jahrsdoerfer developed a scoring system to predict outcomes of middle ear reconstruction. The two absolute criteria for a patient to qualify for surgery are good cochlear function and no imaging evidence of a malformed inner ear; surgery is deferred if the middle ear and mastoid have failed to aerate. Patients should understand that tympanoplasty/canaloplasty may not improve hearing substantially and complications place the auricular construct at risk.

○ **When should bone-anchored hearing aids (BAHA) be placed in patients who are undergoing ear reconstruction?**

It has been recommended that BAHAs should be placed only after ear reconstruction has been completed to avoid compromising the mastoid-region skin used to cover the autologous framework. However, coordinated treatment by otolaryngologist and plastic surgeons, and the development of transcutaneous bone conduction implants (tBCI) make placement possible at any stage during reconstruction—synchronized care also reduces the number of scars.

○ **What are the characteristics of a prominent ear deformity (Fig. 66-3)?**

Prominent ear arises from two main factors: hypertrophy of the concha—recognized as the most significant factor, and effacement of the antihelical fold. Prominence is further influenced by the skull base upon which the ear sits (as most easily demonstrated by the different ear position and prominence in positional plagiocephaly).

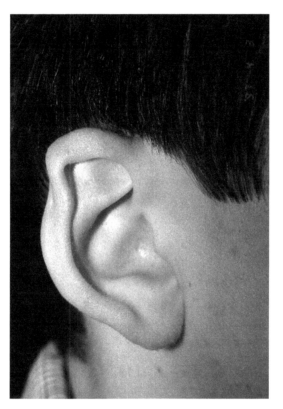

Figure 66-3 Prominent ear deformity.

○ **What is the role of ear taping and splinting in the management of the prominent ear deformity?**

Up to 6 months of age, molding the ear with taping and splinting may improve ear appearance and prevent the need for surgical correction. However, the younger the patient, the more effective the treatment and the shorter the time required for correction.

○ **Why is this limited to the first 3 to 6 months of life?**

Circulating maternal estrogen increases hyaluronic acid in cartilage rendering it more deformable. This probably facilitates passage through the birth canal during delivery but can be exploited to reshape deformities of the ear. While maternal estrogen levels drop within hours of partum, the effect on the cartilage remains longer. Beyond the neonatal period the change from soft to firmer cartilage is less dramatic and splinting will be required for a longer period. Typically beyond 3 months most infants will not tolerate the necessary 24-hour splinting.

○ **What are the primary maneuvers used to better define the effaced antihelical fold and what are the associated complications?**

Procedures can be divided into those that score or thin the antihelix (anterior or posterior surface) and those that accentuate it with sutures. Scoring or abrading the cartilage (particularly the anterior surface) can be associated with sharp and irregular folding. Sutures alone can be associated with suture disruption and loss of correction.

○ **What maneuvers can affect conchal hypertrophy and what are the associated complications?**

The maneuvers for conchal reduction vary from cartilage excision to setback of the conchal bowl. Some authors will also reduce conchal height by lowering the position at which they create the antihelical fold. Conchal setback can be associated with loss of fixation sutures. As in the previous question, efforts to overaccentuate the antihelix to affect the height of the concha can be associated with irregular folds.

○ **What is the effect of conchomastoid sutures?**

Reduction of conchal projection. Conchal reduction can also be achieved by direct excision through an anterior or a posterior incision.

○ **What is the effect of Mustardè sutures?**

Permanent conchoscaphal sutures are placed to recreate the antihelical fold.

○ **Conchomastoid sutures are more commonly associated with what complication?**

Meatus distortion.

○ **What is the most common complication following otoplasty surgery?**

Recurrent deformity with 10% to 25% undergoing revision otoplasty.

○ **What are common unfavorable results of otoplasty?**

These can be divided into undercorrection and overcorrection. Undercorrection is most often secondary to either an insufficient number or inaccurate placement of permanent sutures, or loss of support by resorption of absorbable sutures. Nontechnical causes include unrecognizing underlying skeletal asymmetry, or failure to treat conchal hypertrophy. Overcorrection, mainly in the form of the *telephone ear deformity* results from relative over-resection of skin of the middle third of the ear, resulting in an apparent prominence of the upper and lower thirds. It is accentuated when lobular hypertrophy is not recognized and incompletely treated.

○ **A post otoplasty "pinned back" appearance is attributed to what technical shortcomings?**

A pinned back appearance is due to inadequate resection of the hypertrophic conchal bowl and over accentuation of the antihelix, resulting in lost visibility of the helical rim.

○ **What is cryptotia and how is it treated?**

"Hidden ear" deformity is characterized by the absence of the superior auriculocephalic sulcus and results from overaccentuation of the superior or inferior crus, tipping the upper pole of the ear beneath the adjacent scalp. Correction requires release of abnormal cartilage adhesions on both posterior and anterior surfaces of the ear and coverage of the defect with both auricular and postauricular flaps.

○ **What are the features of the constricted ear (formerly termed both lop ear and cup ear)?**

The four fundamental aspects of the constricted ear include lidding, protrusion, decreased ear size, and low ear position. The majority of constricted ears have decreased radius of curve of the helical rim and some degree of skin deficiency.

○ **What is Stahl's ear?**

Stahl's ear, commonly referred to as "Spock ear," is characterized by either a third crus or abnormal angulation of the superior crus, projecting the helical rim upward or outward. While difficult to correct surgically, this deformity is perhaps the easiest of all ear deformities to correct with neonatal splinting.

● ● ● **REFERENCES** ● ● ●

Bauer BS. Congenital and acquired deformities of the ear. In: Bentz ML, Bauer BS, Zuker RM, eds. *Principles and Practice of Pediatric Plastic Surgery*. St Louis, MO: Quality Medical Publishing; 2008:801–850.

Bauer BS. Reconstruction of microtia. *Plast Reconst Surg*. 2009;124(Suppl 1):14E–26E.

Brent B. Microtia repair with rib cartilage grafts: a review of personal experience with 1000 cases. *Clin Plast Surg*. 2002;29:257–271.

Brent B. The acquired auricular deformity. A systematic approach to its analysis and reconstruction. *Plast Reconstr Surg*. 1977;59: 475–485.

Constantine KK, Gilmore J, Lee K, Leach J Jr. Comparison of microtia reconstruction outcomes using rib cartilage vs porous polyethylene implant. *JAMA Facial Plast Surg*. 2014;16:240–244.

Eriksson E, Vogt PM. Ear reconstruction. *Clin Plast Surg*. 1992;19:637–643.

Lentz AK, Plikaitis CM, Bauer BS. Understanding the unfavorable result after otoplasty: an integrated approach to correction. *Plast Reconstr Surg*. 2011;128:536–544.

Poswillo D. The pathogenesis of the first and second branchial arch syndrome. *Oral Surg Oral Med Oral Pathol*. 1973;35(3):302–328.

Weerda H. *Surgery of the Auricle: Tumors, Trauma, Defects, Abnormalities*. New York, NY: Thieme; 2007.

CHAPTER 67 Congenital Nevi/Tissue Expansion

Stephen Colbert, MD, FACS

• • • CONGENITAL NEVI • • •

○ **Define "congenital."**

Existing at birth.

○ **Does "congenital" imply "hereditary"?**

No.

○ **What is a nevus?**

A chronic benign lesion of the skin or mucosa, commonly known as "mole" or "birthmark". Nevi may be either present at birth (congenital) or appear after birth (acquired).

○ **What is a giant nevus?**

Predicted to be greater than 20 cm in largest diameter in adulthood, correlating in an infant to 6 cm on the head and 9 cm on the body; greater than 1% body surface area on the head and neck, or 2% on the rest of the body; or, of a size that cannot be excised in a single procedure.

○ **What is the incidence of congenital nevi?**

1% to 2%.

○ **What is the incidence of giant nevi?**

For lesions greater than or equal to 9.9 cm, approximately 1 in 20,000.

○ **Nevi results from a proliferation of what cells?**

Melanocytes, of neuroectodermal origin.

○ **In what layer(s) of the skin do nevi occur?**

Dermis and epidermis.

○ **For what cancer are nevi generally considered a risk factor?**

Malignant melanoma.

○ **What is the risk of melanoma in one who has a giant congenital nevus?**

5% to 7% by the age of 60 is the most often reported range; however, reported incidence in the literature ranges from 0% to 42%.

○ **What is an acquired nevus?**

The more common "mole," the occurrence of which begins in childhood and increases rapidly in adolescence and young adulthood.

○ **How are nevi classified by location and histologic pattern?**

Compound, intradermal, and junctional.

○ **What is a compound nevus?**

A nevus with fully formed nests of cells in the epidermis and newly forming cells in the dermis.

○ **What is an intradermal nevus?**

A nevus with nests of cells located exclusively within the dermis; clinically indistinguishable from a compound nevus.

○ **What is a junctional nevus?**

A nevus with nests of cells confined to the dermoepidermal junction; usually presenting as a small, discrete, flat, or slightly raised macule.

○ **How are small congenital nevi managed medically?**

Baseline photography and regular follow-up.

○ **What features of small nevi warrant biopsy?**

Those features suggestive of melanoma: asymmetry, border irregularity, color variegation, and diameter larger than 6 mm; in addition, any nevus that has changed appearance.

○ **At what location(s) are congenital nevi associated with leptomeningeal melanoma?**

Congenital nevi of the head, neck, and trunk, particularly over the spine.

○ **What is a nevus of Ota?**

Pigmented nevus in the distribution of the ophthalmic (V1) and maxillary (V2) division of the trigeminal nerve; usually unilateral, may affect mucosa, associated with development of glaucoma and rare malignant degeneration.

○ **In what demographic segment are nevi of Ota seen?**

Most common in females and Asian populations; occurring in early infancy, approximately 50% congenital, and in early adolescence.

○ **What is the recommended treatment of large congenital nevi?**

Giant nevi should be removed surgically as soon as possible, as there is risk of melanoma even in the first 3 to 5 years of life; nonsurgical or ablative methods are not recommended; surgical excision is staged or involves tissue expansion.

○ **How are small- and medium-sized congenital nevi treated?**

Treatment remains controversial with recommendations ranging from early excision of all nevi to lifetime observation with removal only for specific changes.

● ● ● **TISSUE EXPANSION** ● ● ●

○ **What is the main advantage of using tissue expansion in reconstruction?**

Replacing missing or pathologic tissue with normal-appearing tissue.

○ **What are other advantages?**

Expanded tissue is typically sensate and well vascularized, and final donor defects are minimized.

○ **In what type of situations should tissue expanders be avoided?**

Immediate traumatic or infected fields, open wounds, proximity to malignant tumor, nonexpandable or high-risk tissue such as a skin graft or irradiated tissue.

○ **What are the common disadvantages of tissue expansion?**

Requires two operations, creates an aesthetic deformity during expansion, and may cause transient discomfort during expansion.

○ **What is "creep"?**

Viscoelastic deformation occurring immediately with expansion.

○ **Besides creep, what factors increase dimensions of expanded tissue in the short term?**

Loss of interstitial fluid by pressure, and recruitment of adjacent mobile tissues.

○ **Does stretch of tissue have any effect on cellular proliferation?**

Yes, tension has been shown to induce DNA synthesis and cellular mitosis.

○ **Does expansion affect blood flow in expanding tissue?**

Yes, blood flow increases in expanding tissue; in addition, the placement of an expander functions as a delay for the overlying flap.

○ **What happens to the epidermis during expansion?**

The epidermis thickens.

○ **What happens to the dermis during expansion?**

The dermis thins.

○ **Are these changes in the epidermis and dermis permanent?**

No, such changes have been shown to undergo reversal following expander removal.

○ **What are the risks to fat, muscle, and nerves during expansion?**

Compression could cause atrophy of all of these tissues; in addition, compression of sensory nerves may lead to paresthesias or discomfort.

○ **What tissues are particularly amenable to expansion?**

The scalp and breast; in general, the farther from these tissues, the less successful expansion becomes.

○ **What may happen if an expander is placed beneath an incision?**

Dehiscence and expander exposure.

○ **How should exposure of a tissue expander be treated?**

In general, exposure of an expander is best treated by removal, pocket drainage, and expander replacement at a later date; in selected situations, removal, sterilization, and immediate replacement may be appropriate; in other selected situations, some may consider completion of expansion in the setting of exposure appropriate.

○ **Does tissue expansion require placement of an expandable implant?**

No, techniques such as presuturing, external expanders, and lacing devices allow tissue expansion and ultimate wound closure without placement of internal expanders.

○ **Is placement of incisions for expander insertion important?**

Yes, one of the most critical factors affecting outcome is the placement of the final scar, which is usually affected by placement of the initial incision; in addition, placement of the incision in tissue that is to be expanded may lead to a widened scar or even dehiscence and expander exposure.

○ **What technical error committed during expander placement will likely lead to expansion failure?**

Inadequate development of the pocket where the expander will be placed.

○ **What complications are associated with tissue expanders?**

Seroma formation, transient alopecia during scalp expansion, contour deformities such as dog-ears postoperatively, widened scars, hematoma, infection, expander exposure, expander extrusion, and tissue necrosis.

○ **What is the benefit of a textured surface on a tissue expander?**

Relative immobility due to tissue adherence, maintenance of proper expander orientation, increased capsular compliance, and reduction in capsular contracture.

● ● ● **REFERENCES** ● ● ●

Congenital Nevi

Bittencourt FV, Marghoob AA, Kopf AW, Koenig KL, Bart RS. Large congenital melanocytic nevi and the risk for development of malignant melanoma and neurocutaneous melanocytosis. *Pediatrics*. 2000;106:736–741.

Newman WA. *Dorland's Illustrated Medical Dictionary*. 28th ed. Philadelphia, PA: WB Saunders; 1994;1864–1956.

Fitzpatrick TB, Johnson RA, Wolff K, Suurmond D. *Color Atlas and Synopsis of Clinical Dermatology: Common and Serious Diseases*. 4th ed. New York, NY: McGraw-Hill; 2001.

Gosain AK, Santoro TD, Larson DL, Gingrass RP. Giant congenital nevi: a 20-year experience and an algorithm for their management. *Plast Reconstr Surg*. 2001;108(3):622–631.

Marghoob AA. Congenital melanocytic nevi evaluation and management. *Dermatol Clin*. 2002;20:607–616.

Marghoob AA, Schoenbach SP, Kopf AW, Orlow SJ, Nossa R, Bart RS. Large congenital melanocytic nevi and the risk for the development of malignant melanoma: a prospective study. *Arch Dermatol*. 1996;132:170–175.

Watt AJ, Kotsis SV, Chung KC. Risk of melanoma arising in large congenital melanocytic nevi: a systematic review. *Plast Reconstr Surg*. 2004;113(7):1968–1974.

Tissue Expansion

Concannon MJ, Puckett CL. Wound coverage using modified tissue expansion. *Plast Reconstr Surg*. 1998;102(2):377–384.

De Filippo RE, Atala A. Stretch and growth: the molecular and physiologic influences of tissue expansion. *Plast Reconstr Surg*. 2002;109(7):2450–2462.

Manders EK. Reconstruction using soft tissue expansion. In: Cohen M, ed. *Mastery of Plastic and Reconstructive Surgery*. Boston, MA: Little, Brown and Co; 1994:201–213.

Pasyk K, Argenta L, Austad ED. Histopathology of human expanded tissue. *Clin Plast Surg*. 1987;14:435–445.

CHAPTER 68 Congenital Breast

Samita Goyal, MD

○ **Describe breast development.**

During the sixth week of gestation, ectodermal cells form a primordium along the primitive mammary ridges ("milk lines" that extend from the axilla to the groin). By the 10th week of gestation, the upper and lower aspects of these ridges atrophy; the middle portion of the ridges, located at the level of the fourth interspace, persist and eventually develop into breast tissue. In the fifth month of gestation, the areola develops, and shortly after birth, the nipple appears.

After birth, residual circulating maternal estrogens may cause neonatal gynecomastia which typically involutes as these hormones are metabolized. Thelarche precedes puberty by approximately 1 year and marks the beginning of breast growth. At puberty, estrogens cause ductal and stromal tissue proliferation and progesterones cause alveolar budding and lobular growth. Breast growth is generally completed by 16 to 18 years of age.

○ **Describe chest wall development.**

During the fourth week of gestation, ectodermal cells from the neural crest and somatic cells from the paraxial and lateral plate join and differentiate into forty somites caudal to the head region. These further differentiate into the dermomyotome (dorsal) and sclerotome (ventral), which become the trunk musculature and skeleton, respectively. The sclerotome also differentiates into the vertebral bodies. The sternum develops during the sixth week of gestation separately from the ribs, arising from longitudinal pairings of mesenchymal tissues. Failure of fusion leads to a cleft sternum.

○ **How can congenital breast disorders be generally classified?**

Hypoplastic (athelia, amazia, amastia, unilateral/bilateral hypoplasia, tuberous breast, and Poland syndrome).

Hyperplastic (gynecomastia, hyperplasia, symmastia, polythelia, polymastia, and giant fibroadenoma).

○ **What organ system should always be included in the initial preoperative evaluation of patients with gynecomastia?**

Genitalia may reveal an underlying cause such as testicular tumors, nonpalpable and/or undescended testes. These findings should prompt genetic and/or endocrine evaluation prior to surgery.

○ **What pharmaceutical agents are linked to the development of gynecomastia?**

Cimetidine, digitalis, minocycline, spironolactone, anabolic steroids, haloperidol, opiates, marijuana, phenothiazines, tricyclic antidepressants, progestins, amphetamines, isoniazid, methyldopa, estrogens, diazepam, reserpine, and theophylline.

○ **How is gynecomastia classified?**

There are three grades:

Grade I: small enlargement, no skin redundancy.

Grade IIA: moderate enlargement, no skin redundancy.

Grade IIB: moderate enlargement with skin redundancy.

Grade III: marked enlargement with skin redundancy.

○ **What is the modification of gynecomastia classification for surgical planning?**

Simplify to the three grades:

Grade I: Localized button of tissue localized to areola. Chest not fatty, no skin excess. Simple excision.

Grade II: Diffuse gynecomastia on fatty chest, indistinct tissue edges. Suction lipectomy adjunct to excision.

Grade III: Diffuse gynecomastia with excessive skin, requires skin excision outside areola and/or nipple repositioning.

○ **What are the options for surgical management of gynecomastia?**

Suction-assisted lipectomy or ultrasound-assisted lipectomy only.

Glandular resection through periareolar incision +/− suction-assisted lipectomy.

Skin and glandular resection.

Concentric circle resection.

Pedicled relocation of nipple with skin resection.

Breast amputation with free nipple grafting.

Wise-pattern mastopexy should NOT be performed in gynecomastia.

○ **What is the role of liposuction in gynecomastia?**

Suction-assisted lipectomy is primarily used to improve chest contour by lateral feathering as an adjunct to surgical excision. Although, it can be used as a primary treatment modality in breast tissue that is primarily fatty. Ultrasound-assisted liposuction (UAL) can be used as a primary modality in most patients and is primarily applicable to dense, fibrous tissue. It offers the advantage of minimal external scarring. With the use of UAL, the use of excisional techniques may be reserved for patients with severe gynecomastia with significant skin excess AFTER attempted UAL.

○ **What is the timing of surgical intervention in patients with gynecomastia?**

Surgery should not be offered to patients with gynecomastia for duration of less than 1 year. If gynecomastia persists for more than 1 year, the likelihood of spontaneous resolution is low and surgery may be offered anytime after 1 year. Correctable medical causes such as endocrine imbalance, medications, or tumors preclude surgical intervention.

○ **What is the incidence of gynecomastia in males at puberty?**

Approximately 65% to 75%.

○ **What is the typical time length until spontaneous resolution of gynecomastia in adolescent boys?**

16 to 18 months. Best to wait as long as 2 years prior to intervention. If psychosocial disturbance, may intervene earlier.

○ **What percentage of males with gynecomastia present at puberty have residual gynecomastia at age 17?**

8%.

○ **In which medical condition is gynecomastia associated with an increased incidence of breast cancer?**

Klinefelter syndrome (at least 20 times general population). Breast biopsy is indicated in such cases.

○ **What is the most common complication after correction of gynecomastia?**

Hematoma.

○ **What is the management of gynecomastia in the neonate?**

Requires no therapy, typically resolves in several weeks.

○ **What are the common causes of gynecomastia?**

Increase in estrogens, decrease in androgens, or deficiency in androgen receptors.

○ **What are the multiple disease states in which gynecomastia can be seen?**

Primary testicular failure (Klinefelter, XXY syndrome), secondary testicular failure (orchitis, mumps), endocrine disorders (hyper- or hypothyroidism, adrenocorticohyperplasia), liver disease (most common alcoholic cirrhosis), tumors (lung cancer, testicular cancer, adrenal tumors, pituitary tumors, colon or prostate cancer), congenital syndromes, debilitated disease states (e.g., severe burn).

○ **What tests are generally required by insurance companies prior to approval of gynecomastia surgery?**

Endocrine workup.

○ **How is juvenile breast hypertrophy classified?**

Temporal classification:

Prepubertal hypertrophy: develops before puberty, usually bilateral. Virginal hypertrophy: develops after puberty, either unilateral or bilateral.

Classifications of asymmetry:

Unilateral hyperplasia, bilateral symmetrical hyperplasia, combination of hyperplasia and hypoplasia.

○ **What is the treatment of choice in juvenile breast hypertrophy?**

Reduction mammoplasty. High recurrence rates may require further surgery.

○ **When should surgery be performed in juvenile breast hypertrophy?**

Surgery should be delayed until after puberty, after breast growth has ended.

○ **What is the management of breast enlargement before puberty?**

Rare condition requires search for chromosomal abnormalities, drug, and endocrine workups.

○ **Describe the course of giant fibroadenomas.**

They present during puberty as unilateral, rapidly growing masses. These lesions are benign and discrete, and are thought to occur as a hypersensitivity to physiological circulating levels of gonadal hormones. Diagnosis is confirmed by breast tissue biopsy. If growth is very rapid, surgery may be indicated prior to the completion of the growth due to its large discrepancy in size.

○ **What is the incidence of polythelia?**

Polythelia is the most common congenital breast anomaly that afflicts both boys and girls, with an incidence of 5%.

○ **When should supernumerary nipples be excised?**

In young girls, prior to puberty before accessory breast tissue can form.

○ **Where are accessory mammary structures found most frequently in patients with polymastia?**

The axilla followed by the inframammary region.

○ **Which areas are commonly affected in ectopic polymastia?**

Ectopic polymastia: Breast tissue in areas outside the milk line. Reported in midline, face, ear, neck, back, buttock, posterior or dorsal thigh, scalp, shoulder, and epigastrium.

○ **What associated organ systems are affected in polymastia?**

Renal and thoracic. The incidence of polymastia is lower than polythelia.

○ **What are the incidence and most common location for polythelia (supernumerary nipple)?**

5% and inframammary region (commonly misdiagnosed as nevi).

○ **What is the difference between amastia, amazia, and athelia?**

Amastia: Congenital absence of the breast (nipple–areola complex and glandular tissue).

Amazia: Absence of glandular tissue only.

Athelia: Absence of nipple alone.

○ **What is the primary feature of Poland syndrome?**

Unilateral aplasia or hypoplasia of the pectoralis major muscle (absence of sternal head) and breast hypoplasia.

○ **What is the incidence of Poland syndrome?**

1 in 20,000 to 30,000. Most cases are sporadic and 75% occur on the right side. Some reports of familial cases. Male to female ratio is 3:1.

○ **What is the suggested primary defect in Poland syndrome?**

Subclavian artery disruption sequence resulting in diminished blood supply to affected limb yielding partial loss of tissue in the affected regions.

○ **What are the other associated deformities of Poland syndrome?**

Absence of ribs 2 to 4, hypoplasia of the muscles of the shoulder girdle including the latissimus dorsi, brachysyndactyly, shortening of forearm bones, deficiency of subcutaneous fat, absence of axillary hair, aplasia or hypoplasia of nipple–areola complex.

○ **What study is a useful adjunct in the preoperative workup of patients with Poland syndrome?**

High-resolution CT scan to confirm status of latissimus dorsi and define associated skeletal anomalies.

○ **What are the three aspects of chest wall reconstruction in Poland syndrome?**

Stabilization of chest wall, creation of a soft tissue "fill," breast reconstruction.

○ **What is the surgical management of the breast deformity in male patient with Poland syndrome?**

Latissimus dorsi neuromuscular island flap reconstruction. As early as 5 to 6 years of age. Free latissimus transfer may be considered if the ipsilateral latissimus is not available. Custom-made silicone implant is another alternative.

○ **What is the surgical management of the breast deformity in the female patient with Poland syndrome?**

At age 12 to 13, temporary expander for symmetry during breast development, exchange for permanent implant at the end of breast development. Latissimus dorsi used in cases of inadequate subcutaneous tissue. In adult patients, pedicled TRAM flap may be used, not used in adolescent patients or those considering childbirth.

○ **What percentage of patients with syndactyly of the hand have Poland syndrome?**

10%.

○ **What are the options for skeletal chest wall deformity reconstruction in patients with Poland syndrome?**

No contraindication to single-stage repair. Customized silicone prosthesis placed subcutaneously or beneath latissimus dorsi muscle flap or split-rib grafts; if soft tissue lacking, cover grafts with prosthetic patch or latissimus dorsi muscle flap (preferred), which serves as base for mammary prosthesis. Some cases may require contralateral mastopexy. Free tissue transfer may be required.

○ **What are the components of the tuberous breast deformity?**

Breast hypoplasia (deficiency of base diameter), breast tissue herniation into the areola (leading to a large areola diameter), deficiency of skin envelope, and elevation of the inframammary fold.

○ **What is the classification of the tuberous breast deformity?**

Type I—lower medial quadrant hypoplasia. Type II—lower medial and lateral quadrant hypoplasia. Type III—severe breast constriction.

○ **What is the surgical management of the tuberous breast deformity?**

In most cases, augmentation with a periareolar mastopexy. In severe breast ptosis, augmentation with wise-pattern mastopexy. In severely deficient skin envelope, two-stage reconstruction with tissue expansion.

○ **What are the causes of unilateral hypoplasia?**

Congenital condition or acquired secondary to iatrogenic injury to breast bud.

○ **What is the surgical management of unilateral hypoplasia?**

Delay reconstruction until 13 years if possible. At age 13, a temporary expander is placed for symmetry during breast development, exchanging this for a permanent implant at the end of development. Submusculofascial position is preferred. Nipple–areola reconstruction at completion of expansion.

○ **What is the other anatomic consideration at the time of implant placement in the hypoplastic breast?**

Breast constriction with a shortened and high inframammary fold. Must be addressed at the time of implant placement.

○ **Are congenital breast cases covered by insurance?**

It depends on the individual insurance policies. With appropriate documentation, some cases may be covered by insurance. Some policies consider all congenital breast cases "cosmetic" and do not cover them.

○ **What is pectus excavatum and how is it treated?**

Pectus excavatum is a congenital chest wall deformity leading to a concave curvature of the chest wall, that is, a caved-in appearance. It is usually diagnosed within the first year of life (90% of cases) and typically worsens into adolescence. The most popular surgical intervention was initially described by Ravitch and involves a submammary or vertical midline approach to elevate the pectoralis major muscles from the chest wall and subsequently resect the deformed cartilage. The sternum is then elevated after cutting it transversely, followed by reapproximation of the pectoralis muscles. This is secured in place with a temporary metal strut (Adkins strut), which is removed approximately 6 months later. The Nuss procedure involves placing a retrosternal bar that pushes the sternum anteriorly without any resection of sternal bone. Care is taken to avoid injury to intrathoracic structures during placement, and the bar is left in place for 2 years.

○ **What is pectus carinatum and how is it treated?**

Pectus carinatum is a congenital chest wall deformity that leads to a convex curvature of the chest wall, that is, a bowed-out appearance. It occurs 10% as often as pectus excavatum. It is treated similarly to the Ravitch approach for pectus excavatum. After resection of the deformed sternum, the perichondrial bundles are flattened with reefing sutures. A newer, less invasive approach involving an external prosthesis to flatten the chest wall has been described, but long-term follow-up is yet to be determined.

● ● ● **REFERENCES** ● ● ●

Albanese CT, Rowe MI. Congenital thoracic deformities. In: Benz ML, ed. *Pediatric Plastic Surgery*. 1st ed. Stamford: Appleton & Lange; 1998:730–733.

Borschel GH, Costantino DA, Cederna PS. Individualized implant-based reconstruction of Poland syndrome breast and soft tissue deformities. *Ann Plast Surg*. 2007;59(5):507–514.

Bostwick J. *Plastic and Reconstructive Surgery of the Breast*. St Louis, MO: Quality Medical Publishing; 1990:478.

Caouette-Laberge L, Borsuk D. Congenital anomalies of the breast. *Semin Plast Surg*. 2013;27:36–41.

Georgiade NG, Georgiade GS, Riefkohl R. Esthetic breast surgery. In: McCarthy JG, ed. *Plastic Surgery*. Vol. 6. Philadelphia, PA: WB Saunders; 1990:3839–3840.

Hoehn JG, Georgiade GS. Congenital and developmental deformities of the breast and breast asymmetries. In: Georgiade GS, Riefkohl R, Levin LS, eds. *Plastic, Maxillofacial and Reconstructive Surgery*. 3rd ed. Baltimore, MD: Williams & Wilkins; 1997:715–729.

Jones KL. *Smith's Recognizable Patterns of Human Malformation*. 5th ed. Philadelphia, PA: WB Saunders; 1997:302–303.

Karp NS. Gynecomastia. In: *Grabb and Smith's Plastic Surgery*. 6th ed. Philadelphia, PA: Lippincott Williams & Wilkins; 2007:616–620.

May N, Vasconez LO, Jurkiewicz MJ. Treatment of macromastia in the actively enlarging breast. *Plast Reconstr Surg.* 1977;59:575–578.

Mc Kinney P. Gynecomastia. In: Aston SJ, Beasley RW, Thorne CHM, eds. *Grabb and Smith's Plastic Surgery.* 5th ed. Philadelphia, PA: Lippincott-Raven; 1997:753–757.

Neuman JF. Evaluation and treatment of gynecomastia. *Am Fam Physician.* 1997;55:1835–1844, 1849–1850.

Riefkohl R, Zavitsanos GP, Courtiss EH. Gynecomastia. In: Georgiade GS, Riefkohl R, Levin LS, eds. *Textbook of Plastic, Maxillofacial and Reconstructive Surgery.* Baltimore, MD: Williams & Wilkins; 1997:820–828.

Rohrich RJ, Ha RY, Kenkel JM, Adams WP Jr. Classification and management of gynecomastia: defining the role of ultrasound-assisted liposuction. *Plast Reconstr Surg.* 2003;111:909–923; discussion 924–925.

Sadove AM, van Aalst JA. Congenital and acquired pediatric breast anomalies: a review of 20 years' experience. *Plast Reconstr Surg.* 2005;115:1039–1050.

Simon BE, Hoffman S, Kahn S. Classification and surgical correction of gynecomastia. *Plast Reconstr Surg.* 1973;51(1):48–52.

Skandalakis JE, Gray SW, Ricketts R, et al. The anterior body wall. In: Skandalakis JE, Gray SW, eds. *Embryology for Surgeons: The Embryologic Basis for the Treatment of Congenital Anomalies.* 2nd ed. Baltimore, MD: Williams & Wilkins; 1994:559–563.

Tuerk M. Medications that cause gynecomastia. *Plast Reconstr Surg.* 1993;92:1411.

van Aalst JA, Phillips JD, Sadove AM. Pediatric chest wall and breast deformities. *Plast Reconstr Surg.* 2009;124:38e–49e.

Wood RJ, Bostwick J. Congenital breast deformities. In: Benz ML, ed. *Pediatric Plastic Surgery.* 1st ed. Stamford: Appleton & Lange; 1998:739–746.

CHAPTER 69

Congenital Hand Surgery

Amir H. Taghinia, MD and
Joseph Upton III, MD

○ **What is the OMT classification system?**

The Oberg, Manske, Tonkin classification system is a new system for classification of congenital hand differences. This system was proposed in 2010 and has been recommended to replace the previous IFFSH classification system. The new system reflects deeper clinical and genetic understanding of these conditions. It divides congenital hand differences broadly into three categories: malformations, deformations, and dysplasias.

○ **What is the most common congenital hand anomaly?**

Polydactyly is the most common congenital hand anomaly and it affects approximately 4 to 12 per 1,000 live births.

○ **What are the three types of polydactyly?**

1. Radial polydactyly: Also known as preaxial polydactyly or thumb duplication. Most commonly seen in Caucasian or Asian populations.

2. Central polydactyly: Unusual, comprises only 10% of polydactyly cases. Most often associated with syndactyly (synpolydactyly).

3. Ulnar polydactyly: Also known as postaxial polydactyly. Most commonly seen in African-American or Native American populations.

○   **What classification system is most commonly used for radial polydactyly? What are the types of radial polydactyly?**

The classification system most commonly used is the Wassel classification (Fig. 69-1). Radial polydactyly is classified into six categories based on the level of the polydactyly. The odd numbers indicate polydactyly at the phalanx/metacarpal level, whereas the even numbers indicate polydactyly at the joint level. Type I polydactyly occurs at the distal phalanx, type III at the proximal phalanx, and type V at the metacarpal level. Type II polydactyly occurs at the interphalangeal joint, type IV at the metacarpophalangeal joint level, and type VI at the carpometacarpal (CMC) joint level.

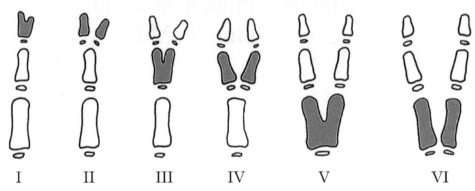

I   II   III   IV   V   VI

Figure 69-1 Wassel classification for radial polydactyly.

○   **What is the most common type of radial polydactyly (thumb duplication)?**

Type IV; polydactyly occurs at the metacarpophalangeal joint level.

○   **What are the different types of ulnar polydactyly? Which of these occurs most commonly?**

There are three types of ulnar polydactyly. Type I is a soft tissue nubbin with a skin bridge. There is a small neurovascular bundle within this bridge. Type II has skeletal connections with the polydactyly typically occurring at the fifth metacarpophalangeal joint level. Type III is duplication of the entire ray. The most common type is type I.

○   **Which thumb partner is typically ablated in reconstruction of radial polydactyly? Why?**

Usually, the ulnar thumb is preserved and the radial partner is ablated. The main reason to keep the ulnar partner is because it preserves the ulnar collateral ligament of the metacarpophalangeal joint. In practice, the best-looking and most functional thumb is preserved.

○   **In type IV radial polydactyly, if the ulnar partner is preserved, reattachment of what structure(s) is important to ensure good long-term function?**

The radial collateral ligament and the insertion of the thenar intrinsic muscles. Preservation of the ulnar partner implies ablation of the radial partners. When the radial partner is removed, the radial collateral ligament and the insertion of the thenar intrinsic muscles onto the radial side should be preserved. Once the radial partner is discarded, these structures need to be reattached to the ulnar partner to restore balance and centralize the metacarpophalangeal joint.

○ **What are the long-term unfavorable outcomes after reconstruction of radial polydactyly?**

Reconstructed thumbs are usually smaller and stiffer than their normal counterparts. Bulges are possible if the bifid metacarpal or phalangeal heads are not shaved. Deviations are possible if the intrinsic muscle tendons are not rebalanced well.

○ **What is syndactyly? What are the different types of syndactyly?**

Syndactyly occurs when the fingers are fused together—"webbed" digits. It is the second most common congenital hand anomaly. Simple syndactyly indicates fusion of the skin only. Complex syndactyly indicates fusion of the bone and skin. Complete syndactyly extends to the fingertips, whereas incomplete syndactyly terminates more proximally (see Fig. 69-2).

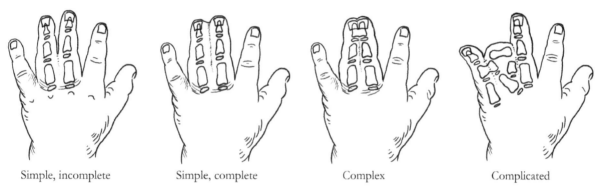

Simple, incomplete   Simple, complete   Complex   Complicated

Figure 69-2 Types of syndactyly.

○ **Which webspace is most commonly involved in syndactyly?**

The third webspace.

○ **What is the embryological timing of digital separation?**

The upper limb bud first forms around 4 weeks of gestation. Bones start to appear in the hand around 5 weeks of gestation. Digital rays start to form around 6 weeks of gestational age. At 7 weeks, loose mesenchyme between digital rays starts to break down and notches appear between the rays. By the end of the eighth week, digital separation is complete.

○ **What is the typical age for syndactyly release? What are the indications for releasing the syndactyly earlier?**

There is controversy about the optimal timing for syndactyly release. The typical age for syndactyly release is between 1 and 2 years, and most authors advocate release around 12 to 14 months of age. Release is performed earlier if the syndactyly is causing abnormal deviation or angulation of the involved digits. A typical scenario is syndactyly of the fourth webspace with bony fusion at the distal phalanx. Ring finger growth is restricted distally by a shorter small finger—thus causing ulnar deviation and possible PIP flexion contracture of the ring finger.

○ **What are the major principles of syndactyly release?**

1. Full-thickness flaps for reconstruction of the commissure—hourglass dorsal flap.
2. Zigzag incisions on the palmar surface to prevent contractures across flexion creases.
3. Full-thickness skin grafts for resurfacing the resultant defects—non–hair-bearing skin from the lower abdomen is advocated.
4. Adequate postoperative immobilization—well-padded long-arm cast.
5. Staged release—do not release both ulnar and radial sides during the same procedure.

○ **What is the proximal limit of syndactyly release (when do you stop releasing the webspace)?**

The bifurcation of the common digital artery is the proximal limit. If the nerve bifurcation is more distal, then the nerve can be internally neurolysed to separate the digital nerves more proximally.

○ **In a complex syndactyly, how can one be sure there will be adequate blood supply to each digit once the syndactyly is released?**

If there is any doubt about vascularity, one can obtain an angiogram preoperatively. The other option is to release the syndactyly in stages. In the first stage, the syndactyly is released partially (i.e., convert to incomplete syndactyly), and in the second stage release is completed.

○ **What is the most common reason for skin graft loss after syndactyly release?**

Inadequate postoperative immobilization. Children are quite active and should be immobilized in a long-arm cast to assure good skin graft take after syndactyly release.

○ **What is "web-creep"?**

This is mild to severe recurrence of the webbing after syndactyly release. This can happen in the long term and is related to a combination of growth and scar contracture at the base of the webspace. Minor procedures may be required (z-plasty) to release the webspace.

○ **What is the best method for surgical release of the first webspace? Other than the skin, what other structure(s) need to be released? What are two commonly used flaps for reconstruction of tight first webspaces?**

The best method for surgical release of the first webspace is a four-flap z-plasty. When releasing the first webspace, it is important to release the tight investing fascia of the first dorsal interosseous and adductor pollicis muscles. The two most commonly used flaps for reconstruction of a tight first webspace are the reverse pedicled radial forearm flap and the groin flap. Other options include the reverse pedicled posterior interosseous flap (which is less reliable) or free fasciocutaneous flaps.

○ **What anatomic feature distinguishes constriction ring syndrome from symbrachydactyly?**

The hand manifestations of constriction ring syndrome and symbrachydactyly can look very similar. Both involve shortened, fused, and/or webbed digits. Symbrachydactyly, formerly called atypical cleft hand, typically affects the hand in the shape of a U—with the central digits/hand being more affected. The major anatomic feature that distinguishes these two entities is that in constriction ring syndrome, the anatomy proximal to the level of the deformation is completely normal. This allows more reliable functional return after reconstruction surgery such as toe transfers.

○ **How is constriction ring of the digits treated?**

Excision of the cutaneous ring and fat/fascia advancement flaps with or without z-plasties.

○ **Outline the classification system for constriction ring syndrome.**

The classification system for constriction ring is shown below:

Type I (mild)—Shallow indentation of skin and soft tissue without distal lymphedema.

Type II (moderate)—Distal lymphedema, acrosyndactyly, and even discontinuous neurovascular or musculotendinous structures, but without vascular compromise.

Type III (severe)—Progressive lymphaticovenous or arterial compromise.

Type IV—Intrauterine amputation.

A type IIIB was introduced by Weinzweig (Plastic and Reconstructive Surgery, 1995). This is a dynamic sub-type which shows progressive swelling along with evolving vascular compromise. Limb salvage can be performed with emergent surgery despite a severe band, thereby, reducing the likelihood of limb loss. These limbs are often left with long-term growth retardation and neurologic deficits.

○ **What are treatment options for short digits (e.g., in constriction ring syndrome or symbrachydactyly)?**

The treatment options are (1) vascularized toe transfers, (2) distraction lengthening, and (3) nonvascularized toe phalanx transfers. Vascularized toe transfers are technically demanding but can provide excellent function and appearance. Distraction lengthening is difficult in the phalanges and prone to complications. Nonvascularized toe phalanx transfers require supple, elastic soft tissues to accommodate the transferred phalanges. None of these options should be entertained if the child has good or excellent function.

○ **What is symphalangism?**

Fused phalanges. The digits are usually short and stiff. The joints are not present or do not bend. There are no flexion/extension creases.

○ **What is clinodactyly?**

Deviated digit (see Fig. 69-3). The deviation is in a radioulnar direction. The most commonly affected digit is the fifth digit where deviation occurs toward a radial direction at the level of the middle phalanx. A "delta" phalanx may cause clinodactyly. A delta phalanx is a condition where the growth plate on one side of the digit does not grow as well as the other side, causing deviation in a radioulnar direction.

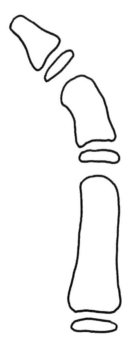

Figure 69-3 Clinodactyly.

○   **What is camptodactyly?**

Bent digit (see Fig. 69-4). This refers to a flexion deformity of a digit in the AP plane. It usually involves the PIP joint of the fifth digit.

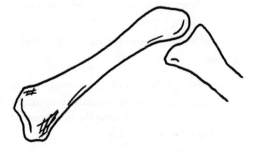

Figure 69-4 Camptodactyly.

○   **What are the possible anatomic anomalies that cause camptodactyly?**

These could be abnormal insertions of intrinsic and extrinsic tendons that cause an imbalance of flexion/extension. The most common variations are abnormal insertions of the intrinsic muscles or flexor digitorum superficialis within the digit. Joint contractures and tight collateral ligaments are usually secondary and not the primary deforming force.

○   **When is it appropriate to release camptodactyly?**

In general, most patients with this condition should be treated with stretching and splinting. Surgical intervention may be appropriate for those with >70 degrees of flexion contracture. However, the results are not satisfactory in the long term and recurrence is common.

○   **What is a congenital trigger thumb?**

Congenital trigger thumb is a condition where the IP joint of the thumb is held in flexion and cannot be passively extended. Focal overgrowth of the flexor tendon is a possible cause. The flexor gets stuck proximal to the A1 pulley causing flexion deformity. A palpable nodule called Notta's node is typically felt at the A1 pulley level. The treatment is surgical release of the A1 pulley. In children younger than 18 months, spontaneous resolution may be seen within 6 months. If the child is older than 2 years, one should entertain release. Steroid injections do not work in children. The most common complication of surgical release is injury to the digital nerves.

○   **What is macrodactyly? When does one amputate versus debulk?**

Large digit. Debulking can be entertained for mild forms of macrodactyly. However, if the finger is very large, has poor range of motion, inhibits hand function, and is insensate (or has poor sensation), then it should be amputated.

○ **What is the classification system for thumb hypoplasia? Describe the five types of thumb hypoplasia?**

The classification system is the Blauth system.

Type I: small thumb with normal joints, hypoplastic intrinsic muscles, and normal function.

Type II: smaller thumb, joints normal with possible ligament instability, more hypoplasia of the intrinsic muscles, possible first webspace deficiency.

Type IIIa: small thumb with laxity of the MP joint collateral ligaments, thenar intrinsic muscles are small and weak, tight first webspace but functional CMC joint—child holds objects against MP head of the thumb.

Type IIIb: similar to type IIIa except metacarpal is incomplete and the CMC joint is not functional—child cannot hold objects with thumb.

Type IV: floating thumb ("pouce flottant")—skin bridge connection to the hand only.

Type V: complete absence of thumb.

○ **What are the treatment options for the different types of thumb hypoplasia?**

Type I: no treatment.

Type II: based on deficiency—possible webspace release with or without ligament reconstruction or opponensplasty.

Type IIIa: webspace release, opponensplasty, and MP joint ligament reconstruction.

Type IIIb, IV, and V: pollicization.

○ **What is the best age in which to perform a pollicization procedure?**

Index finger pollicization remains the ideal restorative procedure for a missing or extremely hypoplastic thumb. While there is no clearly established age for doing this procedure, the surgeon has to balance early intervention for better cortical integration with delayed intervention to allow a technically easier operation due to size of the anatomic structures. Considering these issues, most surgeons agree that the "best" age for pollicization is between 1 and 2 years of age.

○ **What are the options for treatment of a Blauth type IIIb thumb?**

Most surgeons agree that the best reconstructive option for a type IIIb thumb is ablation of the native hypoplastic thumb and index finger pollicization. In addition to severe hypoplasia of the intrinsic and extrinsic muscles, a type IIIb thumb lacks a functional CMC joint. No ligament reconstruction or tendon transfer known can make up for this deficiency. A few authors have reconstructed the CMC joint with a free metatarsophalangeal joint transfer from the toes. Results for this operation have not shown superiority to index finger pollicization.

○ **What are the options for opponensplasty in congenital cases?**

Typically, the flexor digitorum superficialis to the fourth digit is transferred. It is common to use this for type II or IIIa thumbs, because the distal end of the tendon can be used to reconstruct of the radial and ulnar collateral ligaments. In other cases, the abductor digiti minimi can be transferred (Huber transfer).

○ **What is radial club hand?**

Best termed radial longitudinal deficiency, this condition occurs when the radius is shorter than the ulna. There are four types, ranging from mild longitudinal deficiency to complete absence of the radius. The patients have short forearms with radially deviated wrists. Thumb hypoplasia or absence is a common associated finding.

○   **What are other conditions associated with radial or thumb deficiency?**

These manifest as hematologic and/or cardiac anomalies.

1. Holt–Oram syndrome: Autosomal dominant condition with cardiac anomalies (septal defects, conduction deficits such as atrial fibrillation).

2. Fanconi anemia: Bone marrow failure around age 6 to 7.

3. Thrombocytopenia absent radius: Low platelet levels, thumb is usually unaffected.

○   **What are the common hand manifestations of Poland syndrome?**

Hand hypoplasia and brachysyndactyly (short, webbed digits).

○   **What is Apert syndrome?**

Acrocephalosyndactyly. Craniofacial anomalies (midface hypoplasia) and symphalangism with syndactyly of the hands and feet.

• • • **REFERENCE** • • •

Tonkin M, Tolerton S, Quick T, et al. Classification of congenital anomalies of the hand and upper limb: development and assessment of a new system. *J Hand Surg.* 2013;38:1845–1853.

CHAPTER 70 Vascular Anomalies

Javier A. Couto, BS and
Arin K. Greene, MD, MMSc

○ **How are vascular anomalies classified?**

Lesions are divided into tumors and malformations.

Tumors	Malformations
Infantile hemangioma	Capillary
Congenital hemangioma	Lymphatic
Kaposiform hemangioendothelioma	Venous
Pyogenic granuloma	Arteriovenous
	Overgrowth syndromes (e.g., Klippel–Trenaunay)

○ **What is infantile hemangioma?**

A benign tumor of endothelial cells.

○ **How common is infantile hemangioma?**

It is the most common tumor of infancy; 4% to 5% of Caucasians are affected.

○ **What does infantile hemangioma look like?**

Red; but deeper lesions under the skin may appear bluish.

○ **What tissues are affected by infantile hemangioma?**

Skin and/or subcutaneous tissue of the head and neck (60%), trunk (25%), or extremity (15%). The liver is the most common visceral location.

○ **Are there risk factors for infantile hemangioma?**

Yes. The tumor is more common in females (4:1), premature infants, and Caucasians.

○ **Is infantile hemangioma present at birth?**

No, although some infants may have a telangiectatic stain, pale spot, or ecchymotic area.

○ **When is infantile hemangioma first noted?**

Usually, within the first 2 weeks after birth; lesions beneath the skin may not be obvious for a few months.

○ **What is the life cycle of infantile hemangioma?**

It grows for the first 3 to 9 months of age and then slowly regresses.

○ **When does infantile hemangioma stop improving?**

Lesions typically stop involuting by 3.5 years of age.

○ **Does infantile hemangioma completely go away?**

Not usually, in at least 50% of children telangiectasias, damaged skin, destroyed structures, or fibrofatty tissue remains.

○ **Can an infant have multiple infantile hemangiomas?**

Yes, 20% have more than one lesion.

○ **Can multiple lesions be problematic?**

Yes, patients with more than five small, dome-like tumors are at risk for having a hepatic hemangioma.

○ **How is infantile hemangioma diagnosed?**

History and physical examination.

○ **Does infantile hemangioma require treatment?**

No. 90% of lesions are allowed to enlarge and regress without intervention.

○ **When is intervention indicated for a proliferating infantile hemangioma during infancy?**

If a tumor is causing functional problems (i.e., blocking the visual axis or airway), or is at risk for leaving a significant deformity (large lesion on the face).

○ **What is the first-line intervention for a small, localized problematic infantile hemangioma?**

Lesions ≤3 cm in diameter can be injected with corticosteroid (triamcinolone 40 mg/mL) not to exceed 3 mg/kg per injection.

○ **How effective is corticosteroid injection?**

All lesions will stop growing, and two-thirds will become smaller.

○ **What is the intervention for a problematic infantile hemangioma that is too large to inject with corticosteroid?**

Oral pharmacotherapy with either prednisolone (3 mg/kg) or propranolol (2 mg/kg).

○ **What are the advantages and disadvantages of prednisone therapy?**

~100% response rate (10% will stop growing and 90% will become smaller), safe, minimal monitoring, and no long-term side effects.

○ **What are the advantages and disadvantages of propranolol therapy?**

10% nonresponse rate, long duration of treatment, may have greater initial shrinkage of the tumor compared to prednisone, more complicated monitoring for bradycardia, hypotension, hyperkalemia, and hypoglycemia.

○ **Is resection of a problematic infantile hemangioma generally recommended in infancy?**

No. Operative morbidity is high while the tumor is vascular and rapidly growing.

○ **What is the ideal time for operative intervention?**

Between 3 and 4 years of age. At this time the tumor has completed involution, become less vascular, and decreased in size. Resection is still performed before long-term memory and self-esteem begin.

○ **What are the indications for operative intervention?**

Damaged or excess skin, injured anatomic structures, fibrofatty residuum, and residual telangiectasias.

○ **Should laser therapy be used to treat a cutaneous infantile hemangioma during infancy?**

No, laser does not stop the growth of the tumor and increases the risk of ulceration.

○ **Should laser be used to treat an infantile hemangioma after it has involuted?**

Yes, pulse-dye laser can effectively eliminate residual telangiectasias in childhood.

○ **What is a congenital hemangioma?**

A hemangioma that is fully grown at birth and does not enlarge postnatally.

○ **How many types of congenital hemangiomas exist?**

Two; rapidly involuting congenital hemangioma (RICH) and noninvoluting congenital hemangioma (NICH).

○ **How common are they?**

Rare. They comprise less than 1% of all hemangiomas.

○ **Do congenital hemangiomas look like infantile hemangioma?**

No, they are reddish purple, have coarse telangiectasias, and a peripheral halo.

○ **What other features differentiate congenital hemangiomas from infantile hemangioma?**

Congenital hemangiomas have an equal sex distribution, are solitary, most commonly affect the extremities, average 5 cm in diameter, and do not stain positive for the immunohistochemical marker GLUT1.

○ **How is RICH managed?**

Observation. It undergoes complete involution by 14 months of age.

○ **How is NICH managed?**

NICH may be observed or resected. Unlike RICH or infantile hemangioma, it does not regress.

○ **What is kaposiform hemangioendothelioma?**

A benign tumor that can cause Kasabach–Merritt phenomenon (thrombocytopenia, petechiae, and bleeding).

○ **How is kaposiform hemangioendothelioma treated?**

Vincristine or rapamycin.

○ **What is a pyogenic granuloma?**

Pyogenic granuloma is a common pedunculated red lesion that presents at an average age of 6 years, is small (mean diameter 6 mm), and frequently bleeds.

○ **How is pyogenic granuloma treated?**

Definitive treatment is resection. Other methods such as cautery, cryotherapy, or laser have a 50% recurrence rate.

○ **How do vascular malformations differ from vascular tumors?**

Unlike vascular tumors (hemangiomas, kaposiform hemangioendothelioma, pyogenic granuloma), vascular malformations are errors in embryogenesis, and do not have rapidly proliferating endothelium. Although vascular malformations are present at birth, they may not be diagnosed until childhood or adolescence after they have enlarged and/or become symptomatic (Figs. 70-1 and 70-2).

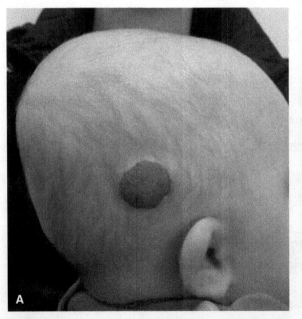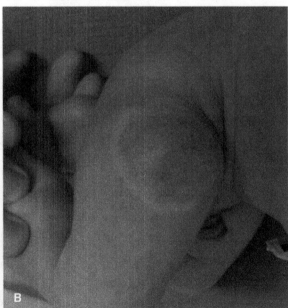

Figure 70-1 Vascular tumors. **A:** Infantile hemangioma. **B:** Congenital hemangioma.

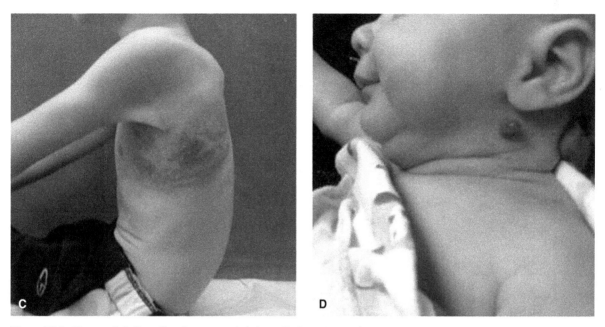

Figure 70-1 *(Continued)* **C:** Kaposiform hemangioendothelioma. **D:** Pyogenic granuloma.

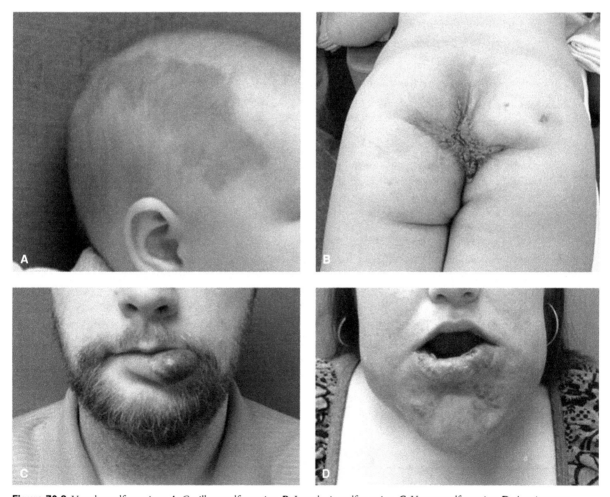

Figure 70-2 Vascular malformations. **A:** Capillary malformation. **B:** Lymphatic malformation. **C:** Venous malformation. **D:** Arteriovenous malformation.

○ **How common are vascular malformations?**

Vascular malformations are much less common than vascular tumors, affecting 0.5% of the population.

○ **What is a capillary malformation?**

The lesion used to be called "port-wine stain." It is an anomaly of dermal capillaries that results in a pink area of skin. Recently, the causative mutation for the lesion has been identified (*GNAQ*).

○ **How is capillary malformation diagnosed?**

The lesion is noted at birth and is diagnosed by history and physical examination.

○ **What is the natural history of capillary malformation?**

The stain darkens and becomes purple. The skin thickens, pyogenic granulomas may develop, and the tissues underneath the stain can become overgrown.

○ **What is the treatment for capillary malformation?**

First-line management is pulse-dye laser to lighten the color of the lesion. Resection is required to improve overgrown tissues.

○ **What is a lymphatic malformation?**

An error in lymphatic development due to a mutation in *PIK3CA*.

○ **How is lymphatic malformation classified?**

Lesions can be macrocystic (>5 mm), microcystic (<5 mm), or combined.

○ **How is lymphatic malformation diagnosed?**

Most lesions can be diagnosed by history and physical examination. However, subcutaneous lymphatic malformations may require ultrasound for diagnosis. Patients frequently undergo MRI to confirm the diagnosis and determine the extent of disease.

○ **What is the morbidity of lymphatic malformation?**

Psychosocial distress, bleeding, leakage of lymph fluid (lymphorrhea), infection, and overgrowth of tissues.

○ **How is lymphatic malformation treated?**

First-line intervention for symptomatic macrocystic lesions is sclerotherapy. Because microcystic lesions have cystic spaces that are too small to sclerose, management is either resection or carbon dioxide laser.

○ **What is sclerotherapy?**

Sclerotherapy involves injecting a scleroscent into a space (e.g., lymphatic cyst, vein). Commonly used scleroscents include doxycycline, sodium tetradecyl sulfate, and ethanol. The scleroscent causes shrinkage of the space, scarring, and improvement in symptoms.

○ **What is a venous malformation?**

An error in venous development, most commonly due to a mutation in *TIE2*.

○ **What are subtypes of venous malformation?**

Glomuvenous malformation is an autosomal dominant lesion that is often small and multiple (due to a mutation in *Glomulin*). Verrucous venous malformation is a hyperkeratotic lesion that typically affects the lower extremity and is caused by a mutation in *MAP3K3*.

○ **How are venous malformations diagnosed?**

Most are diagnosed by history and physical examination. However, subcutaneous venous malformations may require ultrasound for diagnosis. Patients frequently undergo MRI to confirm the diagnosis and determine the extent of disease.

○ **What is the morbidity of venous malformation?**

Lowered self-esteem, pain from phlebothrombosis, and overgrowth of tissues.

○ **How is venous malformation treated?**

First-line therapy is sclerotherapy. Resection is reserved for small lesions or for symptomatic venous malformations that are no longer able to be sclerosed.

○ **What is an arteriovenous malformation?**

An abnormal connection of arteries to veins without an intervening capillary bed.

○ **What are subtypes of arteriovenous malformation?**

Capillary malformation—arteriovenous malformation is an autosomal dominant condition caused by a mutation in *RASA1*; patients typically have circular cutaneous lesions associated with deeper arteriovenous malformations. Patients with a *PTEN* mutation can have arteriovenous malformations.

○ **What is the natural history of arteriovenous malformation?**

The lesion is present at birth and then progresses through four stages: 1 (quiescence), 2 (expansion), 3 (destruction), and 4 (decompensation).

○ **What is the morbidity of arteriovenous malformation?**

Psychosocial distress, pain, ulceration, bleeding, and destruction of tissues.

○ **How is arteriovenous malformation treated?**

First-line management is embolization. Resection is reserved for small lesions or for symptomatic arteriovenous malformations that have failed embolization.

○ **What is embolization?**

Embolization is the delivery of a substance to the nidus of the lesion, causing lesion ischemia, scarring, and improvement in symptoms. Typically, a catheter is inserted into the femoral artery and then is advanced to the nidus of the arteriovenous malformation.

○ **What are the most common vascular malformation overgrowth syndromes?**

CLOVES, Klippel–Trenaunay, Parkes Weber, and Sturge–Weber.

○ **What is CLOVES syndrome?**

Congenital *l*ipomatosis, overgrowth, vascular malformations, epidermal nevi, and scoliosis/skeletal/spinal anomalies. The lesion results from a mutation in *PIK3CA*.

○ **What is Klippel–Trenaunay syndrome?**

Capillary–*l*ymphatic–venous malformation typically of the lower extremity causing overgrowth. The causative mutation is *PIK3CA*.

○ **What is Parkes Weber syndrome?**

Diffuse arteriovenous malformation of the leg causing overgrowth. Patients often have a *RASA1* mutation.

○ **What is Sturge–Weber syndrome?**

Capillary malformation in the V1 trigeminal nerve distribution with either ocular abnormalities and/or leptomeningeal vascular malformation. The condition is due to a mutation in *GNAQ*.

• • • REFERENCES • • •

Boon LM, Enjolras O, Mulliken JB. Congenital hemangioma: evidence of accelerated involution. *J Pediatr.* 1996;128:329–335.

Chang LC, Haggstrom AN, Drolet BA, et al. Hemangioma Investigator Group. Growth characteristics of infantile hemangiomas: implications for management. *Pediatrics.* 2008;122:360–367.

Couto JA, Greene AK. Management of problematic infantile hemangioma using intralesional triamcinolone: efficacy and safety in 100 infants. *J Plast Reconstr Aesthet Surg.* 2014;67:1469–1474.

Couto JA, Maclellan RA, Greene AK. Infantile hemangioma: treatment rate during the proliferating phase. *J Craniofac Surg.* 2014;25: 1933–1934.

Couto RA, Maclellan RA, Zurakowski D, Greene AK. Infantile hemangioma: clinical assessment of the involuting phase and implications for management. *Plast Reconstr Surg.* 2012;130:619–624.

Enjolras O, Mulliken JB, Boon LM, Wassef M, Kozakewich HP, Burrows PE. Noninvoluting congenital hemangioma: a rare cutaneous vascular anomaly. *Plast Reconstr Surg.* 2001;107:1647–1654.

Greene AK. Current concepts of vascular anomalies. *J Craniofac Surg.* 2012;23:220–224.

Greene AK. Management of hemangiomas and other vascular tumors. *Clin Plast Surg.* 2011;38:45–63.

Greene AK, Alomari AI. Management of venous malformations. *Clin Plast Surg.* 2011;38:83–93.

Greene AK, Couto RA. Oral prednisolone for infantile hemangioma: efficacy and safety using a standardized treatment protocol. *Plast Reconstr Surg.* 2011;128:743–752.

Greene AK, Liu AS, Mulliken JB, Chalache K, Fishman SJ. Vascular anomalies in 5,621 patients: guidelines for referral. *J Pediatr Surg.* 2011;46:1784–1789.

Greene AK, Orbach DB. Management of arteriovenous malformations. *Clin Plast Surg.* 2011;38:95–106.

Greene AK, Perlyn CA, Alomari AI. Management of lymphatic malformations. *Clin Plast Surg.* 2011;38:75–82.

Hassanein AH, Mulliken JB, Fishman SJ, Greene AK. Evaluation of terminology for vascular anomalies in current literature. *Plast Reconstr Surg.* 2011;127:347–351.

Maguiness SM, Liang MG. Management of capillary malformations. *Clin Plast Surg.* 2011;38:65–73.

Mulliken JB, Glowacki J. Hemangiomas and vascular malformations in infants and children: a classification based on endothelial characteristics. *Plast Reconstr Surg.* 1982;69:412–422.

Sarkar M, Mulliken JB, Kozakewich HP, Robertson RL, Burrows PE. Thrombocytopenic coagulopathy (Kasabach-Merritt phenomenon) is associated with kaposiform hemangioendothelioma and not with common infantile hemangioma. *Plast Reconstr Surg.* 1997;100:1377–1386.

Section VII RECONSTRUCTION

Wound Healing/Keloids and Negative Pressure Wound Therapy

CHAPTER 71

Christian Kirman, MD, FACS

● ● ● **PRINCIPLES OF WOUND HEALING** ● ● ●

○ **What are the layers of the epidermis and dermis?**

Epidermis (superficial to deep):

1. stratum corneum

2. stratum lucidum

3. stratum granulosum

4. stratum spinosum

5. stratum basalis

Dermis—contains adnexal structures and vasculature

Papillary dermis—superficial, contains vascular tissue

Reticular dermis—deep, contains denser tissue

○ **What are the steps involved in wound healing?**

1. Coagulation: Minutes to hours.

2. Inflammation: 1 to 2 days.

3. Proliferation: 3 to 30 days (depends on bacterial load).

4. Remodeling/differentiation: up to 1 year.

○ **What are the cell types primarily responsible for each of these stages?**

1. Coagulation: platelets.

2. Inflammation: PMNs, macrophages.

3. Proliferation: macrophages, fibroblasts.

4. Remodeling: myofibroblasts (wound contraction), epithelial cells (reepithelialization).

○ **What are the steps involved in epithelialization across a wound?**

Mobilization, migration, mitosis, and differentiation of epithelial cells. The loss and reestablishment of **contact inhibition** initiate and terminate the process.

○ **In a healthy individual, how long does it take for a surgical incision to reepithelialize after closure?**

After a surgical incision is primarily closed, it takes approximately 24 hours for the wound to reepithelialize. After this point, it is not necessary to keep the surgical area dry with an occlusive dressing.

○ **What is the key cell involved in wound remodeling?**

Macrophage. The macrophage is probably the most critical cell in wound healing in general—it initiates the growth factor cascade that results in fibroblast proliferation and thus collagen production.

○ **Which cells are responsible for wound contracture?**

Myofibroblasts: fibroblasts that contain myofibrils permitting contractile activity similar to muscle.

○ **What provides tensile strength to a healing wound?**

Collagen.

○ **Which cells produce collagen in the healing wound, and when does production peak?**

Fibroblasts produce collagen; maximal net collagen production occurs at about 1 to 2 weeks.

○ **How does platelet-derived growth factor (PGDF) affect wound healing?**

PGDF is released by platelets in the inflammatory phase, and attracts macrophages.

○ **How does transforming growth factor-beta (TGF-β) affect wound healing?**

TGF-β is released primarily by macrophages which attracts fibroblasts and is involved with collagen production.

○ **What isomers mediate the profibrotic phenotype of TGF-β?**

TGF-b has three isomers. TGF-β1 and TGF-β2 are profibrotic. TGF-β3 is antifibrotic.

Various fibrotic diseases (such as keloids) might result from aberrant ratios of TGF-β isomers (i.e., increased TGF-β1 and TGF-β2 and decreased TGF-β3).

○ **What is the role of fibroblast growth factor (FGF) in wound healing?**

- FGF-1 and FGF-2 (acidic and basic FGF) are the major proteins in this family and drive rapid proliferation of fibroblasts, epithelial cells, and endothelial cells.
- FGF-7 (keratinocyte growth factor) is a major epidermal growth factor and is involved in dermal–epidermal signaling.
- The sequence of events in wound healing is largely mediated by orchestration of intra- and extracellular regulation of FGF proteins in a defined pattern.

○ **What are the biologic effects of FGF?**

- Fibroblast and epithelial proliferation.
- Collagen production.
- Potent angiogenic factor.

○   **When is a scar fully matured, and how much tensile strength does it achieve?**

Skin incisions have gained approximately 80% of their final strength by 6 weeks, and a scar has its full tensile strength at 12 weeks, at which point it has gained approximately 80% to 90% of its initial tensile strength. Tensile strength doubles approximately every week over the first 4 weeks, secondary to **collagen cross-linking**.

○   **What defines a chronic wound?**

Wounds that fail to heal in 3 months are classified as "chronic wounds."

○   **How does the metalloproteinase level in chronic wounds compare to that in acute wounds?**

In chronic wounds, the metalloproteinase level is increased as compared to that of an acute wound resulting in increased ECM degradation.

○   **What are the different types of collagen?**

There are many types of collagen (more than 10). Critical to wound healing are:

- Type I: most common; in skin, bone, and tendon/ligament.
- Type II: hyaline cartilage.
- Type III: vessel walls; intestine; skin; early scar formation.
- Type IV: basement membrane.
- Type V: fetal and placental tissue.

○   **What is the ratio of type I to type III collagen in normal skin and scars?**

1. Normal skin: 4:1 (i.e., predominantly type I collagen).
2. Immature scar: 2:1.
3. Hypertrophic scar: 2:1.
4. Keloid: 3:1 (varies).
5. Fetal skin: predominantly type III collagen.

○   **Which conditions adversely affect key steps in collagen synthesis?**

1. Vitamin C deficiency (scurvy): inhibits hydroxylation of proline and lysine (required for collagen cross-linking).
2. Colchicine: inhibits secretion of tropocollagen from the cell.
3. Copper deficiency and penicillamine: prevent lysine oxidation (which is necessary for intra- and intermolecular bonding).

○   **What are the detrimental effects of corticosteroids on wound healing?**

Corticosteroids inhibit macrophages, resulting in poor fibroblast stimulation and wound contraction.

○   **What strategy can overcome the effects of steroids?**

Vitamin A (25,000 IU by mouth daily for 3 to 5 days, alternatively 200,000 IU topically three times a day).

○ **How long should you wait before revising a scar?**

One year to allow scar remodeling to complete.

○ **What factors impair wound healing?**

1. Foreign bodies.

2. Infection.

3. Radiated tissue—decreases blood supply.

4. Inadequate blood supply—any cause.

5. Local trauma.

6. Systemic factors (steroid use, obesity, edema, smoking, comorbidities, malnutrition).

○ **What are the escalating strategies that can be used to close a defect (the "reconstructive ladder")?**

• Secondary sintent

• Primary intent

• Skin graft

• Local tissue rearrangement

• Transposition flap

• Free tissue transfer

○ **How do the following tissues differ in healing?**

Bone, Tendon, Nerve, Liver.

Bone healing is accomplished via **osteoinduction, osteoconduction, or osteogenesis. Osteoinduction** refers to precursor cells in the bony tissue being induced to become osteoblasts, often by demineralized bone or bone morphogenic protein (BMP). **Osteoconduction** refers to osteoblasts entering the site, along a nonviable bony scaffold such as cortical grafts or cadaveric bone which is replaced by new bone, by "creeping substitution." **Osteogenesis** refers to healing with vascularized bone grafts or cancellous bone, where osteoblasts survive the transplantation and produce new bone.

Tendons heal by **intrinsic** (minimal inflammation with epitenon cells producing collagen) and **extrinsic** (inflammation, proliferation, remodeling) healing. Extrinsic healing produces adhesions and is increased with immobilization.

Peripheral nerves heal by a combination of degeneration and regeneration. The degenerative process is called Wallerian degeneration and occurs distal to the site of nerve injury.

Hepatic tissue undergoes regeneration.

○ **What adult tissues are able to heal without scarring?**

Bone and liver are the only adult tissues that are able to heal without scar formation. Chronic damage can cause hepatic scarring (cirrhosis).

○ **How are operative wounds classified?**

Class I: Clean—atraumatic, uninfected, no entry into GI/GU/respiratory tract.

Class II: Clean-contaminated—entry into GI/GU/respiratory tract.

Class III: Contaminated—traumatic wounds or gross spillage of enteric contents.

Class IV: Dirty—drainage of abscess or soft tissue infection.

● ● ● TYPES OF WOUNDS ● ● ●

○ **What organisms are associated with bite wounds?**

Cat and dog bites are associated with *Pasteurella multocida* as well as *Staphylococcus* and *Streptococcus* species.

Human bites are associated with *Eikenella corrodens* as well as *Staphylococcus* and *Streptococcus* species and *Bacteroides*.

Bite wounds are typically treated with Augmentin for prophylaxis.

○ **What is the staging of pressure ulcers?**

Stage 1: Skin intact; nonblanching erythema.

Stage 2: Partial-thickness skin loss, abrasions, and blisters included (so into epidermis or dermis).

Stage 3: Full-thickness skin loss with extension into subcutaneous tissue but not through the underlying fascia.

Stage 4: Full-thickness skin loss with extension into muscle, bone, joint, or tendon.

○ **How long does it take for pressure ulcers to arise?**

Early (stage I, nonblanching erythema) pressure ulcer formation can occur within 30 minutes of unrelieved pressure. Partial-thickness skin loss (stage II) can be seen in as little as 2 to 6 hours.

○ **How much pressure is required to cause a pressure sore?**

Unrelieved pressure above 32 mm Hg (capillary arterial pressure) can lead to tissue ischemia and pressure sores.

○ **What are the principles of sacral wound management?**

1. Remove pressure.

2. Maintain hygiene in region (diverting colostomy if needed).

3. Optimize medical issues.

4. Serial wound debridements.

5. Dressing changes (wet-to-dry; enzymatic therapy if necrotic tissue or dilute acetic acid if infected, especially with pseudomonas).

6. Repair with excision and choice of flap once above factors addressed.

○ **In the evaluation of a pressure ulcer, what is the imaging modality of choice for diagnosis of osteomyelitis?**

MRI is the current imaging modality of choice.

Bone biopsy is the gold standard to confirm osteomyelitis.

○ **Where can pressure ulcers occur?**

Anywhere bony prominences exist. In order of prevalence:

1. ischial tuberosity

2. trochanter

3. sacrum

4. calcaneus

5. occiput

6. scapula

○ **What type of flap reconstruction for pressure ulcers is best for ambulatory patients?**

Fasciocutaneous flaps preserve muscle and do not affect ambulation.

○ **What is frostbite, and how is it classified?**

Frostbite occurs with extremely cold temperatures that cause tissue freezing and formation of intracellular ice crystals and microvascular occlusion. After thawing, tissue inflammation and coagulation lead to cell death. It is classified similarly to burns:

First degree: involves epidermis only with hyperemia.

Second degree: involves dermis with blister formation.

Third degree: full-thickness skin and subcutaneous tissue involvement.

Fourth degree: necrosis of deeper tissues such as muscle and bone.

○ **What are the steps of frostbite management?**

1. Resuscitation

2. Rapid rewarming

3. Thrombolytic therapy

4. Watchful waiting

○ **Which animals can potentially transmit rabies?**

Carnivores: dog, cat, raccoon, bat, fox, skunk, coyote. Incidence of rabies from cats is increasing. Exposure alone without a bite can transmit rabies and is an indication for prophylaxis (entering a cave harboring rabid bats).

Rodents do not carry rabies.

○ **How is a rabies exposure managed?**

1. Wash the wound in virucidal agent (dilute Betadine).

2. Rabies immune globulin: give single dose of 20 IU/kg around the wound.

3. Rabies vaccine (human diploid cell vaccine): give five 1-cc doses over a 28-day period (days 0, 3, 7, 14, and 28); intramuscular injection in the deltoid.

4. Give both rabies immune globulin and vaccine to all patients, except for patients with a documented antibody titer, who do not need immune globulin.

○ **Which wounds are "tetanus prone"?**

1. Wounds that are contaminated.

2. Contain devitalized tissue.

3. Are open for more than 6 hours.

4. Are deeper than 1 cm.

○ **What tetanus measures are required for a wound in a "fully immunized" patient?**

A fully immunized patient is one who has received complete tetanus toxoid immunization (3 to 5 doses) with a booster within 5 years of the current injury. If the wound is "tetanus prone," give tetanus toxoid (0.5 mL of adsorbed toxoid intramuscularly). If the wound is not "tetanus prone," do nothing.

○ **What tetanus measures are required for a wound in a patient of unknown or inadequate immunization status?**

These patients need to receive tetanus toxoid for all wounds. In addition, if the patient has received less than two injections of immunization, also give immune globulin (250 units of human tetanus immune globulin).

○ **What organisms are typically associated with necrotizing fasciitis?**

Necrotizing fasciitis is a severe infection that leads to liquefaction necrosis along fascial planes. *Beta-hemolytic streptococci* are commonly associated with this devastating process; however, mixed aerobes and anaerobes can also be found.

○ **What organism is responsible for "gas gangrene"?**

The *Clostridia* species (typically *Clostridium perfringens*) cause gas gangrene. They are obligate anaerobes and so in addition to radical debridement, hyperbaric oxygen has been shown to be beneficial in the treatment of gas gangrene.

⦿ ⦿ ⦿ **KELOIDS** ⦿ ⦿ ⦿

○ **What is the difference between keloids and hypertrophic scars?**

1. Keloids extend beyond the margin of the initial scar, whereas hypertrophic scars do not.

2. Keloids have an increased ratio of types I/III collagen unlike hypertrophic scars.

3. Keloids have larger, thicker, and more irregular collagen fibers than hypertrophic scars.

4. Keloids are commonly found on the face, earlobes, chest, and upper back, whereas hypertrophic scars are commonly found across flexor surfaces.

5. Keloids appear late after initial injury, and can grow indefinitely. Hypertrophic scars arise over the first few weeks, quickly grow, and then regress.

○ **What are the chemical and histological differences between keloids and normal scar tissue?**

Keloids contain elevated levels of TGF-β. In addition, they have increased collagen (especially type III) and vascularity compared with normal tissue. Fibroblasts proliferate faster in keloids than normal tissue.

○ **What are the principles of keloid and hypertrophic scar management?**

1. Excision plus adjuvant therapy (intradermal steroids, silicone gel, radiation therapy).

2. Meticulous tissue handling and closure with intradermal sutures.

3. Pressure earrings/garments.

○ **What are the contraindications to radiation therapy for keloids?**

1. Pediatric patients.

2. Pregnant women.

3. Tissue with underlying visceral structures.

Despite the theoretical risk of neoplastic transformation, fewer than 10 cases of cancer due to radiation therapy for keloids have been reported.

○ **What are the potential side effects of radiation therapy for keloids?**

   1. Hypo- or hyperpigmentation.

   2. Telangiectasias.

   3. Acute skin desquamation.

○ **What is the mechanism of intralesional steroid (triamcinolone acetonide) therapy for keloids?**

   1. Inhibits fibroblast proliferation and collagen production by gene inhibition.

   2. Stimulates collagenase production.

   3. Normalizes collagen ultrastructural organization that is disrupted in keloid nodules.

○ **What is the optimal treatment for earlobe keloids?**

   Surgical excision with or without steroid injection, followed by wearing of magnetic pressure earrings.

○ **Where does scarless wound healing occur?**

   Wound healing occurs without scar in the early mammalian fetus (including human). Levels of <u>hyaluronic acid</u> are significantly higher in fetal skin and appear to correlate with scarless wound healing.

● ● ● WOUND THERAPY/TREATMENT ● ● ●

○ **What diagnosis should be considered in a chronic nonhealing lower extremity wound despite adequate wound care?**

   A <u>Marjolin's ulcer</u> is malignant degeneration of a chronic wound such as a burn or venous stasis ulcer. A biopsy should be performed for diagnosis.

○ **Can a partial-thickness burn scar be left to heal by secondary intention?**

   Generally, partial-thickness burn scars can be given <u>up to 3 weeks</u> to close by secondary intent. If not closed by <u>3 weeks</u>, they need to be grafted to avoid hypertrophic scar formation.

○ **How is burn scar hypertrophy best managed?**

   <u>Pressure garments</u> decrease blood flow to active scars, and decrease collagen fiber production.

○ **During wound therapy with leeches, which bacteria grow in the leech gut?**

   <u>Aeromonas hydrophila</u>. Ciprofloxacin, bactrim, or tetracycline can be used for prophylaxis.

○ **What is the antibacterial mechanism of Acticoat?**

   Acticoat contains <u>silver ions that are directly bactericidal</u>. It needs to be moistened with distilled water prior to application (ions in normal saline will negate the antibacterial effect of Acticoat). It is efficacious against *Pseudomonas*, MRSA, VRE, and some species of yeast.

○ **What are the associated side effects of topical antimicrobial agents?**

Silvadene (silver sulfadiazine)—leukopenia.

Sulfamylon (mafenide acetate)—acidosis (secondary to carbonic anhydrase inhibition).

Silver nitrate—hyponatremia.

Bacitracin—vesicular rash.

○ **What are the clinical indications for Regranex gel (becaplermin, PDGF)?**

Regranex is indicated for lower extremity ulcers:

- of diabetic neuropathy.
- that extend into the subcutaneous tissue.
- that have a good vascular supply.
- that are not infected.

Regranex is not FDA approved for use in ischemic, infected, or superficial wounds, or those that are being closed primarily.

○ **Which biologic dressings contain cultured cells?**

1. TransCyte: a dermal substitute that is composed of cultured neonatal dermal fibroblasts seeded on a silicone/collagen matrix, covered with a nylon sheet.
2. Dermagraft: contains neonatal fibroblasts on a sheet of dexon (polyglycolic acid) or vicryl.
3. Epicyte: a matrix of cultured autologous keratinocytes (i.e., from the same patient).
4. Apligraf: contains both neonatal keratinocytes and fibroblasts; these cells are seeded onto a collagen matrix.

○ **Which other biologic dressings contain dermal matrix?**

1. Biobrane: a nylon sheet covering a silicone layer containing dermal collagen.
2. Integra: a silicone sheet coated with collagen and glycosaminoglycan obtained from bone tendon cartilage.
3. AlloDerm: cadaveric acellular dermis that has been deepithelialized.

○ **Which biologic dressings contain ECM or basement membrane?**

1. Grafix: cryopreserved placental membrane.
2. ACELL: porcine bladder ECM and basement membrane.
3. OASIS: porcine small intestine ECM.

○ **Which wounds are best treated with alginates?**

Highly exudative wounds. Calcium alginate gels are made from seaweed and are hydrophilic, so they can absorb significant amounts of fluid. Alginates prevent tissue maceration, trap bacteria, and can be rinsed off.

○ **How does a split-thickness skin graft initially receive nutrition?**

Plasma imbibition for the first 48 hours until an adequate vascular supply is established. **Inosculation:** Connection of recipient and donor vessels in the graft and recipient bed. **Neovascularization:** Sprouting of new blood vessels.

○   **What are the steps in adherence of a skin graft?**

Phase 1: fibrin phase (first 72 hours).

Phase 2: fibrovascular phase (after 72 hours)—vascular ingrowth and anastomosis.

○   **What dressing is ideal to bolster a split-thickness skin graft?**

A VAC dressing conforms to the wound, holds the skin graft in place for rapid revascularization, and prevents shearing.

○   **What are the causes of skin graft failure?**

1. Hematoma
2. Seroma
3. Infection
4. Shearing forces disrupting skin graft adherence and thus nutrition

○   **What bacterial load is required to cause clinical infection in a split-thickness skin graft?**

10^5 bacteria per cm^3 of tissue.

○   **Which flap type offers the greatest resistance to bacterial infection?**

Musculocutaneous flaps bring in a large proportion of blood supply that best wards off bacterial infection.

○   **What histologic layer mediates skin graft contraction?**

Elastin within the dermis—thicker skin grafts mean more dermis, which means more elastin, and which means more primary or immediate contraction.

Conversely, elastin inhibits delayed (secondary) graft contraction so those grafts without dermis, such as cultured epithelial cells, demonstrate the most delayed contraction.

○   **Hyperbaric oxygen therapy might be beneficial in which clinical situations?**

•   Osteomyelitis
•   Necrotizing infections
•   Ischemia-reperfusion injury
•   Diabetic lower extremity wounds

• • • TISSUE EXPANSION • • •

○   **What are the effects of tissue expansion on flap properties?**

1. Increased tissue surface area, collagen, and ground substance content.
2. Increased vascularity (similar to flap delay).
3. Decreased tensile strength and elasticity (since thinner dermis).
4. Markedly increased sensitivity to epinephrine-induced necrosis.

Tissue expansion results in a net gain of tissue that is due to both stretching of existing tissue and de novo tissue generation.

○ **What growth factor is responsible for increased vascularity in expanded tissue?**

Vascular endothelial growth factor (VEGF) is responsible for angiogenesis by increasing endothelial cell growth and migration.

○ **What are the histologic changes seen following tissue expansion?**

1. Subcutaneous fat atrophies.

2. Dermis becomes thinner.

3. Epidermis becomes thicker, particularly the **stratum spinosum** (increased mitotic activity).

4. Rete ridges become flatter.

○ **What are the tissue zones that result from tissue expansion?**

Tissue expansion results in formation of a capsule surrounding the expander, which is essentially a foreign body reaction. These zones are, from inside to outside, as follows:

Zone A: inner zone, cellular (predominantly macrophages).

Zone B: central zone, fibrous, with fibroblasts and myofibroblasts.

Zone C: transitional zone, with loose collagen.

Zone D: vascular zone.

○ **What is mechanical creep?**

1. A response to constant mechanical force.

2. Collagen realigns and results in a change in tissue elasticity.

3. Interstitial fluid and ground substance are displaced.

4. Depends on viscoelastic properties of skin.

○ **What is stress relaxation?**

Less force is needed to keep tissue stretched to a given length the longer it is held at that length.

○ **Which tissue expansion protocol results in maximal tissue recruitment?**

Cyclic loading: repeated cycles of stretching followed by relaxation.

○ **How can extra tissue be recruited intraoperatively?**

Approximately, 15% to 20% tissue expansion can be gained with a brief 1- to 2-hour session (acute tissue expansion). Clinical studies suggest acute tissue expansion provides tissue of comparable quality to that expanded over a much longer time frame (weeks).

○ **What are the concerns with lower extremity tissue expansion, especially below the knee?**

1. Extensive tissue expansion can cause sural nerve neuropraxia.

2. The region below the knee has relatively limited lymphatic outflow (compared with the trunk), and a tissue expander is at increased risk for cellulitis.

3. Tissue expansion in the lower extremity is particularly problematic in the pediatric population.

○ **What effect does tissue expansion have on hair growth?**

Tissue expansion, such as in the scalp, decreases the telogen, or growth-arrest phase.

○ **How does irradiated tissue differ from normal during tissue expansion?**

Irradiated tissue does not undergo the histologic changes that are seen with normal tissue during tissue expansion. Previous irradiation decreases the net tissue gain from expansion by approximately 25%.

○ **How long do sutures retain tensile strength?**

Catgut—1 week or less.

Monocryl (poliglecaprone 25)—7 to 10 days.

Chromic gut—1 week.

Vicryl, dexon—2 to 4 weeks.

PDS—4 to 6 weeks.

○ **Which conditions associated with impaired wound healing preclude elective rejuvenation surgery?**

• Ehlers–Danlos syndrome: inherited disorder of collagen polymerization, characterized by joint laxity, hyperextensible skin, and poor wound healing.

• Progeria: autosomal recessive disorder (rare) of premature aging, characterized by premature aging, loss of subcutaneous fat, poor wound healing, atherosclerosis.

○ **In which inherited skin disorders is it possible to perform rejuvenation surgery?**

• Cutis laxa: have nonfunctioning elastase inhibitor characterized by coarsely textured drooping skin due to degeneration of dermal elastic fibers.

• Pseudoxanthoma elasticum: associated with increased collagen degradation and deposition of calcium in elastic fibers.

• • • BASICS OF NEGATIVE PRESSURE WOUND THERAPY • • •

○ **What is Negative Pressure Wound Therapy (NPWT)?**

NPWT is a device or wound care apparatus that applies vacuum to a wound surface. It includes a wound–interface material, an adhesive film or drape, and tubing connected to a vacuum source.

○ **When was NPWT first introduced?**

Closed suction drainage has been a long recognized principle of surgery that predates NPWT. However, Morykwas and Argenta first introduced the concept of NPWT in the early 1990s.

○ **What are the indications of NPWT?**

NPWT is indicated in acute, chronic, traumatic, and dehisced wounds; partial-thickness burns; diabetic, pressure, and venous ulcers; flaps and grafts.

○ **What are contraindications to NPWT?**

NPWT is contraindicated in wounds with exposed vasculature, nerves, anastomotic sites and solid organs, malignancy in the wound, untreated osteomyelitis, necrotic tissue present in the wound, and nonenteric or unexplored fistulas.

○ **What is the basic principle of NPWT?**

The exact mechanism of action of NPWT is multifactorial and includes accelerated wound healing by increasing granulation tissue formation, removal of wound fluid, maintenance of moist wound environment, and contracting the wound edges together.

○ **What factors do NPWT effect to increase blood flow in the wound?**

Blood flow is dependent on the pressure applied, distance from the edge, and the tissue type. Blood flow decreases at the wound edge, but immediately increases with vacuum release suggesting that intermittent NPWT may further increase blood flow.

○ **How does NPWT effect wet or draining wounds?**

In patients with large open wounds, serous fluid may accumulate in the wound bed and be efficiently removed by NPWT leading to accelerated wound healing.

○ **What effect does NPWT have on skin surrounding the wound?**

In wounds where the surrounding skin is deformable, such as the abdomen or thigh, it is commonly observed that the wound shrinks considerably when using an NPWT device.

○ **How does NPWT maintain wound homeostasis?**

Covering the wound with a semiocclusive dressing and using foam with insulation qualities minimize evaporation, desiccation, and heat loss.

○ **What complications can occur from NPWT?**

Bleeding and infection have been reported by the FDA in a small number of patients.

In addition, retained foam dressing pieces have also been reported.

○ **Can NPWT be used in patients on anticoagulants or platelet aggregation inhibitors?**

Yes, but extreme caution should be used with patients at higher risk of bleeding or hemorrhage, such as those on anticoagulants or platelet aggregation inhibitors.

• • • CLINICAL USES OF NPWT • • •

○ **How is NPWT applied to wounds?**

An interface material is fitted to the size of the wound and placed on or into the wound bed. The adhesive dressing is placed over the wound. Tubing is connected to the wound through a hole in the adhesive drape and connected to a collection canister and a vacuum source.

○ **What is used for the wound–interface material?**

Many materials can be used including open pore foam, gauze, polyvinyl alcohol sponges, and corrugated polymers. Open pore sponges are most commonly used.

○ **How does the wound–interface material act on the wound?**

The interface material distributes the vacuum throughout the wound and allows for fluid removal. In addition, the wound–interface material causes microdeformations at the wound surface and draws the surrounding skin together.

○ **Can the wound–interface material be hemostatic on the wound?**

The wound–interface materials used in NPWT are not hemostatic and should not be applied to wounds that are bleeding or have a potential to bleed.

○ **Does the wound–interface material have antibacterial properties?**

The commonly used wound–interface materials are inert substances that have no inherent antibacterial properties and should not be applied to grossly infected wounds. There is a silver-impregnated foam that can be used with certain NPWT devices and there are also antibacterial gauze products that can be used with the device.

○ **What happens to the wound if there is no adequate seal to maintain continuous suction on the wound bed?**

There must be an adequate seal to maintain the vacuum or air will leak into the wound causing desiccation.

○ **What pressure is commonly used for NPWT?**

There are no established guidelines on the amount of pressure applied in NPWT. Applying a pressure of 125 mm Hg is most commonly used, but pressures between 60 and 150 mm Hg have also been applied.

○ **What waveforms are commonly used?**

The original work by Morykwas and Argenta showed increased granulation tissue formation with cycling waveforms; however, varying the level of suction can cause pain and may not be well tolerated by patients. Instead, continuous suction is most commonly used.

○ **When is a wound ready for NPWT?**

Wounds may be ready for NPWT after complete debridement of infected and necrotic tissue.

○ **Does NPWT debride wounds?**

NPWT does not debride or remove devitalized tissue in wounds but rather aids to accelerate wound healing.

○ **How often does the wound–interface material need to be changed?**

There are no specific recommendations for changing the wound–interface material. In heavily colonized wounds, the dressing should be changed every 12 to 24 hours, for several days to make sure the wound is clean. Afterward, the dressings are generally changed every 2 to 3 days.

○ **When changing the NPWT dressing, what should be assessed?**

The wound should be assessed for infection, odor, and need for further debridement. In addition, the wound bed should be assessed frequently for duskiness, bruising, and bleeding. The surrounding skin integrity should be monitored for skin breakdown from the adhesive drape and rash secondary to contact dermatitis or fungal infection. Devitalized tissue should be removed as indicated with each dressing change. If the wound is malodorous, the treatment should be stopped for 24 to 48 hours and replaced with saline dressings until the odor has subsided. Then NPWT treatment can be resumed.

○ **How long can NPWT be used on a wound?**

Prolonged use of NPWT beyond 3 months may not be of benefit unless the wound surface area continues to significantly decrease.

○ **When should NPWT be discontinued?**

NPWT should be discontinued if the patient does not tolerate dressing changes or if the wound needs to be frequently assessed for infection. If the wound bed is dusky, bruised, or bleeding, the wound becomes grossly infected, or there is persistent devitalized tissue present, the therapy should be discontinued. The therapy should also be immediately stopped if blood or purulent exudate is noted in the suction canister.

○ **Can NPWT be used in dirty or grossly contaminated wounds?**

NPWT devices should be used with extreme caution in infected wounds. Some clinicians use NPWT devices on infected wounds, and if used, the device should be changed every 12 to 24 hours to avoid worsening infection or sepsis.

○ **Can NPWT be applied to diabetic wounds?**

NPWT has been used as a wound healing therapy after debridement of diabetic foot ulcers. Most of the few randomized diabetic foot ulcer trials compare NPWT to hydrogel, alginate, or gauze—all indicating better wound healing with NPWT.

○ **How does NPWT prepare a wound for surgical closure?**

NPWT prepares the wound bed for surgical closure with skin grafts or tissue substitutes by increasing granulation tissue formation, decreasing the surface area, and possibly increasing blood flow to the wound bed.

○ **What effect does NPWT have on lower extremity wounds?**

NPWT can be used in patients with lower extremity stasis ulcers. In studies of patients with lower extremity ulcers, there was a trend toward less secondary amputations with NPWT applied to the wounds compared to nontreated controls. Patients with lower extremity traumatic injuries, specifically tibia–fibula fractures, treated with NPWT were less likely to require free flap closure of their wounds and were more likely to be closed primarily or with simple skin grafts.

○ **How is NPWT used in the treatment of an open abdomen?**

When the abdominal fascia is left open after a laparotomy, NPWT can be applied in the wound to control infection, manage exudate, and reduce visceral edema. Any exposed viscera should be covered with a nonadherent dressing prior to placement of the NPWT wound–interface material.

○ **How can NPWT be applied to enterocutaneous fistulae?**

The fistula can be isolated and controlled from the surrounding tissues by placing wound–interface material over the fistula. The effluent can be controlled, while the surrounding tissues are protected, the tissues can granulate and the wound can contract around the fistula. Additional therapy must be directed at the underlining cause and control of the fistula.

○ **Can NPWT prevent burn wound progression?**

Early work by Morykwas showed that NPWT prevents tissue injury progression in swine after partial-thickness burns. There have been several small studies since, but no robust clinical trial has been performed to assess the theoretical edema reduction, improved tissue perfusion, or less scarring with NPWT.

○ **Can NPWT be used in chest wall wounds following median sternotomies?**

NPWT allows for wound drainage, chest wall stabilization, and isolation of the chest cavity to prevent contamination, maintenance of a moist environment, granulation stimulation, and increased blood flow to the tissues. After NPWT is used for several days in a deep sternal wound, definitive closure is usually performed with soft-tissue flaps.

○ **How is NPWT used as a bolster for skin grafts?**

The use of NPWT as a bolster for skin grafts has been shown to increase graft take compared with foam bolsters without vacuum. NPWT is generally used for 48 to 72 hours and then removed. A nonadherent material should be applied between the skin graft and wound–interface material.

○ **How is NPWT used to treat lower extremity compartment syndrome?**

NPWT can be applied to open fasciotomy wounds, which decreases the edema and promotes granulation tissue formation allowing these wounds to either completely close in an accelerated manner or contract enough to accept a skin graft.

○ **What role does NPWT have in controlling lymphatic injuries?**

NPWT is effective in controlling lymphocele or lymphatic fistula with complete resolution of the drainage in a mean of 1 to 2 weeks.

● ● ● **REFERENCES** ● ● ●

Argenta LC, Morykwas MJ. Vacuum-assisted closure: a new method for wound control and treatment: clinical experience. *Ann Plast Surg.* 1997;38:563–577.

Attinger CE, Janis JE, Steinberg JS, Schwartz J, Al-Attar A, Couch K. Clinical approach to wounds: debridement and wound bed preparation including the use of dressings and wound-healing adjuvants. *Plast Reconstr Surg.* 2006;117:72S–109S.

Blume PA, Walters J, Payne W, Ayala J, Lantis J. Comparison of negative pressure wound therapy using vacuum assisted closure with advanced moist wound therapy in the treatment of diabetic foot ulcers: a multicenter randomized controlled trial. *Diabetes Care.* 2008;31(4):631–636.

Cothren CC, Moore EE, Johnson JL, Moore JB, Burch JM. One hundred percent fascial approximation with sequential abdominal closure of the open abdomen. *Am J Surg.* 2006;192:238–242.

Fitzpatrick TB. The validity and practicality of sun reactive skin types I–VI. *Arch Dermatol.* 1988;124:869–871.

Goldman R. Growth factors and chronic wound healing: past, present, and future. *Adv Skin Wound Care.* 2004;17:24–35.

Hamed O, Muck PE, Smith JM, Krallman K, Griffith NM. Use of vacuum-assisted closure (VAC) therapy in treating lymphatic complications after vascular procedures: new approach for lymphoceles. *J Vasc Surg*. 2008;48:1520–1523.

Liu W, Wang DR, Cao YL. TGF-beta: a fibrotic factor in wound scarring and a potential target for anti-scarring gene therapy. *Curr Gene Ther*. 2004;4:123–136.

Morkywas MJ, Argenta LC, Shelton-Brown EI, McGuirt W. Vacuum-assisted closure: a new method for wound control and treatment: animal studies and basic foundation. *Ann Plast Surg*. 1997;38:553–562.

Pandya AN, Vadodaria S, Coleman DJ. Tissue expansion in the limbs: a comparative analysis of limb and nonlimb sites. *Br J Plast Surg*. 2002;55:302–306.

Powers CJ, McLeskey SW, Wellstein A. Fibroblast growth factors, their receptors and signaling. *Endocr Relat Cancer*. 2000;7:165–197.

Ratner D. Skin grafting. *Semin Cutan Med Surg*. 2003;22:295–305.

Rumalla VK, Borah GL. Cytokines, growth factors, and plastic surgery. *Plast Reconstr Surg*. 2001;108:719–733.

Saxena V, Hwang CW, Huang S, Eichbaum Q, Ingber D, Orgill DP. Vacuum-assisted closure: microdeformations of wounds and cell proliferation. *Plast Reconstr Surg*. 2004;114:1086–1096.

Sood A, Granick MS, Tomaselli NL. Wound dressings and comparative effectiveness data. *Adv Wound Care*. 2014;3(8):511–529.

Zeng YJ, Xu CQ, Yang J, Sun GC, Xu XH. Biomechanical comparison between conventional and rapid expansion of skin. *Br J Plast Surg*. 2003;56:660–666.

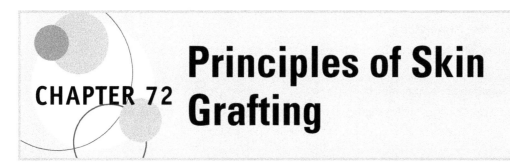

CHAPTER 72 Principles of Skin Grafting

Douglas M. Sammer, MD

○ **What are the two main types of skin graft?**

Split-thickness skin graft (STSG) and full-thickness skin graft (FTSG).

○ **Which parts of skin are included in skin grafts?**

The epidermis and part (STSG) or all (FTSG) of the dermis.

○ **What structures are included with the dermis in both split-thickness and full-thickness skin grafts?**

Adnexal structures including sebaceous glands, hair follicles, sweat glands, and capillaries.

○ **How thick is a "thin" STSG?**

0.005 to 0.012 in.

○ **How thick is an "intermediate" STSG?**

0.012 to 0.018 in.

○ **How thick is a "thick" STSG?**

0.018 to 0.028 in.

○ **What are the advantages of meshing a partial-thickness skin graft?**

Expansion of graft surface area up to six times, better contouring, decreased seroma or hematoma formation beneath the graft.

○ **How does the mesher ratio affect the graft surface area?**

A mesher expansion ratio of 1:1.5 (most commonly used) increases surface area by 50%, a ratio of 1:2 increases surface area by 100%, etc.

○ **What are the disadvantages of meshing?**

Waffled appearance, increased graft contraction (may be an advantage in some situations).

○ **Where should meshing be avoided?**

On the face, hand, or forearm (cosmetically sensitive areas), and over joints, where contracture becomes a problem.

○ **What is the postoperative bolster made of?**

Xeroform, cotton balls, or batting moistened in saline/mineral oil, secured with tie-over sutures or a stapled-on foam dressing.

○ **How long should the bolster stay on postoperatively?**

Five to seven days. Two to three days if the recipient site is contaminated.

○ **What are typical donor sites for STSGs?**

Anterior or lateral thigh in adults, buttock in children (for concealment of scar). The abdomen, back, chest, and scalp are often used if other donor sites are limited.

○ **What is an appropriate donor-site dressing?**

Xeroform gauze dried with a hair-dryer or heat lamp is the traditional dressing. An occlusive semipermeable dressing, such as Opsite or Tegaderm may be used.

○ **What is the advantage of Tegaderm or Opsite for the donor-site dressing?**

Faster healing and pain reduction.

○ **Do the dermis and epidermis regenerate in split-thickness donor sites?**

The donor site epidermis regenerates from the periphery and from adnexal structures, but the dermis does not regenerate. The donor site can be reharvested after it is well healed, if the underlying dermis is thick enough.

○ **How long does a split-thickness donor site take to heal?**

A thin STSG donor site will heal within 1 week, whereas thicker STSG donor sites will take 2 to 3 weeks to heal.

○ **What are the advantages of full-thickness skin grafts?**

Better color, thickness, and texture match with recipient site, decreased contraction.

○ **What are the disadvantages of FTSG?**

Donor site must be closed primarily, limited donor sites, more difficult take compared to split-thickness skin grafts.

○ **What are typical FTSG donor sites?**

Supraclavicular, preauricular, postauricular, volar forearm, and inguinal region.

○ **Why should an FTSG be defatted after harvesting?**

FTSG should be aggressively defatted to improve imbibition and take.

○ **What is a composite graft?**

A graft that includes fat, muscle, or cartilage in addition to skin.

○ **What is the maximum size of a composite graft?**

Variable, but composite grafts that contain cartilage will not take if greater than 1 to 1.5 cm in diameter.

○ **What is the difference between an isograft/autograft, an allograft/homograft, and a xenograft/heterograft?**

Autograft or isograft: from same person, or an identical twin.

Allograft or homograft: from same species.

Xenograft or heterograft: from different species.

○ **What is the purpose of allograft or xenograft?**

Used for temporary coverage of wounds until they are suitable for autografting. Cadaver allograft or more rarely porcine xenografts can be used. Cadaveric allografts do take initially, but are rejected after 10 days. Xenografts are more quickly rejected.

○ **What is the difference between the primary and secondary skin graft contraction?**

Primary contraction is the immediate shrinkage of a skin graft after harvesting, which is due to dermal elastin.

Secondary contraction is the contracture that occurs with healing, and is due to myofibroblast activity.

○ **Do split-thickness or full-thickness skin grafts contract more?**

Primary contraction is greater with thicker skin grafts, whereas secondary contraction is greater with thinner skin grafts.

○ **How does graft thickness affect the ability of the graft to sweat?**

Thicker grafts contain more dermis, and therefore more sweat glands, and will have a greater potential to sweat.

○ **How does graft thickness affect the ability of the graft to grow hair?**

More hair follicles are harvested with thicker grafts, and these will have greater hair growth.

○ **How does graft thickness affect the ability of the graft to develop sensation?**

Thicker grafts contain more neurilemmal sheaths, allowing greater ingrowth of nerve fibers, and greater potential for sensation over time. Thin grafts have less potential for sensation, but may develop sensation more quickly.

○ **What type of sensation develops first in a healing skin graft?**

Pain returns first, then light touch, then hot/cold sensation.

○ **What are the phases of skin graft take?**

Imbibition, inosculation, and revascularization.

○ **What is imbibition?**

The first phase of take, involving the uptake of nutrients from serum in the wound bed by capillary action, lasting 48 to 72 hours.

○   **What is inosculation?**

The second phase of take, involving donor and recipient capillary alignment.

○   **What is revascularization?**

The third phase of take, revascularization occurs through the aligned capillaries, complete at 7 days.

○   **How does revascularization occur?**

Controversial; new recipient site vessels may grow into the graft along the path of graft vessels, new ingrowth may occur randomly, recipient and donor vessels may anastomose, or a combination of the above.

○   **To what type of tissue will a skin graft not take?**

Exposed bone, cartilage, or tendon (unless there is overlying periosteum, perichondrium, or paratenon).

○   **What are the most common causes of failure of skin graft take?**

Hematoma or seroma, poorly debrided or poorly vascularized wound, shearing of the graft, and infection. The most common is hematoma or seroma beneath the graft.

○   **What level of bacterial load in the recipient site precludes skin graft take?**

Skin grafts will not take in wounds with bacterial loads of 10^5 per gram or greater.

○   **What are the two phases of graft adherence?**

The first phase is due to fibrin deposition between the graft and the wound bed, lasting 72 hours. The second phase involves ingrowth of vessels into the graft and production of fibrous tissue.

○   **Once a skin graft is well healed, how should it be taken care of?**

Hand-lotion or cream should be used to prevent desiccation. Skin grafts have decreased sweat and sebaceous glands.

Sweat glands do not function until innervated. Sebaceous gland function is also delayed, although innervation is not required for function.

● ● ● **REFERENCES** ● ● ●

Chang E. Grafts. In: Brown DL, Borschel GH, eds. *Michigan Manual of Plastic Surgery*. Philadelphia, PA: Lippincott Williams & Wilkins; 2004:16–21.

Place MJ, Herber SC, Hardesty RA. Basic techniques and principles in plastic surgery. In: Aston SJ, Beasley RW, Thorne CHM, eds. *Grabb and Smith's Plastic Surgery*. 5th ed. Philadelphia, PA: Lippincott-Raven; 1997:13–26.

Preuss S, Breuing KH, Eriksson E. Plastic surgery techniques. In: Achauer BM, Eriksson E, eds. *Plastic Surgery Indications, Operations, and Outcomes*. St Louis, MO: Mosby; 2000:147–162.

Vasconez HC. Skin grafts. In: Cohen M, ed. *Mastery of Plastic and Reconstructive Surgery*. Boston, MA: Little, Brown and Company; 1994:45–55.

Wolf SE, Herndon DN. Burns and radiation injuries. In: Mattox K, Feliciano D, Moore E, eds. *Trauma*. 4th ed. New York, NY: McGraw-Hill; 2000:1137–1152.

CHAPTER 73 Microsurgery and Flaps

Matthew M. Hanasono, MD

○ **What is a flap?**

Tissue that is either transferred or transplanted with intact circulation.

○ **How are muscle flaps classified by Mathes and Nahai?**

Type I: single vascular pedicle.

Type II: dominant vascular pedicle(s) and minor vascular pedicle(s).

Type III: two dominant pedicles.

Type IV: segmental vascular pedicles.

Type V: dominant vascular pedicle and secondary segmental vascular pedicles.

○ **What is the average tissue survival rate for a microvascular free flap?**

95% or better.

○ **What type of ultrasonography will most reliably image and locate vascular perforators preoperatively?**

Duplex ultrasonography.

○ **What is most likely to improve the survival of the distal portion of a random pattern cutaneous flap?**

Surgical delay prior to flap elevation.

○ **What is the reexploration rate for flap compromise?**

Approximately 10%.

○ **What is the salvage rate for microvascular free flaps that require reexploration for flap ischemia?**

50 to 85%.

○ **What is the maximum warm ischemia time tolerated by muscle flaps?**

Less than 3 hours.

○ **What is the maximum warm ischemia time tolerated by bone flaps?**

Less than 3 hours.

○ **What is the maximum warm ischemia time tolerated by skin and fasciocutaneous flaps?**

Approximately 4 to 6 hours.

○ **What is the warm ischemia time tolerated by jejunal flaps?**

Less than 2 hours.

○ **How can the maximum tolerated ischemia time be increased?**

Cooling of tissues: up to 12 hours of ischemia tolerated for fasciocutaneous tissues, 8 hours for muscle, and 24 hours for bone.

○ **Which results higher flap survival rates, end-to-end or end-to-side anastomoses?**

Most studies demonstrate similar patencies.

○ **Which type of arteriotomy, slit or circular/oval, is more successful?**

Most studies demonstrate similar patencies.

○ **Under what circumstances might an end-to-side anastomosis be advantageous?**

Vessel size discrepancy (larger donor vessel), only one artery or vein available and needed for distal organ/tissue perfusion, limited exposure/availability of similar size donor vessels.

○ **What anastomotic angles are thought to be the most desirable and result in the greatest amount of blood flow to the recipient vessel in an end-to-side anastomosis?**

Based on technical factors and blood flow rates, angles of 45 to 90 degrees result in greater arterial flow than obtuse angles up to 135 degrees.

○ **What methods relieve vasospasm?**

Topical anesthetics (e.g., lidocaine), topical papaverine, topical calcium channel blockers (e.g., verapamil), vessel dilation, adventitial stripping, and sympathetic nerve block (e.g., epidural anesthesia for lower extremity reconstruction).

○ **What is the reason for adventitial stripping?**

To relieve vasospasm and to prevent loose adventitia from being caught in the vessel lumen, a potential trigger for thrombosis.

○ **Which method of adventitial stripping is preferred, blunt or sharp?**

Sharp adventitial stripping is associated with less vessel trauma resulting less vasospasm and improved blood flow to the flap.

○ **What is papaverine?**

Papaverine is an opium alkaloid antispasmodic drug used in the treatment of visceral spasm, vasospasm, and formerly in the treatment of erectile dysfunction. In microvascular surgery, it is applied topically to relieve vasospasm. The mechanism of action is not entirely clear, but it is believed to involve inhibition of the enzyme phosphodiesterase leading to increased levels of cyclic AMP, ultimately leading to vascular smooth muscle relaxation.

○ **What are the characteristics of a viable flap?**

Warmth, pink/perfused color, softness, capillary refill, and detectable pulse (e.g., Doppler).

○ **What are signs of inadequate arterial flow?**

Pale, cool flap with slow (>2 seconds) capillary refill and decreased tissue turgor.

○ **What are signs of inadequate venous flow?**

Cyanotic or dusky flap with fast (<1 second) capillary refill and increased tissue turgor.

○ **What are the most reliable methods of free flap monitoring?**

Clinical observation, Doppler ultrasound flowmetry, pinprick or scratch testing, near-infrared spectroscopy, pulse oximetry, quantitative fluorometry, surface temperature probing.

○ **Besides cost, what is the main disadvantage of using an implantable Doppler probe for free flap monitoring?**

The risk of false positives (loss of Doppler signal when microvascular anastomosis is patent and free flap is viable) due to accidental detachment of the Doppler probe, loosening of the implantable Doppler cuff around the blood vessel, or equipment malfunction. In one study of 20 buried flaps, the implantable Doppler had 100% sensitivity and an 88% false-positive rate. However, other studies have suggested the false-positive rate for the implantable Doppler system is no higher than clinical monitoring.

○ **How is near-infrared spectroscopy used in free flap monitoring?**

In near-infrared spectroscopy monitoring, free flap tissues are exposed to near-infrared light. For each type of tissue, a portion of this light is absorbed and some is reflected back. The detector senses the reflected light and the device uses the ratio of oxyhemoglobin ($HgbO_2$) to deoxyhemoglobin (Hgb) to provide noninvasive real-time measurement of tissue oxygenation. Changes in tissue oxygenation suggest decreased blood flow to the flap and may be secondary to thrombosis of the vascular pedicle. There is some clinical evidence in the literature that a decrease in tissue oxygenation is detected prior to clinical signs that the flap is compromised and may facilitate early reoperation and higher flap salvage rates.

○ **How can buried flaps, such as those used for pharyngeal reconstruction, be monitored?**

A segment of the flap can be pedicled on separate perforating blood vessels and exteriorized. Alternately, an implantable Doppler can be placed on the vein or artery or both, distal to the anastomosis.

○ **How long before a pseudointima forms at the anastomotic site?**

Approximately 5 days.

○ **How long before a new intima forms at the anastomotic site?**

Approximately 1 to 2 weeks.

○ **What types of sutures are typically used for microvascular surgery?**

Nylon or polypropylene sutures ranging from 8-0 to 12-0.

○ **How is the microvascular suture selected?**

Thicker sutures with larger needles are indicated for larger vessels. Thinner sutures with finer needles are indicated for smaller vessels. In general, 9-0 sutures are used for vessels of 2 mm or more in diameter and 10-0 sutures are used for vessels of 1 to 2 mm.

○ **Describe the halving (or "0–180 degrees") technique of microvascular anastomosis.**

The halving technique is probably the most common method of suturing end-to-end anastomoses. The halving technique involves placing the first two sutures 180 degrees apart at 3 and 9 o'clock (or alternately at 6 and 12 o'clock) and adding the intervening sutures using the principle of halves (Fig. 73-1A). The advantage of this technique is that it makes it easy to visualize how to evenly space sutures, making it useful when there is a vessel size mismatch.

○ **Describe the triangulation technique of microvascular anastomosis.**

The triangulation technique, first described by Alexis Carrel, involves placing the first three sutures 120 degrees apart (Fig. 73-1B). This technique decreases the risk of inadvertent inclusion of the opposite wall of the vessel during subsequent sutures placement by retraction of the three initial stay sutures.

○ **Describe the "back wall up" technique of microvascular anastomosis.**

The back wall up technique involves placing the first suture in the middle of the back wall and progressively suturing forward from this point on either side (Fig. 73-1C). It is used for vessels that are especially delicate or that cannot be rotated very much due to short length, but is technically more challenging to take even bites of both vessels so as not to end up with a discrepancy on the front wall.

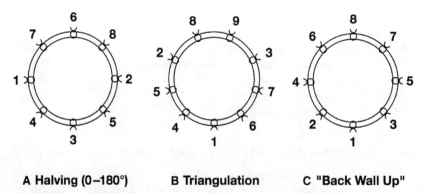

Figure 73-1 Halving (**A**), triangulation (**B**), and "back wall up" (**C**) suture placement techniques for microvascular anastomosis. Numbers indicated the order of suture placement.

○ **In an end-to-end anastomosis, what is the maximum size discrepancy between vessels that can be accommodated?**

Between 2:1 and 3:1.

O   **What are some strategies for performing an anastomosis between vessels with a size mismatch?**

Other than placing sutures farther apart on the larger vessel, strategies include beveling or spatulating the smaller vessel, partially closing or narrowing the larger vessel lumen with sutures, or using an interposition graft that is intermediate in diameter between the two vessels (Fig. 73-2). When the recipient vessel is larger, an end-to-side anastomosis into the recipient vessel can be performed.

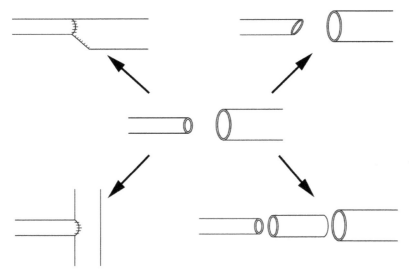

Figure 73-2 Strategies for dealing with a vessel size mismatch include narrowing the larger vessel with sutures, beveling the smaller vessel, using an interposition graft of intermediate diameter, and performing an end-to-side anastomosis when the recipient vessel is larger.

O   **What is "supermicrosurgery"?**

Supermicrosurgery is defined as the microsurgical anastomosis of vessels with a diameter of <0.8 mm.

O   **What are the indications for supermicrosurgery?**

Supermicrosurgical technique is used for lymphovenous bypass in the treatment of lymphedema as well as for free flap transfer based on perforator level microvascular anastomoses (perforator-to-perforator anastomoses).

O   **Under what circumstances can microvascular coupling anastomotic devices generally be used?**

Coupling devices are usually used for minimally discrepant, soft, pliable venous microvascular anastomoses.

O   **Which has superior patency rates, coupled or hand-sewn anastomoses?**

They are similar when used appropriately.

O   **Can coupling devices be used on arteries?**

Yes, but they generally do not work well on thick-walled or inelastic, atherosclerotic vessels.

O   **What is the maximum closing pressure of vascular clips that should be used to minimize damage to vessels?**

30 g/mm^2.

○   **What are some key points when performing an anastomosis for preventing exposure of subendothelium and thereby inducing platelet aggregation?**

Use small needles, avoid repeated needle punctures, equal placement of sutures, avoid tying sutures too loose or too tight, avoid use of too many sutures, which can cause endothelial slough.

○   **How does heparin prevent coagulation?**

Primarily by increasing the action of antithrombin-3, which inactivates thrombin. It also decreases platelet adhesion and inhibits the conversion of fibrinogen to fibrin.

○   **What risks are associated with heparin use?**

In addition to bleeding and hematoma formation, heparin can cause thrombocytopenia. Heparin-induced thrombocytopenia is thought to be caused by antibodies to the complex formed by heparin and platelet factor 4.

○   **How does aspirin function to prevent platelet aggregation?**

Aspirin blocks the endothelial cyclooxygenase pathway with subsequent blockage of thromboxane A2 preventing vasoconstriction and thrombus formation.

○   **Is high-dose aspirin more effective than low-dose aspirin to prevent platelet aggregation?**

No. At low doses, aspirin selectively inhibits thromboxane A2, a platelet aggregator and vasoconstrictor. At high doses, prostaglandin I2, a vasodilator and inhibitor of platelet aggregation are also inhibited. For example, aspirin in doses of 81 and 325 mg has been shown to be more effective in preventing cerebrovascular accidents, myocardial infarction, and death after carotid endarterectomy than doses of 650 and 1,300 mg.

○   **How does dextran work to prevent clotting?**

Dextran is a volume expander that prevents platelet adhesion by increasing the negative electric charge of platelets, erythrocytes, and endothelial cells, resulting in a destabilization of fibrin polymerization. Dextran is also an inactivator of von Willebrand factor, a major contributor to platelet aggregation and adhesion to vessel wall collagen.

○   **What are some possible complications associated with the use of low–molecular-weight dextran?**

Bleeding, pulmonary edema, and allergic reaction including anaphylaxis.

○   **What is the mechanism of the no-reflow phenomenon?**

Ischemia results in cellular swelling in the vascular endothelium with subsequent intravascular platelet aggregation and leakage of intravascular fluid into the interstitial space.

○   **What pharmacologic agents can be used to rescue some free flaps in which anastomotic revision fails to restore flap perfusion or is associated with recurrent thrombosis?**

Thrombolytic agents such as streptokinase, urokinase, tissue plasminogen activator.

○   **How do thrombolytic agents work?**

Thrombolytic agents, such as streptokinase, urokinase, and tissue plasminogen activator, function by directly or indirectly activating plasminogen to form plasmin, which cleaves fibrin in clots as well as fibrinogen and coagulation factors V, VIII, IX, XI, and XII.

○ **What are the risks associated with using streptokinase?**

In addition to bleeding and hematoma formation, streptokinase is antigenic and can result in an allergic response (6% incidence) with a 0.1% incidence of anaphylactic reaction. Streptokinase can also result in a "lytic state," causing diffuse bleeding when administered in high doses. Unlike streptokinase, urokinase and tissue plasminogen activator do not appear to be antigenic.

○ **What is the mechanism of thrombosis in microvascular anastomosis?**

Exposure of subendothelial collagen-containing surfaces to which platelets adhere eventually leading to fibrin deposition, vasospasm, stenosis, and thrombosis, causing loss of blood flow.

○ **What is Virchow's triad?**

Virchow's triad refers to risk factors for thrombosis and includes stasis, intimal injury, and hypercoagulability.

○ **Besides a technical error in the microvascular anastomosis, what are other causes of free flap vascular thrombosis?**

Causes of free flap thrombosis include: infection, pedicle compression, kinking, or twisting, thermal or traction injury during flap harvest or to the recipient blood vessel, hypercoagulable disorder, and, possibly, hypotension or vasospasm.

○ **Can a microvascular free flap be successful in a hypercoagulable patient?**

Yes, patients with inherited hypercoagulable disorders (thrombophilias) can successfully undergo microvascular free flap surgery, though probably with lower success rates and need for prophylactic anticoagulation. In one series of 58 patients with various thrombophilias, the free flap success rate was 80%.

○ **Why is bipolar electrocautery preferable to monopolar electrocautery in the control of bleeding from or around a recipient or donor blood vessel used in microvascular free tissue transfer?**

Bipolar cautery damages tissue, including endothelium and media, over a much more limited distance (approximately 1–2 mm) compared to unipolar cautery.

○ **Why is the number of sutures placed in an anastomosis critical?**

Too few sutures result in excessive bleeding and thrombus formation; too many result in increased damage to the endothelium and thrombus formation.

○ **Which anastomotic technique demonstrates greater success rates, interrupted suture placement or continuous sutures?**

In experienced hands, similar success rates are observed.

○ **What is the Acland (vessel strip) test?**

The Acland test is used to confirm antegrade vascular flow through the venous anastomosis. Two jeweler forceps are used to gently occlude the vessel distal to the venous anastomosis. Blood is milked out of the vessel between the forceps by gently sliding the distal forceps along the vessel without injuring in, resulting in a segment of collapsed vessel between the proximal and distal forceps. Releasing the proximal forceps should result in filling of the collapsed vessel segment if the anastomosis is patent.

○ **Does smoking tobacco increase free flap failure rate?**

In nondigital flaps, most retrospective studies demonstrate similar (nondigital) flap survival and thrombosis rates between smokers and nonsmokers, although smokers have a higher incidence of healing complications at the flap interface and at the donor site.

○ **What happens to vein grafts when they are used to bridge intra-arterial gaps?**

There is ingrowth of smooth muscle cells and creation of a neointima that results in significant thickening of the vein wall. Also, graft length decreases by 26% to 30% when used as an intra-arterial or intravenous graft.

○ **In addition to excellent vascular and neural anastomoses what other factor determines the success of functional free skeletal muscle transfer?**

Reestablishment of the correct resting tension since very small decreases in resting tension can markedly reduce the power and amplitude of muscle contraction.

○ **Name some commonly used donor sites for free osseous and osseocutaneous flaps.**

Rib, fibula, iliac crest, second metatarsal, radius, calvarium, scapula.

○ **In what ways are vascularized bone transfers superior to nonvascularized bone grafts?**

Vascularized bone grafts demonstrate earlier incorporation, bone hypertrophy, mechanical strength to failure, osseous mass retention, and resistance to local infection.

○ **What techniques can be used to prolong ischemia time in limb replantation?**

Cooling and AV shunting.

○ **What are the major contraindications to replantation?**

Concomitant life-threatening injury, multiple segmental injuries to the amputated part, severe crushing or avulsion of the tissues, extreme contamination, inhibiting systemic illness (small vessel disease, diabetes mellitus, etc.), prior surgery or trauma to the amputated part precluding replantation.

○ **How do leeches function to relieve venous congestion?**

By secreting hirudin, a selective thrombin inhibitor that is injected into the hosts tissue as they feed on host blood.

○ **What pathogenic bacterium do leeches commonly transmit?**

Aeromonas hydrophila.

○ **What antibiotics should be used in the prophylaxis or treatment of bacterial infections associated with the use of leeches?**

Ciprofloxacin, tetracycline, trimethoprim-sulfamethoxazole, or second- and third-generation cephalosporins.

○ **Does the order of anastomosis and microvascular clamp removal affect the survival of free flaps?**

There are no significant differences in flap survival based on the order of anastomosis or microvascular clamp removal seen in an animal model, although early, transient venous congestion does develop if the artery is anastomosed first and the clamp on the artery is removed prior to venous anastomosis and clamp removal.

○ **Can loupe magnification be safely used for microvascular anastomoses?**

High-power loupes have been used for anastomosing vessels greater than 1 mm in diameter with success rates comparable to those achieved using a microscope.

○ **Can microvascular surgery be successfully performed in children?**

Yes. A success rate of 93% has been observed in children younger than 15 years, despite smaller blood vessel size.

○ **Can microvascular surgery be successfully performed in the elderly?**

Yes. Age has not been found to be an independent predictor of flap loss in several studies. However, older age is frequently associated with medical comorbidities, including cardiac and peripheral vascular disease, as well as development of other complications related to long surgeries.

○ **What is the role of computed tomography angiography (CTA) in free flap surgery?**

CTA can be used to visualize fasciocutaneous and myocutaneous perforators, which can be helpful in flap design, minimizing the incision length and allowing the surgeon to more precisely center the flap skin paddle to ensure adequate perfusion. CTA may also be useful in selecting a specific perforator to supply blood to the flap skin paddle, allowing the surgeon to ligate other perforators and pedicle side branches knowing that the flap will remain well perfused. CTA has been most commonly used for deep inferior epigastric perforator flaps, but has also been described in anterolateral thigh and fibula free flaps.

● ● ● **FLAPS** ● ● ●

○ **What is the vascular supply and classification of the sartorius muscle?**

Superficial femoral artery and vein, type IV—segmental.

○ **What is the vascular supply of the gastrocnemius muscle?**

Sural vessels.

○ **The lateral arm flap is supplied by what artery?**

Posterior radial collateral artery.

○ **The arterial pedicle to the radial forearm flap arises between what two muscles?**

Brachioradialis and flexor carpi radialis.

○ **What are the indications of leech therapy?**

Venous congestion.

○ **What method of flap monitoring is most reliable?**

Clinical observation.

○ **What flap receives its motor innervation from the obturator nerve?**

Gracilis.

○ **What is the dominant vascular supply of the gracilis flap?**
Ascending branch of the medial circumflex artery.

○ **The rectus femoris receives its blood supply from what source?**
Lateral circumflex femoral artery.

○ **What organism is associated with medicinal leeches?**
Aeromonas hydrophila (Gram-negative rod).

○ **What artery provides the primary blood supply to a groin flap?**
Superficial circumflex iliac artery.

○ **The gluteal thigh flap is supplied by what vessel?**
Inferior gluteal artery.

○ **The periosteal perforators of the peroneal artery will be found bordering what aspect of the fibula.**
Posteromedial.

○ **The parascapular flap is based on what vessel?**
Circumflex scapular artery.

○ **Which nerve provides sensation to the lateral arm flap?**
Posterior brachial cutaneous nerve (C5–6).

○ **The venous outflow of the reverse radial forearm flap depends on what vessel?**
Radial venae comitantes.

○ **The fibula flap is based on what vessel?**
Peroneal vessels.

○ **The fibula and radial forearm osteocutaneous flap can provide up to what length of bone?**
25 and 10 cm, respectively.

○ **What is the dominant vascular supply to the vastus lateralis muscle?**
Descending branch of the lateral femoral circumflex artery.

○ **Which muscles comprise the borders of the triangular space?**
Triceps (lateral), teres major (inferior border), and teres minor (superior).

○ **What vessel traverses the triangular space?**
Circumflex scapular artery.

○ **The gracilis muscle is immediately posterior to what muscle?**
Adductor longus muscle.

○ **Name the three subtypes of fasciocutaneous flaps according to Cormack–Lamberty.**
Type A: Multiple perforators
Type B: Solitary perforator
Type C: Segmental perforator

○ **Name the three subtypes of fasciocutaneous flaps according to Nahai–Mathes.**
Type A: Direct cutaneous perforator
Type B: Septocutaneous perforator
Type C: Musculocutaneous perforator

○ **Describe the arc of rotation of a flap.**
The range of reach of the flap when transposed at its point of rotation (usually the vascular pedicle).

○ **What is the vascular supply of the temporoparietal fascia flap?**
Superficial temporal artery and vein.

○ **The saphenous artery originates from what artery?**
Genicular.

○ **What is the secondary vascular supply of the gracilis flap?**
Superficial femoral artery and vein.

○ **The paramedian forehead flap is based on what vessel?**
Supratrochlear.

○ **What is the source of free radicals in the ischemic flap?**
Xanthine oxidase.

○ **What is the blood supply of the deltopectoral flap?**
First, second, and third perforating branches of the internal mammary artery.

○ **The posterior thigh flap involves transfer of what three muscles?**
Biceps femoris, semimembranosus, and semitendinosus muscles.

○ **What are the main functions of the gluteus maximus muscle?**
Extension of the hip joint and adductor of the thigh.

○ **The deep inferior epigastric artery arises from what artery?**
External iliac.

○ **What is the dominant pedicle to the latissimus dorsi muscle?**
Thoracodorsal.

○ **Where does the gluteus maximus muscle insert?**
Greater trochanter of the femur.

○ **What is the blood supply to the trapezius flap?**
Transverse cervical artery.

○ **What is an angiosome?**
Composite area of tissue supplied by the same source artery.

○ **Which gastrocnemius muscle has a longer reach?**
Medial head.

○ **What is the blood supply to the soleus muscle?**
Popliteal.

○ **The radial forearm neurosensory flap is innervated by what nerve(s)?**
Lateral and medial antebrachial cutaneous nerves.

○ **The great toe flap and second toe flap are based on what vessel?**
First dorsal metacarpal artery and venae comitantes.

○ **What is the blood supply of the external oblique?**
Lateral cutaneous branches of the inferior eight posterior intercostal arteries.

○ **What are the muscles that define the boundaries of the quadrangular (quadrilateral) space?**
Long head of the triceps (medial), teres major (inferior), and teres minor (inferior), humerus (lateral).

○ **What structures traverse the quadrangular (quadrilateral) space?**
Posterior circumflex humeral vessels and axillary nerve.

○ **Which is more lateral, the quadrangular space or the triangular space?**
The quadrangular space is more lateral (makes sense since the humerus is one of its borders).

○ **What are the two dominant pedicles of the omental flap?**
The right and left gastroepiploic artery and vein.

○ **Can the anterolateral thigh flap be neurotized?**
Yes, from the lateral femoral cutaneous nerve.

○ **What is the origin and insertion of the gracilis muscle?**

The pubic symphysis and the medial tibial condyle.

○ **The forehead flap is based on what vessel?**

Superficial temporal artery and vein.

○ **The random pattern flap is based on what blood supply?**

Subdermal plexus.

○ **What is the appropriate length-to-width design ratio of a random pattern flap?**

2 to 1.5.

○ **What is the blood supply of the nasolabial flap?**

Angular artery (from facial artery).

○ **What is the dominant vascular pedicle to the pectoralis major flap?**

Pectoral branch of the thoracoacromial artery and venae comitantes.

○ **What is the origin of the pectoralis major muscle?**

The medial half of the clavicle, the anterior surface of the sternum, the cartilaginous portions of the upper seven ribs, and the aponeurosis of the external oblique muscle.

○ **The vascular pedicle to the anterolateral thigh flap traverses what muscles?**

Vastus lateralis and rectus femoris muscles.

○ **What is the function of the rectus femoris muscle?**

Hip flexion and knee extension.

○ **What is the blood supply of the abductor digiti minimi flap?**

Deep palmar artery (from ulnar artery) and venae comitantes.

○ **The reverse sural flap depends on what blood supply?**

The median superficial sural artery.

○ **What is the origin of the tensor fascia lata flap?**

Anterior 5 cm of the outer portion of the iliac crest and ASIS.

○ **What is the blood supply of the tensor fascia lata flap?**

Ascending branch of the lateral circumflex femoral artery.

○ **What is the course of the radial collateral artery to the lateral arm flap?**

Courses through the lateral intermuscular septum between the brachialis and lateral head of the triceps muscle.

○ **What is the innervation of the trapezius muscle?**

Spinal accessory nerve (XI).

● ● ● **REFERENCES** ● ● ●

Acland RD. Microvascular anastomosis: a device for holding stay sutures and a new vascular clamp. *Surgery.* 1974;75:185–187.

Ahn CY, Shaw WW, Berns S, Markowitz BL. Clinical experience with the 3M microvascular coupling anastomotic device in 100 free-tissue transfers. *Plast Reconstr Surg.* 1994;93:1481–1484.

Braga A, Lineaweaver WC, Whitney TM, Follansbee S, Buncke HJ. Sensitivities of *Aeromonas hydrophila* cultured from medicinal leeches to oral antibiotics. *J Reconstr Microsurg.* 1990;6:135–137.

Bui DT, Cordeiro PG, Hu QY, Disa JJ, Pusic A, Mehrara BJ. Free flap reexploration: indications, treatment, and outcomes in 1193 free flaps. *Plast Reconstr Surg.* 2007;119:2092–2100.

Burget GC, Menick FJ. *Aesthetic Reconstruction of the Nose.* St Louis, MO: Mosby; 1994.

Chang LD, Buncke G, Slezak S, Buncke HJ. Cigarette smoking, plastic surgery, and microsurgery. *J Reconstr Microsurg.* 1996;12:467–474.

Corbitt C, Skoracki RJ, Yu P, Hanasono MM. Free flap failure in head and neck reconstruction. *Head Neck.* 2014;36:1440–1445.

Cordeiro PG, Santamaria E. Experience with the continuous suture microvascular anastomosis in 200 consecutive free flaps. *Ann Plast Surg.* 1998;40:1–6.

Cormack GC, Lamberty BG. A classification of fascio-cutaneous flaps according to their patterns of vascularization. *Br J Plast Surg.* 1984;37:80–87.

Devaraj VS, Kay SP, Batchelor AG, Yates A. Microvascular surgery in children. *Br J Plast Surg.* 1991;44:276–280.

Disa JJ, Polvora VP, Pusic AL, Singh B, Cordeiro PG. Dextran-related complications in head and neck microsurgery: do the benefits outweigh the risks? A prospective randomized analysis. *Plast Reconstr Surg.* 2003;112:1534–1539.

Frey M, Gruber H, Freilinger G. The importance of the correct resting tension in muscle transplantation: experimental and clinical aspects. *Plast Reconstr Surg.* 1983;71:510–518.

Godina M. Preferential use of end-to-side arterial anastomoses in free flap transfers. *Plast Reconstr Surg.* 1979;64:673–682.

Goldberg JA, Pederson WC, Barwick WJ. Salvage of free tissue transfers using thrombolytic agents. *J Reconstr Microsurg.* 1989;5:351–356.

Hanasono MM, Butler CE. Prevention and treatment of thrombosis in microvascular surgery. *J Reconstr Microsurg.* 2008;24:305–314.

Hong JP, Koshima I. Using perforators as recipient vessels (supermicrosugery) for free flap reconstruction of the knee region. *Ann Plast Surg.* 2010;64:291–293.

Hood JM, Lubahn JD. Bipolar coagulation at different energy levels: effect on patency. *Microsurgery.* 1994;15:594–597.

Johnson PC, Barker JH. Thrombosis and antithrombotic therapy in microvascular surgery. *Clin Plast Surg.* 1992;19:799–807.

Jones NF, Jarrahy R, Song JI, Kaufman MR, Markowitz B. Postoperative medical complications—not microsurgical complications—negatively influence the morbidity, mortality, and true costs after microsurgical reconstruction for head and neck cancer. *Plast Reconstr Surg.* 2007;119:2053–2060.

Jones NF. Intraoperative and postoperative monitoring of microsurgical free tissue transfers. *Clin Plast Surg.* 1992;19:783–797.

Khouri RK, Shaw WW. Monitoring of free flaps with surface-temperature recordings: is it reliable? *Plast Reconstr Surg.* 1992;89:495–499.

Lin SJ, Nguyen MD, Chen C, et al. Tissue oximetry monitoring in microsurgical breast reconstruction decreases flap loss and improves rate of flap salvage. *Plast Reconstr Surg.* 2011;127:1080–1085.

Lineaweaver WC, Buncke HI. Complications of free flap transfers. *Hand Clin.* 1986;2:347–351.

Lohman R, Siemionow M, Lister G. Advantages of sharp adventitial dissection for microvascular anastomoses. *Ann Plast Surg.* 1998;40:577–585.

Mathes SJ, Nahai F. Classification of the vascular anatomy of muscles: experimental and clinical correlation. *Plast Reconstr Surg.* 1981;67:177–187.

Mathes SJ, Nahai F. *Clinical Atlas of Muscle and Musculocutaneous Flaps.* St Louis, MO: CV Mosby Company; 1979.

Mathes SJ, Nahai F. *Reconstructive Surgery: Principles, Anatomy & Technique.* Quality Medical Publishing; 1997.

Mitchell GM, Zeeman R, Rodegers IW, Pribaz JJ, O'Brien BM. The long-term-fate of microvenous autografts. *Plast Reconstr Surg.* 1988:82:473–479.

Nguyen MQ, Crosby MA, Skoracki RJ, Hanasono MM. Outcomes of flap salvage with medicinal leech therapy. *Microsurgery.* 2012;32:351–357.

Nunley A, Koman LA, Urbaniak JR. Arterial shunting as an adjunct to major limb revascularization. *Ann Surg.* 1981;193:271–273.

Reus WF 3rd, Colen LB, Straker DJ. Tobacco smoking and complications in elective microsurgery. *Plast Reconstr Surg.* 1992;89: 490–494.

Rhee RY, Donayre CE, Ouriel K, Neschis DG, Shortell CK. Low dose heparin therapy: in vitro verification of antithromonbotic effect. *J Vasc Surg.* 1991;14:628–634.

Rosenberg JJ, Fornage BD, Chevray PM. Monitoring buried free flaps: limitations of the implantable Doppler and use of color duplex sonography as a confirmatory test. *Plast Reconstr Surg.* 2006;118:109–113.

Rosenberg RD. Actions and interaction of antithrombin and heparin. *N Engl J Med.* 1975;292:146–151.

Rozen WM, Chubb D, Whitaker IS, Acosta R. The efficacy of postoperative monitoring: a single surgeon comparison of clinical monitoring and the implantable Doppler probe in 547 consecutive free flaps. *Microsurgery.* 2010;30:105–110.

Serletti JM, Higgins JP, Moran S, Orlando GS. Factors affecting outcome in free-tissue transfer in the elderly. *Plast Reconstr Surg.* 2000;106:66–70.

Seuter F. Inhibition of platelet aggregation by acetylsalicylic acid and other inhibitors. *Haemostasis.* 1976;5:85–95.

Shenaq SM, Klebuc MJ, Vargo D. Free-tissue transfer with the aid of loupe magnification: experience with 251 procedures. *Plast Reconstr Surg.* 1995;95:261–269.

Spector JA, Draper LB, Levine JP, Ahn CY. Routine use of microvascular coupling device for arterial anastomosis in breast reconstruction. *Ann Plast Surg.* 2006;56(4):365–368.

Taylor GI, Palmer JH. The vascular territories (angiosomes) of the body: experimental study and clinical applications. *Br J Plast Surg.* 1987;40:113–141.

Tolhurst DE, Haeseker B, Zeeman RJ. The development of the fasciocutaneous flap and its clinical applications. *Plast Reconstr Surg.* 1983;71:597–606.

Wang TY, Serletti JM, Cuker A, et al. Free tissue transfer in the hypercoagulable patient: a review of 58 flaps. *Plast Reconstr Surg.* 2012;129:443–453.

Weiland AJ, Phillips TW, Randolph MA. Bone grafts: a radiologic, histologic, and biomechanical model comparing autografts, allografts, and free vascularized bone grafts. *Plast Reconstr Surg.* 1984;74:368–379.

Weinstein PR, Mehdorn HM, Szabo Z. Microsurgical anastomosis: vessel injury, regeneration, and repair. In: Serafin D, Buncke HJ Jr, eds. *Microsurgical Composite Tissue Transplantation.* St Louis, MO: CV Mosby; 1979:111–144.

Wieslander JB. Endothelialization following end-to-end and end-in-end (sleeve) microarterial anastomoses. A scanning electron microscopic study. *Scand J Plastic Reconstr Surg.* 1984;18:193–199.

Wilson CS, Albert BS, Buncke HJ, Gordon L. Replantation of the upper extremity. *Clin Plast Surg.* 1983;10:85–101.

Zhang F, Pang Y, Buntic R, et al. Effect of sequence, timing of vascular anastomosis, and clamp removal on survival of microsurgical flaps. *J Reconstr Microsurg.* 2002;18:697–702.

Zhang L, Moskovitz M, Piscatelli S, Longaker MT, Siebert JW. Hemodynamic study of different angled end-to-side anastomoses. *Microsurgery.* 1995;16:114–117.

CHAPTER 74 Perforator Flaps

Ming-Huei Cheng, MD, MBA, FACS and Jung-Ju Huang, MD

○ **What is the arterial source of a perforator flap?**

Either septocutaneous branch or musculocutaneous branch passing through muscle to nourish the fasciocutaneous flap from its mother vessel.

○ **What is an angiosome?**

The angiosomes of the body are distinct vascular territories that are composed of muscle and the overlying skin and the adipose tissues. The angiosomes define the anatomical borders from which tissues are available for composite transfer.

○ **How are the cutaneous vessels defined according to their course?**

They are defined as septocutaneous and myocutaneous vessels. Septocutaneous vessels course either between the tendons or muscles following the intermuscular septa. Myocutaneous perforators penetrate through the muscle to nourish the subcutaneous tissue.

○ **What is the anatomical basis for perforator-based skin flap design and harvest?**

The size, length, direction, and connections of the cutaneous perforators provide basis of flap design. At least one adjacent anatomical cutaneous vascular territory can be captured with safety when based on a particular perforator.

○ **What is the contribution of Taylor and Daniel to the evolution of the perforator flap surgery?**

These authors were the first who attempted to harvest skin flaps on the septocutaneous and myocutaneous perforators that they had identified during their vascular anatomy studies on cadavers. They mapped the vascular anatomy of the skin and identified an average of 374 dominant cutaneous vessels of 0.5 mm or greater in diameter, and introduced the angiosome concept for further perforator flap surgery.

○ **What is a true perforator flap?**

A "true" perforator flap relies on perforator vessels from a given source vessel that must first penetrate a muscle before piercing the deep fascia to reach the skin.

○ **What are the advantages of the perforator flaps?**

1. Less donor site morbidity.

2. Muscle sparing and allows thin flap harvesting.

3. Versatility in design to include as little or as much tissue as required.

4. Improved postoperative recovery of the patient.

5. Increased versatility in flap design and more economic flap application, including chimeric flap design or harvesting more than one flap basing on the same mother vessel.

○ **What is the definition of a reliable perforator vessel?**

The reliable perforator is defined as a perforator that sprouts from the carrier muscle with a "visible" pulsation, usually greater than 1 mm in diameter. A reliable perforator is believed to have the ability to expand its perfusion over its territory after the perforator flap elevation.

○ **How are the perforator vessels identified?**

Currently, the most practical, simple, safe, speedy, and inexpensive method is the use of handheld Doppler ultrasound probe. Other techniques include computed tomographic angiography, magnetic resonance imaging angiography, and color-flow duplex scanning.

○ **How are the axial artery and perforators discriminated with the Doppler probe?**

The axial artery has a unidirectional pulsating course whereas there is no evident pulsating sound around the perforator.

○ **What are the available preoperative tools to identify the exact location of the perforators?**

The available and reliable image studies include multidetector-row helicon computed tomography angiography and magnetic resonance imaging.

○ **What is the most common consequence when a tiny perforator is selected?**

Marginal flap necrosis beyond the territory of the perforators.

○ **What are the requirements for an acceptable perforator flap donor site?**

1. Predictable and consistent blood supply;

2. At least one large perforator with the diameter greater than 1 mm;

3. Sufficient pedicle length;

4. Primary closure of the donor site with the absence of excessive wound tension.

5. Provision of similar soft-tissue volume that matches the recipient defect

6. Donor site with well-hidden scar is more favorable

○ **What are the most commonly used perforator flaps?**

Anterolateral thigh perforator flap, deep inferior epigastric perforator (DIEP) flap, super gluteal artery perforator flap, inferior gluteal artery perforator flap, thoracodorsal perforator flap, tensor fascia lata perforator flap, medial plantar perforator flap, deep circumflex iliac perforator flap, superficial circumflex iliac artery perforator flap, medial sural artery perforator flap, transverse gracilis perforator flap, internal mammary artery perforator flap, profunda artery perforator flap, anterior obturator artery perforator flap, lumbar artery perforator flap, intercostal artery perforator flap, and submental artery perforator flap.

○ **What is a free-style free flap?**

An anatomic region that is not the traditional flap territory with the appropriate size, color, and pliability is selected, and the skin perforators in that region are mapped using a Doppler probe. Mapped perforators are dissected toward source vessels to provide adequate vessel length and size. By applying the concept of free-style free flap, small- or moderate-sized flap can be designed and harvested from almost any part of the body as long as the donor site appearance is acceptable to the patient.

○ **What is the main advantage of a free-style free flap?**

The advantage of this concept is that it provides the surgeon an extra sense of freedom and variability when approaching a flap harvest and choosing the recipient site. Once perforators can be identified, any area of the body can serve as donor site for flap harvesting. There is no limitation on the flap selection and more flaps can be harvested for reconstruction, even in areas that had been used as flap donor site before.

○ **What are the most common causes of the perforator thrombosis?**

Stretching, twisting, drying, compression of the perforator and technical error.

○ **What are the strategies to reexplore a thrombosed perforator flap?**

1. Explore early.
2. Resect the thrombosed vessel segment and reanastomose with or without vein graft. Vessels with damaged intima should be resected as much as possible.
3. Open the vessels and squeeze the proximal vessel to evacuate the thrombus. Thrombus can also be suctioned out gently with smooth needle and manually applied suction force with syringe.
4. Do not inject any solution from the cut end since this maneuver may cause migration and plugging of thrombus into the smaller perforators.
5. Relieve the tension from the flap.
6. Inject few thrombolytic agents, such as urokinase, streptokinase from the donor artery and drain it out from the donor vein in an attempt of thrombolysis.
7. Systemic infusion of low-dose heparin 2,500 to –5,000 units/day.
8. If the flap remained unperfused, the whole pedicle should be checked under microscope.
9. Inappropriate flap inset can cause twist of the pedicle and subsequent thrombus formation. All the stitches can be released to make sure the flap is inset in appropriate manner.

○ **What are the principles in "thinning" of a perforator flap?**

1. Preserve the fat and the fascia within a circle of 1 cm diameter around the perforator;
2. Use loupes or microscope to perform the procedure;
3. Perform thinning when there is circulation in the flap, either before division of pedicle or after restoration of blood circulation.

○ **What is "supermicrosurgery" as a technique?**

Supermicrosurgery technique involves division of the perforator flap pedicle above the deep fascia and anastomosing small vessels that are less than 1 mm (0.5–0.7 mm) using 12-0 nylon with a greater magnification microscope. It allows free transfer of flaps on vessels harvested without breaching deep fascia, the so-called "perforator-to-perforator" free flap transfer. The technique of supermicrosurgery has also been expanded in lymphatic surgeries, such as lymphatico-lymphatical anastomosis or lymphaticovenous anastomosis with various anastomosis techniques for lymphedema treatment.

○ **What are the advantages in applying supermicrosurgery technique in perforator flap surgery?**

The donor site morbidity is reduced since the fascia remains intact and the muscle is not dissected. Flap harvest can be performed quickly without intramuscular dissection. Besides, only a short vascular pedicle is taken without sacrificing perfusion to the surrounding tissues.

○ **What are disadvantages to apply supermicrosurgery technique in perforator flap surgery?**

The primary disadvantage is the short and small pedicle rendering the inset and the difficulty of performing anastomosis on tiny diameter vessels on a short pedicle.

○ **What is the "supermicrosurgery" impact on management of extremity lymphedema?**

Multiple lymphaticovenular anastomoses on a single limb were reported to improve the lymphedema significantly. It also serves as prophylactic procedures in patients receiving lymph node dissection with the potential risk of developing lymphedema in the future.

○ **List the perforator flaps and their accompanying nerves that can be harvested as a sensate flap.**

Thoracodorsal perforator flap—lateral branch of the intercostal nerve

Medial plantar artery perforator flap—medial plantar nerve

Anterolateral thigh flap—lateral femoral musculocutaneous nerve

Deep inferior epigastric perforator flap—sensory branch of the intercostal nerve

Superior gluteal artery perforator flap (SGAP)—super and middle gluteal nerve

○ **What is a pedicled perforator flap?**

By applying the concept of perforator flap into regional reconstruction, a perforator flap close to the defect is dissected and transferred by meticulous intramuscular dissection of the perforator without division and reanastomosis of the vascular pedicle. One of the recently highly applied areas was the perineal reconstruction using perforator flaps from the medial and posterior thigh, such as the, gracilis perforator flap (medial circumflex femoral artery perforator flap), profunda artery perforator flap, anterior obturator perforator flap, gluteal artery perforator flap and more distant pedicle perforator flap, such as pedicle ALT flap and pedicle DIEP flap.

○ **What are the advantages of pedicled perforator flap?**

The microsurgical anastomosis is eliminated and the potential risk of flap loss diminished. A perforator flap is designed close to the defect and can be based on traditional flap design, like rotation, transposition, advancement and interposition/island flaps and transposed to the recipient site based on the perforator. Many of the traditional used reconstruction method can be modified to a more reliable and more versatile manner, such as converting the gracilis myocutaneous flap to gracilis perforator flap to vulvar reconstruction. Traditional flaps can be designed with improvement of providing an axial and reliable blood supply. Owing to the preservation of the perforator, the traditional pedicle flap length-to-width rule is no longer needed.

○ **List examples of pedicled perforator flap in head and neck reconstruction.**

1. Submental artery perforator flap
2. Facial artery musculomucosal flap
3. Temporoparietal artery perforator flap
4. Internal mammary artery perforator flap

○ **Who described the anterolateral thigh flap?**

Song et al. described it as a septocutaneous perforator flap in 1984.

○ **What is the source artery of the ALT perforator flap?**

Septocutaneous or musculocutaneous perforators derived from the descending, oblique or transverse branch of lateral circumflex femoral system.

○ **What is the landmark for the perforators in the anterolateral thigh region?**

A line is drawn from anterior superior iliac spine to the lateral border of the patella and the perforators are usually located in a circle 3 cm around the midpoint of this line.

○ **What is the ratio of septocutaneous versus myocutaneous perforators in the anterolateral thigh perforator flap?**

In different reported series, only 12% to 33% of the patients were reported to have septocutaneous vessels while 67% to 88% had myocutaneous perforators only.

○ **What can be the maximum dimension of an anterolateral thigh perforator flap?**

8 × 20 cm.

○ **What are the advantages of thinning anterolateral thigh perforator flaps?**

1. Uniformly thin and pliable flaps become available especially for reconstruction of oral cavity, neck, hand and fingers, axilla, forearm, and anterior tibial area, when the flap is thicker than required.
2. Avoids secondary defatting or liposuction procedure.
3. Improved sensory recovery.
4. Early range-of-motion training when used in hands and fingers and better and quicker postoperative functional recovery in buccal and tongue reconstruction.

○ **What is the upper width limit of the anterolateral thigh flap that can be usually closed primarily?**

Although the laxity is important for this issue, generally up to 8 cm defect can be closed primarily.

○ **What are the variations in the anatomy of the anterolateral thigh flap?**

Variations occur in 2% of the cases.

1. Absence of any perforator to the skin.
2. Small perforator.
3. Perforator pedicle that contains an artery but no vein.
4. Artery not going with the vein side by side.

○ **What is the technical management when anatomical variations are encountered during elevation of anterolateral thigh flap?**

1. Try to dissect a perforator from the transverse branch in the upper thigh or use the tensor fascia lata perforator flap.
2. Use an anteromedial thigh flap or flaps from the medial thigh, such as profunda artery perforator flap or gracilis perforator flap.
3. Convert to ALT myocutaneous flap if the skin flap is not totally detached from the vastus lateralis (VL) muscle.
4. Shift to the opposite thigh or other donor sites with similar flap character, such as TAP flap or V-RAM or DIEP flap.

○ **What are the main application areas of the anterolateral thigh flap?**

Head and neck reconstruction, esophagus reconstruction, chest empyema with bronchocutaneous fistula, abdominal wall reconstruction, pelvic reconstruction, upper and lower extremity reconstruction.

○ **How is the decision made if an anterolateral thigh perforator flap should be used pedicled or as a free flap in abdominal wall reconstruction?**

This depends on the location of the defect and length of the pedicle. The flap is raised first without division of the pedicle. If simple transposition is enough, microvascular anastomosis can be saved. If not, the recipient vessels should be explored. The most sizable recipient vessels could be the deep inferior epigastric artery and vein.

○ **What are the advantages of using an ALT flap for head and neck reconstruction?**

1. Long pedicle (12.01 ± 1.05 cm) with sufficient diameter (2.0–2.5 mm)
2. Pliable and wide flap territory
3. Allows for two-team approach during tumor ablation surgery
4. Feasibility to design as either a single skin paddle for one-layer defect reconstruction or double-skin paddle for through-and-through defects
5. Moderate/changeable flap thickness with traditional ALT flap harvesting, thinning procedure, and the incorporation of the VL muscle as myocutaneous flap.
6. Possibility for thinning.
7. Possibility to harvest as a chimeric flap or composite flap along with the neighboring tissues, including the vastus lateralis muscle, fascia of the tensor fascia lata, and iliac crest for bony reconstruction.
8. Potentially sensate by including the lateral femoral cutaneous nerve.
9. Inconspicuous scar over the donor site.

○ **What are the contraindications of the anterolateral thigh flap?**

The absolute contraindications are severe atherosclerosis, previous injury, and injury in the thigh region. Obesity is the relative contraindication.

○ **Describe the thigh flaps according to their source artery.**

1. ALT flap—descending branch of the lateral femoral circumflex artery (LCFA)
2. Medial thigh flap—a branch from the LCFA or descending branch of LCFA
3. Proximal two-thirds of lateral thigh skin—transverse branch of the LCFA
4. Skin at the medial thigh—medial femoral circumflex artery and profunda (deep) femoral artery
5. Skin at posterolateral thigh—third or fourth perforator from the deep femoral artery
6. Inferior gluteal thigh flap—inferior gluteal artery
7. Posterior popliteal thigh flap—a branch of the popliteal artery

○ **Compare the tensor fascia lata perforator flap and anterolateral thigh flap.**

The most remarkable difference is the anatomy of the vessels. The descending branch of the LCFA that supplies the anterolateral thigh flap runs longitudinally in the intermuscular septum between the rectus femoris and vastus lateralis muscle, whereas the transverse or ascending branch of the TFL flap runs laterally. Tensor fascia lata flap has a shorter pedicle, and the subcutaneous tissue is thicker.

○ **Which perforator flaps are available for breast reconstruction?**

Deep inferior epigastric perforator (DIEP) flap, thoracodorsal artery perforator (TAP) flap, superior and inferior gluteal artery perforator flap, profunda artery perforator flap (PAP), anterolateral thigh flap (ALT).

○ **What is the blood supply of the DIEP flap?**

Perforating vessels originating from the deep inferior epigastric artery.

○ **What are the advantages of DIEP flap over TRAM flap?**

The rectus abdominis muscle with fascia is preserved in DIEP flap, which results in less donor site morbidity and shorter recovery period.

○ **What are the contraindications for the DIEP flap?**

Midline abdominal scar, previous liposuction, inadequate subcutaneous tissue, and obesity.

○ **What are the most significant risk factors of fat necrosis in the DIEP flap?**

Radiotherapy and smoking.

○ **What are risk factors for flap failure in DIEP flap?**

Tobacco use, small-sized perforators, venous congestion in contralateral lateral zone (Zone IV).

○ **What are the indications for bilateral breast reconstruction with bilateral DIEP flaps?**

1. Bilateral prophylactic mastectomies.
2. Therapeutic and contralateral prophylactic mastectomies.
3. Postexplantation of bilateral implants due to rupture or capsular contractures.
4. Bilateral subcutaneous mastectomies post foreign-body injection.

○ **Which vein is considered as a "lifeboat" and spared during the harvest of DIEP flap?**

The ipsilateral and contralateral superficial inferior epigastric veins.

○ **What are alternative perforator flap for breast reconstruction if abdominal tissue is not available and their advantages and disadvantages?**

Anterolateral thigh perforator flap: easy flap harvesting with long/sizable pedicle, with significant donor site scar, Thoracodorsal artery perforator flap: long and sizable pedicle but need to change position during surgery and the volume is inadequate, Superior gluteal artery perforator flap and inferior gluteal artery perforator flap: adequate flap volume but very difficult perforator and pedicle dissection and need to change position during surgery, profunda artery perforator flap: ease of flap dissection, but relatively inadequate flap volume.

○ **What is the main indication of the traditional gluteus maximus myocutaneous flap?**

Since the gluteus maximus myocutaneous flap has a thick subcutaneous layer and can be raised as a pedicled flap, it is an excellent tool to cover large sacral midline defects and obliterate the dead space and presents as a good option for sacrum pressure ulcer treatments in young patients with good health status.

○ **What are the disadvantages of the traditional gluteal maximus myocutaneous flap?**

The exposure of the donor vessels is difficult, the vascular pedicle is short, and the flap dissection is challenging.

○ **What are the advantages of SGAP flap over superior gluteus maximus myocutaneous flap?**

The SGAP flap provides a better intraoperative exposure and a longer vascular pedicle, the scar is well hidden and contour deformities are minimized. In SGAP flap, the anatomical and functional integrity of the muscle is preserved; therefore, exposure of any nerves or bony eminences is avoided, postoperative pain is decreased and hospitalization period is shortened.

○ **What are the preferred recipient vessels in breast reconstruction with SGAP flap?**

The axillary vessels should not be used for SGAP flap in breast reconstruction since the pedicle length is often insufficient to allow the flap insetting medially. The preferred recipient vessels are either the perforators of the internal mammary vessels at the second or third intercostals space or the internal mammary vessels themselves between the second to the fourth intercostal junction.

○ **Who first described the use of SGAP flap in breast reconstruction?**

In 1995, Allen and Tucker first reported the use of the SGAP flap in breast reconstruction.

○ **What are the indications of SGAP flap in breast reconstruction?**

SGAP flap can be used for total and partial breast reconstruction and is indicated in patients who have an athletic body habitus or who had previous abdominal surgeries that preclude the use of free DIEP flap, such as midline abdominal scar, multiple abdominal surgeries, abdominoplasty.

○ **Who first described the thoracodorsal artery perforator flap?**

Angrigiani et al. in 1995.

○ **What are the various compositions of the thoracodorsal artery perforator flap?**

Dermoadiposal flap, a composite or chimeric fashion flap including bone or regional muscle flap or a flow-through pattern flap.

○ **What are the advantages of the thoracodorsal artery perforator flap over scapular and parascapular flaps?**

Thoracodorsal artery perforator flap has a longer pedicle and a relatively thinner subcutaneous tissue.

○ **What are the application areas of the thoracodorsal perforator flap?**

Because the thoracodorsal perforator flap is a large and thin flap without hair, it can be used effectively for resurfacing the skin and soft-tissue defect over the hand or thumb, pretibia, and foot, as well as after release of burn scar contracture, resection of malignant skin lesions or radiation ulcers. It is also suitable of facial resurfacing in the head and neck cancer surgery and is a good option in breast reconstruction in selected patients. A pedicled perforator flap can be designed for reconstruction of partial breast deformity after radiation, and chest wall reconstruction.

Recently, the flap has been modified with the use of the perforators from its descending branch close to the anterior axillary line. With this modification, the surgeons can harvest the flap without turning the patient during surgery. It allows more efficient surgeries with two team approach and reduces operation time.

○ **What are the advantages of the thoracodorsal perforator flap?**

Large flap size, well-hidden donor scar, a long and reliable pedicle and variable tissue compositions.

○ **What are the disadvantages of the thoracodorsal perforator flap?**

Longer operation time because of changing position if the perforators from the transverse branch are to be used, relatively narrow flap can be harvested with donor site primary closure comparing to the ALT flap.

○ **Describe the anatomical location of the perforators of the medial sural artery perforator flap.**

Most of the perforators located 9 to 18 cm from the popliteal crease in the medial calf area, and the numbers range from one to four.

○ **What are the advantages of the medial sural artery perforator flap?**

1. Thin and pliable.
2. Less hair bearing.
3. Long and sizable vascular pedicle.
4. Volume can be adjusted by the inclusion of part of the gastrocnemius muscle.
5. The plantaris tendon can be harvested at the same time for tendon repair or used as a sling.
6. The location allows a two-team approach in head and neck reconstruction.

○ **What are the drawbacks of medial sural artery perforator flap?**

1. Donor site scar widening and contour deformity.
2. Donor site cannot be closed primarily if the flap is greater than 5 cm in width.

○ **Describe the anatomic location of the deep circumflex iliac perforator (DCIP) artery.**

The perforator is usually 1 to 2 cm above the iliac crest and 5 cm posterior to the anterior superior iliac crest.

○ **How is the skin paddle of the DCIP flap designed?**

The skin paddle is designed over the perforator and centered at the longitudinal axis of the upper border of the anterior part of the iliac crest.

○ **What are the advantages of DCIP flap over standard iliac crest osseocutaneous flap?**

1. Easier contouring.
2. Eliminates the need for secondary debulking procedure.
3. Minimal sacrifice of the abdominal muscles and reduced the donor site morbidity.

○ **Describe the anatomic location of the medial plantar perforator vessels.**

The medial plantar system emerges through the septum between the abductor hallucis muscle and the flexor digitorum brevis and sends several perforators through this intermuscular septum into the medial plantar skin.

○ **What are the main application areas of the medial plantar perforator flap?**

The flap provides thick, glabrous skin and is especially suitable for the repair of a finger pulp, volar surfaces of the digits, palm or foot plantar defects.

○ **Describe the anatomical location and flap design of an SCIA flap?**

Before surgery, a line connecting the anterior superior iliac supine and groin crease is made. The superficial circumflex iliac artery gives perforators along this line. Usually multiple perforators can be identified.

○ **What are the advantages of SCIA flap?**

A concealed donor site scar is obtained. Basically, all the perforators are septocutaneous without the requirement of intramuscular flap dissection. The flap is thin and hairless, suitable for recipient sites requiring thin flap for reconstruction.

○ **What are the disadvantages of SCIA flap?**

Small pedicle vascular size, moderate pedicle length.

○ **Propose clinical applications of SCIA flap?**

Dorsal foot reconstruction, lower leg defect reconstruction, and hemi-tongue reconstruction.

○ **Describe the anatomical feature and flap design of the profunda artery perforator (PAP) flap**

The PAP flap is nourished by perforators from the profunda femoral artery. Profunda artery gives four branches after the lateral and medial circumflex artery. The first and second branches give perforators supplying the fasciocutaneous tissue of the posterior medial thigh. The perforators pass through the adductor magnus muscle or the intermuscular septum between the gracilis muscle and adductor magnus muscle as septocutaneous branches. Before surgery, the gracilis muscle is marked and perforators can be mapped with handheld Doppler from the intermuscular septum or adductor magnus muscle.

○ **What are the advantages of the PAP flap?**

The PAP flap locates medial thigh, giving a well-concealed scar. The flap is soft with abundant tissue. Multiple perforators are available, giving the possibility of chimeric flap design or harvesting multiple independent flaps at the same time.

○ **Propose clinical applications of the PAP flap.**

Breast reconstruction, pedicle PAP flap for perineal reconstruction, soft-tissue reconstruction, such as head and neck, extremities.

○ **Propose perforator-based free flaps for one-stage repair of an ischemic finger with pulp defect.**

Free medial plantar perforator flap, free perforator-based ulnar forearm flap.

○ **What are the advantages of the medial plantar perforator flap?**

1. Minimal donor site morbidity.

2. Possibility of primary defatting.

3. Availability of two venous drainage systems (concomitant and cutaneous venous systems).

4. Good color and texture match with the finger skin.

5. Concealed location of the donor site.

6. Ease in flap elevation.

○ **Where is the most common location of perforators of the IMA perforator?**

The largest and most commonly found internal mammary artery perforator has been reported to be in the second and third intercostal spaces.

○ **What is the vascular pedicle of the IMA perforator flap?**

Internal mammary artery and vein.

○ **What is the advantage of the IMA perforator flap?**

1. Freedom of arc of rotation to the chest wall and neck.

2. Reliable blood supply from the internal mammary vessels.

3. Similar skin texture and color to the neck.

4. Primary closure of donor site.

5. Being able to preserve the pectoralis muscle myocutaneous flap for further application in repeated recurrent head and neck cancer reconstruction.

○ **What is a chimeric flap?**

A chimeric flap has separate components with separate vascular supplies that are attached to a common source vessel, either by artificial anastomosis or as a natural structure.

○ **What is a perforator-based chimeric flap?**

Skin paddles or different tissue components can be elevated based on at least two perforators from different vascular systems, which can be merged or anastomosed to a final source pedicle.

○ **What are the advantages of using a chimeric flap?**

Easy three-dimensional insetting, acceptable aesthetic appearance, reduced donor site morbidity, precise flap design, shorter operation time, and requirement of one pair of recipient vessels.

○ **What are the disadvantages of using a chimeric flap?**

The possible variations of perforators, a learning curve, easy twisting of perforators and/or pedicle and sometimes the need for a second venous drainage or shifting to double flaps.

○ **Which flaps are available to be harvested as chimeric flap?**

Anterolateral thigh flap, thoracodorsal artery perforator flap, medial sural artery perforator flap and profunda artery perforator flap

○ **Propose a flap for one-stage reconstruction of wide and through-and-through cheek defect involving the oral commissure.**

The anterolateral thigh chimeric flap with vastus lateralis for volume augmentation, and tensor fascia lata for mouth angle suspension.

● ● ● **REFERENCES** ● ● ●

Allen RJ, Haddock NT, Ahn CY, Sadeghi A. Breast reconstruction with the profunda artery perforator flap. *Plast Reconstr Surg.* 2012;129:16e–23e.

Allen RJ, Treece P. Deep inferior epigastric perforator flap for breast reconstruction. *Ann Plast Surg.* 1994;32(1):32–38.

Allen RJ, Tucker C Jr. Superior gluteal artery perforator free flap for breast reconstruction. *Plast Reconstr Surg.* 1995;95(7):1207–1212.

Angrigiani C, Grilli D, Siebert J. Latissimus dorsi musculocutaneous flap without muscle. *Plast Reconstr Surg.* 1995;96(7):1608–1614.

Blondeel PN, Van Landuyt K, Hamdi M, Monstrey SJ. Soft tissue reconstruction with the superior gluteal artery perforator flap. *Clin Plast Surg.* 2003;30(3):371–382.

Blondeel PN. One hundred free DIEP flap breast reconstructions: a personal experience. *Br J Plast Surg.* 1999;52(2):104–111.

Blondeel PN. The sensate free superior gluteal artery perforator (S-GAP) flap: a valuable alternative in autologous breast reconstruction. *Br J Plast Surg.* 1999;52(3):185–193.

Callegari PR, Taylor GI, Caddy CM, Minabe T. An anatomic review of the delay phenomenon: I. Experimental studies. *Plast Reconstr Surg.* 1992;89(3):397–407; discussion 417–418.

Celik N, Wei FC. Technical tips in perforator flap harvest. *Clin Plast Surg.* 2003;30(3):469–472.

Chen HC, Tang YB. Anterolateral thigh flap: an ideal soft tissue flap. *Clin Plast Surg.* 2003;30(3):383–401.

Chijiwa T, Arai K, Miyazaki N, Igota S, Yamamoto N. Making of a facial perforator map by thermography. *Ann Plast Surg.* 2000;44(6):596–600.

Geddes CR, Morris SF, Neligan PC. Perforator flaps: evolution, classification, and applications. *Ann Plast Surg.* 2003;50(1):90–99.

Gedebou TM, Wei FC, Lin CH. Clinical experience of 1284 free anterolateral thigh flaps. *Handchir Mikrochir Plast Chir.* 2002;34(4):239–244.

Gill PS, Hunt JP, Guerra AB, et al. A 10-year retrospective review of 758 DIEP flaps for breast reconstruction. *Plast Reconstr Surg.* 2004;113(4):1153–1160.

Goh TLH, Park SW, Cho JY, Choi JW, Hong JP. The search for ideal thin skin flap: superficial cifcumflex iliac artery perforator flap—a review of 210 cases. *Plast Reconstr Surg.* 2015;135:592–601.

Guerra AB, Metzinger SE, Bidros RS, et al. Bilateral breast reconstruction with the deep inferior epigastric perforator (DIEP) flap: an experience with 280 flaps. *Ann Plast Surg.* 2004;52(3):246–252.

Guerra AB, Metzinger SE, Lund KM, Cooper MM, Allen RJ, Dupin CL. The thoracodorsal artery perforator flap: clinical experience and anatomic study with emphasis on harvest techniques. *Plast Reconstr Surg.* 2004;114(1):32–41; discussion 42–43.

Guerra AB, Soueid N, Metzinger SE, et al. Simultaneous bilateral breast reconstruction with superior gluteal artery perforator (SGAP) flaps. *Ann Plast Surg.* 2004;53(4):305–310.

Hallock GG. Doppler sonography and color duplex imaging for planning a perforator flap. *Clin Plast Surg.* 2003;30(3):347–357, v–vi.

Hallock GG. Simultaneous transposition of anterior thigh muscle and fascia flaps: an introduction to the chimera flap principle. *Ann Plast Surg.* 1991;27(2):126–131.

Hamdi M, Blondeel P, Van Landuyt K, Tondu T, Monstrey S. Bilateral autogenous breast reconstruction using perforator free flaps: a single center's experience. *Plast Reconstr Surg.* 2004;114(1):83–89; discussion 90–92.

Huang JJ, Chang NJ, Chou HH, et al. Pedicle perforator flaps for vulvar reconstruction – new generation of less invasive vulvar reconstruction with favorable results. *Gynecol Oncol.* 2015;137:66–72.

Huang WC, Chen HC, Wei FC, Cheng MH, Schnur DP. Chimeric flap in clinical use. *Clin Plast Surg.* 2003;30(3):457–467.

Inoue T, Kobayashi M, Harashina T. Finger pulp reconstruction with a free sensory medial plantar flap. *Br J Plast Surg.* 1988;41(6): 657–659.

Kao HK, Chang KP, Chen YA, Wei FC, Cheng MH. Anatomical basis and versatile application of the free medial sural artery perforator flap for head and neck reconstruction. *Plast Reconstr Surg.* 2010;125(4):1135–1145.

Kaplan JL, Allen RJ, Guerra A, Sullivan SK. Anterolateral thigh flap for breast reconstruction: review of the literature and case reports. *J Reconstr Microsurg.* 2003;19(2):63–68.

Kim JT. Latissimus dorsi perforator flap. *Clin Plast Surg.* 2003;30(3):403–431.

Kimata Y, Uchiyama K, Ebihara S, et al. Versatility of the free anterolateral thigh flap for reconstruction of head and neck defects. *Arch Otolaryngol Head Neck Surg.* 1997;123(12):1325–1331.

Kimata Y. Deep circumflex iliac perforator flap. *Clin Plast Surg.* 2003;30(3):433–438.

Kimura N, Satoh K, Hasumi T, Ostuka T. Clinical application of the free thin anterolateral thigh flap in 31 consecutive patients. *Plast Reconstr Surg.* 2001;108(5):1197–1208; discussion 1209–1210.

Kimura N, Satoh K, Hosaka Y. Tensor fasciae latae perforator flap. *Clin Plast Surg.* 2003;30(3):439–446.

Koshima I, Fukuda H, Yamamoto H, Moriguchi T, Soeda S, Ohta S. Free anterolateral thigh flaps for reconstruction of head and neck defects. *Plast Reconstr Surg.* 1993;92(3):421–428; discussion 429–430.

Koshima I, Moriguchi T, Soeda S, Kawata S, Ohta S, Ikeda A. The gluteal perforator-based flap for repair of sacral pressure sores. *Plast Reconstr Surg.* 1993;91(4):678–683.

Koshima I, Nanba Y, Tsutsui T, Takahashi Y. Medial plantar perforator flaps with supermicrosurgery. *Clin Plast Surg.* 2003;30(3): 447–455, vii.

Koshima I, Saisho H, Kawada S, Hamanaka T, Umeda N, Moriguchi T. Flow-through thin latissimus dorsi perforator flap for repair of soft-tissue defects in the legs. *Plast Reconstr Surg.* 1999;103(5):1483–1490.

Kroll SS, Schusterman MA, Reece GP, Miller MJ, Robb G, Evans G. Abdominal wall strength, bulging, and hernia after TRAM flap breast reconstruction. *Plast Reconstr Surg.* 1995;96(3):616–619.

Kroll SS, Sharma S, Koutz C, et al. Postoperative morphine requirements of free TRAM and DIEP flaps. *Plast Reconstr Surg.* 2001;107(2):338–341.

Lee BT, Lin SJ, Bar-Meir ED, Borud LJ, Upton J. Pedicled perforator flaps: a new principle in reconstructive surgery. *Plast Reconstr Surg.* 2010;125(1):201–208.

Lee HB, Tark KC, Rah DK, Shin KS. Pulp reconstruction of fingers with very small sensate medial plantar free flap. *Plast Reconstr Surg.* 1998;101(4):999–1005.

Massey MF, Spiegel AJ, Levine JL, et al. Perforator flaps: recent experience, current trends, and future directions based on 3974 microsurgical breast reconstructions. *Plast Reconstr Surg.* 2009;124(3):737–751.

Morris SF, Taylor GI. Predicting the survival of experimental skin flaps with a knowledge of the vascular architecture. *Plast Reconstr Surg.* 1993;92(7):1352–1361.

Peek A, Müller M, Ackermann G, Exner K, Baumeister S. The free gracilis perforator flap: anatomical study and clinical refinements of a new perforator flap. *Plast Reconstr Surg.* 2009;123(2):578–588.

Rand RP, Cramer MM, Strandness DE Jr. Color-flow duplex scanning in the preoperative assessment of TRAM flap perforators: a report of 32 consecutive patients. *Plast Reconstr Surg.* 1994;93(3):453–459.

Rowsell AR, Eisenberg N, Davies DM, Taylor GI. The anatomy of the thoracodorsal artery within the latissimus dorsi muscle. *Br J Plast Surg.* 1986;39(2):206–209.

Saad A, Sadeghi A, Allen RJ. The anatomic basis of the profunda femoris artery perforator flap: a new option for autologous breast reconstruction – a cadaveric and computer topography angiogram study. *J Reconstr Microsurg.* 2012;28:381–386.

Safak T, Klebuc MJ, Mavili E, Shenaq SM. A new design of the iliac crest microsurgical free flap without including the "obligatory" muscle cuff. *Plast Reconstr Surg.* 1997;100(7):1703–1709.

Shieh SJ, Chiu HY, Yu JC, Pan SC, Tsai ST, Shen CL. Free anterolateral thigh flap for reconstruction of head and neck defects following cancer ablation. *Plast Reconstr Surg.* 2000;105(7):2349–2357; discussion 2358–2360.

Song YG, Chen GZ, Song YL. The free thigh flap: a new free flap concept based on the septocutaneous artery. *Br J Plast Surg.* 1984;37(2):149–159.

Taylor GI, Daniel RK. The anatomy of several free flap donor sites. *Plast Reconstr Surg.* 1975;56(3):243–253.

Taylor GI, Palmer JH. The vascular territories (angiosomes) of the body: experimental study and clinical applications. *Br J Plast Surg.* 1987;40(2):113–141.

Taylor GI, Townsend P, Corlett R. Superiority of the deep circumflex iliac vessels as the supply for free groin flaps. Clinical work. *Plast Reconstr Surg.* 1979;64(6):745–759.

Taylor GI. The angiosomes of the body and their supply to perforator flaps. *Clin Plast Surg.* 2003;30(3):331–342, v.

Verpaele AM, Blondeel PN, Van Landuyt K, et al. The superior gluteal artery perforator flap: an additional tool in the treatment of sacral pressure sores. *Br J Plast Surg.* 1999;52(5):385–391.

Wallace CG, Kao HK, Jeng SF, Wei FC. Free-style flaps: a further step forward for perforator flap surgery. *Plast Reconstr Surg.* 2009;124 (6 suppl):e419–e426.

Wei FC, Jain V, Suominen S, Chen HC. Confusion among perforator flaps: what is a true perforator flap? *Plast Reconstr Surg.* 2001; 107(3):874–876.

Wei FC, Kao HK, Jeng SF, Wei FC. Have we found an ideal soft-tissue flap? An experience with 672 anterolateral thigh flaps. *Plast Reconstr Surg.* 2002;109(7):2219–2226; discussion 2227–2230.

Wei FC, Mardini S. Free-style free flaps. *Plast Reconstr Surg.* 2004;114(4):910–916.

Wong C, Saint-Cyr M, Arbique G, et al. Three- and four-dimensional computed tomography angiographic studies of commonly used abdominal flaps in breast reconstruction. *Plast Reconstr Surg.* 2009;124(1):18–27.

Wong C, Saint-Cyr M, Rasko Y, et al. Three- and four-dimensional arterial and venous perforasomes of the internal mammary artery perforator flap. *Plast Reconstr Surg.* 2009;124(6):1759–1769.

CHAPTER 75

Vascular Composite Allotransplantation

Ingrid Ganske, MD and
Bohdan Pomahac, MD

• • • NOMENCLATURE • • •

○ **What is an allograft?**

Tissue transplantation between unrelated individuals of the same species.

○ **What is an autograft?**

Donor tissue, such as a skin graft, that comes from the same patient.

○ **What is the term for a graft that comes from a genetically identical donor, such as an identical twin?**

Isograft.

○ **What is a xenograft?**

A cross species graft, such as porcine skin grafts used as temporary skin substitutes or porcine or bovine acellular dermal matrices.

○ **What is the difference between orthotopic and heterotopic transplants?**

Orthotopic transplants are transferred into an anatomically similar site, whereas heterotopic transplants are transferred into a site different from their origin.

• • • HISTORY • • •

○ **When was the first human organ transplantation?**

Dr. Joseph Murray performed the first solid organ transplantation, a kidney, in 1954, between identical twin brothers.

○ **What types of composite tissue allotransplantations have been performed?**

Hand, lower extremities, face, abdominal wall, knee, flexor tendon apparatus, nerve, larynx, skeletal muscle, tongue, trachea, scalp, uterus, penis.

• • • IMMUNOLOGY • • •

○ **Which antigens are the most immunogenic?**

Major histocompatability complex (MHC) antigens. In humans, these are human leukocyte antigens (HLAs). HLAs reside on the surface of cells. HLA class I antigens are expressed on all nucleated cells, and class II antigens are only expressed on antigen presenting cells (APCs) such as B lymphocytes, monocytes, macrophages, dendritic cells (DCs), endothelial cells, and activated T cells.

○ **What is hyperacute rejection?**

ABO incompatibility and antibody incompatibility result in hyperacute rejection, which is mediated by the humoral immune system and occurs within minutes of transplantation.

○ **What is acute rejection?**

Acute rejection is caused by the direct pathway of allorecognition, in which donor APCs migrate to host lymphoid tissue and activate T cells. These T cells migrate to the graft and mediate graft rejection. Acute rejection occurs within weeks to months following transplant, and periodically at various time points later.

○ **What is chronic rejection?**

Chronic rejection occurs months to years after transplantation. It is contributed to by both direct and indirect pathways of allorecognition, although the indirect pathway is thought to be of greater significance in the pathogenesis of chronic graft rejection. In the indirect pathway, host APCs present processed donor antigens to host T cells. Intimal hypertrophy leading to lumen obliteration and ischemia are typical, as well as sclerotic skin changes.

○ **Which is the most common type of rejection?**

Acute rejection. Chronic rejection in vascular composite allotransplantation (VCA) is just being defined.

○ **Which tissue type is most antigenic?**

Skin and vascular endothelium is thought to be the most antigenic and immunoreactive tissue in VCA.

The vascularized muscle component of limb allografts may induce a cell-mediated response greater than the skin; however, muscle as a single component is less antigenic than skin.

○ **Which tissue types are least antigenic?**

Cartilage and tendon are the least antigenic. Bone represents lower immunogenicity than skin and muscle.

○ **Which tissue type is best to monitor for rejection?**

The skin is also an easily monitored tissue (versus solid organs), so it is the most sensitive indicator of acute rejection in that it is clearly visible and can be easily evaluated by both patient and physician. Therefore, this tissue type is most appropriate to be monitored and biopsied.

○ **What are the main groups of immunosuppressive medications?**

1. Steroids (prednisone)

2. Cytotoxic drugs (cyclophosphamide, methotrexate, azathioprine)

3. Fungal or bacterial products (cyclosporine, tacrolimus/FK506, mycophenolate mofetil, and sirolimus)

4. Antilymphocyte and antithymoglobulin

○ **What is the mechanism of steroids?**

Steroids with anti-inflammatory actions, such as prednisone, inhibit NF-kB transcription factor, which inhibits cellular activation and cytokine production.

○ **What is the mechanism of cytotoxic drugs?**

Cyclophosphamide, methotrexate, and azathioprine interfere with DNA replication and kill the proliferating lymphocytes activated by alloantigens.

○ **What is the mechanism of cyclosporine and FK 506?**

Cyclosporine and FK506 inhibit calcineurin activation and IL-2 gene transcription, which interferes with T-cell activation pathways. Cyclosporine is a metabolic extract from the fungus Tolypocladium inflatum gamus discovered in the 1970s that has revolutionized the field of visceral organ transplantation and has been shown to prolong limb allograft survival in experimental studies. FK506 is a macrolide lactone antibiotic isolated from soil fungus.

○ **What is the mechanism of mycophenolate mofetil?**

It is derived from the fungus Penicillium stoloniferum and inhibits inosine monophosphate dehydrogenase, which is necessary for production of guanine monophosphate needed for B and T lymphocyte proliferation.

○ **Which immunosuppressive medications have not been shown to impair wound healing?**

Antilymphocyte agents, such as lymphocyte immune globulin, antithymoglobulin (ATG), and monoclonal antibodies against T-cell receptors such as basiliximab.

○ **What are common side effects of immunosuppressive medications?**

Renal toxicity, blood glucose disturbances, opportunistic infections. Skin malignancies can also occur long term.

○ **What is tolerance?**

The specific absence of a destructive immune response to a transplanted tissue in the absence of immunosuppression. The key element of this definition is "specific," because the recipient must remain capable of response to other antigens. Tolerance can be developed by central or peripheral mechanisms.

○ **What is central tolerance?**

In the thymus, alloreactive T cells that develop in response to bone marrow–derived APC are deleted. In rodents, deletion of T cells can be induced by introducing donor antigens into the thymus by intrathymic injection. Other studies have examined mixed hematopoietic bone marrow transplantations. This frequently involves total body irradiation for the recipient, followed by donor bone marrow transplantation (deplete of donor T cells) to induce mixed chimerism.

○ **What is peripheral tolerance?**

Mechanisms of peripheral tolerance include T-cell nonresponsiveness, induction of T-suppressor cells, and T-cell deletion. Monoclonal antibodies and DCs play a role in stimulating peripheral tolerance.

○ **What are the important viral serologies to crossmatch?**

Hepatitis B, hepatitis C, cytomegalovirus, Epstein–Barr virus, and human immunodeficiency virus.

○ **What is graft-versus-host disease?**

An entity occurring in bone marrow transplant patients. T cells present in the graft attack the tissues of the recipient, perceiving the host tissues as antigenically foreign. Acute GVHD is observed in the first 3 months; the chronic form is later. Clinical manifestations include damage to the liver, skin, mucosa, GI tract.

● ● ● **ETHICS** ● ● ●

○ **What are the primary ethical dilemmas with reconstructive transplantation?**

Reconstructive transplantation is performed in healthy patients who have a normal life expectancy, and requires lifelong immunosuppression, which induces medical issues, and may even shorten life expectancy.

○ **What are the specific risk–benefit concerns with upper extremity transplantation?**

Justifications for upper extremity transplantation include both functional and self-image improvement. Transplanted hands have been reported to perform better than prosthesis; however, prosthetic technology is a rapidly improving field. There is a general consensus that bilateral amputees are good candidates for transplantation.

In addition, chronic rejection, which is common in all organ transplants, results in fibrosis and potentially leads to decreased function in the long term.

○ **What are specific ethical concerns for facial allotransplantation?**

Transfer of appearance from deceased donor; though a significant concern, we have learned that it does not occur. Selection of patients—who is and who is not a good candidate? All recipients must undergo thorough psychiatric prescreening.

Salvage plan in case facial allograft loss occurs; typically this involves autologous skin grafts or flap reconstruction. Salvage might leave the patient in a functional and aesthetic state worse than pretransplantation. In addition, donor harvest must be expedient and well-planned so that it does not impact vital organ harvest from the same donor.

● ● ● **REFERENCES** ● ● ●

Barth RN, Rodriguez ED, Mundinger GS, et al. Vascularized bone marrow-based immunosuppression inhibits rejection of vascularized composite allografts in nonhuman primates. *Am J Transplant.* 2011;11(7):1407–1416.

Harrison JH, Merrill JP, Murray JE. Renal homotransplantation in identical twins. *Surg Forum.* 1956;6:432–436.

Hui-Chou HG, Nam AJ, Rodriguez ED. Clinical facial composite tissue allotransplantation: a review of the first four global experiences and future implications. *Plast Reconstr Surg.* 2010;125:538–546.

Lee WP, Yaremchuk MJ, Pan YC, Randolph MA, Tan CM, Weiland AJ. Relative antigenicity of components of a vascularized limb allograft. *Plast Reconstr Surg.* 1991;87(3):401–411.

Lee WPA, Butler P, Mathes D. Transplantation in plastic surgery. In: Mathes SJ, Hentz VR, eds. *Plastic Surgery.* 2nd ed. Philadelphia, PA: WB Saunders; 2006:269–292.

Madani H, Hettiaratchy S, Clarke A, Butler PE. Immunosuppression in an emerging field of plastic reconstructive surgery: composite tissue allotransplantation. *J Plast Reconstr Aesthet Surg.* 2008;61(3):245–249.

Murray JE. Organ transplantation (skin, kidney, heart) and the plastic surgeon. *Plast Reconstr Surg.* 1971;47(5):425–431.

Pomahac B, Bueno EM, Sisk GC, Pribaz JJ. Current principles of facial allotransplantation: the Brigham and Women's Hospital Experience. *Plast. Reconstr Surg.* 2013;131:1069–1076.

Sarhane KA, Khalifian S, Ibrahim Z, et al. Diagnosing skin rejection in vascularized composite allotransplantation: advances and challenges. *Clin Transplant.* 2014;28(3):277–285.

Sarhane KA, Tuffaha SH, Broyles JM, et al. A critical analysis of rejection in vascularized composite allotransplantation: clinical, cellular and molecular aspects, current challenges, and novel concepts. *Front Immunol.* 2013;4:406.

Siemionow MZ, Kulahci Y, Bozkurt M. Composite tissue allotransplantation. *Plast Reconstr Surg.* 2009;124:e327–e329.

Silverman RP, Banks ND, Detolla LJ, et al. A heterotopic primate model for facial composite tissue transplantation. *Ann Plast Surg.* 2008;60(2):209–216.

Starzl TE. Immunosuppressive therapy and tolerance of organ allografts. *N Engl J Med.* 2008;358(4):407–411.

Whitaker IS, Duggan EM, Alloway RR, et al. Composite tissue allotransplantation: a review of relevant immunological issues for plastic surgeons. *J Plast Reconstr Aesthet Surg.* 2008;61(5):481–492.

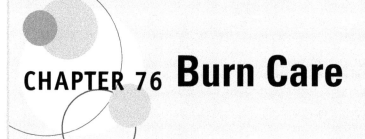

CHAPTER 76 Burn Care

Nicole L. Nemeth, MD, FACS

○ **What is the first step in management of a burn victim?**

Primary survey—maintain airway patency, breathing, circulation. (Just like the ABCs of any trauma.)

Secondary survey—identify associated life-threatening injuries and remove burned clothing and jewelry.

○ **What are the ABA criteria for transfer to a specialized burn center?**

1. Partial-thickness burns involving greater than 10% total body surface area (TBSA)

2. Burns that involve the face, hands, feet, genitalia, perineum, or major joints

3. Third-degree burns in any age group

4. Electrical burns, including lightning injury

5. Chemical burns

6. Inhalation injury

7. Burn injury in patients with preexisting medical disorders that could complicate management

8. Any patients with traumatic injury in which the burn injury poses the greatest risk of morbidity or mortality

9. Any burned children if the hospital initially receiving the patient does not have qualified personnel or equipment for children

10. Any patient with burns that require special social, emotional, or long-term rehabilitative intervention

○ **What methods are used to estimate burn size?**

Lund and Brower chart—most accurate, accounts for body proportions by age group.

Wallace's "Rule of Nines"—head and neck (9%), anterior torso (18%), posterior torso (18%), each upper extremity (9%), each lower extremity (18%), and perineum (1%).

"Patient's Palm" method—the patient's palm is roughly equivalent to 1% of the TBSA.

○ **When should fluid resuscitation begin in a burn victim?**

Fluid resuscitation should begin immediately. Resuscitation for burns >20% TBSA in an adult is based on the Parkland formula. Resuscitation requirements are calculated based on the time of injury, not the time of presentation.

○ **What is the Parkland formula?**

4 mL × weight (kg) × %TBSA = total volume of Lactated Ringer's (LR) to be given over the first 24 hours.

○ **At what rate should fluid resuscitation begin for a 70-kg man with second- and third-degree scald burns to the anterior torso and the anterior aspect of both lower extremities, now 2 hours postinjury?**

This patient has about 18% TBSA to the anterior torso and 9% TBSA to each anterior lower extremity (18 + 9 + 9 = 36% TBSA).

4 mL × 70 kg × 36% = 10,080 cc of LR over first 24 hours.

Half of volume is given over the first 8 hours; the remainder is given over the next 16 hours.

10,080 ÷ 2 = 5,040 mL needed within the first 8 hours.

5,040 ÷ 6 = 840 mL/hr (the total fluid requirements for the first 8 hours will be given within 6 hours since the patient presented in a delayed fashion).

○ **For this patient, at what rate should fluid resuscitation continue over the next 16 hours?**

5,040 ÷ 16 = 315 cc/hr.

○ **At what rate should fluid resuscitation begin for a 70-kg man now 24 hours after flash flame exposure, with an 18% area of first-degree burn to the posterior torso?**

No fluid resuscitation is instituted for first-degree burns of any etiology.

○ **How are the resuscitation requirements determined for children?**

Based on body surface area:

Galveston Shriners Burns Institute formula: 5,000 mL/m^2/BSA burn + 2,000 mL/m^2/total BSA = total LR for first 24 hours.

○ **What is the single best monitor of fluid resuscitation?**

Urine output (0.5 mL/kg/hr for adults; 1.0–2 mL/kg/hr for children).

○ **By what percent does inhalation injury increase fluid resuscitation requirements?**

40% to 75% (~2 cc/kg/%TBSA).

○ **What is the fluid regimen for patients with myoglobinuria or hemoglobinuria?**

Discontinue LR and begin normal saline with sodium bicarbonate.

○ **What osmotic diuretic may be added to assist in clearing the urine of these pigments?**

Mannitol.

○ **Which burn patients should receive tetanus immunization?**

10% TBSA burn injury should receive 0.5 cc of tetanus toxoid; if unknown immunization history or >10 years since last booster, add 250 units of immunoglobulin.

○ **What are the depth classifications of burn injury?**

First degree—involves epidermis only.

Second degree—involves partial thickness of dermis.

Third degree—involves full thickness of dermis and all adnexal structures.

Fourth degree—involves underlying muscle, bone, or tendon.

○ **What is the clinical appearance of a partial-thickness versus full-thickness burn wound?**

A partial-thickness wound bed usually will be pink and moist underneath blisters, with intact sensation. A full-thickness injury will appear dry and insensate, and may be white, leathery, or charred depending on the depth of involvement.

○ **In what order do different sensory modalities return in a healed burn wound?**

Pain (first), light touch, temperature, vibration (last).

○ **What are the three histologic zones of burn injury?**

Zone of necrosis—area of tissue necrosis due to destruction from burn injury.

Zone of ischemia—surrounds zones of necrosis; can convert to zone of necrosis because of inadequate tissue perfusion.

Zone of hyperemia—surrounds zone of ischemia; usually reversible injury (heals).

○ **What intervention prevents the progression of a zone of ischemia to a zone of necrosis?**

Adequate fluid resuscitation with perfusion of ischemic tissue.

○ **When should escharotomies be performed?**

For deep, circumferential extremity burns with decreased or absent pulses or deep burns involving the torso that impair ventilation.

○ **How should escharotomy incisions be planned?**

Release of eschar should occur immediately at the bedside using a Bovie electrocautery.

Midaxial incisions release eschar of extremities.

Axial incisions along the flanks that connect across the midline to release the chest/torso.

Unilateral midaxial incisions on the digits on the radial surface of the small finger and thumb; escharotomy incisions on the index, long, and ring finger generally should be placed on the ulnar surface.

○ **If perfusion to a distal extremity does not improve after an escharotomy is performed, what is the next step in management?**

Fasciotomy.

○ **What is the cardiovascular response to a burn injury?**

Cardiac output (CO) initially decreases and systemic vascular resistance (SVR) increases.

After the first 24 to 48 hours, the heart rate and CO increase and SVR decreases.

○ **How are red blood cells affected by burn injury?**

Their $T_{1/2}$ is shortened.

○ **What are some causes of early renal insufficiency in burned patients?**

Hypovolemia, vasoconstriction due to catecholamine release, myoglobinuria, nephrotoxic medications.

○ **What is the cause of Curling's ulcer?**

A decrease in splanchnic blood flow and gut motility (ileus) place burn patients at risk for Curling's ulcer usually involving the stomach or proximal small bowel. Appropriate prophylaxis is usually instituted to prevent mucosal erosion.

○ **Which muscle relaxant should be avoided in burned patients?**

Succinylcholine—causes marked hyperkalemia.

○ **What is the immunologic response to thermal injury?**

Decreased lymphocytes, macrophages, immunoglobulins, and lysosomal enzymes.

○ **What is the hypermetabolic response?**

After an early "ebb" phase, a more prolonged period of protein catabolism, lipolysis, tachycardia, increased urinary output, increased oxygen consumption, nitrogen loss, and elevated body temperature ensues.

○ **What are the hormonal manifestations of the hypermetabolic response?**

Increased levels of cortisol, catecholamines, and glucagons; there is an overall increase in the blood glucose level.

○ **What are signs and symptoms of inhalation injury?**

Facial burns, singed nasal hairs, carbonaceous sputum, hypoxemia with or without an elevated carbon monoxide (CO) level, hoarseness, stridor.

○ **What is an accurate and practical test for diagnosing an inhalation injury?**

Fiberoptic bronchoscopy.

○ **Why is the early diagnosis of inhalation injury critical?**

Inhalation injury will increase the fluid requirements for resuscitation, may lead to airway edema and respiratory distress, and can significantly increase the risk for mortality.

○ **How can parenchymal thermal lung injury be detected?**

^{133}Xenon lung scan.

○ **What is CO poisoning considered the "great imitator?"**

The symptoms of CO poisoning mimic those of the flu. Carboxyhemoglobin levels as low as 10% can cause headache, dizziness, nausea, and dyspnea. Higher levels can lead to chest pain, tachycardia, seizures, loss of conscious and death.

○   **What is the treatment of carbon monoxide poisoning?**

Hyberbaric oxygen (usually delivered at 2.5–3 atmospheres of pressure) is administered in a hyperbaric oxygen chamber for patients with elevated carboxyhemoglobin levels upon arrival at most burn centers. In pregnant patients, the threshold for treatment can be for levels as low as 10%, since fetal hemoglobin has an higher affinity for CO.

○   **What is the $T_{1/2}$ of carbon monoxide at room air and on 100% oxygen?**

~4 hours on room air, ~45 minutes on 100% oxygen (at sea level).

○   **What is the initial treatment of suspected inhalation injury?**

100% oxygen via face mask or nasal cannula.

○   **What is a low-voltage versus a high-voltage electrical exposure?**

Low voltage—<1,000 volts, mostly cutaneous manifestations of burn injury.

High voltage—>1,000 volts, extent of injury usually involves deeper structures (based on resistance of different tissues to passage of current).

○   **How does a lightning injury differ from a high-voltage electrical accident?**

Lightning injuries result in a "flashover" and do not tend to cause devastating internal thermal injuries.

○   **What is the most common cause of death in a lightning victim?**

Cardiopulmonary arrest.

○   **Which tissue has the greatest amount of resistance and therefore produces the most heat?**

Bone.

○   **Which tissues have the least resistance to electrical current?**

Nerves, blood vessels, muscle.

○   **What are emergent management considerations for electrical injury?**

Evaluate for associated injuries, including cervical spine or extremity fractures, pneumothorax, neurologic changes, cardiac arrhythmias.

Escharotomy or fasciotomy alone or in combination (for compartment syndrome) and nerve decompression (e.g., release of Carpal tunnel, Guyon's canal) may also be warranted emergently.

○   **What are long-term management considerations for a patient with an electrical injury?**

Debridement of all nonviable tissue, especially muscle; involved extremities may require amputation.

Cataracts may present with a slow and progressive onset years after the injury.

○   **How are low-voltage electrical oral commissure burns managed?**

Conservative local wound and splinting with a mouth spreader to prevent microstomia.

○ **What is a known complication of the use of a mouth spreader splint?**

Hemorrhage from the superficial labial artery with sloughing of the eschar (5–7 days).

○ **What are the first steps in management of a chemical burn?**

Disrobe patient, early irrigation of affected area with copious amounts of plain water, identify offending agent, identify and treat systemic toxicity.

○ **Why should a chemical burn NOT be treated with a neutralizing agent?**

The heat generated can induce a thermal injury.

○ **Which causes a deeper burn: acids or alkalis?**

Alkalis.

○ **What are some commonly encountered alkali agents?**

Lime, bleach, sodium hydroxide, potassium hydroxide (usually agents found in household cleaning products).

○ **What are the mechanisms by which alkali chemicals induce tissue injury?**

1. Fat saponification.
2. Water extraction from cells.
3. Formation of hydroxide ion-containing alkaline proteinates, leading to deeper tissue penetration.

○ **What are examples of some commonly encountered acidic agents?**

Acetic acid, hydrochloric acid, hydrofluoric acid (HF), trichloroacetic acid.

○ **By what mechanisms do acid chemicals induce tissue injury?**

Hydrolysis of proteins, generation of heat in contact with skin.

○ **How does HF differ in its mechanism of injury?**

Free fluoride ions complex with bivalent cations (Ca^{++}, Mg^{++}) to form insoluble salts, thereby depleting the available Ca^{++} and Mg^{++} in circulation.

○ **What can be applied topically to chelate fluoride ions and reduce pain?**

2.5% calcium gluconate in a water-soluble gel.

○ **If pain relief is refractory to topical calcium gluconate, what is the next step in management?**

Subcutaneous injection of 10% calcium gluconate.

○ **How are phosphorous and phosphoric acid similar to HF?**

They bind calcium ions.

○ **What can be applied topically to impede oxidation and burn injury from phosphorous compounds?**

0.5% copper sulfate solution—on contact, copper sulfate forms a black film that delineates the area of phosphorus injury.

○ **What is the mechanism of tissue injury from frostbite?**

Thrombosis of microvasculature and extracellular ice crystal formation causing cellular damage.

○ **What is the initial treatment of an appendage with frostbite?**

Rapid rewarming (water bath at 104–108°F) for 20 to 40 minutes until reperfusion occurs.

○ **What are other potential modalities for treatment of frostbite?**

Ibuprofen, intravenous heparin, thrombolytics.

○ **How soon should surgical debridement of involved tissue be performed for frostbite?**

After full demarcation of necrosis, weeks to months later. Local wound care is the mainstay of treatment otherwise.

○ **What is the basic tenet of surgical treatment for burn wounds?**

Wounds that will not heal within 2 weeks should be excised and skin grafted.

○ **Which wounds tend to require excision and autografting?**

Deep partial-thickness and full-thickness burn wounds.

○ **What is the "overlay" grafting method?**

The use of widely expanded (4:1 meshed) split-thickness autograft with a meshed, unexpanded homograft overlay (used for patients with large burns and minimal donor sites).

○ **What is the most common side effect of silver sulfadiazine (Silvadene)?**

Transient leukopenia.

○ **What is the most common side effect of mafenide acetate (Sulfamylon)?**

Carbonic anhydrase inhibition or hyperchloremic metabolic acidosis.

○ **What are the side effects of silver nitrate solution?**

Electrolyte leaching, methemoglobinemia, silver discoloration of tissues.

○ **What is Acticoat?**

Antimicrobial silver-coated barrier dressing.

○ **What is Biobrane?**

Knitted nylon mesh bonded to a thin silicone membrane with a porcine collagen matrix.

○   **How does TransCyte compare to Biobrane?**

Both are temporary skin replacement products—TransCyte has a polymer membrane with newborn human fibroblasts cultured onto a porcine collagen nylon mesh.

○   **What is Integra?**

Bilaminate membrane—outer silicone layer and inner dermal layer made up of bovine type I collagen that is cross-linked with shark glycosaminoglycans and chondroitin-6-sulfate.

○   **What are some advantages and disadvantages of using Integra for wound closure or contracture release?**

The disadvantages are the need for a second surgery to remove the outer silicone layer, the risk of collecting fluid under the Integra, and infection.

The advantage is the creation of a "neodermis" and the ability to take a very thin (~0.005 in) split-thickness skin graft.

○   **When should the outer silicone layer be removed?**

Approximately 21 days.

○   **How does AlloDerm differ from allograft?**

AlloDerm is acellular cadaver skin that incorporates as a neodermis and can also be grafted with a much thinner skin graft.

Allograft is cadaveric homograft. It is not acellular so an eventual immune response is to be expected.

○   **What is xenograft?**

From the root word *xenos* (the Greek word for "foreign"), xenograft refers to tissue that is transplanted from one species to a different species. In burn care, the most commonly used xenograft is porcine skin for temporary wound coverage.

○   **What is CEA?**

Cultured epithelial autograft—keratinocytes cultured in a laboratory setting over 3 to 4 weeks from a single punch biopsy of patient's normal skin.

Utilized for near total 100% TBSA burns that require excision and grafting.

○   **How is a skin graft perfused within the first 24 to 48 hours?**

By plasmatic imbibition; the graft becomes vascularized by inosculation over a period of 3 to 4 days.

○   **What is plasmatic imbibition?**

Plasmatic imbibition is the passive transport of nutrients from the wound bed to the graft.

○   **What is inosculation?**

Inosculation is the establishment of anastomoses between graft and recipient blood vessels. Revascularization is complete by 7 days.

○ **What is neovascularization?**

The ingrowth of durable, new vessels into the skin graft.

○ **What is primary versus secondary contraction?**

Primary contraction is the passive immediate recoil of a skin graft after graft harvest.

Secondary contraction is the shrinkage of the graft that occurs during the healing process due to the action of myofibroblasts. Increasing amounts of deep dermis included in thicker grafts are comparatively more resistant to secondary contraction than a graft that includes less dermis.

○ **In what order do skin grafts undergo increasing amounts of primary contraction?**

Meshed split thickness, thin split thickness, thick split thickness, full thickness. How do you remember this? MORE DERMIS = MORE ELASTIN = MORE PRIMARY CONTRACTION.

○ **What is the depth of harvest for each type of split-thickness skin graft?**

Thin split-thickness skin graft: ≈0.005 to 0.012 in thick

Medium split-thickness skin graft: ≈0.012 to 0.018 in thick

Thick split-thickness skin graft: ≈0.018 to 0.030 in thick

○ **What quality of the skin graft determines the degree of primary contraction?**

Elastin present in increasing amounts with the thickness of the dermal component provides a greater potential for primary contraction.

○ **What is an important aspect of burn rehabilitation/reconstruction that begins during the acute phase of the injury?**

Early range of motion, mobilization, and proper positioning/splinting.

○ **How should burned areas be splinted?**

Neck in slight extension, shoulder abducted, elbow in full extension, hand in intrinsic plus position, hips in extension/abduction, knees in full extension, and foot in neutral position/90 degrees of dorsiflexion.

○ **What is the best way to preserve the most normal appearance in facial burn coverage?**

Using medium- or full-thickness skin grafts and grafting within facial aesthetic units. Full-thickness skin grafts require closure at the donor site (either primary or with split-thickness skin grafting), and tend not to be used in the acute phase of burn coverage.

○ **How can the reconstruction of burn alopecia be managed?**

Excision and primary closure (for small, concentrated defects).

Tissue expansion (defects up to 50% of the scalp).

Scalp rotational flaps (larger defects, with or without tissue expansion).

○ **What is the approach to operative management of an anterior neck contracture with lower lip and lower eyelid ectropion?**

Usually, the neck undergoes surgical release first, followed by the lower lip and lower eyelids. Lower lip and lower eyelid ectropion may improve or resolve after release of the anterior neck.

○ **What is the preferred skin graft technique for upper versus lower eyelid ectropion reconstruction?**

The upper eyelid is released with a split-thickness skin graft (for mobility), whereas the lower eyelid is released with a full-thickness skin graft (for support).

○ **What are examples of flaps commonly used in burn reconstruction?**

Z-plasty, V-to-Y, 5 flap plasty (also known as, "Jumping Man").

Scalp rotational flaps.

Advancement of neck and facial flaps after tissue expansion.

Pedicled or free tissue transfer for release of burn scar contracture (scapular/parascapular, thoracoepigastric, anterolateral thigh, latissimus dorsi).

○ **How can one predict the length of postexpansion tissue gain for use in an advancement flap for adjacent wound coverage or resurfacing?**

The predicted length of tissue gain can be calculated by the expander dimensions. The advancement length is calculated by subtracting the base diameter from the circumference of the fully expanded implant.

○ **What are exfoliating "burns?"**

Certain infectious and autoimmune conditions, such as scalded skin syndrome, pemphigus vulgaris, bullous pemphigoid, erythema multiforme, Stevens–Johnson syndrome, and toxic epidermal necrolysis, can lead to blistering and desquamation and are often treated in a burn center.

○ **How are the different exfoliating "burns" diagnosed and differentiated?**

Skin biopsy, clinical presentation, and history of known offending agent or medication.

● ● ● **REFERENCES** ● ● ●

Brou JA, Robson MC, McCauley RL, et al. Inventory of potential reconstructive needs in the patient with burns. *J Burn Care Rehabil.* 1989;10:555–560.

Hansen SL, Voigt DW, Wiebelhaus P, Paul CN. Using skin replacement products to treat burns and wounds. *Adv Skin Wound Care.* 2001;14(1):37–44.

Herndon D, ed. *Total Burn Care.* 2nd ed. London, UK: WB Saunders; 2002.

Nguyen TT, Gilpin DA, Meyer NA, Herndon DN. Current treatment of severely burned patients. *Ann Surg.* 1996;223(1):14–25.

Press B. Thermal, electrical, and chemical injuries. In: Aston SJ, Beasley RW, Thorne C, eds. *Grabb and Smith's Plastic Surgery.* 5th ed. Philadelphia, PA: Lippincott-Raven; 1997:161–189.

Sheridan RL. Burns. *Crit Care Med.* 2002;30(11 Suppl):S500–S514.

CHAPTER 77 Ear Reconstruction

William W. Dzwierzynski, MD, FACS,
Elizabeth A. O'Connor, MD, and
Jenna Cusic, MD

○ **Identify the anatomy of the ear (Fig. 77-1).**

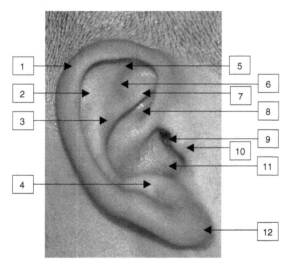

1. Helix
2. Scapha
3. Antihelix
4. Antitragus
5. Posterior crus antihelix
6. Triangular fossa
7. Anterior crus antihelix
8. Cymba of concha
9. External auditory meatus
10. Tragus
11. Cavum of concha
12. Lobule

Figure 77-1 Anatomy of the ear.

○ **Which embryologic structures give rise to the ear?**

The first two branchial arches give rise to six hillocks that form the ear.

The first arch forms the malleus, incus, and anterior hillocks (1–3).

The second arch forms the stapes and posterior hillocks (4–6).

○ **What structures arise from the anterior (1–3) hillocks?**

The tragus, root helix, and superior helix.

○ **What structures arise from the posterior (4–6) hillocks?**

The antihelix, antitragus, and lobule.

○ **What ear structures are formed from the first branchial groove?**

The external auditory canal and concha.

○ **What is the average length of the ear?**

The average length is 6 cm. Approximately 90% of the growth occurs by 5 years of age.

○ **What is the angle of protrusion of the ear?**

25 to 30 degrees.

○ **What is the vascular supply of the ear?**

The ear is supplied by branches of the <u>external carotid artery:</u>

1. The lateral ear is supplied by the superficial temporal and posterior auricular arteries.

2. The medial ear is supplied by the posterior auricular and posterior occipital arteries.

3. The triangular fossa and scapha are supplied by the helical branch of the superficial temporal artery.

4. The concha is supplied by septal perforators of the posterior auricular artery.

○ **What is the vascular supply to the ear cartilage?**

The cartilage is an avascular structure, which is supplied by the surrounding perichondrium and soft tissue.

○ **What is the lymphatic drainage of the ear?**

The lymphatic drainage may vary, although it generally follows embryologic development:

1. The superolateral ear and anterior external auditory meatus drain to the parotid nodes.

2. The superomedial ear and posterior external auditory meatus drain to the mastoid nodes.

3. The inferior ear and lower external auditory meatus drain to the superficial cervical nodes.

4. The concha and meatus drain to the preauricular nodes.

○ **Describe the innervation of the ear.**

   1. The auriculotemporal branch (V2) supplies the superolateral ear.

   2. The great auricular branch (C2–3) supplies the inferolateral and inferomedial ear.

   3. The lesser occipital branch (C2–3) supplies the superomedial ear.

   4. The auditory ("Arnold's") branch (X) supplies the concha and external auditory canal.

○ **How do you anesthetize the ear?**

Anesthesia of the ear, except the concha and external auditory canal, can be performed with a ring block around the base of the ear. Anesthesia to the concha and external auditory canal must be performed with local infiltration.

○ **What is the treatment for ear burns?**

The primary goal is to prevent chondritis. Topical <u>mafenide</u> is used for dressing changes. The eschar is left in place as a biologic dressing. Defects with intact perichondrium will heal in, while others will require late excision and repair.

○ **What is the treatment for frostbite of the ear?**

Topical mafenide is used for burns and frostbite. It is highly soluble, which allows penetration of eschar and cartilage. Sulfonomides are carbonic anhydrase inhibitors, which can lead to <u>metabolic acidosis.</u>

○ **What is the management of an ear hematoma?**

Ear hematomas are treated by aspiration or incision and drainage. Bolster dressing is applied to prevent reaccumulation. Hematoma forms between the cartilage and perichondrium of the ear. This disrupts the vascular supply to the cartilage, which may become necrotic or infected. Clotted blood forms a fibrotic mass that deforms the overlying tissue. This is known as a "cauliflower," "boxer's," or "wrestler's" ear.

○ **What are the most common malignancies of the ear?**

   1. Squamous cell cancer: 50% to 60%

   2. Basal cell cancer: 30% to 40%

   3. Melanoma: 1% to 2%

○ **What are the causes of a prominent ear?**

   1. Underdeveloped antihelical fold, leading to protrusion of the scapha and helical rim, causing prominence in the upper to middle 1/3.

   2. Prominent concha, causing middle 1/3 prominence.

   3. Protruding earlobe, causing lower 1/3 prominence.

○ **What is a constricted ear?**

Abnormally small ears which may appear prominent due to the inadequate circumference of the helical rim, leading the auricle to cup forward.

○ **What is a Stahl's ear?**

An ear with a third crus, in addition to the anterior and posterior crus of triangular fossa (Fig. 77-2).

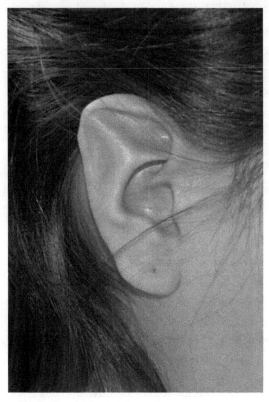

Figure 77-2 Example of a Stahl's ear. See Color insert.

○ **What is cryptotia?**

The upper pole of the helix is buried beneath the temporal skin.

○ **Auricular cartilage has notable plasticity in the immediate newborn period due to what?**

Circulating maternal estrogens, which peak at day 3 and return to baseline at week 6.

○ **What treatment may take place of or precede surgical intervention in newborns with ear deformities such as constricted ears?**

Ear molding, which takes advantage of the early ear plasticity. Results are most successful with earlier intervention, ideally prior to 6 weeks of age.

○ **What are the otoplasty goals?**

From the front view the helical rim should be visible and not hidden behind the antihelix, and from the rear view the helical rim should be straight, not "C" shaped.

○ **How are defects of skin and perichondrium repaired?**

Primary closure is used for small defects. The cartilage may be removed and a skin graft applied onto the medial skin. Local skin flaps such as bipedicled flaps from the medial ear may be used.

○   **What is the Antia–Buch reconstruction technique?**

Antia–Buch technique of helical rim advancement can be used for defects up to 2.5 cm. The helical rim is separated from the scapha through an incision in the helical sulcus. This extends from the lower edge of the defect to the upper lobule, including skin, perichondrium, and cartilage. The posteromedial skin is left intact, whereas the chondrocutaneous flap is advanced. V-Y advancement of the root helix and trimming scaphal cartilage allow for additional coverage (see Fig. 77-3).

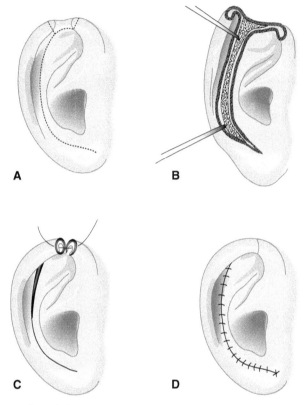

Figure 77-3 The Antia–Buch reconstruction technique.

○   **How are helical rim defects greater than 3 cm treated?**

The Converse tunnel procedure is used for helical rim defects greater than 3 cm. A cartilage strut is tunneled under postauricular skin. Three weeks later, the strut is lifted on an anteriorly based flap and inset into the defect.

○   **Describe the tubed pedicle technique.**

The tubed pedicle technique is used for helical reconstruction. A bipedicled flap is elevated and fashioned into a tube. This is sewn to the edge of the defect. A second stage is performed to elevate the flap.

○   **What are reconstructive options for the conchal bowl and helical root?**

1. Healing by secondary intention.

2. Full-thickness skin grafts can be placed onto perichondrium.

3. If the perichondrium is not present, the cartilage should be excised and skin graft placed onto medial ear skin.

○   **How large of a defect can be closed primarily (i.e., Tanzer's excision)?**

A defect of 2 cm or less can be closed using a wedge excision technique with star-shaped pattern to allow for closure without excessive excision of the helical rim. This is commonly referred to as a Tanzer's excision.

○ **What is a Banner flap?**

This is a postauricular flap from the superior auriculocephalic sulcus. It is used in conjunction with a cartilage graft for upper one-third defects.

○ **What are the reconstructive options for defects of the middle one-third of the ear?**

1. Defects limited to helical rim are closed by Antia–Buch technique.

2. Wedge excision with primary closure (i.e., Tanzer's excision) (<2 cm).

3. Cartilage graft with postauricular or temporoparietal flap/skin graft (i.e., Dieffenbach's flap or Converse tunnel technique) (>2 cm).

4. Contralateral chondrocutaneous composite flap (>2 cm).

○ **What is a Dieffenbach flap?**

This is a postauricular flap with contralateral cartilage support, which is used to reconstruct defects of the middle one-third. Cartilage graft is sutured into the defect with postauricular skin advanced over for skin coverage. The flap is then divided 2 to 3 weeks later (see Fig. 77-4).

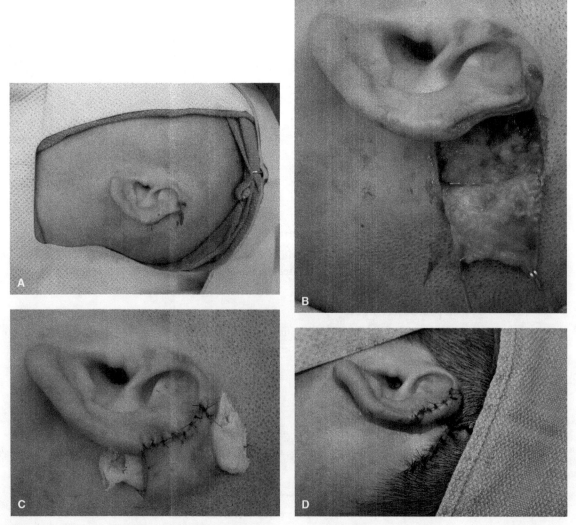

Figure 77-4 Example of a Dieffenbach flap.

○ **Is cartilage required for lobular reconstruction?**

Although the lower ear is not composed of cartilage, reconstruction with cartilage provides better support. Wedge excision and primary closure can be performed by defects <50%. Local preauricular and postauricular flaps with cartilage struts are used for defects >50%.

○ **What is a split earlobe and how is this treated?**

Split earlobe results from a traumatic earring injury or heavy earring use. Straight line closure will result in a notched earlobe. A wedge excision and zigzag repair can prevent notching.

○ **Describe the use of the temporoparietal fascial flap in ear reconstruction.**

This superficial temporal fascia flap is based on the superficial temporal vessels. It is tunneled to the ear for cartilage coverage and covered with skin graft. It is a thin and pliable flap that preserves external topography. This is used when local skin flaps are not available.

○ **What is the management of partial ear amputation?**

Partial amputation even with a wide small pedicle has good prognosis with debridement and primary closure. Partial amputation with a narrow pedicle and a large amount of cartilage to support has a poor prognosis with primary repair.

○ **Describe the approach to total ear amputation.**

Cartilage banking or the "pocket principle" is rarely used at this time due to cartilage degradation and deformity. Microvascular replantation should be attempted. If this is not possible, staged reconstruction should be performed.

○ **What should be done if no sufficient venous outflow can be established for an ear replantation?**

Leech therapy.

○ **Do patients with microtia have hearing difficulties?**

Most patients have atresia of the external auditory canal, tympanic membrane, and the middle ear ossicles resulting in conductive hearing loss. The inner ear is derived from a separate embryologic tissue than the middle and external ear.

○ **At what age is ear reconstruction generally pursued?**

This is debated and may be as early as 5 years, or at age 9 to 10, when the opposite ear (and the framework) for modeling the reconstruction reaches adult size, and patients harbor enough rib cartilage to harvest.

○ **What are the options for total ear reconstruction?**

1. Autogenous reconstruction
2. Composite autogenous/alloplastic reconstruction with alloplastic framework
3. Prosthetic

○ **Describe autogenous ear reconstruction.**

Ear reconstruction involves multiple stages, number, order, and complexity depending on the technique. Brent's technique is a modification of Tanzer's technique and involves four stages. It is simpler and with less risk of complications. Nagata's technique involves two stages and has the potential for a more optimal aesthetic result, yet may be more challenging. A framework is created using the contralateral ear as a model, and contralateral or ipsilateral (depending on the technique) costal cartilages 6 to 8 or 5 to 9 for the structure. This is placed in a subcutaneous pocket. The cartilage framework is then lifted with the overlying skin and the posterior defect is covered with a skin graft and rotated into anatomic position.

○ **What determines the shape of the reconstructed ear?**

The cartilage framework, but also the available options of tissue for coverage. The framework may need to be adapted in consideration of any limitations of abnormal skin coverage.

● ● ● **REFERENCES** ● ● ●

Allison GR. Anatomy of the external ear. *Clin Plast Surg.* 1978;5:419–422.

Antia NH, Buch VI. Chondrocutaneous advancement flap for the marginal defect of the ear. *Plast Reconstr Surg.* 1967;39:472–477.

Bos EJ, Scholten T, Song Y, et al. Developing a parametric ear model for auricular reconstruction: a new step towards patient-specific implants. *J Craniomaxillofac Surg.* 2015;43:390–395.

Boutros SG, Thorne CH. Chapter 53. Reconstruction of acquired ear defects. In: Guyron B, Erikkson E, Persing JA, eds. *Plastic Surgery: Indications and Practice.* China: Elsevier; 2009:717–726.

Brent B. Reconstruction of traumatic ear deformities. *Clin Plast Surg.* 1978;5:437–445.

Brent B. The acquired auricular deformity. A systematic approach to its analysis and reconstruction. *Plast Reconstr Surg.* 1977;59: 475–485.

Cheney ML, Hadlock TA, Quatela VC. In: Baker SR, ed. *Local Flaps in Facial Reconstruction.* Philadelphia, PA: Elsevier; 2007:581–624.

Doft M, Goodkind A, Diamond S, DiPace J, Kacker A, LaBruna A. The newborn butterfly project: a shortened treatment protocol for ear molding. *Plast Reconstr Surg.* 2015;135(3):577e–583e.

Elsahy NI. Acquired ear defects. *Clin Plast Surg.* 2002;29:175–186.

Elsahy NI. Reconstruction of the ear after skin and cartilage loss. *Clin Plast Surg.* 2002;29:201–212.

Elsahy NI. Reconstruction of the ear after skin and perichondrium loss. *Clin Plast Surg.* 2002;29:187–200.

Firmin, F. State-of-the-art autogenous ear reconstruction in cases of microtia. In: Staudenmaier R. *Aesthestics and Functionality in Ear Reconstruction. Adv Otorhinolaryngol.* Basel, Switzerland: Karger; 2010;25–52.

Gosain A, Kumar A, Huang G. Prominent ears in children younger than 4 years of age: what is the appropriate timing for otoplasty? *Plast Reconstr Surg.* 2004;114(5):1042–1054.

Gosman AA, Reece EM. Ear reconstruction. In: Janis JE, ed. *Essentials of Plastic Surgery.* St Louis, MO: Quality Medical Publishing; 2007:314–323.

Lo J, Tsang W, Yu J, Ho O, Ku P, Tong M. Contemporary hearing rehabilitation options in patients with aural atresia. *Biomed Res Int.* 2014;2014:761579.

Menick FJ. Reconstruction of the ear after tumor excision. *Clin Plast Surg.* 1990;17:405–415.

Songcharoen S, Smith RA, Jabaley ME. Tumors of the external ear and reconstruction of defects. *Clin Plast Surg.* 1978;5:447–457.

Thorne CH. Chapter 30. Otoplasty and ear reconstruction. In: Thorne CH, Beasley RW, Aston SJ, Bartlett SP, Gurtner GC, Spear SL, eds. *Grabb & Smith's Plastic Surgery.* 6th ed. Philadelphia, PA: Lippincott Williams & Wilkins; 2007:297–312.

Turpin IM. Microsurgical replantation of the external ear. *Clin Plast Surg.* 1990;17:397–404.

Wilkes G, Wong J, Guilfoyle R. Microtia reconstruction. *Plast Reconstr Surg.* 2014;134(3):464e–479e.

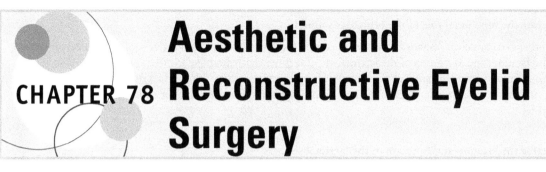

Aesthetic and Reconstructive Eyelid Surgery

CHAPTER 78

Farzad R. Nahai, MD

○ **What makes up the anterior, middle, and posterior lamellae of the eyelid?**

The three lamellae or "layers" of the eyelid are anatomical divisions that help with the understanding of lid function and lid surgery.

The <u>anterior lamella</u> is defined as the skin and underlying orbicularis muscle.

The <u>middle lamella</u> is the orbital septum and accompanying fatty pads.

The <u>posterior lamella</u> is the conjunctiva and levator apparatus and corresponding lower lid retractors.

○ **Describe the surface anatomy findings of the aged eyelid and the underlying structures responsible.**

Four key features are apparent on the surface examination of the aged eyelid: contour irregularities, the lid crease, lid position, and rhytids.

<u>Contour irregularities</u> that are often apparent are because of protruding periorbital fat pads; principally the medial upper fat pad and the lower lid fat pads.

An elevated <u>lid crease</u> represents stretch or dehiscence of the levator apparatus from the tarsal plate and is often a tell-tale sign of lid ptosis.

<u>Lower lid position</u> that is descended away from the corneoscleral limbus is indicative of lower lid laxity and poor canthal support. Often a negative canthal tilt (downward slope of a line drawn from the medial canthus to the lateral canthus) and scleral show (a viewable strip of white sclera between the lower corneoscleral limbus and lid border) are present as well. Upper lid position that encroaches on the upper corneoscleral limbus raises suspicion that ptosis is present.

Brow strain and horizontal forehead <u>rhytids</u> often accompany lid ptosis and dermatochalasis.

○ **What are the analogous structures in the upper and lower eyelid?**

The levator aponeurosis is specific to the upper eyelid and is analogous to the capsulopalpebral fascia of the lower lid.

○ **Describe the anatomy of the orbicularis oculi muscle.**

The orbicularis oculi muscle is a complex array of concentrically oriented muscles with origins medial to the medial canthus and insertions lateral to the lateral canthus. Further differentiation is made based on the location relative to the underlying lid structures; oriented in a concentric manner from outside to in they are the <u>orbital</u> orbicularis, <u>preseptal</u> orbicularis, and <u>pretarsal</u> orbicularis. Further divisions (based on function and innervation) can be made, principally the inner canthal orbicularis and the extracanthal orbicularis.

○ **Describe the functional role of the orbicularis muscle.**

The orbicularis muscle is responsible for eyelid closure (both passive blink and active squint), corneal protection, and lubrication, and as a pump of the lacrimal sac. The inner canthal orbicularis (that orbicularis which resides within 1 cm of the medial canthus) is responsible for passive involuntary blink; the extracanthal orbicularis (that orbicularis which resides outside the inner canthal portion) is responsible for voluntary protective forceful blinking.

○ **Describe the location and function of the lacrimal sac.**

The lacrimal sac resides lateral and posterior to the base of the nasal sidewall within the lacrimal crest. The upper portion of the sac is wrapped on its anterior and posterior aspects by the anterior and posterior medial heads of the orbicularis muscle, hence the muscle's pump action on it. The lacrimal system is a conduit for the passage of tears from the eye (exiting via the upper and lower canalicular systems) into the nasal sinus. Obstruction within this low-pressure system can result in epiphora (excess tearing) or mucocele.

○ **What is Whitnall's tubercle?**

Whitnall's tubercle is minor bony spur on the inner aspect of the lateral orbital rim that represents the bony insertion point of the lateral canthal tendon.

○ **What nearby anatomic structure helps locate Whitnall's tubercle?**

Eisler's fat pad is a minor fat pad located superficial to and immediately above Whitnall's tubercle immediately under the orbital septum. Identifying Eisler's fat pad is one method of locating the insertion of the lateral canthal tendon.

○ **What is Bell's phenomenon?**

This is the reflex upward rotation of the globe during lid closure. This acts as a further protective mechanism of the cornea. It is present in most patients but not in all.

○ **How many fatty compartments are there in the upper eyelid? Describe them. How can they be told apart?**

There are two separate fatty pads in the upper eyelid, the nasal or medial pad and the central pad. Both reside directly under the orbital septum and superficial to the levator apparatus. The medial fatty pad is located above the medial canthus and can be identified by its whitish-yellow color. The central fatty pad is more centrally located approximating the level of the medial corneoscleral limbus and is deeper yellow in color.

○ **How many fatty compartments are there in the lower eyelid? How can they be told apart?**

In contrast to the upper eyelid, the lower eyelid has three fatty compartments; the nasal (or medial), central, and lateral fatty pads. Similarly, the medial fatty pad is more whitish-yellow in color and the other two are deeper yellow.

○ **What structure divides the medial from the central fatty pad in the lower eyelid?**

The inferior oblique muscle divides the medial from the central fatty pad in the lower eyelid. It is because of this location that it is at high risk for injury during lower lid procedures. Extreme caution should be exercised when manipulating the central or medial fatty pads to avoid injury to this extraocular muscle.

○ **What is the most commonly injured muscle in upper lid blepharoplasty?**

The superior oblique. It resides deep and medial to the medial fat pad.

○ **Describe the innervation of the orbicularis muscle.**

The differing function of the orbicularis is based on its anatomic location and is reflected in its differing nerve input.

The extracanthal orbicularis muscle is primarily responsible for purposeful, voluntary, and forceful lid closure. This portion of the muscle is innervated by branches of the frontal and zygomatic branches of the facial nerve.

The inner canthal orbicularis (that portion of the muscle in proximity to the medial canthus) is responsible for involuntary lid closure and blinking. This muscle is primarily driven by buccal branch innervation. Injury to the buccal branch or inner canthal orbicularis can severely affect proper lid function and corneal lubrication and protection. The extracanthal orbicularis is more expendable.

○ **What is the difference between *blepharochalasis* and *dermatochalasis*?**

Blepharochalasis is characterized by intermittent inflammation of the eyelid with exacerbations and remissions of eyelid edema. This process results in a stretching and subsequent atrophy of the eyelid tissue and over time recurrent episodes and aged appearance. There is typically no associated pain or erythema and it primarily affects young women. *Dermatochalasis* is defined as an excess of skin of the eyelids that is congenital or age related.

○ **What are three common presenting findings in upper lid ptosis?**

Depressed lid position, brow strain, and a high-riding or absent lid crease.

○ **What are the degrees of levator function?**

Levator function is expressed as the distance between excursion of upper lid margin from full down gaze to full up gaze without brow movement. Excellent (>10 mm), good (8–10 mm), fair (5–7 mm), or poor (1–4 mm). The proper procedure for ptosis repair is often based on levator function.

○ **What are the common methods of ptosis repair?**

Fasanella–Servat procedure is an example of a transconjunctival approach to ptosis repair. Levator advancement is an example of open transcutaneous ptosis repair. Lid suspension to the brow with either fascia or a silicone sling is an example of a procedure used for severe ptosis with minimal levator function.

○ **What are the differences between the Asian eyelid and the Occidental eyelid?**

Asian eyelids are marked by the presence of epicanthal folds and lack of pretarsal show. The lid crease is significantly lower relative to the ciliary margin than that of Caucasian eyelids (4–6 mm compared with 8–10 mm). The insertion of the orbital septum relative to the tarsus is lower in Asian eyelids, thus periorbital fat is typically seen lower in the eyelid and closer to the lid crease compared with Caucasians. The Asian lid crease may or may not obscure the medial canthus.

○ **What are the goals of Asian eyelid surgery?**

The "double eyelid surgery" focuses on establishing a modicum of visible pretarsal lid and developing a lid fold that is seen separately from the lid margin, preserving the epicanthal fold. Incisions are made within the lid at the desired level of fold creation, excess fat is removed, and fixation sutures are placed to control the height of the lid crease. It is critical to maintain a low lid crease and the epicanthal fold, lest a Caucasian eyelid result occurs.

○ **What are the surgical options for minimal upper lid ptosis repair with good levator function?**

For minimal ptosis, Müeller muscle conjunctival resection or the Fasanella–Servat procedure is proposed.

○ **What are the options for moderate ptosis with fair levator function?**

Shortening of the levator palpebrae or levator muscle advancement is proposed.

○ **What is the treatment for severe ptosis with poor levator function?**

For severe ptosis with a levator function <5 mm, a brow/frontalis suspension is indicated.

● ● ● RECONSTRUCTION ● ● ●

○ **What are the fundamental dictums of eyelid reconstruction?**

Reconstruction of any lid defect must take into account *lining, support,* and *coverage. Lining* refers to the conjunctiva that will protect the cornea, *support* refers to the rigid tarsus and medial and lateral canthal tendons, and *coverage* is the skin and muscle that cover everything. Basically, the three lamellar layers of the eyelid are considered and each one must be accounted for in the reconstruction.

○ **How are lid defects of less than 25% of the total lid width repaired?**

In general, upper and lower eyelid defects that are less than 25% the total width of the lid can be repaired by primary closure. It is important that portion of the defect that contains the tarsal plate be made at a right angle relative to the ciliary margin. This will facilitate a closure that minimizes any contour irregularity or notching along the lid margin. The remaining portion of the defect outside the tarsus is managed based on the presentation. In cases with poor lower lid laxity, consideration must be given to a concomitant lid support procedure such as a canthopexy or canthoplasty.

○ **How are lid defects between 25% and 50% of the total lid width repaired?**

Lid defects between 25% and 50% the total length of the lid must incorporate the import or rotation of new tissue for reconstruction. Primary lid closure is not feasible in these situations. An assessment must be made as to whether the defect is "shallow and wide" or "deep and narrow." Shallow and wide defects of the lower eyelid can often be repaired by recruitment of lower eyelid and midface tissue, similar to vertical vector aesthetic lower lid procedures. Deep and narrow defects of the lower eyelid will require rotation and advancement of laterally based tissue. For the lower eyelid, a Tenzel flap, a laterally based rotation advancement flap, is commonly used. Lateral canthal support must be performed as well. A common flap for the upper eyelid is the Tripier flap, an axially based upper eyelid myocutaneous flap.

○ **How are lid defects that are greater than 50% of total lid length repaired?**

Shallow and wide defects of the lower eyelid may still be reconstructed with midface advancement although a cartilage graft is often needed to reconstruct the tarsal plate. Lateral canthal support must also be performed with intact tissue or imported tissue in the form of the graft or local tissue such as a turn over temporal fascial flap or turn over lateral orbital wall periosteal flap. Total eyelid reconstruction requires a "lid-sharing" technique; a Hewes flap (from the upper lid) to reconstruct the lower eyelid or a Cutler-Beard flap (from the lower eyelid) to reconstruct the upper eyelid.

○ **What is a *Hewes* flap? What is a *Hughes* flap?**

These are both conjunctival lid-sharing flaps from the upper eyelid that include a portion of the tarsal plate. These flaps are best for wide and deep lower lid defects, typically greater than 5 mm in height. The Hewes flap preserves an attachment to the lateral canthal tendon when needed for lower lid reconstruction (best for defects that include the lateral aspect of the lower lid); the Hughes flap does not, it is purely the tarsus and the conjunctiva, no canthal tendon. (A helpful way to differentiate the two, Hewes with an "e" like tendon with an "e.") These flaps are maintained on their upper lid pedicle for 4 to 6 weeks before separation and inset. Both of these flaps will require some sort of coverage by either a rotational flap or a skin graft.

○ **What is a *Cutler-Beard* flap?**

This is a full-thickness flap of skin, muscle, conjunctiva, and/or cartilage from the lower lid used to reconstruct large full-thickness upper lid defects. This lid-sharing flap is maintained on its lower lid pedicle for 4 to 6 weeks before separation and inset.

○ **What is a Mustardé flap?**

This is medially based facial flap utilized for very large lower lid and malar defects that cannot be reconstructed with the above-listed techniques. A Mustardé flap is a large rotation advancement flap made up of the entire cheek and lower face. The releasing incision is made over the zygomatic arch, continues caudally in front of the ear, and extends down into the neck where the back cut is made.

• • • UPPER LID COSMETIC • • •

○ **What is an "A-frame" deformity?**

The A-frame deformity can be the result of aging or aggressive periorbital fat removal in the upper eyelid. The youthful upper eyelid has a smooth arched contour. The A-frame deformity is a peak-shaped depression of the medial portion of the upper eyelid similar to an A-frame, or two segments meeting at a right angle, thus disrupting the smooth arch. Hollowing of the upper eyelid from age-related fat atrophy or overresection of the medial aspect of the central fat pad can lead to an A-frame deformity.

○ **Describe the anatomic features that make up the upper lid crease.**

The upper lid crease is a result of the dermal insertion of the tarso-levator muscle as it terminates and inserts onto the tarsal plate. Fibers extend from the upper aspect of the tarsal plate, penetrate the pretarsal orbicularis, and terminate on the dermis of the eyelid skin. The location of these fibers extending into the dermis determines the location of the lid crease.

○ **How are the central and medial fatty pads of the upper lid identified?**

The central and medial fatty pads of the upper eyelid reside deep to the orbital septum. Interpad septae separate the two and they differ in color, the medial fatty pad is a pale whitish-yellow and the central fat pad is straw yellow in color.

○ **What is the open sky technique in upper lid blepharoplasty?**

This describes a method of upper lid blepharoplasty that removes excess skin, muscle, and orbital septum en bloc.

○ **Describe the general principles behind upper lid markings for blepharoplasty.**

In general, markings are made to preserve the upper lid crease and levator attachments to the dermis, preserve adequate skin for eyelid closure, and maintain a smooth fold arch. The actual amount of skin and muscle removed from each lid may differ based on patient presentation so it is important to remember that markings are often based on *what skin is left behind* rather than what skin is removed. In general, the skin resected medially is done more conservatively while one can remove more skin laterally.

○ **Can an upper lid blepharoplasty and a ptosis repair be done at the same time?**

Yes, this is considered a transcutaneous ptosis repair. After the removal of the excess skin and muscle, the tarsal plate and levator muscle can be readily exposed and repaired by tarso-levator advancement.

○ **What is lagophthalmos and how is it avoided during blepharoplasty?**

Lagophthalmos is an inability to close the eyelid fully. This increases the risk of corneal exposure and damage. There are three main causes associated with eyelid surgery:

1. excessive upper lid skin removal

2. injury to the buccal branch of the facial nerve that innervates the inner canthal orbicularis muscle responsible for blinking

3. poor lateral canthal support resulting in fish mouth eyelid closure

These complications are avoided by:

1. careful measurement of upper eyelid markings prior to resection and preserving a critical amount of upper lid skin

2. avoiding dissection within the soft tissues of the lower lid medial to the level of the medial corneoscleral limbus

3. performing canthoplasty/pexy and proper lateral canthal support in open lower lid procedures

○ **Can a protruding upper medial fatty pad be treated without incising the lid skin?**

Yes, by performing a transconjunctival upper lid blepharoplasty. This technique accesses the upper medial fat pad through an upper lid conjunctival incision above and medial to the medial horn of the tarsal plate. This procedure is indicated in the patient without upper lid skin excess but a bulging medial fat pad alone.

● ● ● **LOWER LID COSMETIC** ● ● ●

○ **What type of patient will get the best result from a transconjunctival lower lid blepharoplasty?**

Transconjunctival lower lid blepharoplasty addresses excess periorbital fat by means of fat resection and/or fat redraping. The best candidates to have only their fat addressed are typically younger patients who have fat protrusion with normal skin tone and minimal wrinkles, and normal lid tone and lid position. In addition, a transconjunctival approach can be combined with a skin pinch on the surface or skin resurfacing by means of chemical peel or laser.

○ **What layers in what order are transected during a transconjunctival lower lid blepharoplasty in order to reach the orbital fat?**

Beginning from the conjunctiva the layers are as follows: lid conjunctiva, capsulopalpebral fascia, and orbital septum. The preseptal approach is preferred as more precise fat resection can be performed and the fat does not obstruct the view and access to orbital rim. In the direct approach, the capsulopalpebral fascia and septum are bypassed and the lower lid retractors are divided to directly access the periorbital fat.

○   **What are the benefits of the lower lid transconjunctival approach?**

No visible external scar, quick recovery, less risk for complications such as lower lid malposition (Fig. 78-1).

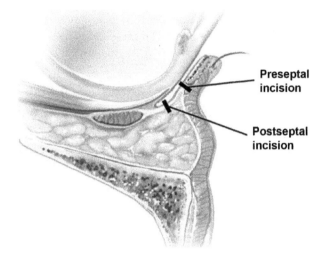

Figure 78-1 Reproduced with permission from Nahai F. *The Art of Aesthetic Surgery: Principles & Techniques*. St Louis, MO: Quality Medical Publishing, Inc.; 2005:729.

○   **What are the limits of the lower lid transconjunctival approach?**

Only effective at fat removal or repositioning. Can be a challenging dissection. Will not treat the skin. Access to the lateral fat pad can be difficult.

○   **What are the findings that indicate a lower lid blepharoplasty patient who is at high risk for postoperative lid malposition?**

Lower lid laxity (displacement of the lid more than 10 mm from the globe), poor snap test, exophthalmos, prior lid surgery, scleral show, Grave's disease, negative vector midface. If these findings are present, canthal anchoring is considered <u>mandatory</u> during lower lid blepharoplasty.

○   **What are some of the non-surgical options for lower lid rejuvenation?**

Fine crepe like lines, that in general do not respond well to surgery can be improved significantly with chemical peels or laser resurfacing. Lower lid fatty pad prominence and a deep periorbital groove can be treated with hyaluronic acid gel fillers. The younger the patient and the less overall signs of ageing around the eyelid, the more effective the nonsurgical options are.

○   **What is a skin-muscle flap and how is it developed during a lower lid procedure?**

The skin-muscle flap refers to the flap of lower eyelid skin and underlying orbicularis muscle that is elevated to access the orbital septum and orbital fat. The easiest method to dissect and develop the skin muscle flap is through a subciliary lid incision preserving pretarsal orbicularis and staying within the preseptal plane. This dissection can be brought to the level of the orbital septum and further into the midface if indicated. A portion of the skin and muscle is typically resected during lower lid blepharoplasty to achieve an aesthetic result.

○ **What is the orbitomalar ligament and what is achieved by releasing it?**

The orbitomalar ligament is a dense extension of fibers from the periosteum of the orbital rim that extends to and through the orbicularis muscle and terminates in the dermis of the overlying lid skin. It is the landmark demarcation between the lower lid and the midface. Releasing the orbitomalar ligament enhances lower lid skin and muscle mobility in a cephalad vector, blunts the lid cheek junction, facilitates reduction of malar festoons, accommodates fat redraping, and provides a gateway to the midface.

○ **What is the difference between a *canthoplasty* and a *canthopexy*?**

Both of these are suture techniques employed to strengthen the lateral canthus and support the lower eyelid, both terms are also referred to as canthal anchors. A *canthopexy* is a tightening lateral canthal anchoring procedure that corrects laxity of the lateral canthal tendon without tendon release or partial resection. A *canthoplasty* is a more aggressive means of lateral canthal anchoring that involves division of the lateral canthal tendon and/or lower lid margin shortening by wedge resection with permanent repositioning.

○ **Where is the correct placement for a canthopexy/plasty suture?**

A lateral canthal anchor suture used in canthoplasty or canthopexy should result in proper lid position, lid tension, and lid shape. Most often the suture should be placed several millimeters deep to the surface of the orbital rim on the inner aspect of the lateral orbital wall within the periosteum at the mid-pupillary line (this approximates the location of Whitnall's tubercle). Slight alterations to this position are made for enopthalmos and exophthalmos. The bite on the lid margin is within the posterior lamella where the tarsal plate and canthal tendon reside.

○ **How is "fat redistribution" performed and what are its benefits?**

When transposition of eyelid fat is indicated, periorbital fat must be released from the overlying orbital septum and interpad septa. During dissection it is important to keep the pedicle to the fat intact. The fat is then positioned into the desired location (i.e., over the orbital rim or into the tear trough) and secured based on the surgeon's preference. Options for securing the fat included suturing to the periosteum, suturing to the local fascia or muscle, or transcutaneous sutures that are clipped later.

○ **When fat resection is performed, how does the surgeon know when to stop?**

Fat resection in the lower eyelid is indicated if there is a significant excess of fat and there is no plan to transpose the fat over the rim. In these cases, medial, central, and lower eyelid fat should be treated so that a smooth contour is achieved in the final result. A safe point at which fat resection is adequate enough to achieve a desirable result is to contour the fat level with the inferior orbital rim. Excessive fat removal can lead to orbital hollowing.

○ **How are retrobulbar hematomas diagnosed?**

Retrobulbar hematoma is a rare complication of blepharoplasty caused by bleeding deep to the orbital septum that occurs within the rigid enclosure of the bony orbit. A small amount of blood in a small rigid space can cause symptoms and severe damage rapidly. Patients with retrobulbar hematomas typically complain of rapid onset, worsening, severe, and lancinating pain in the globe and orbit. This is often associated with severe proptosis and diminished visual acuity. As compression on the central retinal artery and optic nerve progresses, temporary or permanent blindness can occur. Such complaints are assumed to be and treated as a retrobulbar hematoma until proven otherwise.

○ **How are retrobulbar hematomas treated?**

Ideally a retrobulbar hematoma is diagnosed early and treated as an emergency. Patients with retrobulbar hematomas typically complain of rapid onset, worsening, severe, lancinating pain in the globe and orbit. Any complaints in the postoperative time period of increasing pain, proptosis, and loss of vision should be considered and treated as a retrobulbar hematoma until proven otherwise.

Treatment involves immediate release of the sutures, canthotomy, operative exploration, evacuation of blood, proper hemostasis, control of hypertension, and intravenous corticosteroids and acetazolamide to decrease swelling. Strongly consider ophthalmologic consultation to assess vision and the globe. Once the situation is under control, the canthus and surface incisions can be closed.

○ **What are the potential causes of diplopia or blurry vision after eyelid surgery?**

There are many potential causes of double vision or blurry vision after eyelid surgery: periorbital swelling, dry eyes, ophthalmic ointments, permanent or temporary injury of the extraocular muscles (principally the superior oblique or inferior oblique muscles), corneal exposure, corneal abrasion, and infection. Persistent diplopia or blurry vision (lasting more than 3–4 weeks) deserves a formal workup and consultation with an ophthalmologist.

○ **What is chemosis and how is it treated?**

Chemosis is an inflammatory edematous phenomenon that occurs within the scleral portion of the conjunctiva of the globe. Akin to a blister, chemosis is believed to be the result of local trauma, exposure, and temporary lymphatic drainage obstruction secondary to eyelid surgery. Treatment options include topical steroid containing drops or ointments, lubricating compounds, tarsorrhaphy sutures, patching and compression, and conjunctivectomy.

○ **How is lower lid malposition or ectropion acutely treated?**

Mainly taping and massage, tarsorrhaphy sutures in severe cases with exposure and lack of Bell's phenomenon. Application of obliquely oriented strips of tape can offer some support to the lateral canthus and oppose the cicatricial force causing the ectropion. Massage helps reduce swelling that affects lid position and function. More advanced management options include injections of dilute triamcinolone and 5-flurouracil to control and slow down the internal scar process, and injections of hyaluronic acid gels fillers to create an internal support structure for the lower lid.

○ **How is persistent lid malposition or ectropion treated?**

This is variable based on the degree of malposition. Options range from canthopexy/plasty alone, canthopexy/plasty and spacer graft, or canthopexy/plasty and spacer graft and midface recruitment. In the severe or recurrent cases, a fascial sling, skin graft, or local flaps may be needed. The Patipa finger displacement test can be used to help decide which procedures may be necessary.

● ● ● **REFERENCES** ● ● ●

Codner MA, Wolfli JN, Anzarut A. Primary transcutaneous lower blepharoplasty with routine lateral canthal support. a comprehensive 10-year review. *Plast Reconstr Surg.* 2008;121(1):241–250.

Difrancesco LM, Codner MA, McCord CD. Upper eyelid reconstruction. *Plast Reconstr Surg.* 2004;114(7):98e–107e.

Eser Y, Potochy J, Spira M, Shenaq SM. *A Differential Approach to the Midface Lift: An Anatomic and Clinical Study.* Seattle, WA: 81st Annual Meeting of the American Association of Plastic Surgeons; 2002.

Finsterer J. Ptosis: causes, presentation, and management. *Aesthetic Plast Surg.* 2003;27:193–204.

Glatt HJ. Transconjunctival flap supplementation: an approach to the reconstruction of large lower eyelid defects. *Ophthal Plast Reconstr Surg.* 1997;13:90–97.

Jacobs S. Prophylactic lateral canthopexy in lower blepharoplasties. *Arch Facial Plast Surg.* 2003;5:267–271.

Jelks G, Jelks E. Blepharoplasty. In: Peck GC, ed. *Complications and Problems in Plastic Surgery.* 5th ed. New York, NY: Gower Medical Publishing; 1992:18–19.

Lelli GR, Lisman RD. Blepharoplasty complications. *Plast Reconstr Surg.* 2010;125(3):1007–1017.

McCord C, Nahai FR, Codner MA, Nahai F, Hester TR. Use of porcine acellular dermal matrix (Enduragen) grafts in eyelids: a review of 69 patients and 129 eyelids. *Plast Reconstr Surg.* 2008;122(4):1206–1213.

McCord CD Jr, Ellis DS. The correction of lower lid malposition following lower lid blepharoplasty. *Plast Reconstr Surg.* 1993;92(6): 1068–1072.

Pacella SJ, Nahai FR, Nahai F. Transconjunctival blepharoplasty for upper and lower eyelids. *Plast Reconstr Surg.* 2010;125(1):384–392.

Patipa M. Transblepharoplasty lower eyelid and midface rejuvenation: part I. Avoiding complications by utilizing lessons learned from the treatment of complications. *Plast Reconstr Surg.* 2004;113(5):1459–1468.

Patipa M. Transblepharoplasty lower eyelid and midface rejuvenation: part II. Functional applications of midface elevation. *Plast Reconstr Surg.* 2004;113(5):1469–1474.

Shin YH, Hwang K. Cosmetic lateral canthoplasty. *Aesthetic Plast Surg.* 2004;28:317–320.

Tyers AG, Collin JRO. Levator aponeurotic repair. In: *Colour Atlas of Ophthalmic Plastic Surgery.* Oxford: Butterworth-Heinemann, 1998:130–139.

Weinfeld AB, Burke R, Codner MA. The comprehensive management of chemosis following cosmetic lower blepharoplasty. *Plast Reconstr Surg.* 2008;122(2):579–586.

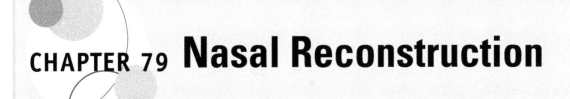

CHAPTER 79 Nasal Reconstruction

Brian M. Parrett, MD and
Julian J. Pribaz, MD

○ **What are the aesthetic subunits of the nose and what is the subunit principle?**

The alae, the columella, the soft triangles, the tip, the sidewalls, and the dorsum. The basic tenet of the subunit theory explains that if a defect encompasses more than 50% of a given subunit, a better aesthetic result will be achieved by complete excision and replacement of the subunit with suitable tissue.

○ **What are the differences in skin quality between the different nasal subunits?**

The skin of the dorsum and sidewalls tends to be thin and smooth, whereas the skin of the tip and alae is denser and more sebaceous.

○ **What are the three principles that guide reconstruction of any full-thickness nasal defect?**

A satisfactory reconstruction must provide nasal **lining**, structural **framework (cartilage or bone)**, and aesthetically appropriate skin **coverage**.

○ **What are the potential donor sites for full-thickness skin grafting of nasal defects and why are skin grafts not the best treatment option for most nasal defects?**

Preauricular, postauricular, and supraclavicular skin provide the best color and quality match for nasal skin. Skin grafts can result in color and contour deformities and the possibility of secondary contracture in the nose.

○ **What nasal regions have the best and worst aesthetic results when allowed to heal by secondary intention?**

The best results with secondary intention are on the medial canthal area and glabella. The worst results are on the nasal tip.

○ **What are common donor sites for reconstructing the cartilaginous and bony framework of the nose?**

The nasal septum, auricular conchal cartilage, and rib cartilage provide cartilage grafts. For bone grafts, split cranial (from the parietal skull), rib or iliac crest may be used.

○ **What are the best methods to prevent cartilage warping?**

Perichondrium should be removed from nasal cartilage grafts to prevent warping or curling. To prevent warping, the cartilage graft should be designed symmetrically and allowed to sit at least 30 minutes prior to insertion.

○ **What is the blood supply to the dorsal nasal flap and what nasal regions can it reconstruct best?**

The angular artery (terminal segment of the facial artery) provides blood supply to this flap. The dorsal nasal flap is best used for midline dorsal defects less than 2.0 cm.

○ **What are the two most versatile local flaps for reconstruction of the ala?**

The bilobed flap is best used for defects less than or equal to 1.5 cm in diameter and the nasolabial flap is best used for defects >1.5 to 3 cm in diameter. In addition, central tip and medial defects are more likely treated with a bilobed flap and lateral alar defects are more likely treated with a staged nasolabial flap.

○ **What are the two best options for reconstruction of a full-thickness alar rim defect?**

A composite graft from the ear for defects less than 1.5 cm and a staged nasolabial flap for defects greater than 1.5 cm.

○ **What are key steps in the use of composite grafts?**

The graft recipient site should ideally be allowed to heal by secondary intention prior to graft placement. The defect is then recreated with the goal to maximize graft contact with vascularized tissue, that is, turnover of scar tissue. The graft should be designed so that no portion is greater than 1 cm from a vascularized recipient site wound edge. Postoperative cooling with iced saline compresses over the graft can improve survival.

○ **How do you best design a bilobed flap and what is the total rotation?**

A proper design, known as the Zitelli modification, should limit the total rotation about the pivot point to 90 to 100 degrees (45–50 degrees per lobe), with the smaller second flap placed in the loose skin of the nasal dorsum or sidewall (Fig. 79-1).

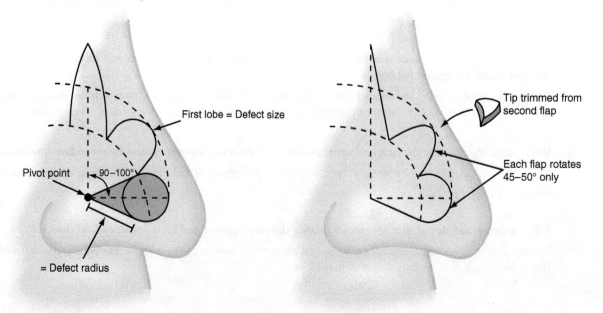

Figure 79-1 Zitelli's design for the bilobed flap. A triangular excision is needed between the pivot point and the defect to avoid dog-ear formation. Diameter of first lobe is equal to that of the defect; the second lobe is made smaller. Wide undermining just above the periosteum is needed keeping the nasal muscles within the flaps; avoid subcutaneous dissection.

○   **What is the blood supply of the nasolabial flap?**

Tributaries of the facial artery and its angular branch, which perforate the levator labii muscle near the ala and radiate across the cheek. The flap can be inferiorly or superiorly (more common) based and often requires two stages (division 3 weeks later).

○   **What is the ideal donor tissue for larger defects of the nasal tip and alae?**

A forehead flap is best used for defects >3 cm, especially when multiple subunits are involved.

○   **What is the blood supply of the forehead flap and when should the second stage (division and inset) be performed?**

The supraorbital and supratrochlear arteries provide blood supply; the commonly used paramedian forehead flap is supplied by the supratrochlear vessels primarily. The supratrochlear vessels exit the orbit over the periosteum, pass through corrugator muscles and, 2 cm above the supraorbital rim, pierce the frontalis muscle and then run vertically in subcutaneous fat close to the dermis. The second stage (flap division) should be performed 3 to 4 weeks after the first stage.

○   **What are the stages of, and the advantages of, the three-stage forehead flap?**

Many surgeons are now using the three-stage forehead flap. The first stage is forehead flap elevation and inset with minimal to no flap thinning. The second stage 3 to 4 weeks later involves re-elevating the distal flap, thinning it considerably, and shaping the underlying framework with addition of cartilage grafts if needed. The third stage is division of the pedicle and flap inset 3 to 4 weeks after the second stage. This is useful in smokers or in major (near total) nasal reconstructions as no flap thinning in the first stage avoids flap necrosis and contour irregularities. In full-thickness defects, it allows skin graft placement or a folded flap for lining reconstruction in the first stage and then cartilage graft placement in the second stage.

○   **What is the approach for an adequately sized forehead flap that leaves too large a forehead defect for primary closure?**

The donor site defect can be easily treated with healing by secondary intention with dressing changes. Do not place a skin graft as it leads to poor aesthetic results.

○   **When must framework be supplied?**

Anytime the inherent cartilaginous architecture of the nose is compromised.

○   **The alar wings do not normally contain cartilage; why must they be supported by cartilage when reconstructed?**

To resist the centripetal contractile forces of a healing tissue flap and subsequent alar notching and retraction.

○   **What are the principles guiding selection of adequate nasal lining?**

Adequate vascular supply, sufficient pliability to conform to a concave contour, and appropriate thinness to avoid airway obstruction.

○ **What are options for nasal lining?**

Redundant skin folded over from the coverage flap, skin graft on the undersurface of a flap, mucoperichondrial flaps from the septum, rotational or advancement flaps from residual vestibular lining, facial artery musculomucosal flaps, or free flaps for larger defects.

○ **What is the blood supply to the septal mucoperichondrial flaps?**

When based inferiorly, a septal branch of the superior labial artery that enters the nasal septum lateral to the nasal spine provides blood supply. The hinge flap design is based on the dorsum of the septum and supplied via the anterior ethmoidal vessels.

○ **What is the role of free microvascular tissue transfer in nasal reconstruction?**

Free flaps (mainly the radial forearm) are used for total or subtotal, multilayered nasal reconstruction. In this scenario, free flaps are used for nasal lining in the first stage. Although quite bulky, the robust vascular supply of the free flap results in negligible contraction of the tissue, which is carefully thinned in subsequent procedures and then covered with cartilage grafts and a forehead flap for skin coverage. Burget and Walton have detailed their work in the difficult area of subtotal or total nasal reconstruction.

• • • REFERENCES • • •

Burget GC, Menick FJ. The subunit principle in nasal reconstruction. *Plast Reconstr Surg.* 1985;76:239–247.

Burget GC, Walton RL. Optimal use of microvascular free flaps, cartilage grafts, and a paramedian forehead flap for aesthetic reconstruction of the nose and adjacent facial units. *Plast Reconstr Surg.* 2007;120:1171–1207.

Menick FJ. Nasal reconstruction. *Plast Reconstr Surg.* 2010;125:138e–150e.

Parrett BM, Pribaz JJ. An algorithm for treatment of nasal defects. *Clin Plast Surg.* 2009;36:407–420.

Zitelli JA. The bilobed flap for nasal reconstruction. *Arch Dermatol.* 1989;125:957–959.

CHAPTER 80

Mandibular Reconstruction

Melissa M. Poh, MD and
Matthew M. Hanasono, MD

* * * **GENERAL** * * *

○ **What is the anatomy of the mandible?**

The mandible consists of two bony halves fused in the midline (symphysis). Each hemimandible consists of a condyle, neck, ramus, angle, and body. The masseter, temporalis, and medial pterygoid muscles close the mouth.

The lateral pterygoid muscle protracts the mandible and opens the mouth. The digastric, mylohyoid, geniohyoid, and genioglossus muscles also help open the mouth.

○ **What is the blood supply to the mandible?**

The inferior alveolar artery, which is a terminal branch of the maxillary artery. It courses within the mandible along with the inferior alveolar nerve. The mandibular periosteum also provides additional blood supply.

○ **What nerve supplies sensation to the mandible?**

The inferior alveolar nerve, which enters the mandible on the lingual side of the ramus through the mandibular foramen. It travels through the mandible supplying sensation to the teeth, then a branch (mental nerve) exits the mandible at the mental foramen to supply sensation to the lower lip. Lower lip cancers can invade the mandible by perineural spread along the mental and inferior alveolar nerves, in addition to involving the mandible by direct extension.

○ **What is the function of the mandible?**

The mandible is essential for normal mastication, swallowing, and speech. It also sets the proportions and aesthetic contours of the lower face.

○ **What are the goals of mandibular reconstruction?**

1. Reestablish facial balance and symmetry.

2. Create a surface for mastication or dental restoration.

3. Prevent deviation of jaw leading to malocclusion.

4. Provide a stable wound that does not result in orocutaneous fistula.

○ **What are the common indications for mandibular reconstruction?**

1. Primary bone tumor (e.g., osteosarcoma).

2. Tumor involving adjacent structures (e.g., squamous cell carcinoma of floor of the mouth).

3. Osteoradionecrosis.

4. Traumatic defects.

○ **What is the most common malignancy involving the mandible?**

Squamous cell carcinoma arising from the oral mucosa and invading the mandibular bone is the most common malignancy.

○ **What is ameloblastoma?**

Ameloblastoma is the most common odontogenic tumor. It is a locally aggressive, slow-growing epithelial neoplasm. The tumor is painless and causes gradual jaw expansion producing facial asymmetry. It is usually benign although rare malignant variants exist.

○ **What are the options for mandibular reconstruction?**

1. Vascularized bony flaps such as a free fibular, iliac crest, scapula, or radial forearm osseous or osteocutaneous flap.

2. Pedicled pectoralis major muscle flap with or without reconstruction plate, or rib graft.

3. Nonvascularized bone graft.

4. Soft-tissue free flaps such as anterolateral thigh flap, rectus abdominis myocutaneous.

5. Primary closure.

○ **When can nonvascularized bone grafts be used in mandibular reconstruction?**

In small (<5 cm) isolated bony defects with good soft-tissue coverage and no history or need for radiation.

○ **What are the most common complications associated with the use of a reconstruction plate and soft tissue?**

1. Plate exposure.

2. Plate fracture or fatigue.

3. Screw loosening.

4. Infection.

○ **What are the major risk factors of reconstruction plate extrusion?**

1. Anterior location.

2. Pre- or postoperative radiation.

○ **What is the Andy Gump deformity?**

Resection of the anterior segment of the mandible, which leads to loss of oral competence, difficulties with speech and mastication and loss of chin projection.

○ **When might soft-tissue flaps be considered for mandibular reconstruction?**

1. Posterior/lateral defects.

2. Sick or elderly patients who cannot tolerate a lengthy operation.

3. No bony options because of previous surgery/trauma or medical comorbidities.

○ **What are the typical pedicle lengths for the fibula, iliac crest, and scapula flaps?**

1. Fibula: 6 to 8 cm, but can be lengthened if fibula is removed from proximal pedicle.

2. Iliac crest: 6 to 8 cm.

3. Scapula: 4 cm, up to 14 cm if subscapular artery is included.

4. Radial forearm: up to 20 cm.

○ **How are the bony flaps fixed to the native mandible?**

With a reconstruction plate or miniplates. Studies have not shown any difference in rates of malunion or other complications.

○ **What are the advantages and disadvantages of use of miniplates?**

Advantages:

1. More precise application of hardware to bone flap.

2. Low profile and, therefore, avoids adding bulk to external surface of the bone.

3. Ease of selective removal should the need arise (e.g., extrusion).

4. Provides adequate stability.

Disadvantage:

1. Requires steeper learning curve to shape bone flap.

○ **What are the advantages and disadvantages of use of a reconstruction plate for flap fixation?**

Advantages:

1. Can be used as a template to help shape the bone flap.

2. Strong rigid fixation.

Disadvantages:

1. Plate can be bulky and hence palpable in patients with minimal soft-tissue coverage.

2. Stress shielding can lead to load bearing and subsequent bony resorption and osteopenia.

○ **What is the minimal length of an osteotomized segment?**

Ideally at least 1.5 cm to ensure an adequate periosteal blood supply to the segment.

○   **What is osteoradionecrosis (ORN) of the mandible?**

A necrotic wound in irradiated bone that persists for 3 to 6 months without healing. The period of highest risk for ORN is the first 3 years after radiation therapy and most cases occur at radiation doses greater than 60 Gy.

○   **What are the indications of resection and reconstruction of ORN?**

1. Pain.
2. Fistula.
3. Fracture.
4. Exposed bone.

○   **What must be excluded prior to diagnosing ORN?**

Recurrent cancer.

○   **What is the optimal method of treatment for ORN of the mandible that has failed conservative treatment?**

Resection of necrotic mandible and reconstruction with a free flap to bring well-vascularized tissue into the irradiated area.

○   **What is the role of hyperbaric oxygen in the treatment of ORN?**

The use of hyperbaric oxygen is controversial. It is frequently used to treat ORN; however, the practice is not supported by randomized clinical trials. It may be helpful for small lesions, following surgical debridement.

○   **What is bisphosphonate related osteonecrosis of the jaws (BRONJ)?**

Similar to ORN, patients who receive intravenous bisphosphonate for cancer or, much less commonly, oral bisphosphonates for osteoporosis, are at risk for developing necrosis of the mandible and maxilla.

○   **What is the pathophysiology of BRONJ?**

Although not completely understood, bisphosphonates are known to cause apoptosis of mature osteoclasts and osteoclast progenitor cells as well as strongly inhibit osteoblastic activity and cause a reduction in bone vascularity. The net effect appears to be an overall reduction in bone resorption and turnover, but also a reduced ability to heal, possibly resulting in osteonecrosis in some patients.

○   **How is BRONJ treated?**

Early-stage BRONJ is treated with oral hygiene care, antibiotic mouthwash, and oral antibiotics. Many patients respond to this treatment. Once BRONJ becomes advanced, with pathologic fracture, fistula, or osteolysis extending to the inferior mandibular border, surgical debridement or mandibular resection is indicated.

○ **What are some options for reconstructing composite mandibular defects that include a through-and-through cheek defect (see Figs. 80-1 to 80-3)?**

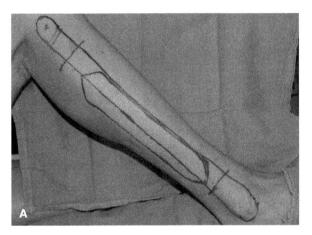

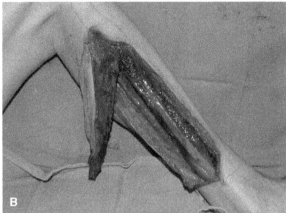

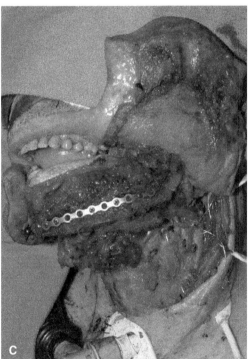

Figure 80-1 Right fibula osteocutaneous free-flap skin markings (**A**), and completed harvest (**B**) showing preservation of 7 cm of proximal and distal bone and design of skin paddle centered over the posterior border of the fibula, where the perforating blood vessel emerges from the posterior intermuscular septum. Fibula free flap after osteotomies, inset, and fixation with a titanium reconstruction plate for a mandibular defect (**C**).

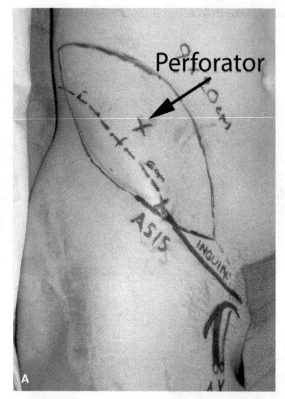

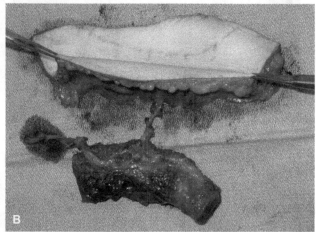

Figure 80-2 Iliac crest osteocutaneous free-flap skin markings (**A**), and completed harvest (**B**) showing outline of skin paddle over first perforator and harvest of bone beginning at or just lateral to the anterior superior iliac spine (ASIS).

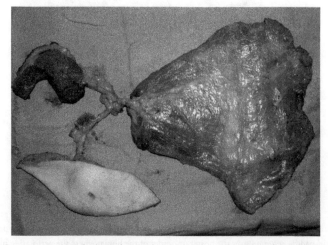

Figure 80-3 A chimeric free flap including scapular bone, latissimus dorsi muscle, and parascapular skin flaps all based on the subscapular artery and vein.

1. Combine a fibula osteocutaneous free flap with a pectoralis major myocutaneous pedicled flap (PMC).

2. Combine a fibula osteocutaneous free flap with a second soft-tissue free flap, such as the anterolateral thigh (ALT) free flap.

3. Use a 2-skin paddle fibula free flap based on separate cutaneous perforators arising from the peroneal artery.

4. Use a chimeric fibula free flap and soleus muscle free flap, both based on the peroneal artery (the soleus muscle can be skin grafted or allowed to mucosalize spontaneously if used to close the intraoral defect).

5. Use of a chimeric free flap based on the subscapular system (e.g., scapular bone–parascapular cutaneous–latissimus dorsi myocutaneous chimeric free flap) or the deep circumflex iliac artery system (e.g., iliac crest osteocutaneous–internal oblique muscle free flap).

○ **What are the options of condylar reconstruction?**

1. Excise and reinsert the native condyle as a nonvascularized graft as long as the condyle is disease free.

2. Shape the end of fibular segment, cover it with excess periosteum or fascia, and insert it into the joint.

3. Free medial femoral condyle flap.

4. Use a costochondral graft.

5. Prosthetic condyle.

6. No reconstruction.

○ **What is the risk of condylar implants?**

1. Erosion into the middle cranial fossa.

2. Joint dislocation.

3. Sensorineural hearing loss due to migration of the prosthesis into the epitympanum, resulting in destruction of the cochlea.

○ **Who is a candidate for primary osseointegration?**

Patients who undergo vascularized bony reconstruction for trauma, benign tumors, osteomyelitis, ORN or low-malignancy tumors that do not require postoperative radiation.

○ **What is the minimum width of bone required for dental implants?**

6 mm. At least 1 mm of healthy bone must surround the implant to ensure adequate osseointegration.

○ **What is the minimum vertical bone height for dental implants?**

7 to 10 mm.

○ **Which bony flaps can be used for osseointegrated implants?**

Fibula, iliac crest, and scapula.

○ **How are computer-aided design and computer-generated models useful in mandibular reconstruction?**

These technologies, which involve planning bony free-flap reconstructions on a computer, then creating accurate physical models using three-dimensional printers, can help to guide the surgery. Computer-generated cutting guides can also be used to assist with osteotomy placement and custom-made titanium reconstruction plates can be manufactured, eliminating the need for plate bending. All of these technologies contribute to improving accuracy and reducing operative time in mandibular reconstruction.

• • • **FIBULA** • • •

○ **What is the blood supply to the fibula?**

Peroneal vessels, which branch off the tibioperoneal trunk.

○ **What length of bone can harvested?**

Generally, between 22 and 26 cm in an adult patient.

○ **What is the blood supply to the cutaneous portion of the osteocutaneous fibula graft?**

Perforators from the peroneal artery that travel at least partially within the posterior intermuscular septum, which separates the deep and superficial posterior compartments.

○ **Where are perforators typically located on the leg?**

Most commonly they arise within the middle third of the lower leg, though they may be located more proximal or distal.

○ **What muscles are dissected off of the fibula during harvest?**

The peroneus brevis and longus, extensor digitorum longus, extensor hallucis longus, tibialis posterior, and flexor hallucis longus muscles.

○ **What nerve can be included to provide sensation to the skin paddle of the osteocutaneous fibula flap?**

Lateral sural cutaneous nerve.

○ **What muscle can be harvested with the fibula for use in composite mandibular reconstruction?**

Soleus or flexor hallucis longus muscles.

○ **How much proximal and distal fibula should be preserved?**

1. Approximately 4 to 6 cm from the fibular head to protect the common peroneal nerve wrapping around the fibular head.
2. Approximately 6 to 8 cm proximal to the lateral malleolus to avoid ankle joint instability (Fig. 80-1).

○ **What are the contraindications to using a free fibula flap for mandibular reconstruction?**

Nonpalpable pulses in foot or other evidence on physical examination of arterial insufficiency (e.g., nonhealing ulcers, hairless, shiny skin, symptoms of claudication) and/or venous stasis (e.g., edema, purplish discoloration). If there is any question to the adequacy of blood flow to the foot, then a CT angiogram, MR angiogram, or conventional arteriogram should be obtained.

○ **Is routine preoperative angiography of the lower extremity necessary prior to harvesting a free fibula flap?**

No. Several studies demonstrate that if the patient has a normal physical examination then angiography adds no benefit and is unnecessary. However, if the patient has abnormal examination or a history of lower extremity vascular trauma, then an angiogram or CTA is justified.

○ **What is the average width of the lateral surface of the fibula?**

About 18 mm in males and 13 mm in females.

○ **What is a double-barreled fibula?**

To more closely approximate the height of the mandible (mean height of 34 mm in males and 31 mm in females), an osteotomy can be performed where the distal half is turned 180 degrees to be stacked on the proximal half.

○ **What is the donor morbidity for a fibular osteocutaneous flap?**

1. Prolonged leg swelling.

2. Paresthesias.

3. Pain after prolonged walking.

4. Difficulty in squatting.

5. Great toe stiffness or contractures.

○ **What is peronea arteria magna and what is the incidence?**

A single dominant arterial inflow to the distal lower extremity that comes from the peroneal artery. The incidence is up to 5%.

● ● ● ILIAC CREST ● ● ●

○ **What is the blood supply to the iliac crest bone flap?**

Deep circumflex iliac vessels.

○ **What is the length of bone that can be harvested from the iliac crest?**

Approximately 14 to 16 cm.

○ **What muscle can be harvested with the iliac crest?**

The internal oblique muscle supplied by the ascending branch of the DCIA. It is important to repair the muscle defect to minimize risk for postoperative hernia/bulge.

○ **What are the disadvantages to using the iliac crest for mandibular reconstruction?**

1. Relatively short pedicle length, which may necessitate use of vein grafts.

2. The skin paddle can be bulky and unreliable.

3. Donor-site morbidity including pain with ambulation, gait disturbance, lateral femoral cutaneous nerve injury, and abdominal bulges/hernia formation.

○ **How can donor site morbidity be reduced?**

Harvest a split-thickness iliac bone, taking just the inner table. Performing a perforator dissection of the blood vessels supplying the skin paddle, to minimize the amount of muscle harvested with the flap (Fig. 80-2).

● ● ● SCAPULA ● ● ●

○ **What is the blood supply to the scapula?**

Circumflex scapular artery, which branches from the subscapular artery, and supplies the lateral and medial borders of the scapula. Some authors have also described using the angular branch of the thoracodorsal artery, which supplies the scapular angle or tip.

○ **How do you find the circumflex scapular artery?**

The circumflex scapular artery travels through the triangular space, which is formed by the teres major, teres minor and the long head of the triceps muscle, and is located about two-fifths of the distance from the scapular spine to the scapular tip. It curves around the lateral scapular border, giving off several branches that supply the lateral scapular bone, before dividing into horizontal and vertical branches, which supply the scapular and parascapular cutaneous flaps. The horizontal branch also supplies the medial scapular bone, although the primary blood supply to this part of the scapula is the dorsal scapular artery.

○ **How do you find the angular artery?**

The angular artery arises from the thoracodorsal artery, usually the latissimus dorsi branch, but occasionally from the serratus anterior branch or more proximal to the branching of the thoracodorsal into these branches. It travels deep to the latissimus dorsi muscle within a fat pad to supply the scapular angle or tip.

○ **What is the bone length that can be harvested from the scapula?**

Up to 14 cm of bone can be harvested from either the lateral or the medial edge of the scapula. The lateral bone flap, which is based on the vertical branch off of the circumflex scapular artery, has a shorter pedicle but provides thick, corticocancellous bone that may be usable for dental implants. The medial bone flap, which is thinner, is based on the horizontally oriented cutaneous branch of the circumflex scapular artery and is associated with less postoperative shoulder stiffness.

○ **What is the advantage of the scapular flap?**

The ability to design several flaps based on a single vascular axis (also known as chimeric flaps). Because the subscapular artery ultimately supplies the latissimus dorsi and serratus anterior muscles (via the thoracodorsal artery) and the parascapular skin paddle and the scapular skin and bone (by the circumflex scapular artery), reconstructions using several tissue types can be performed with a chimeric flap, requiring only a single arterial and venous anastomosis (Fig. 80-3).

○ **What are the disadvantages of the scapular flap?**

The need to reposition the patient for harvest and closure of donor site prior to performing the anastomosis. Some patients may note a degree of shoulder stiffness and rotator cuff weakness.

● ● ● RADIAL FOREARM ● ● ●

○ **What is the blood supply to the radial forearm flap?**
Radial artery.

○ **What preoperative test is absolutely necessary if a radial forearm flap is planned?**
Allen's test.

○ **Between the insertions of what two muscles on the radius, should the osteotomies be made when harvesting the bone?**
The brachioradialis and the pronator teres muscles.

○ **What is the length of bone that can be harvested from the radius?**

Up to 10 cm and 40% of the cross section of the radius.

○ **What is the fracture rate with using the osteocutaneous radial forearm flap?**

12% to 20%. This rate has decreased to with the use of prophylactic plating of the radius after the bony flap is harvested.

○ **What nerve needs to be preserved during the flap harvest?**

Superficial radial nerve, which is a sensory nerve to the dorsal thumb and first finger.

○ **Where is the superficial radial nerve located?**

The superficial radial nerve is located lateral to the radial artery, beneath the brachioradialis muscle. It pierces the deep fascia about 7 cm proximal to the wrist and divides into lateral and medial branches.

○ **What is the limitation to the radial osteocutaneous forearm flap in mandibular reconstruction?**

The bone harvested is thin and cannot usually tolerate osteotomies or accept dental implants.

○ **What nerve can be included in the harvest to provide a sensate flap?**

Lateral antebrachial cutaneous nerve, which is a branch from the musculocutaneous nerve.

○ **What is the most common complication related to the donor site?**

Failure of the skin graft to take over the tendons, which can be minimized by performing a suprafascial dissection and preserving paratenon over the tendons.

● ● ● REFERENCES ● ● ●

Ang E, Black C, Irish J, et al. Reconstructive options in the treatment of osteoradionecrosis of the craniomaxillofacial skeleton. *Br J Plast Surg.* 2003;56:92–99.

Bahr W. Blood supply of small fibula segments: an experimental study on human cadavers. *J Craniomaxillofac Surg.* 1998;26:148–152.

Boyd JB, Mulholland RS, Davidson J, et al. The free flap and plate in oromandibular reconstruction: long-term review and indications. *Plast Reconstr Surg.* 1995;95:1018–1028.

Celik N, Wei FC, Chen HC, et al. Osteoradionecrosis of the mandible after oromandibular cancer surgery. *Plast Reconstr Surg.* 2002;109:1875–1881.

Chang EI, Clemens MW, Garvey PB, Skoracki RJ, Hanasono MM. Cephalometric analysis for microvascular head and neck reconstruction. *Head Neck.* 2012;34:1607–1614.

Chang YM, Santamaria E, Wei FC, et al. Primary insertion of osseointegrated dental implants into fibula osteoseptocutaneous free flap for mandibular reconstruction. *Plast Reconstr Surg.* 1998;102:680–688.

Cordeiro PG, Disa JJ, Hidalgo DA, Hu QY. Reconstruction of the mandible with osseous free flaps: a 10-year experience with 150 consecutive patients. *Plast Reconstr Surg.* 1999;104:1314–1320.

Disa JJ, Cordeiro PG. The current role of preoperative arteriography in free fibula flaps. *Plast Reconstr Surg.* 1998;102:1083–1088.

Forrest C, Boyd B, Manktelow R, Zuker R, Bowen V. The free vascularized iliac crest tissue transfer: donor site complications associated with eighty-two cases. *Br J Plast Surg.* 1992;45:89–93.

Frodel JL Jr, Funk GF, Capper DT, et al. Osseointegrated implants: a comparative study of bone thickness in four vascularized bone flaps. *Plast Reconstr Surg.* 1993;92:449–455; discussion 456–458.

Gurlek A, Miller MJ, Jacob RF, Lively JA, Schusterman MA. Functional results of dental restoration with osseointegrated implants after mandible reconstruction. *Plast Reconstr Surg.* 1998;101:650–655; discussion 656–659.

Hanasono MM, Militsakh ON, Richmon JD, Rosenthal EL, Wax MK. Mandibulectomy and free flap reconstruction for bisphosphonate-related osteonecrosis of the jaws. *JAMA Otolaryngol Head Neck Surg.* 2013;139:1135–1142.

Hanasono MM, Skoracki RJ. Computer-assisted design and rapid prototype modeling in microvascular mandible reconstruction. *Laryngoscope.* 2013;123:597–604.

Hanasono MM, Skoracki RJ. The scapular tip osseous free flap as an alternative for anterior mandibular reconstruction. *Plast Reconstr Surg.* 2010;125:164e–166e.

Hidalgo DA, Pusic AL. Free flap mandibular reconstruction: a 10-year follow-up study. *Plast Reconstr Surg.* 2002;110:438–449; discussion 450–451.

Hidalgo DA. Condyle transplantation in free flap mandible reconstruction. *Plast Reconstr Surg.* 1994;93:770–781; discussion 782–783.

Horiuchi K, Hattori A, Inada I, et al. Mandibular reconstruction using the double barrel fibular graft. *Microsurgery.* 1995;16:450–454.

Kroll SS, Robb GL, Miller MJ, Reese GP, Evans GR. Reconstruction of posterior mandibular defects with soft tissue using the rectus abdominis free flap. *Br J Plast Surg.* 1998;51:503–507.

Lutz BS, Wei FC, Ng SH, Chen IH, Chen SH. Routine donor leg angiography before vascularized free fibula transplantation is not necessary: a prospective study of 120 clinical cases. *Plast Reconstr Surg.* 1999;103:121–127.

Mariani PB, Kowalski LP, Magrin J. Reconstruction of large defects postmandibulectomy for oral cancer using plates and myocutaneous flaps: a long-term follow-up. *Int J Oral Maxillofac Surg.* 2006;35:427–432.

Militsakh ON, Werle A, Mohyuddin N, et al. Comparison of radial forearm with fibula and scapula osseocutaneous free flaps for oromandibular reconstruction. *Arch Otolaryngol Head Neck Surg.* 2005;131:571–575.

Nahabedian MY, Tufaro A, Manson PN. Improved mandible function after hemimandibulectomy, condylar head preservation, and vascularized fibular reconstruction. *Ann Plast Surg.* 2001;46:506–510.

Ohsaki M, Maruyama Y. Anatomical investigations of the cutaneous branches of the circumflex scapular artery and their communications. *Br J Plast Surg.* 1993;46:160–163.

Patel A, Maisel R. Condylar prostheses in head and neck cancer reconstruction. *Arch Otolaryngol Head Neck Surg.* 2001;127:842–846.

Robey AB, Spann ML, McAuliff TM, Meza JL, Hollins RR, Johnson PJ. Comparison of miniplates and reconstruction plates in fibular flap reconstruction of the mandible. *Plast Reconstr Surg.* 2008;122:1733–1738.

Rosson GD, Singh NK. Devascularizing complications of free fibula harvest: peronea arteria magna. *J Reconstr Microsurg.* 2005;21:533–538.

Seikaly H, Chau J, Li F, et al. Bone that best matches the properties of the mandible. *J Otolaryngol.* 2003;32:262–265.

Shpitzer T, Gullane PJ, Neligan PC, et al. The free vascularized flap and the flap plate options: comparative results of reconstruction of lateral mandibular defects. *Laryngoscope.* 2000;110:2056–2060.

Thoma A, Levis C, Young JE. Oromandibular reconstruction after cancer resection. *Clin Plast Surg.* 2005;32:361–375.

Urken ML, Buchbinder D, Costantino PD, et al. Oromandibular reconstruction using microvascular composite flaps: a report of 210 cases. *Arch Otolaryngol Head Neck Surg.* 1998;124:46–55.

Urken ML, Buchbinder D, Weinberg H, Vickery C, Sheiner A, Biller HF. Primary placement of osseointegrated implants in microvascular mandibular reconstruction. *Otolaryngol Head Neck Surg.* 1989;101:56–73.

Villaret DB, Futran NA. The indications and outcomes in the use of osseocutaneous radial forearm free flap. *Head Neck.* 2003;25:475–481.

Waits CA, Toby EB, Girod DA, Tsue TT. Osteocutaneous radial forearm free flap: long-term radiographic evaluation of donor site morbidity after prophylactic plating of radius. *J Reconstr Microsurg.* 2007;23:367–372.

Wax MK, Winslow CP, Hansen J, et al. A retrospective analysis of temporomandibular joint reconstruction with free fibula microvascular flap. *Laryngoscope.* 2000;110:977–981.

Wei FC, Celik N, Yang WG, Chen IH, Chang YM, Chen HC. Complications after reconstruction by plate and soft tissue free flap in composite mandibular defects and secondary salvage with osseocutaneous flap. *Plast Reconstr Surg.* 2003;112:37–42.

Wei FC, Chen HC, Chuang CC, Noordhoff MS. Fibular osteoseptocutaneous flap: anatomic study and clinical application. *Plast Reconstr Surg.* 1986;78:191–200.

Yu P, Chang EI, Hanasono MM. Design of a reliable skin paddle for the fibula osteocutaneous flap: perforator anatomy revisited. *Plast Reconstr Surg.* 2011;128:440–446.

Zoumalan RA, Hirsch DL, Levine JP, Saadeh PB. Plating in microvascular reconstruction of the mandible: can fixation be too rigid? *J Craniofac Surg.* 2009;20:1451–1454.

CHAPTER 81

Scalp and Calvarial Reconstruction

David M. Adelman, MD, PhD, FACS and Matthew M. Hanasono, MD

○ **What are the five layers of the scalp?**

Skin, subcutaneous fat, galea aponeurotica, loose areolar tissue, and pericranium (remembered by the mnemonic: SCALP).

○ **What fascial structure connects the frontalis muscle anteriorly to the occipitalis muscle posteriorly?**

The galea aponeurotica.

○ **What is the significance of the temporal line of the calvarium?**

It is the line along which the deep temporal fascia fuses with the pericranium.

○ **What is the pericranium?**

The pericranium is the periosteum of the calvarial bones.

○ **Which region of the scalp offers the greatest mobility?**

The parietal region, located over the temporoparietal fascia.

○ **What blood vessels supply the scalp?**

The paired supratrochlear, supraorbital, superficial temporal, posterior auricular, and occipital blood vessels.

○ **Which arteries are branches of the internal carotid artery? Which are branches of the external carotid artery?**

The supratrochlear and supraorbital arteries arise from the ophthalmic artery, which is the first branch of the internal carotid artery. The others are branches of the external carotid artery.

○ **What is the sensory innervation of the scalp?**

The paired supratrochlear (V1) and supraorbital (V1) nerves, which supply forehead and frontoparietal scalp; the zygomaticotemporal (V2) nerve, which supplies the region lateral to the brow and the temporal region; the auriculotemporal (V3) nerve, which supplies the lateral scalp; and the greater occipital (C2) and lesser occipital (C2–3) nerves, which supply the occipital region.

○ **Where are the temporal branches of the facial nerve located?**

On the deep surface of the temporoparietal fascia within the loose areolar tissue, along an imaginary line that connects the ear lobe to a point 1.5 cm above the lateral eyebrow (Pitanguy line).

○ **What are the three layers of the calvarium?**

Outer table, diploic space, and inner table.

○ **What are the bones of the calvarium, and by which process are they formed during development?**

The frontal, parietal, and temporal bones are formed by intramembranous ossification. The occipital and sphenoid bones are formed by endochondral ossification.

○ **By what age is calvarial growth complete?**

Calvarial growth is generally complete by 7 years of age.

○ **What is aplasia cutis congenita?**

Aplasia cutis congenita is a rare congenital disorder characterized by a localized absence of skin, dermal appendages, and, in some cases, subcutaneous tissues. Although it may occur anywhere on the body, the majority occurs on the scalp. In 15% to 30% of cases, aplasia cutis congenita may be associated with defects of the underlying skull or dura, exposing the brain and sagittal sinus, which can be life threatening.

○ **How is aplasia cutis congenita treated?**

The best treatment strategy remains a subject of debate. Small wounds that do not involve dura, brain, or sagittal sinus exposure can be managed conservatively with moist dressings. When the dura with enlarged veins, the brain, or the sagittal sinus are exposed, emergency coverage with skin grafts, allografts, or flap reconstruction may be indicated to prevent bleeding and infection. Many calvarial defects exhibit spontaneous bone growth, while others may need delayed cranioplasty.

○ **Do all scalp defects require reconstruction?**

No. Some partial-thickness defects may be left to heal by secondary intention. However, contracture may result, and the scar may have limited or no hair growth.

○ **What factors may preclude use of local flaps for scalp reconstruction?**

Wounds in which tension-free, broadly based flaps cannot be created. Also, prior radiation, surgery or infection, as well as tobacco use, corticosteroid use, or diabetes mellitus may result in flap loss or impaired wound healing and are relative contraindications.

○ **Which scalp wounds are most amenable to primary closure?**

Small scalp defects, usually less than 3 cm in diameter. Wide undermining is usually required since the scalp tissues have limited elasticity. Galeal scoring may be a useful adjunct.

○ **Which scalp wounds are most amenable to skin grafting?**

Those with a well-vascularized base for accepting the graft, such as those with intact fascia or pericranium.

○ **How can skin graft survival onto calvarial bone be improved?**

Burring of the outer table until the vascularized diploic space is reached. Galeal, temporoparietal fascia, or pericranial flaps may also be rotated over calvarial bone prior to skin graft placement and will improve graft survival.

○ **What are the drawbacks of skin grafting for scalp reconstruction?**

Potential graft loss, especially when radiation is given, alopecia, poor color and thickness match, shiny appearance, and breakdown following even relatively minor trauma.

○ **What are the potential benefits of acellular biologic matrices for scalp reconstruction?**

Unlimited supply, no donor site morbidity, can be placed on minimally perfused surfaces, and may decrease need for flap reconstruction.

○ **What are the potential downsides to using an acellular biologic matrix for scalp reconstruction?**

May require skin grafting as a second procedure, requires a vascularized wound bed, alopecia, and prone to infection prior to becoming vascularized.

○ **What are the benefits of tissue expansion in scalp reconstruction?**

Tissue expansion can facilitate closure of wounds involving up to 50% of the scalp with hair-bearing tissue.

○ **What are the drawbacks of tissue expansion in scalp reconstruction?**

Frequent complications (up to 25%), including expander extrusion and infection, particularly in previously radiated tissues. Several weeks may be needed for healing and expansion after initial placement, making this a suboptimal technique for primary reconstruction when adjuvant therapy is indicated. A noticeable decrease in hair density may also occur.

○ **In what situations might tissue expansion of the scalp be contraindicated?**

When there is inadequate time to perform expansion and final reconstruction before giving adjuvant therapy. Tissue expansion is also contraindicated in wounds that are open, infected, or irradiated, or do not have stable calvarial coverage, as well as in patients who cannot tolerate staged reconstruction.

○ **In what plane are tissue expanders placed when used in scalp reconstruction?**

In the subgaleal space.

○ **By how much should the scalp be expanded?**

The expanded scalp should be at least 20% larger than size of defect to allow for tissue recoil. Multiple tissue expanders are sometimes needed to achieve this degree of expansion.

○ **What is the benefit of galeal scoring when using local flaps for scalp reconstruction?**

Although galeal scoring results in only modest improvements in flap length (1.67 mm per galeal incision according to a study by Raposio et al.), it significantly decreases wound tension (up to 40% according to the same study).

○ **How is galeal scoring performed?**

Galeal scoring is performed perpendicular to the line of maximal tension. Incisions are made through the galea but not deeper to avoid blood vessel transection and vascular compromise of flap.

○ **What are the principles of local flap design for scalp reconstruction?**

Flaps should try to incorporate at least one major scalp vessel and need to be 3 to 5× the diameter of the defect to close without tension. Skin grafts can be used to cover the flap donor site provided there is intact periosteum but will result in an area of alopecia (Fig. 81-1).

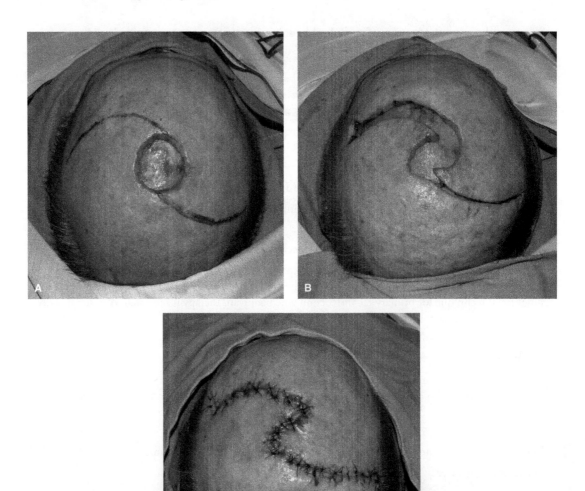

Figure 81-1 Small- to moderate-sized scalp defect (**A**), closed with broadly based local scalp flaps (**B**), and final result (**C**).

○ **What regional flaps are used in scalp reconstruction?**

Temporoparietal fascia flaps and temporalis muscle flaps may be used for defects in the temporal region; trapezius and latissimus dorsi muscle or myocutaneous flaps may be used for defects in the occipital region.

○ **What are pericranial flaps typically used for?**

Anterior pericranial flaps supplied by the deep branches of the supraorbital and supratrochlear blood vessels are often used in skull base surgery when a defect has been created between the paranasal sinuses and the anterior cranial fossa. The flap is delivered through a calvarial defect, such as one created during a frontal craniotomy, and placed along the anterior cranial floor. The nasal side of the flap usually mucosalizes spontaneously. In other cases, pericranial flaps are elevated and rotated over exposed calvarial bone after scalp resection and used as a vascularized bed for skin graft coverage.

○ **What is the blood supply to the pericranium?**

The blood supply to the pericranium is via the middle meningeal and intracranial circulation to the calvarial bone. As a result, disruption of blood supply to the scalp does not result in calvarial bone necrosis.

○ **What are the common indications for free flap reconstruction of the scalp?**

Large size, full-thickness scalp defects, and prior surgery or radiation treatment, which limits vascularity and pliability of local flaps (Fig. 81-2).

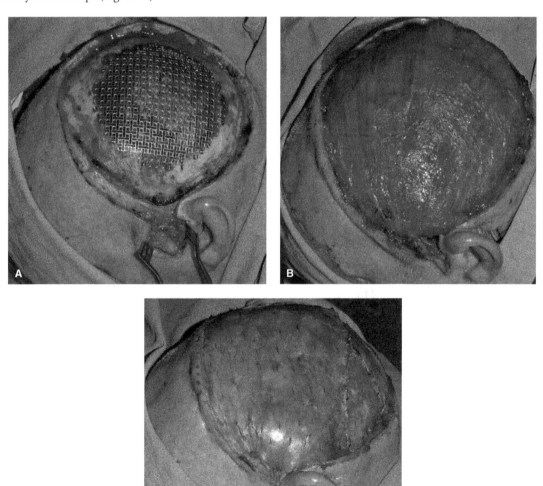

Figure 81-2 Large size full-thickness scalp defect including a full-thickness calvarial defect reconstructed with titanium mesh (**A**), latissimus dorsi muscle free flap anastomosed to the superficial temporal vessels (**B**), and final result after coverage with an unmeshed split-thickness skin graft (**C**).

○ **What factors are important in selecting a free flap for scalp reconstruction?**

Defect size, vascular pedicle length, flap size, thickness and tissue type, donor site morbidity, and surgeon preference.

○ **What free flaps are commonly used in scalp reconstruction?**

1. Latissimus dorsi muscle/myocutaneous flap: thin, broad flap for large defects; the muscle flap may be covered with an unmeshed skin graft with good aesthetic outcomes, particularly in bald patients.

2. Serratus anterior muscle flap: thin, small muscle with a long vascular pedicle; lower three slips of muscle may be harvested without significant scapular winging.

3. Radial forearm fasciocutaneous flap: small flap with a long vascular pedicle; may be more durable than a muscle flap with skin graft; relatively poor donor site appearance.

4. Omental flap: can cover a large surface area; irregular contour; requires laparotomy.

5. Rectus abdominis muscle/myocutaneous flap: long but narrower than the latissimus dorsi muscle flap; can be harvested with two-team approach; myocutaneous flap is usually overly thick.

6. Anterolateral thigh flap: can be a fasciocutaneous or myocutaneous flap; may be overly thick in some patients; has potential to cover a large defect, but will require skin grafting of the donor site.

○ **Which recipient vessels are commonly used in free flap scalp reconstruction?**

The superficial temporal vessels are preferred by many surgeons. The facial vessels are often second choices, but their use often requires interpositional vein grafts.

○ **What are the key points of postoperative care following free flap scalp reconstruction?**

Besides flap monitoring, elevation of the head to minimize edema, patient positioning to minimize pressure and shear forces on the flap or skin graft, use of closed suction drains to prevent seromas, and head positioning to prevent compression or kinking of the vascular pedicle.

○ **What steps are necessary to prepare for scalp replantation?**

The avulsed scalp must be cleansed, shaved, and debrided; arteries and veins must be found in the avulsed scalp, as well as sensory nerves, if possible; recipient vessels and nerves must be prepared; vein grafts are harvested; and broad-spectrum antibiotics are given.

○ **How many microvascular anastomoses are necessary for successful scalp replantation?**

This is controversial. However, anastomoses of one artery and two veins are usually recommended. Medicinal leeches may help in cases of venous congestion.

○ **What are the indications for calvarial reconstruction?**

To provide protective coverage of intracranial contents and to restore contour.

○ **What are the advantages of autologous bone in calvarial reconstruction?**

No foreign-body reaction, lower incidence of graft loss, and exposure and infection can sometimes be managed without graft removal.

○ **What are the disadvantages of autologous bone in calvarial reconstruction?**

Limited amount of available graft material, and donor site morbidity.

○ **What are the common sources of autologous bone for calvarial reconstruction and their advantages/disadvantages?**

Split calvarial bone: may be harvested from same operative field as defect, usually from the parietal region where skull is thickest and not over midline to avoid injury to the sagittal sinus; limited size of available graft; risk of violating the dura during harvest.

Iliac crest bone: larger quantity of bone than the calvarium; donor site pain, impaired gait, high rate of hematomas, and deformity or hernia if full-thickness bone is used.

Rib: large defects may be reconstructed by harvesting multiple ribs and splitting them; may destabilize the chest wall, especially if adjacent ribs are harvested; risk for pneumothorax during harvest; may result in undesirable washboard-like contour.

○ **What are the advantages of alloplastic calvarial reconstruction?**

Unlimited amount of material, may be sized and contoured as needed, and no donor site morbidity.

○ **What are the disadvantages of alloplastic calvarial reconstruction?**

Requires well-vascularized coverage, usually requires removal after exposure or infection, some materials result in heat or cold intolerance, and some cause radiographic artifacts.

○ **What are some common materials used for alloplastic calvarial reconstruction?**

1. Titanium: durable with minimal foreign body reaction, may experience cold intolerance, radiopaque, and causes artifacts on radiographic imaging.
2. Methyl methacrylate: durable, easily contoured; radiolucent; hardening process is exothermic.
3. Calcium hydroxyapatite: often used in combination with titanium mesh, may allow for some osteoconduction (bone ingrowth), hardening process is isothermic, and can be brittle.
4. Polyetheretherketone: highly durable, radiolucent, and must be custom made.

○ **How are infected calvarial reconstructions best managed?**

Usually by a two-staged approach. The first stage consists of debridement or removal of the infected bone or implant, antibiotic treatment, and scalp reconstruction with well-vascularized tissue. Reconstructive flap is re-elevated and calvarial reconstruction is performed at a second stage. Without rigid protection of the brain, care must be taken to avoid injury between stages.

● ● ● **REFERENCES** ● ● ●

Antonyshyn O, Gruss JS, Zuker R, Mackinnon SE. Tissue expansion in head and neck reconstruction. *Plast Reconstr Surg.* 1988;82:58–68.

Arnold PG, Rangarathnam CS. Multiple-flap scalp reconstruction: orticochea revisited. *Plast Reconstr Surg.* 1982;69:605–613.

Bilkay U, Kerem H, Ozek C, Erdem O, Songur E. Alopecia treatment with scalp expansion: some surgical fine points and a simple modification to improve the results. *J Craniofac Surg.* 2004;15:758–765.

Blake GB, MacFarlane MR, Hinton JW. Titanium in reconstructive surgery of the skull and face. *Br J Plast Surg.* 1990;43:528–535.

Chao AH, Yu P, Skoracki RJ, DeMonte F, Hanasono MM. Microsurgical reconstruction of composite scalp and calvarial defects in cancer: a 10-year experience. *Head Neck.* 2012;34:1759–1764.

Chicarilli ZN, Ariyan S, Cuono CB. Single-stage repair of complex scalp and cranial defects with the free radial forearm flap. *Plast Reconstr Surg.* 1986;77:577–585.

Grigg R. Forehead and temple reconstruction. *Otolaryngol Clin North Am.* 2001;34:583–600.

Gurlek A, Alaybeyoglu N, Demir CY, Aydoğan H, Bilen BT, Oztürk A. Aesthetic reconstruction of large scalp defects by sequential tissue expansion without interval. *Aesthetic Plast Surg.* 2004;28:245–250.

Hanasono MM, Goel N, DeMonte F. Calvarial reconstruction with polyetheretherketone implants. *Ann Plast Surg.* 2009;62(6): 653–655.

Hoffman JF. Management of scalp defects. *Otolaryngol Clin North Am.* 2001;34:571–582.

Hudson DA, Arasteh E. Serial tissue expansion for reconstruction of burns of the head and neck. *Burns.* 2001;27:481–487.

Hussussian CJ, Reece GP. Microsurgical scalp reconstruction in the patient with cancer. *Plast Reconstr Surg.* 2002;109:1828–1834.

Ioannides C, Fossion E, McGrouther AD. Reconstruction for large defects of the scalp and cranium. *J Craniomaxillofac Surg.* 1999; 27:145–152.

Lee EI, Chao AH, Skoracki RJ, Yu P, DeMonte F, Hanasono MM. Outcomes of calvarial reconstruction in cancer patients. *Plast Reconstr Surg.* 2014;133:675–682.

Leedey JE, Janis JE, Rohrich RJ. Reconstruction of acquired scalp defects: an algorithmic approach. *Plast Reconstr Surg.* 2005;116: 54e–72e.

Lesavoy MA, Dubrow TJ, Schwartz RJ, Wackym PA, Eisenhauer DM, McGuire M. Management of large scalp defects with local pedicle flaps. *Plast Reconstr Surg.* 1993;91:783–790.

Lipa JE, Butler CE. Enhancing the outcome of free latissimus dorsi muscle flap reconstruction of scalp defects. *Head Neck.* 2004;26: 46–53.

Losken A, Carlson GW, Culbertson JH, et al. Omental free flap reconstruction in complex head and neck deformities. *Head Neck.* 2002;24:326–331.

Lutz BS, Wei FC, Chen HC, Lin CH, Wei CY. Reconstruction of scalp defects with free flaps in 30 cases. *Br J Plast Surg.* 1998;51: 186–190.

Manson PN, Crawley WA, Hoopes JE. Frontal cranioplasty: risk factors and choice of cranial vault reconstructive material. *Plast Reconstr Surg.* 1986;77:888–904.

McCarthy JG, Zide BM. The spectrum of calvarial bone grafting: introduction of the vascularized calvarial bone flap. *Plast Reconstr Surg.* 1984;74:10–18.

Menders EK, Schenden MJ, Furrey JA, Hetzler PT, Davis TS, Graham WP 3rd. Skin expansion to eliminate large scalp defects. *Plast Reconstr Surg.* 1984;74:493–507.

Newman MI, Hanasono MM, Disa JJ, Cordeiro PG, Mehrara BJ. Scalp reconstruction: a 15-year experience. *Ann Plast Surg.* 2004;52:501–506.

Orticochea M. New three-flap scalp reconstruction technique. *Br J Plast Surg.* 1971;124:184–188.

Ozkan O, Coskunfirat OK, Ozgentas HE, Derin A. Rationale for reconstruction of large scalp defects using the anterolateral thigh flap: structural and aesthetic outcomes. *J Reconstr Microsurg.* 2005;21:539–545.

Pinar YA, Govsa F. Anatomy of the superficial temporal artery and its branches: its importance for surgery. *Surg Radiol Anat.* 2006;28:248–253.

Raposio E, Nordstrom RE, Santi PL. Undermining of the scalp: quantitative effects. *Plast Reconstr Surg.* 1998;101:1218–1222.

Seery GE. Surgical anatomy of the scalp. *Dermatol Surg.* 2002;28:581–587.

Silberstein E, Vasileios P, Landau D, et al. Aplasia cuts congenita: clinical management and a new classification system. *Plast Reconstr Surg.* 2014;134:766e–774e.

Temple CL, Ross DC. Scalp and forehead reconstruction. *Clin Plast Surg.* 2005;32:377–390.

Terkonda RP, Sykes JM. Concepts in scalp and forehead reconstruction. *Otolaryngol Clin North Am.* 1997;30:519–539.

Tolhurst DE, Carstens MH, Greco RS, Hurwitz DJ. The surgical anatomy of the scalp. *Plast Reconstr Surg.* 1991;87:603–612.

Ueda K, Harashina T, Inoue T, Tanaka I, Harada T. Microsurgical scalp and skull reconstruction using a serratus anterior myo-osseous flap. *Ann Plast Surg.* 1993;31:1014.

Van Rappard JH, Molenaar J, Van Doorn D, Sonneveld GJ, Borghouts JM. Surface-area increase in tissue expansion. *Plast Reconstr Surg.* 1988;82:833–839.

CHAPTER 82 Lip Reconstruction

Scott L. Hansen, MD, FACS and
Hani Sbitany, MD, FACS

○ **What is the function of the lips?**

Establishment of oral competence (function of orbicularis oris muscle), modulation of the spoken word, facial expression, as well as a role in social relationships.

○ **What is cheiloscopy?**

The study of lip prints. Lip prints have a unique topographic pattern, just like a fingerprint pattern.

○ **What are the critical and unique anatomic landmarks of the lip?**

Philtral columns, philtral groove, Cupid's bow and tubercle for the upper lip; the vermilion (white roll or mucocutaneous junction); and oral commissures.

○ **Where is Cupid's bow located?**

Found on the upper lip, Cupid's bow is the area of vermilion border at the base of the two philtral columns.

○ **When do the lips begin to develop embryologically?**

At 4 to 5 weeks of gestation.

○ **What are the important processes that occur during embryologic development of the lips?**

The two medial nasal prominences fuse with the maxillary prominences to form the upper lip. The mandibular prominence contributes to lower lip development. Failure of neural crest cell migration (as early as day 22) results in variable clefting of the upper lip.

○ **Discuss the perioral subunit principle of the lips.**

Burget and Menick described the lateral subunit, bordered by the philtral column, nasal sill, alar base and nasolabial fold, as well as the medial subunit, which represents one-half of the philtrum.

○ **What is the subunit principle?**

When the majority of a subunit has been lost, replacement of the entire subunit with like tissue yields the best aesthetic reconstruction.

○ **What is the blood supply to the lip?**

Is derived from the facial artery, branching into both the inferior and superior labial artery.

○ **What muscle planes does the facial artery travel within?**

Deep to the platysma, risorius, and zygomaticus major and minor muscles and superficial to the buccinator and levator anguli oris.

○ **Where does the inferior labial artery branch from the facial artery?**

2.6 cm lateral and 1.5 cm inferior to the oral commissure.

○ **The facial artery terminates into what artery in the midface?**

It becomes the angular artery, forming branches to the nasal ala and anastomosing with the dorsal nasal artery. The facial and labial arteries communicate with the subdermal plexus through a dense population of musculocutaneous perforators.

○ **What is the lymphatic drainage pattern of the lips?**

The upper lip and lateral lower lip drain primarily to the submandibular lymph nodes. The remaining lower lip drains to the submental nodes.

○ **What is the motor innervation to the lips?**

The facial nerve, whose buccal and marginal mandibular branches supply the perioral musculature on their undersurface.

○ **What muscles of facial expression are innervated on their superficial surface?**

The buccinator, levator anguli oris, and mentalis.

○ **What is the sensory innervation to the lips? What innervates the upper lip?**

Maxillary and mandibular divisions of the fifth cranial nerve. The infraorbital nerve, which is a terminal branch of the maxillary nerve, innervates the upper lip. The lower lip and chin receive sensory innervation from branches of the mandibular nerve (mental nerve).

○ **Where does the inferior alveolar nerve travel?**

The inferior alveolar nerve, a branch of the mandibular nerve, travels through the body of the mandible and exits from the mental foramen.

○ **What landmarks are used for an infraorbital nerve block?**

The nerve exits the infraorbital foramen 4 to 7 mm below the inferior orbital rim on a vertical line that descends from the medal limbus of the iris.

○ **What is the course of the infraorbital nerve and what does it supply?**

It travels beneath the levator labii superioris and superficial to the levator anguli oris to supply the lateral nasal sidewall, ala, columella, medial cheek, and upper lip.

○ **What landmarks are used to find the mental foramen?**

It is located below the apex of the second mandibular bicuspid but has 6 to 10 mm of lateral variability.

○ **What territory does the mental nerve supply?**

The lower lip skin down to the labiomental fold. The nerve is located in the submucosa as it exits the foramen and frequently is visible in this location.

○ **What are the steps for performing a mental nerve block?**

The lower lip is pulled out, and with tension, the mental nerve can be visualized on stretch in the mucosa on each side. It is just lateral to the canine, using this technique. It is injected with local anesthetic in the mucosa, and not at the mental foramen.

○ **Which nerve block anesthetizes the central chin?**

Inferior alveolar nerve block.

○ **What are the goals of lip reconstruction?**

Reconstruction of skin and oral mucosa, re-establishment of the vermilion, maintenance of an adequate stomal diameter, maintenance of sensation, and to restore normal oral sphincter function (competence).

○ **What are the limits of primary closure of the lower lip in terms of tissue loss? What about the upper lip?**

Up to one-third of lower lip loss may be tolerated with primary closure before microstomia and oral incompetence become a concern. Up to 25% tissue loss of the upper lip allows for reasonable primary closure.

○ **What is the minimal functional diameter of the oral stoma?**

3 cm.

○ **What is the difference between primary closure of the upper lip as opposed to the lower lip?**

The unique anatomic landmarks of the upper lip (Cupid's bow, philtral columns) make the upper lip less amenable than the lower lip for primary closure.

○ **How is primary closure performed?**

Precise layered closure should be suture specific. Fast-absorbing material (4-0 or 5-0 chromic gut) in the buccal mucosa (which heals rapidly). The orbicularis oris is repaired with large bites of a long-absorbing (vicryl or PDS) suture or permanent suture (clear nylon). Interrupted, buried sutures of fine vicryl (5-0) may be used for dermal approximation, followed by a running or interrupted monofilament suture (e.g., 6-0 nylon) in the skin.

○ **How does one treat vermilion lesions?**

The vermilion should be handled with care. Discrepancies of 1 mm can be detected at a conversational distance. Lesions near the vermilion border must be excised with a vertical ellipse.

○ **In what direction are horizontal lesions of the vermilion excised?**

Transversely.

○ **At what angle should incisions of the vermilion cross the mucocutaneous line?**

90-degree angle.

○ **What technique may be used when incising across the vermilion?**

When crossing the vermilion with an incision, the fine anatomic borders of the uninvolved, marginal vermilion should be tattooed with dye prior to local infiltration. This allows for proper alignment when closing. Again, the incision should cross the vermilion border at a 90-degree angle.

○ **Where are sutures placed when closing a vermilion lesion?**

Sutures are placed on the surrounding lip skin, and never on the vermilion directly. Inflammation from sutures on the vermilion border may distort this line.

○ **Where are the majority of malignancies of the lip—the upper or lower?**

95% of lip cancers involve the lower lip (more sun-exposed).

○ **What histologic types are most lip malignancies?**

90% of all lip cancers are squamous cell carcinoma (SCC). Other, rarer subtypes (sebaceous carcinoma, adenoid cystic carcinoma, acinic cell carcinoma, and Merkel cell carcinoma) may also occur.

○ **Which lesion represents a precursor to SCC?**

Keratoacanthoma, which looks clinically similar to SCC.

○ **Lip cancers make up what percentage of all oral carcinomas?**

25%.

○ **What margins should one take when excising lip malignancies?**

In one prospective study (72 consecutive patients with primary stage I/II SCC of the lower lip), full-thickness excision with 3-mm margins yielded a 89.9% tumor-free specimen rate with a 2.8% recurrence rate after a 5-year median follow-up. 3- to 5-mm margins appear to be sufficient in most series.

○ **What techniques may be used when excising an SCC from the lower lip?**

A flared W-plasty, single-barrel, or double-barrel incision (in contrast to conventional V-excisions) aid in wider margins and avoidance of crossing the labiomental fold.

○ **What general principles apply in lip reconstruction?**

A wide variety of flaps are available for reconstitution of the upper and lower lips. Two main strategies are available: rotation-advancement of remaining uninvolved lip peripheral to the defect and lip-switch flaps.

○ **What is the reconstructive technique of lip-switching?**

The concept is based on the dual blood supply to the lips from the facial artery and using tissue from one lip to reconstruct the other lip.

○ **What is an Abbé flap based upon and what is it used for?**

More commonly from the lower lip, it is based upon the coronal branch of the inferior labial artery, and is used to close a paramedian or philtral defect.

○ **How is an Abbé flap designed?**

Designed so that it measures one-half the width of the upper lip defect. A secondary division of the pedicle is performed at 3 weeks postelevation.

○ **How does the Estander flap differ from the Abbé flap?**

The Estlander's derivation of the Abbé flap involves a triangular designed flap, based on the superior labial artery. It provides coverage for lateral lower lip defects involving the commissure.

○ **What is the Gillies fan flap used for?**

As a rotational advancement flap, the Gillies fan flap donates upper lip and cheek tissue to close large central lower lip tissue losses (>50%). Several modifications of this original concept have been established. McGregor (1983) initially described a rectangular-shaped musculocutaneous flap similar to Gillies, but with a more narrow base and thus without the distortion at the oral commissure present in its predecessor. Typically, the width of the flap is the same as the vertical defect height and the length of the flap is equivalent to the width of the defect in addition to the width of the flap.

○ **What is unique about the Karapandzic flap?**

Originally described in 1974, this is an innervated orbicularis oris (composite) flap. Used to repair midline upper and lower lip defects, this flap is elevated by semicircular incisions camouflaged within the nasolabial folds, and mobilized based on neurovascular pedicles consisting of trigeminal and facial motor and sensory supply. This flap provides a functionally competent oral sphincter. Other innervated composite flaps incorporate levator anguli oris or depressor anguli oris for muscle units. Each of these flaps can restore up to 50% defects unilaterally and may be raised bilaterally to restore total lip defects.

○ **What type of defect is reconstructed with a Webster–Bernard flap?**

Very large (>80%) defects of the lower lip can be reconstructed with the Webster–Bernard flap. This involves medial advancement of cheek tissue to recreate the lower lip. The vermilion is then reconstructed with a mucosal flap.

○ **What is the preferred reconstructive technique following a full-thickness excision of the central 75% of the upper lip?**

Bilateral Karapandzic flaps with an Abbé flap. The Karapandzic flaps allow for transfer of innervated upper lip skin and musculature, while the Abbé flap allows for reconstruction of the central philtrum.

○ **Which flap is preferred for reconstruction of a full-thickness tumor resection from the left lateral lower lip and left commissure?**

Estlander flap.

○ **The facial artery myomucosal (FAMM) flap consists of what layers of tissue and structures?**

Oral mucosa, submucosa, buccinator muscle, facial artery, and venous plexus. As such, this flap is idea for reconstructing defects of the wet vermillion. This flap is not used for large, full-thickness defects of the lower lip.

○ **When local or regional flaps are not available, what is the next step in lip reconstruction?**

Free flap options are available for total lip reconstitution, but are plagued by bulky reconstruction, the failure to restore a competent oral sphincter, and aesthetic limitations.

○ **For each flap (Abbé, Bernard–Burow, Estlander, Gillies, Karapandzic) describe the advantages and disadvantages.**

Abbé flap: Ideal for central defects of the upper lip (philtral). Color match and rapid reinnervation are well described. Pedicled flap configuration (requiring secondary division), minor secondary vermilion discrepancies, and upper lip asymmetries are all negative characteristics.

Modified Bernard–Burow flap: Postoperative scars are camouflaged with natural creases along alar base and sill. Displacement of philtral columns and distortion of nasolabial fold contribute to disfavor of this flap.

Estlander flap: Optimal for reconstruction of lateral lower commissural defects. Adverse effect of microstomia and ablation of the natural fold of the oral commissure are potential outcomes.

Gillies fan flap: Designed for large lower lip defects (>50%), it has a generous arc of rotation. Similar to the Estlander flap, this flap may reduce the aperture of the mouth. It also disrupts and displaces the modiolus. Finally, distortion of the lip and lack of neural supply can lead to severe aesthetic deformities and oral incompetence.

Karapandzic flap: Neurovascular rotational flap provides reconstruction with a competent oral sphincter. Similar to the Gillies and Estlander flaps, distortion and displacement of the modiolus occurs.

○ **What is the primary difference between the Karapandzic and Gillies flaps?**

Both are advancement flaps of the lower lip tissue, used to reconstruct lower lip central defects. However, the Karapandzic flap involves dissection and preservation of facial nerve branches, thus resulting in a functional reconstruction.

○ **What are the potential complications of lip reconstruction?**

The main complication post lip reconstruction is microstomia. Other complications, such as philtral or commissural obliteration, nerve injury, and oral incompetence can also occur.

○ **What are the major muscles which elevate the upper lip?**

The levator labii superioris, zygomaticus major, and levator angulii oris.

○ **What muscles depress the lower lip and angle of the mouth?**

The depressor labii inferioris and depressor anguli oris.

○ **What muscle elevates the central lower lip?**

Mentalis muscle.

○   **What is the most common etiology of commissure wounds?**

Electrical burns. Frequently observed in children between the ages 1 and 4 years.

○   **What is the early management of commissure electrical burns?**

While some believe in immediate excision and closure is warranted, most proceed with conservative therapy, including topical antibiotics, and allowing the wound to demarcate.

○   **What is the most common complication in the acute phase of commissure healing?**

Bleeding from the labial artery, which usually occurs 24 to 48 hours after the injury.

○   **What regional flap can be used to reconstruct a hair-bearing, complete upper lip defect?**

Temporal frontal scalp flap based on the superficial temporal vessels or a submental flap based on the submental artery, a branch of the facial artery.

○   **What free flap would be most appropriate to reconstruct a complete lower lip defect?**

The radial forearm flap which is thin, pliable, and has a long, reliable vascular pedicle. The palmaris longus tendon can be incorporated into the flap to provide a sling.

● ● ● **REFERENCES** ● ● ●

Anvar BA, Evans BC, Evans GR. Lip reconstruction. *Plast Reconstr Surg.* 2007;120(4):57e–64e.

Baumann D, Robb G. Lip reconstruction. *Semin Plast Surg.* 2008;22(4):269–280.

Burget GC, Menick FJ. Aesthetic restoration of one-half of the upper lip. *Plast Reconstr Surg.* 1986;78(5):583–593.

Campbell JP. Surgical management of lip carcinoma. *J Oral Maxillofac Surg.* 1998;56:955–961.

Canady JW, Thompson SA, Bardach J. Oral commissure burns in children. *Plast Reconstr Surg.* 1996;97:738–744; discussion 745; 746–755.

de Visscher JG, Gooris PJ, Vermey A, Roodenberg JL. Surgical margins for resection of squamous cell carcinoma of the lower lip. *Int J Oral Maxillofac Surg.* 2002;31:154–157.

de Visscher JG, van der Waal I. Etiology of cancer of the lip. A review. *Int J Oral Maxillofac Surg.* 1998;27:199–203.

Dupin C, Metzinger S, Rizzuto R. Lip reconstruction after ablation for skin malignancies. *Clin Plast Surg.* 2004;31(1):69–85.

Godek CP, Weinzweig J, Bartlett SP. Lip reconstruction following Mohs' surgery: the role for composite resection and primary closure. *Plast Reconstr Surg.* 2000;106(4):798–804.

Langstein HN, Robb GL. Lip and perioral reconstruction. *Clin Plast Surg.* 2005;32(3):431–445.

Lesavoy MA, Smith AD. Lower third face and lip reconstruction. In: Mathes SJ, ed. *Plastic Surgery.* 2nd ed. Philadelphia, PA: W. B. Saunders; 2006:799–858.

McGregor IA. Reconstruction of the lower lip. *Br J Plast Surg.* 1983;36:40–47.

Schulte DL, Sherris DA, Kasperbauer JL. The anatomical basis of the Abbé flap. *The Laryngoscope.* 2001;111:382–386.

Tobin GR, O'Daniel TG. Lip reconstruction with motor and sensory innervated composite flaps. *Clin Plast Surg.* 1990;17(4):623–632.

Wei FC, Tan BK, Chen IH, Hau SP, Liau CT. Mimicking lip features in free-flap reconstruction of lip defects. *Br J Plast Surg.* 2001; 54:8–11.

Zide BM. Deformities of the lips and cheeks. In: McCarthy JG, ed. *Plastic Surgery.* Philadelphia, PA: W. B. Saunders; 1990:2009–2037.

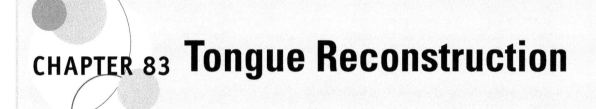

CHAPTER 83 Tongue Reconstruction

Pieter G. L. Koolen, MD and
Samuel J. Lin, MD, MBA, FACS

○ **How much of the tongue lies within the oral cavity?**

The anterior two-thirds of the tongue. The posterior limit of the oral cavity superiorly is the junction of the hard and soft palates and inferiorly the sulcus terminalis of the tongue.

○ **What are other terms for the posterior third of the tongue?**

The pharyngeal tongue or tongue base.

○ **Where are the circumvallate papillae and the fungiform papillae located?**

The circumvallate papillae lie immediately anterior to the sulcus terminalis. The fungiform papillae are scattered on the upper surface of the tongue anterior to the circumvallate papillae.

○ **What separates the oral and pharyngeal portions of the tongue?**

The sulcus terminalis.

○ **Where on the tongue is the foramen cecum?**

The apex of the sulcus terminalis.

○ **Which structure migrates through the foramen cecum of the tongue during embryological development?**

The thyroid.

○ **Which embryological structures fuse to form the tongue?**

The median tongue bud (tuberculum impar) and two distal tongue buds form the oral tongue. The hypobranchial eminence becomes the pharyngeal tongue.

○ **Describe the surface anatomy of the tongue.**

The oral tongue has an apex, which touches the incisors, a dorsum (the upper surface), and a smooth ventral surface, which is contiguous with the oral floor and gingiva. The tongue base is more vertical in orientation and contiguous with the glossoepiglottic folds.

○ **What nerves provide general sensation to the tongue?**

Oral: lingual nerve. Pharyngeal: glossopharyngeal nerve.

○ **Which cranial nerves transmit taste sensation?**

Cranial nerves (CN) VII, IX, and X; all contain special sensory taste afferent fibers.

○ **What is the course of the chorda tympani nerve?**

Taste fibers leave the lingual nerve and are conveyed via the chorda tympani. It carries taste sensory fibers from the anterior two-thirds of the tongue to the intratemporal facial nerve. With the lingual nerve, the chorda tympani travels from the ventral surface of the tongue to the lingual sulcus, where it is caudal to the submandibular duct; then superiorly, to the lingual border of the mandible near the third molar. The chorda tympani leaves the lingual nerve at the medial border of the lateral pterygoid and traverses the middle ear, joining CN VII in the facial canal.

○ **Where are taste buds located?**

Tongue, soft palate, palatoglossal arches, posterior surface of the epiglottis (CN X), and posterior oropharynx.

○ **How many taste buds are there on each papilla?**

Approximately 3, 250 and 1,200 taste buds are found on the fungiform, vallate, and foliate papillae, respectively. Filiform papillae have no taste buds.

○ **What are the four types of taste?**

Salty, sweet, sour, and bitter.

○ **Where on the tongue is salty taste sensed?**

The entire tongue surface can sense salty taste. There is a strong misconception that there is a "taste map." In fact every taste can be sensed in all regions of the tongue.

○ **What other sensation is important in recognizing flavors?**

Olfaction. Patients who cannot smell may complain of lack of taste sensation.

○ **Describe the musculature of the tongue.**

The musculature of the tongue is divided into two functional halves by a fibrous septum. The extrinsic muscles, styloglossus, hyoglossus, and genioglossus together control the position of the tongue. They connect the tongue to the hyoid, mandible, and styloid processes. The palatoglossus assists in tongue elevation but is usually considered primarily to be a muscle of the palate. The intrinsic muscles shape the tongue by controlled contractions of transverse, longitudinal, and vertical fibers either side of the midline septum.

○ **What provides motor supply to the muscles of the tongue?**

The hypoglossal nerve.

○ **What is the function of the genioglossus muscle?**

The anterior fibers of genioglossus retract the tongue tip. The bulk action of genioglossus is to protrude the tongue anteriorly and inferiorly.

○ **What is the blood supply of the tongue?**

The lingual artery, arising from the external carotid artery, provides inflow. Drainage is via venae comitantes into the internal jugular vein.

○ **What is the lymphatic drainage of the tongue?**

The oral tongue lymphatics drain into the respective cervical nodal basin bilaterally. The level II nodes are most commonly affected by tongue cancer metastases, but levels I and III are also at high risk. Hence, the most commonly performed elective neck dissection for tongue cancer is a selective neck dissection of levels I, II, and III (also referred to as a supraomohyoid neck dissection).

○ **What are the most important functions of the tongue?**

Airway protection, swallowing (deglutition), tasting, articulating speech, and tongue finger function. Additionally, the tongue assists chewing by repeatedly presenting the food bolus to the teeth.

○ **What use is the "finger function" of the tongue?**

The ability of the tongue to form a firm tip that is useful for clearing the oral sulci, manipulating a food bolus, and cleaning the lips and dentition.

○ **What are the phases of swallowing?**

There are voluntary and involuntary phases of swallowing. First, in the voluntary (oral) phase of swallowing, the apex of the tongue is pressed against the palate. The intrinsic muscles move food posteriorly into the oropharynx by elevating sequential portions of the tongue to the palate. The tongue base is positioned superiorly and posteriorly, forming a food platform in readiness for the involuntary phase. Concurrently the hyoid bone is moved superiorly.

During the involuntary (pharyngeal), phase the palatopharyngeal sphincter seals the nasopharynx, while the larynx and pharynx are elevated. The tongue base and pharyngeal constrictors force the food bolus inferiorly over the posteriorly arched epiglottis and closed laryngeal inlet.

○ **What is the most common tongue malignancy?**

Squamous cell carcinoma of the tongue.

○ **How are lingual cancers staged?**

The American Joint Committee on Cancer method for planning treatment, estimating prognosis, and comparing research of oral cavity and oropharyngeal cancers involves categorizing tumors according to the tumor size (Tis, T1, T2, T3, or T4), nodal metastases (N0, N1, N2, N3), and presence of distant metastases (Mx, M0, M1). Once the three tumor characteristics (TNM) are known, the tumor can be given a stage I to IV. Oral tongue cancer staging differs from pharyngeal tongue only with respect to the T4 definitions, because the adjacent structures that might be invaded vary.

T1: tumor less than 2 cm in maximum dimension.

T2: tumor 2 to 4 cm.

T3: tumor more than 4 cm.

T4: tumor invades adjacent structures.

○ **What are the relative survival rates for various stages of tongue cancer?**

According to the National Cancer Institute of the United States National Institutes of Health, the 5-year relative survival rate for cancers localized to the primary site (tongue) is approximately 77%, for those that have spread to regional lymph nodes or extended directly beyond the primary site is approximately 55%, and for cancers that have already metastasized at diagnosis is approximately 29%. The relative survival rate measures the survival of the cancer patients in comparison to the general population to estimate the effect of cancer.

○ **What part of the tongue is most frequently affected first by malignancy?**

The midlateral aspect of the tongue.

○ **What is an oral glossectomy?**

The resection of the tongue tip and up to half of the tongue base is called an oral glossectomy. Other defects include subtotal hemiglossectomy (a wide local excision that is smaller than a hemiglossectomy), hemiglossectomy (divided into either an oral or extended hemiglossectomy), and total glossectomy.

○ **What are the priorities in lingual reconstruction?**

Immediate wound closure, prevention of orocervical fistula, obliteration of dead space lingual to the mandible, maintenance/restoration of tongue function, coverage of major vessels, and uncomplicated wound healing.

○ **How much of the tongue is required to maintain tongue function?**

A portion of at least 20% to 30% of the lateral tongue is required for some residual tongue function. It is critical that the chosen reconstruction does not tether residual tongue function.

○ **How is residual tongue function maintained with reconstruction?**

The most important factor in preserving function is maintaining residual tongue mobility by avoiding tethering. Reconstruction methods that may lead to tethering of the residual tongue include primary closure, skin grafting, or poorly designed regional or distant flaps. Correctly planned reconstruction provides sufficient flap size for coverage of the defect with the tongue in all ranges of movement. In addition, the flap should cover adjacent floor of mouth, pharyngeal, or palate defects as required.

○   **Why is the volume of a free flap important in reconstructing subtotal or total tongue defects?**

The presence of bulk in a flap supports the ventral tongue, preventing prolapse or contralateral shifting of the residual tongue. Bulk helps direct oral contents and secretions laterally toward the oropharynx and allows the neotongue to contact the palate, which is important for speech and swallowing.

○   **What are the options for reconstructing lingual defects?**

Primary closure, skin grafts, and local, regional, or distant flaps. Common free flaps for tongue reconstruction include radial forearm, lateral arm, rectus abdominis myocutaneous, and anterolateral thigh.

○   **Which free flaps can be used to provide general sensation to the reconstructed tongue?**

Radial forearm, anterolateral thigh, and lateral arm are three commonly used flaps for tongue reconstruction, which may be innervated to provide sensation.

○   **Do noninnervated flaps used for tongue reconstruction regain sensation?**

Yes. Ninety percent of noninnervated fasciocutaneous free flaps placed on an unscarred bed in the oral cavity regained at least some sensory modalities, likely the result of axonal sprouting into the flap. Sensory upgrading of the flap may occur secondary to the large cortical representation of the tongue in the sensory homunculus.

○   **Do innervated free flaps for tongue reconstruction regain normal sensation?**

No. Flaps are unable to taste because they lack taste buds. However, patients rarely complain about loss of taste (likely because taste buds are almost ubiquitous within the buccal cavity). General sensory function of an innervated free flap approaches that of the normal tongue and is superior to the donor site sensation.

○   **Do innervated flaps function better than noninnervated flaps?**

No studies to date have compared tongue function in innervated versus noninnervated flaps. Innervated flaps gain general sensation sooner postoperatively than noninnervated flaps. However, sensation may not be important for tongue function.

○   **What factors affect sensory recovery in flaps used for tongue reconstruction?**

Postoperative radiation and the use of a recipient nerve other than the lingual or inferior alveolar nerve negatively impact the sensory recovery of innervated free flaps for tongue reconstruction. Age, smoking, and the size of the defect do not seem to influence the return of sensation.

○   **How does the provision of radiation therapy affect the choice of reconstruction?**

While radiation therapy unfortunately diminishes the wound-healing capabilities of tissues, it does, however, improve the survival of patients. The choice of reconstruction, therefore, needs to withstand the effects of radiation as much as possible. Prior irradiation not only adversely affects wound healing but also makes the dissection of tissue planes and of recipient vessels for microvascular transfer significantly more difficult than in a nonirradiated field. Postoperative radiation increases scarring, may cause xerostomia, and may affect the swallowing mechanism, making a freely (untethered) mobile reconstruction even more critical to successful tongue function. Chemotherapy compounds the effects of radiation. In general, the presence of radiation changes or of a plan to deliver postoperative radiotherapy should strongly encourage the use of a microvascular reconstruction, which can import liberal volumes of nonirradiated tissue with its own blood supply. It should also be remembered that tissues subjected to postoperative irradiation would invariably shrink, meaning that a reconstruction must overcorrect tongue volume to compensate.

○ **What is the effect of a palatal build-down prosthesis on tongue function?**

A prosthesis placed over the palate in an attempt to achieve tongue–palate contact has a negative impact on function because the patient will lose important sensory feedback from the palate. (Palatal sensation might explain how noninnervated flaps are able to function similar to reinnervated flaps.)

○ **What are the important determinates of functional outcome following tongue reconstruction?**

The primary predictor of postoperative function is defect size, with larger defects associated with poorer outcomes. Postoperative radiotherapy and midline defects correlate with worse functional results. Reconstructions that maintain tongue mobility and bulk give patients better speech and swallowing.

○ **What are the advantages of the radial forearm free flap for tongue reconstruction?**

Large surface area available; thin, pliable tissue; long pedicle if required; technically easy to harvest; several useful variants: neurofasciocutaneous, osseofasciocutaneous, and tendofasciocutaneous.

○ **What are the disadvantages of the radial forearm free flap?**

Lack of bulk for large tongue defects and the donor site morbidity, which includes sensory changes and poor cosmesis.

○ **What are the advantages of the suprafascial dissection for a radial forearm free flap?**

Fewer donor site complications: decreased rate of skin graft loss, less delayed healing, decreased incidence of tendon exposure.

○ **What options exist for reconstructing total or subtotal tongue defects?**

Primarily free flaps: anterolateral thigh, rectus abdominis myocutaneous, latissimus dorsi, jejunum.

○ **For total tongue defects, can the tongue muscles be reconstructed?**

No. Currently, the tongue muscles are too complex to reconstruct. Functioning gracilis may be transferred in either a longitudinal or a transverse orientation, with the goal of providing only elevation of the neotongue when required. Too few studies exist to comment on the utility of functioning muscle transfers in tongue reconstruction.

○ **Are there problems associated with using muscle flaps for tongue reconstruction?**

Noninnervated muscle flaps undergo atrophy and over time may not provide enough bulk in reconstruction of large defects. The reinnervation of musculocutaneous flaps is worse than that of noninnervated fasciocutaneous flaps.

○ **Can the tongue be transplanted from a cadaveric donor?**

Yes. In 1999, tongue transplantation was demonstrated as technically feasible in a canine model. In 2003, the first tongue transplantation in humans was performed in Vienna to reconstruct an oncological defect involving the total tongue with infiltration of the mandible and floor of mouth (T4N2bM0). The patient was immunosuppressed immediately postoperatively and thereafter. Resection margins were free of tumor but recurrence occurred after 12 months and the patient died 1 month later. At 10 months, the patient had regained sensation to the left tongue but not independent motor function; however, the patient was able to swallow saliva and small amounts of pulpy foods, and speak intelligibly. Since then, a composite transplantation of tongue with mandible and floor of mouth has been achieved in late 2009 in Spain. Composite tissue allotransplantation for oncological defect reconstruction remains highly controversial.

● ● ● **REFERENCES** ● ● ●

Avery CM, Pereira J, Brown AE. Suprafascial dissection of the radial forearm flap and donor site morbidity. *Int J Oral Maxillofac Surg.* 2001;30:37–41.

Bannister LH. Alimentary system. In: Williams PL, ed. *Gray's Anatomy.* 38th ed. Toronto, ON, Canada: Churchill-Livingstone; 1999: 1683–1733.

Bastian RW, Riggs LC. Role of sensation in swallowing function. *Laryngoscope.* 1999;109:1974–1977.

Berry M, Bannister LH, Standring SM. Nervous system. In: Williams PL, ed. *Gray's Anatomy.* 38th ed. Toronto, ON, Canada: Churchill-Livingstone; 1999:901–1397.

Boyd B, Mulholland S, Gullane P, et al. Reinnervated lateral antebrachial cutaneous neurosome flaps in oral reconstruction: are we making sense? *Plast Reconstr Surg.* 1994;93:1350–1359; discussion 1360–1362.

Chang SC, Miller G, Halbert CF, Yang KH, Chao WC, Wei FC. Limiting donor site morbidity by suprafascial dissection of the radial forearm flap. *Microsurgery.* 1996;17:136–140.

Collins P. Embryology and development. In: Williams PL, ed. *Gray's Anatomy.* 38th ed. Toronto, ON, Canada: Churchill-Livingstone; 1999:91–341.

de Bree R, Hartley C, Smeele LE, Kuik DJ, Quak JJ, Leemans CR. Evaluation of donor site function and morbidity of the fasciocutaneous radial forearm flap. *Laryngoscope.* 2004;114(11):1973–1976.

Evans GRD, Kroll SS. Intraoral soft tissue reconstruction. In: Schusterman MA, ed. *Microsurgical Reconstruction of the Cancer Patient.* Philadelphia, PA: Lippincott-Raven; 1997:13–23.

Greene FL, Balch CM, Page DL, et al. *AJCC Cancer Staging Handbook.* 6th ed. New York, NY: Springer-Verlag; 2002.

Haughey BH. Tongue reconstruction: concepts and practice. *Laryngoscope.* 1993;103:1132–1141.

Haughey BH, Beggs JC, Bong J, Genden EM, Buckner A. Microneurovascular allotransplantation of the canine tongue. *Laryngoscope.* 1999;109:1461–1470.

Horner MJ, Ries LA, Krapcho M, et al. *SEER Cancer Statistics Review, 1975–2006.* Bethesda, MD: National Cancer Institute; 2009, http://seer.cancer.gov/csr/1975–2006/, based on November 2008 SEER data submission, posted to the SEER web site

Huang CH, Chen HC, Huang YL, Mardini S, Feng GM. Comparison of the radial forearm flap and the thinned anterolateral thigh cutaneous flap for reconstruction of tongue defects: an evaluation of donor-site morbidity. *Plast Reconstr Surg.* 2004;114(7): 1704–1710.

Imanishi Y, Isobe K, Nameki H, et al. Extended sigmoid-shaped free jejunal patch for reconstruction of the oral base and pharynx after total glossectomy with laryngectomy. *Br J Plast Surg.* 2004;57:195–202.

Kermer C, Watzinger F, Oeckher M. Tongue transplantation: 10-month follow-up. *Transplantation.* 2008;85:654–655.

Kimata Y, Sakuraba M, Hishinuma S, et al. Analysis of the relations between the shape of the reconstructed tongue and the postoperative functions after subtotal or total glossectomy. *Laryngoscope.* 2003;113:905–909.

Kuriakose MA, Loree TR, Spies A, Meyers S, Hicks WL Jr. Sensate radial forearm free flaps in tongue reconstruction. *Arch Otolaryngol Head Neck Surg.* 2001;127:1463–1466.

Kveton JF, Bartoshuk LM. Taste. In: Bailey BJ, Calhoun KH, eds. *Head and Neck Surgery—Otolaryngology.* 2nd ed. Philadelphia, PA: Lippincott-Raven, 1998:609–626.

McConnell FM. Analysis of pressure generation and bolus transit during pharyngeal swallowing. *Laryngoscope.* 1988;98:71–78.

Murakami R, Tanaka K, Kobayashi K, et al. Free groin flap for reconstruction of the tongue and oral floor. *J Reconstr Microsurg.* 1998;14:49–55.

Nicoletti G, Soutar DS, Jackson MS, Wrench AA, Robertson G. Chewing and swallowing after surgical treatment for oral cancer: functional evaluation in 196 selected cases. *Plast Reconstr Surg.* 2004;114:329–338.

Nicoletti G, Soutar DS, Jackson MS, Wrench AA, Robertson G, Robertson C. Objective assessment of speech after surgical treatment for oral cancer: experience from 196 selected cases. *Plast Reconstr Surg.* 2004;113:114–125.

Salibian AH, Allison GR, Armstrong WB, et al. Functional hemitongue reconstruction with the microvascular ulnar forearm flap. *Plast Reconstr Surg.* 1999;104:654–660.

Salibian AH, Allison GR, Rappaport I, Krugman ME, McMicken BL, Etchepare TL. Total and subtotal glossectomy: function after microvascular reconstruction. *Plast Reconstr Surg.* 1990;85(4):513–524; discussion 525–526.

Santamaria E, Wei FC, Chen IH, Chuang DC. Sensation recovery on innervated radial forearm flap for hemiglossectomy reconstruction by using different recipient nerves. *Plast Reconstr Surg.* 1999;103:450–457.

Soutar DS, McGregor IA. The radial forearm flap in intraoral reconstruction: the experience of 60 consecutive cases. *Plast Reconstr Surg.* 1986;78:1–8.

Swartz WM, Banis JC. Intraoral reconstruction. *Head and Neck Microsurgery*. Baltimore, MD: Williams & Wilkins; 1992.

Urken ML, Moscoso JF, Lawson W, Biller HF. A systematic approach to functional reconstruction of the oral cavity following partial and total glossectomy. *Arch Otolaryngol Head Neck Surg*. 1994;120:589–601.

Vriens JP, Acosta R, Soutar DS, Webster MH. Recovery of sensation in the radial forearm free flap in oral reconstruction. *Plast Reconstr Surg*. 1996;98:649–656.

Yoleri L, Mavioglu H. Total tongue reconstruction with free functional gracilis muscle transplantation: a technical note and review of the literature. *Ann Plast Surg*. 2000;45:181–186.

Yousif NJ, Dzwierzynski WW, Sanger JR, Matloub HS, Campbell BH. The innervated gracilis musculocutaneous flap for total tongue reconstruction. *Plast Reconstr Surg*. 1999;104(4):916–921.

CHAPTER 84
Chest and Abdominal Wall Reconstruction

Eugene Y. Fukudome, MD and
Donald J. Morris, MD, FACS

• • • THORACIC RECONSTRUCTION • • •

○ **What is the most common intrathoracic problem that requires intervention by a plastic surgeon?**

Empyema (collection of pus within the pleural space). This can be secondary to problems such as bronchopleural fistula or esophageal perforation, and a thoracic surgeon may enlist the help of a plastic surgeon in managing these difficult problems.

○ **What is a bronchopleural fistula, and what is the cause?**

A bronchopleural fistula is a communication between a bronchus and the pleural cavity that is usually caused by postoperative necrosis of the bronchial stump following lung resection. A bronchopleural fistula can also result from necrotizing pneumonia or necrosis of the bronchial wall secondary to radiation.

○ **What are the important principles in the successful management of an empyema resulting from a bronchopleural fistula or esophageal perforation?**

1. Assessment and optimization of the patient's overall medical condition and nutrition status.

2. Appropriate antibiotics based on culture and sensitivity data.

3. Resection and/or debridement of the bronchopleural fistula or esophageal perforation back to healthy tissue, and closure.

4. Obliteration of dead space and reinforcement of any bronchial or esophageal repairs with well-vascularized tissue. Typically a flap is required.

5. Adequate drainage after reconstruction.

○ **How do you obliterate intrathoracic dead space?**

Larger, bulkier muscle flaps (pectoralis major, latissimus dorsi) or omentum is used to fill the hemithorax. Often, an intercostal muscle flap is used to bolster a bronchial or esophageal repair, and a muscle flap can be transposed into the chest through the intercostal muscle flap donor site. Alternatively, a rib resection can be performed to allow transposition of the muscle into the chest.

○ **What are the common acquired chest wall problems that require intervention by a plastic surgeon?**

Chest wall defects resulting from tumor resection, trauma, or wounds resulting from radiation, severe infection, and surgical complications.

○ **What are the important goals and principles in the successful management of these chest wall problems?**

1. Resection of the tumor with adequate margins.

2. Debridement of all devitalized/damaged issue.

3. Optimization of respiratory mechanics by the creation of an airtight pleural space with a stable chest wall such that negative intrathoracic pressure can be generated during inspiration.

4. Protect intrathoracic organs and prevent problems such as lung hernia and diaphragmatic hernia.

5. Recruitment of well-vascularized soft-tissue coverage of the defect that will allow for adjuvant radiation therapy if indicated.

6. Re-establish a cosmetically acceptable chest wall contour.

○ **Describe the differences between nonrigid, semirigid, and rigid reconstruction of the chest wall.**

Nonrigid methods of reconstruction include soft-tissue flaps such as muscle and musculocutaneous flaps. While this method does recruit well-vascularized tissue, there is minimal contribution to the structural integrity of the chest wall. Paradoxical chest wall motion may be a significant problem to these patients postreconstruction.

Semirigid methods typically refer to a situation where mesh is used to span a skeletal defect, and the mesh is sutured in place under tension. Synthetic (polypropylene and polytetrafluoroethylene [PTFE]) or bioprosthetic mesh can be used depending on the clinical situation.

Rigid fixation involves the use of foreign bodies such as polymethylmethacrylate "sandwiched" between synthetic mesh such as polypropylene. Autologous forms of rigid fixation can include rib and fascia grafts, but these have largely been replaced by synthetic products. Absence of bacterial contamination, and well-vascularized, nonradiated soft-tissue coverage is critical when using foreign material for rigid fixation of the chest wall because infection will require removal of the construct with loss of the entire reconstruction.

○ **When is rigid reconstruction of the chest wall indicated, and when is nonrigid reconstruction sufficient?**

Universally accepted guidelines based on high-quality data do not exist, but various authors have provided the following guidelines:

Size-based criteria: chest wall defects larger than 5 cm, or defects involving 4 or more ribs should undergo rigid reconstruction.

Location-based criteria: chest wall defects involving the apex and posterior chest wall do not require rigid fixation, except when the tip of the scapula may become impacted in the defect. In this case, semirigid fixation should be considered. Anterior and lateral defect should be considered for rigid reconstruction.

○ **What are the problems associated with rigid reconstruction of the chest wall?**

Rigid fixation is associated with higher rates of surgical site infection. When infection occurs, reoperation and removal of foreign material are indicated, either acutely, or after a delay period to first allow for fibrosis. In either case, this may lead to a delay in any planned chemotherapy or radiation therapy. Rigid reconstruction may also result in more chronic pain. The risks and benefits of rigid fixation of the chest wall must be carefully considered for each individual patient.

○ **How does radiation therapy impact reconstruction of the chest wall?**

Radiation-induced fibrosis may result in enough stiffening of the chest wall to prevent paradoxical respiratory movement so that rigid reconstruction may be unnecessary. It is also prudent to avoid placement of a foreign body in a radiated field. Radiation therapy also mandates the use of well-vascularized healthy tissue for reconstruction.

○ **What are the common flaps used for thoracic reconstruction?**

The latissimus dorsi, pectoralis major, rectus abdominis, and serratus anterior muscles are commonly used. The omental flap also has several applications. Intercostal muscle flaps play a role in re-enforcement of bronchial, tracheal, and esophageal repairs. Free tissue transfers are less commonly used, but may be required.

○ **What is the blood supply of the latissimus dorsi muscle?**

The thoracodorsal artery, arising from the subscapular artery, is the primary blood supply of the latissimus dorsi muscle. The latissimus dorsi flap can also be based on posterior intercostal perforators and used as a turnover flap to address defects in the mid-back region. For thoracic surgery patients who have previously undergone a posterolateral thoracotomy, the latissimus dorsi muscle is often divided, making the distal portion of the muscle unusable for reconstruction unless a muscle-sparing thoracotomy was used.

○ **What is the blood supply of the serratus anterior muscle?**

The serratus branch off the thoracodorsal artery from the subscapular system supplies the serratus anterior muscle.

○ **What is the blood supply of the pectoralis major muscle?**

The pectoral branch of the thoracoacrominal artery is the primary blood supply of the pectoralis major muscle. The pectoralis major muscle can also be based on internal mammary artery (IMA) perforators and used as a turnover flap for sternal wound closure.

○ **What is the blood supply of the rectus abdominis muscle?**

Although the primary blood supply of the rectus abdominis muscle is the deep inferior epigastric artery, for chest wall reconstruction, this flap is typically based on the superior epigastric artery, originating from the IMA. In cases where the IMA has been divided, a rectus abdominis muscle flap can be raised based on intercostal and subcostal vessels. A previous subcostal incision, however, is a contraindication to a superiorly based rectus abdominis flap.

○ **What is the blood supply of the greater omentum?**

The right and left gastroepiploic arteries supply the greater omentum. The omental flap can be based on either the right or left gastroepiploic artery.

• • • STERNAL RECONSTRUCTION • • •

○ **How frequently does dehiscence of median sternotomy wounds occur?**

1% to 5% of median sternotomy wounds will dehisce.

○ **What are the common sternal and mediastinal problems that require intervention by a plastic surgeon?**

Infection: Postoperative complications such as poststernotomy infections and mediastinitis. In addition, the sternoclavicular joint may become infected from hematogenous seeding from a distant source.

Exposures: Major vessels, pericardium and its contents, vascular grafts, and other critical hardware such as ventricular assist devices may become exposed and require coverage.

○ **What are some risk factors for sternal wound infection?**

Diabetes, COPD, obesity, smoking, renal failure, peripheral vascular disease, IMA harvest (bilateral harvest is higher risk than unilateral harvest), prolonged hospital course, ICU course or ventilator support, and use of intra-aortic balloon pump.

○ **What are the different presentations of sternal wound infections?**

Sternal wound infections can present in three relatively distinct ways as categorized by Pairolero.

Type I infections occur within several days and present with serosanguineous drainage.

Type II infections occur a few weeks postoperatively and present with cellulitis, osteomyelitis, mediastinitis, and drainage of pus.

Type III infections occur months later and present with osteomyelitis, chondritis, and a chronically draining sinus tract.

○ **How are sternal wound infections managed?**

Sternal wounds must be managed in conjunction with the cardiac surgeon, and any operative debridement should occur in a cardiac surgery suite with cardiac anesthesia in an event that any mediastinal structures are injured.

Type I infections typically are handled by irrigation, minimal debridement, and re-closure, and are usually handled by the cardiac surgeon.

Type II and III infections are managed by following the principles of chest wall reconstruction. Irrigation and drainage of the infection is critical, and devitalized tissue must be debrided. Cartilage is relatively poorly vascularized, and when infected, must be debrided as well. When the patient is medically as optimized as possible, reconstruction is undertaken using healthy well-vascularized tissue to obliterate the dead space and close the wound. Carefully selected patients who have a low bacterial burden, well-vascularized bone, and no dead space may be candidates for sternal osteosynthesis.

○ **What is the main cause of failure of reconstruction of a dehisced/infected median sternotomy wound?**

Inadequate debridement.

○ **Are sternal infections typically managed as a single-stage operation consisting of thorough debridement with immediate coverage, or in a multi-staged manner?**

Single-stage debridement and closure has been reported, but the debridement must be aggressive to ensure *all* devitalized soft tissue, bone, and cartilage is removed. More commonly, a staged approach is used. A staged approach allows for repeated assessment of the wound and tissue, and allows culture and sensitivity data to be finalized to ensure proper antibiotic choice. Negative pressure wound therapy, such as the VAC device, facilitates a staged approach because the VAC device can promote the formation of healthy granulation tissue, protect the mediastinal contents, and stabilize the sternum and allow for extubation prior to definitive reconstruction.

○ **Is there a role for rigid sternal fixation in the management of sternal reconstruction?**

Many surgeons are reluctant to place any hardware for rigid sternal fixation in the setting of recent sternal infection; therefore, soft-tissue-only reconstruction is typical. Although rigid sternal fixation is not necessary, an unstable sternum may result in chronic pain, paradoxical movement, and respiratory impairment. To address these problems related to sternal instability, some authors have successfully performed rigid internal fixation in carefully selected patients with an adequately debrided wound, low bacterial burden, and well-vascularized bone. This approach requires further study, but may represent a future approach to this problem. In addition, primary sternal plating at the time of cardiac surgery (rather than traditional wire cerclage) may be indicated in patients that are high risk for wound complications (diabetes, COPD, obesity, renal failure, immunosuppression, etc.).

○ **What are the common flap choices for sternal reconstruction?**

Pectoralis major, omentum, and rectus abdominis.

○ **Describe the multiple ways in which the pectoralis major muscle can be used for sternal reconstruction?**

One or both pectoralis major muscles can be used.

When the internal mammary artery was used for CABG (usually the left IMA), this muscle can be used as an advancement or transposition flap, based on the thoracoacromial artery. The muscle can be dissected free from the chest wall as well as the overlying skin, can be released from the humerus to increase mobility, and can also be split to cover superior and inferior defects. The muscle can also be left attached to the skin as a musculocutaneous flap, and this is often the better option as it avoids devascularizing the anterior chest skin. If the IMA is preserved, the muscle can be used as a turnover flap, based on the IMA perforators.

○ **Describe the various ways an omental flap can be harvested for sternal reconstruction?**

The omental flap can be harvested through a transdiaphragmatic approach and brought up into the mediastinum. Alternatively, the omentum can be harvested through an upper midline laparotomy incision, but should be placed into the mediastinum using a transdiaphragmatic course to avoid an upper midline ventral hernia. Laparoscopic harvest of the omentum is also described as a minimally invasive approach.

○ **Is there a flap which is "best" for sternal reconstruction?**

The pectoralis muscle is probably the most commonly used flap and is often considered to be the "first-line." However, a recent meta-analysis of the topic failed to show that a muscle flap was superior to an omental flap.

○ **Describe flap selection in upper, middle, and lower third back wound reconstruction.**

Trapezius muscle flap (upper), latissimus muscle flap (middle), gluteus muscle flap, and superior or inferior gluteal artery perforator flaps (lower). Paraspinous muscle should be considered for advancement or turnover to cover exposed spinal hardware.

○ **What is the most common organism identified in sternal infections/mediastinitis?**

Staphylococcus species.

○ **Should debridement and flap coverage be performed in one stage, or should flap coverage be performed in a delayed fashion after debridement and dressing changes or closed drainage?**

Studies indicate that aggressive debridement and immediate flap coverage has a very high success rate (approximately 95%) and avoids the drawbacks of delayed closure, such as multiple operations and prolonged exposure of mediastinal contents.

○ **What are other advantages of flap closure of infected/dehisced sternal wounds?**

Decreased hospital stay and cost.

● ● ● RECONSTRUCTION OF THE ABDOMINAL WALL ● ● ●

○ **Describe the anatomy of the musculofascial layers of the abdominal wall, including the lineal alba, arcuate line, and semilunar lines.**

The anterior abdominal wall is made up of paired rectus abdominis muscles, and pyramidalis muscles. Lateral to the rectus abdominis muscles, the abdominal wall has three muscle layers: (1) external oblique, (2) internal oblique, and (3) transversus abdominis. The aponeurosis of these muscles fuse lateral to the rectus abdominis muscles to create the semilunar lines. Above the arcuate line, the rectus abdominis muscle has an anterior sheath (composed of the external oblique and part of the internal oblique aponeurosis) and a posterior sheath (composed of part of the internal oblique and transversus abdominis aponeurosis). Below the arcuate line, there is only an anterior sheath composed of the aponeurosis from the three muscles. Finally, the muscular aponeuroses form the midline linea alba that separate the left and right rectus muscles.

○ **Describe the blood supply of the abdominal wall.**

The abdomen is supplied by the superior epigastric artery, the deep inferior epigastric artery (zone 1), superficial branches of the circumflex iliac and external pudendal vessels (zone II), and intercostal, subcostal and lumbar arteries (zone III of Huger's classification). The laterally based vessels are found between the internal oblique and transverse abdominis muscles along with the nerves.

○ **What are the common abdominal wall problems that require intervention by a plastic surgeon?**

Most commonly, midline abdominal wall defects due to incisional hernias with retraction of the muscles laterally. There may actually not be any tissue loss per se, but the defect is due to loss of domain. There may be loss of healthy skin due to multiple operations complicated by infection or fistulae. Significant abdominal wall defects can also result from tumor resection.

○ **What are the goals of abdominal wall reconstruction?**

Protect intra-abdominal organs, restore musculofascial integrity and function, prevent recurrent herniation, and provide stable soft-tissue coverage with an acceptable contour.

○ **What are the critical components to assess when evaluating abdominal wall defects?**

While the size of the defect is important, it is also critical to accurately assess the skin, musculofascial layer, and intra-abdominal domain. In addition, the location of the defect will impact reconstructive options, and must be assessed.

○ **What are some options for management of skin and soft-tissue defects of the abdominal wall?**

Closure, typically with undermining, healing by secondary intention (with dressing changes or negative-pressure wound therapy), skin grafting, local or regional flaps, tissue expansion, or in rare cases, free tissue transfer.

○ **What are some options for management of abdominal wall defects involving the musculofascial layers?**

Closure, typically with component separation, fascia grafts, flaps containing fascia, or with the use of implanted mesh (this should only be considered when there is adequate skin coverage overlying the mesh).

○ **Describe the components separation technique.**

In an anterior component separation, the external oblique aponeurosis is incised lateral to the semilunar line, and the avascular plane between the external oblique and internal oblique muscle is dissected to allow medial advancement of the complex consisting of the rectus abdominis muscle with its surrounding sheath and the internal oblique and transversus abdominis muscles. A posterior component separation deep to the transversus abdominis muscles can also be utilized including the posterior rectus sheath.

○ **What distances are gained by performing a components separation?**

On each side, an estimated length gain is 3 to 5 cm at the epigastrium, 7 to 10 cm at the umbilical region, and 1 to 3 cm at the suprapubic region.

○ **Describe some modifications of a standard components separation?**

Minimally invasive techniques can be used to limit undermining, and preserve perforating vessels to the skin. These modifications may reduce dead space and ischemia, and may reduce postoperative wound complications.

○ **What role can tissue expansion play in abdominal wall reconstruction?**

Tissue expanders can be placed subcutaneously to increase the amount of skin available. They can also be placed in the avascular plane between the external and internal oblique muscles to facilitate fascial expansion and closure.

○ **Describe the different types of mesh, and how these can be used to reconstruct the abdominal wall.**

Implantable mesh is either synthetic or biologic. Biologic mesh is derived from either human or animal material (dermis or other), while synthetic material can be manufactured from various materials, and has been classified as macroporous (polypropylene), microporus (expanded polytetrafluoroethylene or ePTFE), or composite. Polypropylene's macroporous structure allows for tissue in-growth, but may cause adhesions of the mesh to bowel, whereas ePTFE's microporus structure does not allow in-growth. While adhesions are minimized, the mesh is never incorporated, but heals with capsule formation, and has no resistance to infection. Once contaminated, this type of mesh must be removed. Composite meshes combine more than one material and are designed for intraperitoneal use with less risk of bowel adhesion formation. Mesh can be placed as either an overlay or underlay to bolster the primary fascial closure (with or without component separation), or as a bridged repair where the mesh spans a gap in the fascia.

○ **What are the characteristics of an optimal abdominal wall reconstruction?**

Hernia recurrence rates are lowest when fascial closure is achieved, and mesh is used to bolster the repair as an underlay. Wrinkles in the mesh should be avoided, and the mesh should underlap the musculofascial layer. Dead space must be obliterated, and drains should be placed. A bridged repair is inferior, and is associated with a high failure rate. Mesh underlay appears to be superior to mesh overlay. Typical recommendations are to avoid synthetic mesh in contaminated fields and to avoid placing polypropylene in an intraperitoneal location; however, high-quality studies to address these issues are lacking, and the optimal use for each type of mesh is yet to be determined.

○ **What are the reconstructive options for the ventral hernia repair in a heavily contaminated case?**

Fascia closure should be strived for usually by addition of bilateral external oblique component separation. Many surgeons feel that in heavily contaminated cases, synthetic mesh is contraindicated, and that it may be necessary to use a bridging biologic mesh if the fascia cannot be closed; however, there is a high rate of postoperative seroma formation and a high failure rate, and future operations are likely. Further studies are needed to determine an optimal reconstructive strategy.

○ **What are the challenges in performing abdominal wall reconstruction in patients who also have an enterocutaneous fistula?**

The presence of an enterocutaneous fistula predisposes these patients to malnutrition as well as electrolyte abnormalities. These patients will require a bowel resection and anastomosis in addition to abdominal wall reconstruction, and an anastomotic leak in the early postoperative period may result in early fistula recurrence, or may also present as life-threatening abdominal sepsis. The clinician must maintain vigilance when caring for these complex patients.

○ **What are some intraoperative maneuvers that could be useful during a difficult case?**

Preoperative mechanical bowel preparation, gastric decompression, paralysis, and avoidance of nitrous oxide are essential. Some surgeons advocate monitoring peak inspiratory pressure and bladder pressure to avoid postoperative abdominal compartment syndrome or similar problems. Abdominal compartment syndrome can be lethal and therefore must be avoided. With peak inspiratory pressures increasing more than 10 mm from baseline, one must consider a bridging mesh to avoid this complication.

○ **What is the role for flaps in abdominal wall reconstruction?**

While component separation is very effective for central midline musculofascial defects, it is much less useful for superior or inferior midline defects, or lateral defects. In these cases, regional flaps may provide a reconstructive solution.

○ **Name some flaps that can be used for abdominal reconstruction?**

Lower abdominal defects can be repaired with a tensor fascia lata flap, rectus femoris flap, or anterolateral thigh flap. These flaps have been reported to reach the supraumbilical position. Vastus lateralis, or gracilis flaps can also be used for lower defects. A subtotal thigh flap can provide a significant amount of tissue for large defects. The latissimus dorsi muscle can be used for upper lateral defects. Often, these defects are reconstructed with mesh and the flap is used to cover the mesh with well-vascularized tissue.

○ **How do you manage an abdominal wall desmoid tumor?**

Abdominal wall desmoid tumors should be managed in conjunction with a general surgeon. Recent studies have shown that many of these can be treated with oral agents such as non steriodal antiinflammatories, thereby avoiding surgery in some patients. While these are benign tumors that do not metastasize, they are locally aggressive and have a tendency to recur. An en bloc full-thickness wide local excision should be performed with negative pathological margins to minimize the risk of recurrence. Due to the large defect size resulting from an aggressive resection, abdominal wall reconstruction can be a challenge, but should follow the principles outlined above. Abdominal wall desmoid tumors do not require chemotherapy or radiation.

● ● ● **REFERENCES** ● ● ●

Albino FP, Patel KM, Nahabedian MY, Sosin M, Attinger CE, Bhanot P. Does mesh location matter in abdominal wall reconstruction? A systematic review of the literature and a summary of recommendations. *Plast Reconstr Surg.* 2013;132(5):1295–1304.

Althubaiti G, Butler CE. Abdominal wall and chest wall reconstruction. *Plast Reconstr Surg.* 2014;133(5):688e–701e.

Arnold PG, Pairolero PC. Chest-wall reconstruction: an account of 500 consecutive patients. *Plast Reconstr Surg.* 1996;98(5):804–810.

Arnold PG, Pairolero PC. Intrathoracic muscle flaps: a 10-year experience in the management of life-threatening infections. *Plast Reconstr Surg.* 1989;84(1):92–98; discussion 99.

Bakri K, Mardini S, Evans KK, Carlsen BT, Arnold PG. Workhorse flaps in chest wall reconstruction: the pectoralis major, latissimus dorsi, and rectus abdominis flaps. *Semin Plast Surg.* 2011;25(1):43–54.

Berri RN, Baumann DP, Madewell JE, Lazar A, Pollock RE. Desmoid tumor: current multidisciplinary approaches. *Ann Plast Surg.* 2011;67(5):551–564.

Cicilioni OJ Jr, Stieg FH 3rd, Papanicolaou G. Sternal wound reconstruction with transverse plate fixation. *Plast Reconstr Surg.* 2005;115(5):1297–1303.

Cohen M. Reconstruction of the chest wall. In: Cohen M, ed. *Mastery of Plastic and Reconstructive Surgery.* Boston, MA: Little, Brown and Company; 1994:1248–1267.

Gottlieb LJ, Pielet RW, Karp RB, Krieger LM, Smith DJ Jr, Deeb GM.. Rigid internal fixation of the sternum in postoperative mediastinitis. *Arch Surg.* 1994;129(5):489–493.

Hanna WC, Ferri LE, McKendy KM, Turcotte R, Sirois C, Mulder DS. Reconstruction after major chest wall resection: can rigid fixation be avoided?. *Surgery.* 2011;150(4):590–597.

Hawn MT, Snyder CW, Graham LA, Gray SH, Finan KR, Vick CC. Long-term follow-up of technical outcomes for incisional hernia repair. *J Am Coll Surg.* 2010;210(5):648–655.

Huger WE Jr. The anatomic rationale for abdominal lipectomy. *Am Surg.* 1979;45(9):612–617.

Itani KM, Rosen M, Vargo D, et al. Prospective study of single-stage repair of contaminated hernias using a biologic porcine tissue matrix: the RICH Study. *Surgery.* 2012;152(3):498–505.

Ko JH, Wang EC, Salay DM, Paul BC, Dumanian GA. Abdominal wall reconstruction: lessons learned from 200 "components separation" procedures. *Arch Surg.* 2009;144(11):1047–1055.

Krpata DM, Stein SL, Eston M, et al. Outcomes of simultaneous large complex abdominal wall reconstruction and enterocutaneous fistula takedown. *Am J Surg.* 2013;205(3):354–358; discussion 358–359.

Mahabir RC, Butler CE. Stabilization of the chest wall: autologous and alloplastic reconstructions. *Semin Plast Surg.* 2011;25(1):34–42.

Mathes SJ, Steinwald PM, Foster RD, Hoffman WY, Anthony JP. Complex abdominal wall reconstruction: a comparison of flap and mesh closure. *Ann Surg.* 2000;232(4):586–596.

Montgomery A. The battle between biological and synthetic meshes in ventral hernia repair. *Hernia.* 2013;17(1):3–11.

Pairolero PC, Arnold PG, Harris JB. Long-term results of pectoralis major muscle transposition for infected sternotomy wounds. *Ann Surg.* 1991;213(6):583–589; discussion 589–590.

Ramirez OM, Ruas E, Dellon AL. "Components separation" method for closure of abdominal-wall defects: an anatomic and clinical study. *Plast Reconstr Surg.* 1990;86(3):519–526.

Raman J, Lehmann S, Zehr K, et al. Sternal closure with rigid plate fixation versus wire closure: a randomized controlled multicenter trial. *Ann Thorac Surg.* 2012;94(6):1854–1861.

Roche NA, Van Landuyt K, Blondeel PN, Matton G, Monstrey SJ. The use of pedicled perforator flaps for reconstruction of lumbosacral defects. *Ann Plast Surg.* 2000;45(1):7–14.

Rohrich RJ, Lowe JB, Hackney FL, Bowman JL, Hobar PC. An algorithm for abdominal wall reconstruction. *Plast Reconstr Surg.* 2000;105(1):202–216.

Rosenthal AH. Thoracic and abdominal reconstruction. In: Brown DL, Borschel GH, eds. *Michigan Manual of Plastic Surgery.* Philadelphia, PA: Lippincott Williams & Wilkins; 2004:344–348.

Roth DA. Thoracic and abdominal wall reconstruction. In: Aston SJ, Beasley RW, Thorne CH, eds. *Grabb and Smith's Plastic Surgery.* 5th ed. Philadelphia, PA: Lippincott-Raven; 1997:1023–1029.

Saulis AS, Dumanian GA. Periumbilical rectus abdominis perforator preservation significantly reduces superficial wound complications in "separation of parts" hernia repairs. *Plast Reconstr Surg.* 2002;109(7):2275–2280; discussion 2281–2282.

Seyfer AE. Chest wall reconstruction. In: Achauer BM, Eriksson E, eds. *Plastic Surgery Indications, Operations, and Outcomes.* St Louis, MO: Mosby; 2000:547–562.

Singh K, Anderson E, Harper JG. Overview and management of sternal wound infection. *Semin Plast Surg*. 2011;25(1):25–33.

Souza JM, Dumanian GA. An evidence-based approach to abdominal wall reconstruction. *Plast Reconstr Surg*. 2012;130(1):116–124.

Tsukushi S, Nishida Y, Sugiura H, et al. Non-rigid reconstruction of chest wall defects after resection of musculoskeletal tumors. *Surg Today*. 2015;45(2):150–155.

van Wingerden JJ, Lapid O, Boonstra PW, de Mol BA. Muscle flaps or omental flap in the management of deep sternal wound infection. *Interact Cardiovasc Thorac Surg*. 2011;13(2):179–187.

Ventral Hernia Working Group, Breuing K, Butler CE, et al. Incisional ventral hernias: review of the literature and recommendations regarding the grading and technique of repair. *Surgery*. 2010;148(3):544–558.

Vyas RM, Prsic A, Orgill DP. Transdiaphragmatic omental harvest: a simple method for sternal wound coverage. *Plast Reconstr Surg*. 2013;131(3):544–552.

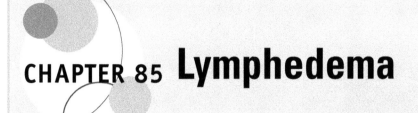

CHAPTER 85 Lymphedema

Arin K. Greene, MD, MMSc and
Sumner A. Slavin, MD

○ **What is lymphedema?**

Accumulation of protein-rich fluid in the interstitial space due to lymphatic dysfunction.

○ **How common is lymphedema?**

Approximately 150 million people are affected worldwide.

○ **What structures are most commonly involved?**

The extremities, followed by the genitalia.

○ **Does lymphedema affect the superficial or deep areas of the extremity?**

Only the subcutaneous tissues are involved.

○ **What is the natural history of lymphedema?**

Adipose and fibrous tissues are produced which cause enlargement of the limb.

○ **How is lymphedema classified?**

Primary or secondary.

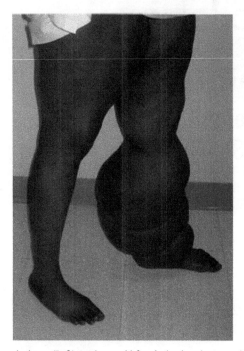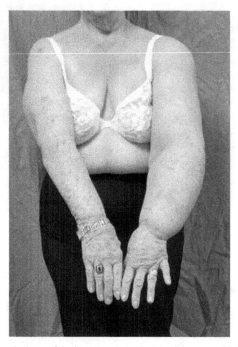

Types of lymphedema. (**Left**) A 24-year-old female developed primary lymphedema of the lower extremity during adolescence. (**Right**) A 70-year-old female with upper extremity lymphedema following mastectomy, axillary lymphadenectomy, and radiation for breast cancer.

○ **What is primary lymphedema?**

Lymphedema that results from a congenital malformation of the lymphatic system.

○ **How common is primary lymphedema?**

Rare. The prevalence is approximately 1:100,000.

○ **When does primary lymphedema present?**

Males usually present in infancy, females typically develop swelling in adolescence.

○ **What structures are most commonly affected by primary lymphedema?**

Lower extremities (90%), genitalia (16%), and upper extremities (10%).

○ **Is there a genetic cause of primary lymphedema?**

Yes, mutations in *VEGFR3*, *FOXC2*, *SOX18*, and *CCBE1* cause some familial/syndromic forms of lymphedema.

○ **What is Milroy disease?**

Lymphedema of one or both lower extremities present at birth, with either a family history of disease or a mutation in *VEGFR3*.

○ **What is Meige disease?**

Lymphedema of one or both lower extremities presenting in adolescence with a family history of the disease; a genetic mutation has not been identified.

○ **What is secondary lymphedema?**

Lymphedema that results from injury to the lymphatic system.

○ **What is the most common cause of lymphedema worldwide?**

Parasitic infection (filariasis), causing lower extremity lymphedema.

○ **What is the most common cause of lymphedema in developed countries?**

Upper extremity lymphedema secondary to axillary lymphadenectomy and radiation treatment for breast cancer.

○ **What percentage of women with breast cancer who have axillary lymphadenectomy and radiation develop lymphedema?**

Approximately 33%.

○ **How long after axillary lymphadenectomy and radiation does it take for lymphedema to become clinically evident?**

3 to 24 months.

○ **How is lymphedema diagnosed?**

More than 90% of patients are diagnosed by history and physical examination.

○ **What conditions are most commonly confused with lymphedema?**

Lipedema, venous stasis, systemic causes of edema (cardiac, renal, hepatic disease), posttraumatic swelling, Klippel–Trenanuay syndrome, Parkes–Weber syndrome, and hemihypertrophy.

○ **Can obesity cause lymphedema?**

Yes, when a patient's body mass index exceeds 60 kg/m^2 lower extremity lymphatic dysfunction occurs (obesity-induced lymphedema).

○ **What test can confirm the diagnosis of lymphedema?**

Lymphoscintigraphy is 92% sensitive and 100% specific for lymphedema.

○ **Is CT or MRI useful to diagnose lymphedema?**

No, they are less accurate than lymphoscintigraphy and have nonspecific findings.

○ **Can a biopsy diagnose lymphedema?**
No, histopathology shows nonspecific inflammation.

○ **What is the most common complication of lymphedema?**
Cellulitis.

○ **What other problems result from lymphedema?**
Difficulty with daily activities, inability to wear proper-fitting clothing, and psychosocial morbidity.

○ **Is lymphedema curable?**
No, it is a chronic, progressive condition.

○ **What is the first-line treatment for lymphedema?**
Compression using either elastic stockings, a pneumatic pump, or bandaging.

○ **Are there drugs available to treat lymphedema?**
No.

○ **Is blood pressure monitoring and venepuncture harmful to a lymphedematous limb?**
No, but the nonaffected extremity should be used if possible.

○ **When is operative intervention for lymphedema indicated?**
Significant morbidity despite maximal conservative treatment.

○ **What are the two categories of operative intervention for lymphedema?**
Excisional or physiological procedures.

○ **What are excisional procedures?**
Operations that remove lymphedematous tissue.

○ **What are physiological procedures?**
Operations that attempt to restore lymph drainage.

○ **Which is superior, excisional, or physiological procedures?**
Excisional procedures are more effective and predictable. They can also be used for moderate and severe disease.

○ **What is the first-line excisional procedure for extremity lymphedema?**
Suction-assisted lipectomy.

○ **What is the second-line operative procedure for severe extremity lymphedema with significant skin excess?**

Staged skin and subcutaneous excision.

○ **What is the Charles procedure?**

Circumferential removal of skin, subcutaneous tissue, and fascia followed by skin grafting of the underlying muscle.

○ **Is the Charles procedure effective?**

Yes, but it is rarely used because it has significant postoperative morbidity.

○ **What are the most common physiological procedures performed?**

Lymphaticovenous anastomosis and vascularized lymph node transfer.

○ **What are the advantages and disadvantages of lymphaticovenous anastomosis?**

The procedure generally is reserved for patients with early disease before subcutaneous fibro-adipose tissue develops. Improvement is variable and patients usually require the continued use of compression garments.

○ **What are the advantages and disadvantages of vascularized lymph node transfer?**

The procedure generally is reserved for individuals with early lymphedema before fibro-adipose hypertrophy occurs. Improvement is variable. Patients are at risk for lymphedema at the site where lymph nodes are harvested; the rate has been reported to be as high as 23%.

• • • REFERENCES • • •

Brorson H, Svensson H. Liposuction combined with controlled compression therapy reduces arm lymphedema more effectively than controlled compression therapy alone. *Plast Reconstr Surg.* 1998;102:1058–1067; discussion 1068.

Brorson H, Ohlin K, Olsson G, Nilsson M. Adipose tissue dominates chronic arm lymphedema following breast cancer: an analysis using volume rendered CT images. *Lymphat Res Biol.* 2006;4:199–210.

Chang DW, Suami H, Skoracki R. A prospective analysis of 100 consecutive lymphovenous bypass cases for treatment of extremity lymphedema. *Plast Reconstr Surg.* 2013;132:1305–1314.

Gloviczki P, Calcagno D, Schirger A, et al. Noninvasive evaluation of the swollen extremity: experiences with 190 lymphoscintigraphic examinations. *J Vasc Surg.* 1989;9:683–689; discussion 690.

Greene AK, Grant FD, Slavin SA. Lower-extremity lymphedema and elevated body-mass index. *N Engl J Med.* 2012;366:2136–2137.

Greene AK, Slavin SA, Borud L. Treatment of lower extremity lymphedema with suction-assisted lipectomy. *Plast Reconstr Surg.* 2006;118:118e–121e.

Koshima I, Nanba Y, Tsutsui T, Takahashi Y, Itoh S. Long-term follow-up after lymphaticovenular anastomosis for lymphedema in the leg. *J Reconstr Microsurg.* 2003;19:209–215.

Maclellan RA, Couto RA, Sullivan JE, Grant FD, Slavin SA, Greene AK. Management of primary and secondary lymphedema: analysis of 225 referrals to a center. *Ann Plast Surg.* 2015;75:197–200.

Maclellan RA, Greene AK. Lymphedema. *Semin Pediatr Surg.* 2014;23:191–197.

Maegawa J, Yabuki Y, Tomoeda H, Hosono M, Yasumura K. Outcomes of lymphaticovenous side-to-end anastomosis in peripheral lymphedema. *J Vasc Surg.* 2012;55:753–760.

Miller TA. Charles procedure for lymphedema: a warning. *Am J Surg.* 1980;139:290–292.

Miller TA, Wyatt LE, Rudkin GH. Staged skin and subcutaneous excision for lymphedema: a favorable report of long-term results. *Plast Reconstr Surg.* 1998;102:1486–1498; discussion 1499–1501.

O'Brien BM, Mellow CG, Khazanchi RK, Dvir E, Kumar V, Pederson WC. Long-term results after microlymphaticovenous anastomoses for the treatment of obstructive lymphedema. *Plast Reconstr Surg*. 1990;85:562–572.

Schook CC, Mulliken JB, Fishman SJ, Alomari AI, Grant FD, Greene AK. Differential diagnosis of lower extremity enlargement in pediatric patients referred with a diagnosis of lymphedema. *Plast Reconstr Surg*. 2011;127:1571–1581.

Schook CC, Mulliken JB, Fishman SJ, Grant FD, Zurakowski D, Greene AK. Primary lymphedema: clinical features and management in 138 pediatric patients. *Plast Reconstr Surg*. 2011;127:2419–2431.

Vignes S, Blanchard M, Yannoutsos A, Arrault M. Complications of autologous lymph-node transplantation for limb lymphoedema. *Eur J Vasc Endovasc Surg*. 2013;45:516–520.

CHAPTER 86

Lower Extremity Reconstruction—Soft-Tissue Concepts

Todd A. Theman, MD and Matthew L. Iorio, MD

○ **What are the boundaries of the femoral triangle?**

- Proximally—inguinal ligament.

- Laterally—sartorius.

- Medially—adductor longus.

- Floor—iliacus, psoas, pectineus, and adductor longus.

○ **Which muscles of the lower extremity are located in the superficial posterior compartment? What is the innervation and function of each? Superficial posterior compartment?**

- Gastrocnemius, innervated by posterior tibial nerve, functions in plantar flexion.

- Plantaris (as for gastrocnemius).

- Soleus (as for gastrocnemius).

○ **Deep posterior compartment?**

- Flexor hallucis longus/posterior tibial nerve/toe flexion.

- Tibialis posterior/posterior tibial nerve/inversion and plantar flexion of ankle.

- Flexor digitorum longus (as for flexor hallucis longus).

○ **Lateral compartment?**

- Peroneus brevis/superficial peroneal nerve/ankle eversion.

- Peroneus longus (as for brevis).

○ **Anterior compartment?**
  • Tibialis anterior/deep peroneal nerve/ankle dorsiflexion.
  • Extensor digitorum longus/deep peroneal nerve/toe extension.
  • Extensor hallucis longus/deep peroneal nerve/toe extension.
  • Peroneus tertius/deep peroneal nerve/ankle eversion and weak dorsiflexion.

○ **In which compartments do the trifurcated arteries travel in the lower extremity?**
  Anterior tibial artery—anterior compartment.
  Posterior tibial artery—deep posterior compartment.
  Peroneal artery—deep posterior compartment.

○ **What nerve may accompany the lesser saphenous vein and what does it innervate?**
  The **sural nerve** provides sensation to the skin over the posterolateral lower extremity, the lateral heel, and the lateral border of the foot. It is found between the Achilles tendon and lateral malleolus and up to 25 cm can be harvested.

○ **The plantar surface of the foot may be divided into four layers. Which muscles may be found in the most superficial layer?**
  • Flexor digitorum brevis.
  • Abductor hallucis.
  • Abductor digiti quinti.

○ **What nerves provide sensation to the foot and what are their respective dermatomes?**
  • Posterior tibial nerve—plantar midfoot and heel
  • Sural nerve—lateral midfoot
  • Saphenous nerve—medial ankle
  • Superficial peroneal nerve—dorsal distal foot
  • Deep peroneal nerve—first web space

○ **Which tendon of the lower extremity is the preferred donor for grafting and which nerve is most at risk during harvest?**
  Plantaris tendon. It is present in approximately 80% of lower limbs. Dissection begins just posterior to the medial malleolus, placing the posterior tibial nerve at risk.

○ **What findings are indicative of compartment syndrome?**
  • Palpable firmness of compartment, pallor, pain on passive extension is compartment-specific:
    • Anterior: pain on passive plantar flexion and foot eversion, toe flexion.
    • Lateral: pain on passive dorsiflexion and foot inversion.
    • Superficial posterior: pain on passive ankle dorsiflexion with knee extended.
    • Deep posterior: pain on passive ankle dorsiflexion, toe extension.
  • Compartmental pressures >35 mm Hg (or differential pressure <30)
    • Pulselessness is a very late finding as venous and lymphatic flow through the compartment will occlude prior to compression of arterial flow. A differential pressure is obtained by subtracting the compartmental pressure from the patient's diastolic pressure.

○ **How do you treat a compartment syndrome of the lower extremity?**

Fasciotomies. Medial and lateral longitudinal incisions should allow adequate exposure to incise intermuscular septae, thereby releasing all four compartments. Remember that fasciotomies will also be appropriate for expected severe elevation in compartment pressures that are associated with crush injury, electrical burn, massive fluid resuscitation, and reperfusion injury.

○ **What is the procedure of choice for reconstruction of small-to-medium defects of the plantar surface of the foot?**

V-Y plantar advancement flap. The plantar skin and fascia should be incised congruently to maintain intact the vessels perforating the fascia from the medial and lateral plantar arteries.

○ **What would you do to reconstruct a more extensive defect of the plantar foot in an ambulatory patient?**

Provide soft-tissue coverage that is durable and tolerant of shear forces experienced with ambulation. A muscle flap with a skin graft has been shown to perform well for such reconstructions.

○ **What additional measures should be considered when reconstructing the plantar surface of the foot?**

If the plantar surface is insensate, the patient should be educated on being vigilant and meticulous in caring for the foot. Custom orthotics with a metatarsal bar should decrease metatarsal head pressure and shearing and compression forces on the reconstructed foot.

○ **What is the Gustilo classification system for tibial injury?**

Gustilo classification

I		Low-energy, simple bone fracture, clean wound <1 cm.
II		Moderate comminution and contamination, wound >1 cm, moderate soft-tissue damage.
III		High energy, comminution of the fracture, wound >1 cm, extensive soft-tissue damage, highly contaminated.
	A	Adequate soft-tissue cover.
	B	Inadequate soft-tissue coverage, extensive periosteal stripping.
	C	Arterial injury requiring repair for salvage.

○ **What is the Byrd classification system for tibial injury?**

Byrd classification.

I	Low-energy fracture, oblique or spiral fracture with clean-cut laceration <1 cm.
II	Medium-energy trauma, displaced or comminuted fracture with laceration >2 cm, myocutaneous contusion.
III	High-energy trauma, severely displaced or comminuted fracture, segmental fracture or bone defect, laceration >2 cm, myocutaneous soft-tissue loss.
IV	High-energy bursting trauma, crushing or avulsion with arterial damage (that requires repair).

○ **What muscles can be used to reconstruct the soft tissue over the proximal one-third of the tibia?**

Medial gastrocnemius (medial sural artery and venae comitantes). The medial hemi-gastrocnemius is the larger and longer of the two and is more commonly used.

Lateral gastrocnemius (lateral sural artery and venae comitantes).

○ **What muscle can be used to reconstruct the soft tissue over the middle one-third of the tibia?**

Soleus (the proximal muscle is supplied by branches of the peroneal artery while the distal muscle is supplied by posterior tibial artery perforators). Modifications of this muscle may be made, such as a hemisoleus for greater arc of rotation. A split tibialis anterior muscle flap may also be used for long, thin defects.

○ **What flaps can be used to reconstruct the soft tissue over the distal one-third of the tibia?**

Free muscle or fasciocutaneous flaps. The choice of flap will depend upon the extent of soft-tissue injury, necessary pedicle length, and the surgeon's familiarity. While a free tissue transfer for a distal one-third open tibial fracture is the classic answer, there are possibilities of local flaps, such as a distally based hemisoleus flap or propeller flap.

○ **The anterolateral thigh (ALT) flap has become a workhorse of lower extremity soft-tissue reconstruction. What landmarks are used to mark the flap, what is the pedicle, and what muscle is sometimes harvested with the flap?**

The meridian of an ALT flap is along a line drawn from the ASIS to the superolateral border of the patella with the hip internally rotated. The descending branch of the lateral circumflex femoral artery (branch of profunda femoris) is the pedicle. The perforators may traverse the vastus lateralis muscle, which can be harvested also. Mark the midpoint of this line and perforators are usually found 5 cm proximal and distal to this midpoint and 1 to 2 cm medial to the line.

○ **Within what timeframe should an osteocutaneous defect of the tibia receive definitive soft-tissue reconstruction?**

Ideally within 72 hours, after which the total complication, rate including infections and flap loss, increases dramatically. Inadequate soft-tissue or bone debridement is the common cause of postoperative failure, and while early soft-tissue coverage is important, it should not be at the expense of adequate debridement.

○ **A reverse-flow sural artery flap is used to reconstruct a calcaneus wound. To best preserve the vascularity of this flap, the distal dissection of the pedicle should terminate where?**

5 cm above the lateral malleolus, in order to not divide peroneal artery perforators that supply the flap. Partial flap loss is the most common complication.

○ **What factors favor amputation over lower extremity salvage/reconstruction?**

- Insensate plantar surface of foot (particularly in adults with a nerve gap).
- Ischemia time >6 hours or crush mechanism.
- Multi-level injury in the ipsilateral limb.
- Loss of plantar flexion.
- Severe comorbid illness or condition precluding reconstruction.

The literature remains divided on whether reconstruction or amputation is associated with better long-term functional outcomes, return to work, and cost, so treatment decisions remain individualized. Absent plantar sensation does not preclude reconstruction, as approximately 50% of patients with an intact nerve will regain plantar sensation at 2 years. While a low initial injury severity score is associated with salvage, a high score does not predict amputation and is not associated with long-term functional outcomes.

○ **You are asked to emergently evaluate a newborn with a threatened lower limb. You find a congenital constriction ring with severe distal lymphedema, progressive cyanosis, and clubfoot. What is the next step in management?**

Congenital constriction bands present along a spectrum from shallow soft-tissue depression to constriction ring with distal lymphedema and acrosyndactyly (fusion of distal parts), progressive lymphatic or arteriovenous compromise, and congenital amputation. They are frequently associated with prematurity, low birth weight, and clubfoot. Limb-length discrepancies are common in infancy. The rare case of a deep constriction ring with progressive neurologic arteriovenous compromise necessitates emergency limb salvage. The etiology is early amnion rupture and oligohydramnios.

Correction of the deformity involves excision of the constriction ring, reconstruction of underlying absent structures (tendon, nerve), correction of limb length discrepancy with lengthening or contralateral epiphysiodesis, and adipofascial flaps and/or local transposition flaps to fill the contour deformity.

● ● ● REFERENCES ● ● ●

Askins G, Ger E. Congenital constriction band syndrome. *J Pediatr Orthop.* 1988;8:461–466.

Francel TJ, Vander Kolk CA, Hoopes JE, Manson PN, Yaremchuk MJ. Microvascular soft-tissue transplantation for reconstruction of acute open tibial fractures: timing of coverage and long-term functional results. *Plast Reconstr Surg.* 1992;89:478–487; discussion 488–489.

Godina M. Early microsurgical reconstruction of complex trauma of the extremities. *Plast Reconstr Surg.* 1986;78(3):285–292.

Gustilo RB, Mendoza RM, Williams DN. Problems in the management of type III (severe) open fractures: a new classification of type III open fractures. *J Trauma.* 1984;24:742–746.

Hasegawa M, Torii S, Katoh H, Esaki S. The distally based superficial sural artery flap. *Plast Reconstr Surg.* 1994;93:1012–1020.

Kasabian AK, Karp NS. Lower extremity reconstruction. In: Aston SJ, Beasley RW, Thorne CH, eds. *Grabb and Smith's Plastic Surgery.* 5th ed. Philadelphia, PA: Lippincott-Raven; 1997:1031–1048.

May JW Jr, Rohrich RJ. Foot reconstruction using free microvascular muscle flaps with skin grafts. *Clin Plast Surg.* 1986;13:681–689.

Thorne CH, Siebert JW, Grotting JC, et al. Reconstructive surgery of the lower extremity. In: McCarthy JG, ed. *Plastic Surgery.* Philadelphia, PA: WB Saunders; 1990:4029–4092.

Warren AG, Brorson H, Borud LJ, Slavin SA. Lymphedema: a comprehensive review. *Ann Plast Surg.* 2007;59:464–472.

CHAPTER 87 Lower Extremity Reconstruction— Orthopedic Concepts

Pieter G.L. Koolen, MD,
John B. Hijjawi, MD, FACS, and
Samuel J. Lin, MD, MBA, FACS

○ **How many compartments exist in the thigh and leg? Which muscles, nerves, and blood vessels lie in which compartments?**

Thigh (Table 87-1)

Table 87-1

Compartment	Motor Nerve	Blood Supply	Muscles
Anterior	Femoral (L2-4)	Femoral	Quadriceps femoris, sartorius iliopsoas, pectineus
Medial	Obturator (L2-4)	Profunda femoris Obturator	Gracilis, adductor longus Adductor brevis, adductor magnus, Obturator externus
Posterior	Sciatic (L4-S3)	Profunda femoris (branches)	Biceps femoris, semitendinosus Semimembranosus Adductor magnus

Lower Leg (Table 87-2)

Table 87-2

Compartment	Motor Nerve	Blood Supply	Muscles
Anterior	Deep peroneal	Tibialis anterior	Tibialis anterior Extensor digitorum longus Extensor hallucis longus Peroneus tertius
Lateral	Superficial peroneal	Peroneal	Peroneus longus Peroneus brevis
Superficial posterior	Tibialis (branches)	Tibialis posterior (branches)	Gastrocnemius Plantaris Soleus
Deep posterior	Tibialis	Tibialis posterior	Popliteus Flexor digitorum longus Flexor hallucis longus Tibialis posterior

○ **Which nerves supply sensation to the foot?**

• Dorsum: superficial peroneal except the first web which is supplied by the deep peroneal.

• Sole: medial and lateral plantar from the posterior tibial.

○ **What are the biomechanical effects of the foot that make reconstruction potentially suboptimal?**

Normal gait requires the foot to transition from a flexible structure to a rigid structure as the hindfoot makes contact and forces are transitioned to the forefoot. The forefoot's unique osteoligamentous structures facilitate this conservation of energy. Current flap techniques cannot replicate the biomechanics of the intact foot.

○ **What percentage of patients with diabetes mellitus develops heel ulcers?**

15%.

○ **What are the possible biomechanical effects on the foot of patients with diabetes mellitus?**

• Reduced subtalar joint mobility.

• Limited first metatarsal mobility.

○ **What is a Charcot foot?**

It is acute or gradual arthropathy of the foot that most commonly occurs in patients with diabetes. It was originally described in patients with syphilis. The pathophysiology of the disease has not been definitively elucidated but it may involve trivial microtrauma that affects the joints of the foot. Another theory attributes autonomic changes that lead to increased osteopenia of the bones. Swelling, erythema, pain, and ulceration (40%) may develop that mimics infection. Collapse of the osseoligamentous structures of the foot leads to derangements in pressure points on the foot.

○ **What is the most common location of bony sarcomas of the lower extremity?**

Proximal tibia.

○ **What are the most common complications of limb salvage for these sarcomas?**

- Wound healing (skin flap necrosis).
- Wound infection.
- Nerve palsy.
- Hardware failure.

○ **What are the treatment options of resectable bony sarcomas of the distal femur and proximal tibia?**

- Amputation.
- Reconstruction with oncologic appliance and soft-tissue flap.
- Rotationplasty (children).

○ **Why is it necessary to perform flap coverage of the knee oncologic appliance for tumors of the distal femur/proximal tibia?**

Wound complication rates of over 50% have been reported with prosthesis placement without flap coverage. Malignant lesions in this region require resection of adjacent soft tissue, skeletonization of neurovascular structures, and development of large subcutaneous flaps. This leads to an increased risk of implant exposure and infection without the use of adjunctive flap coverage.

○ **What is a Girdlestone procedure?**

Described in the 1940s, it is resection of the femoral head and neck for severe infection of the hip. Although the procedure is uncommon in the modern era, it is still employed for severe stage IV trochanteric pressure ulcers complicated by osteomyelitis. The vastus lateralis muscle flap may be employed to interpose in the dead space created by the resection.

○ **What are the ambulatory implications of a Girdlestone procedure?**

The leg will be shorter and require the patient to be dependent on walking aids, such as a walker or crutch.

○ **What are the possible clinical circumstances of a peroneal nerve injury?**

- Fracture of a tibia or fibula.
- Sharp injury.
- Severe adduction injury of the knee.
- Gunshot wound.
- Iatrogenic (ganglion resection, fibula harvest).

○ **Why should tourniquet placement directly below the knee (proximal leg) be avoided?**

Peroneal nerve palsy with compression at the head of the fibula may develop. Place the tourniquet above the knee. Avoid tourniquets in patients with vascular bypass grafts across the region of tourniquet control.

○ **If the common peroneal nerve is disrupted, what are the treatment options?**

- Primary repair of nerve in the low-energy or sharp injury with or without nerve graft. This can be performed immediately or within weeks after the injury.

- Tibialis posterior transfer. Since an equinovarus deformity inevitably develops despite use of a kick-up brace, muscle balancing with early tendon transfer may be advantageous.

○ **What is Gustilo's classification of open tibial fractures as modified in 1998?**

- I: "with cutaneous defect <1 cm, clean, little soft-tissue injury"

- II: "laceration >1 cm, no extensive soft-tissue injury, no flaps or avulsions" moderate crush injury and comminution of bone and contamination.

- III: extensive soft-tissue damage with muscle and sometimes n/vasc, high contamination "included are high-energy, industrial, segmental, and severe comminution."
  - IIIA: "extensive soft-tissue lacerations, high-energy injury but cover available."
  - IIIB: "soft-tissue loss and periosteal stripping, massive contamination, bone comminution or loss."
  - IIIC: any injury with arterial injury requiring repair regardless of soft-tissue damage degree.

○ **In general, which injuries in the Gustilo's classification require soft-tissue flaps?**

Gustilo IIIB and IIIC injuries usually require flap coverage.

○ **After a limb-threatening lower extremity injury (Gustilo type IIIB), is the functional outcome better after limb salvage or early amputation?**

They have equivalent functional outcomes at 2 and 7 years after the injury.

○ **For Gustilo IIIB fractures of the tibial shaft, what is the recommended form of fixation?**

Intramedullary nailing is the treatment of choice for most of these injuries. There is controversy whether the nail should be placed with or without intramedullary reaming. External fixation may be used initially, especially in patients presenting with highly contaminated wounds.

○ **What is the amputation rate for Gustilo grade IIIC tibial fracture?**

87%.

○ **The classification using the mangled extremity severity score (MESS, Johansen 1990) classifies patients according to which of the four criteria?**

- Shock.
- Ischemia.
- Age.
- Skeletal/soft-tissue damage.

○ **Do limb injury severity scores such as the MESS correlate with function after limb salvage?**

No. When prospectively evaluated, a low score has been shown to indicate a high likelihood of successful limb salvage; however, high scores are poorly predictive of function and should be used cautiously.

○ **What factors best correlate with functional outcome after a limb-threatening lower-extremity injury?**

Socioeconomic and demographic factors have the best correlation with eventual outcome. Factors associated with a poorer outcome include lower education level, economic status, older age, female gender, nonwhite race, smoking, poor self-efficacy, and being involved in a lawsuit. A major complication also correlates with a poorer outcome.

○ **Should absent plantar sensation be used as an indication for early amputation?**

No, over 50% of patients presenting with an insensate foot after a lower extremity injury regain plantar sensation and eventual sensory function is similar to other patients with severe lower extremity injuries. A visualized disruption of the tibial nerve may be considered an indication for amputation in an adult.

○ **What percentage of patients with a limb-threatening lower extremity injury return to employment?**

58% return to employment within 7 years of the injury.

○ **What percentage of patients with a limb-threatening lower extremity injury regain a functional status within population norms?**

34% eventually recover an overall functional status within the normal range for the population as measured by the Sickness Impact Profile.

○ **After a limb-threatening lower extremity injury (Gustilo type IIIB), which treatment has a higher associated cost: early amputation or limb salvage?**

At 2 years, postinjury medical costs are similar between the two groups. While patients treated with limb salvage have higher costs associated with rehospitalizations for acute care, those treated with amputation have higher costs associated with rehabilitation. When considering the prosthesis-associated costs, the patients treated with amputation have a higher overall cost at 2 years. Over the course of a lifetime, it is projected that the costs associated with an amputation are triple those of limb salvage, making reconstruction a cost-effective treatment.

○ **How does one assess bony viability when surgically treating a patient with osteomyelitis?**

Assess for the presence of punctate bleeding from the bone after debridement (the paprika sign). This is most commonly done using a burr and the presence of bleeding from the bone indicates viability.

○ **According to Godina, patients requiring free-flap reconstruction for tibial coverage are classified as reconstructed:**

Early (<72 hours), delayed (>72 hours and <3 months), or late (>3 months).

○ **Microvascular failure and infection was commonest in which group?**

Delayed group.

○ **Microvascular success and absence of infection was commonest in which group?**

Early group.

○ **What are the reconstructive options for a large (>5 cm) bony gap/defect in the tibia?**

These defects may be treated with acute shortening and subsequent lengthening or bone transport using a ring external fixator frame (Ilizarov frame). A free vascularized bone transfer (typically a free fibula graft) is another option. More recently the induced membrane technique of Masquelet has become popular as well. This involves placement of a temporary polymethyl methacrylate (PMMA) cement spacer with subsequent cancellous bone grafting.

○ **Ilizarov distraction osteogenesis distracts approximately at what rate?**

0.25 mm distraction × 4/day.

○ **After the desired length of bone is achieved, how long is the Ilizarov frame left on?**

For the same length of time as the distraction to allow <u>consolidation</u>.

○ **What is the ideal length that should be preserved for a below-knee amputation?**

Optimally 12 to 15 cm as measured from the knee joint line. Residual limbs that are too short are more difficult to fit with a prosthesis and may functionally act similar to a through knee amputation rather that a BKA. Residual limbs that are too long may have compromised soft-tissue coverage. If the residual limbs are too long, it may also compromise prosthesis options because some of the most advanced prosthetics are 10 inches in length and require adequate shortening of the limb in order to be used.

○ **What is a Lisfranc amputation?**

Amputation through the level of the transmetatarsal joints.

○ **What is a Symes amputation?**

Amputation just above the ankle joint.

○ **What are the first signs in compartment syndrome?**

General pain and tingling in the limb out of proportion with the injury with **pain on passive extension** of the involved muscle groups.

○ **What is the normal tissue pressure?**

2 to 7 mm Hg.

○ **At what tissue pressure is one concerned of compartment syndrome?**

An absolute pressure of 30 mm Hg or within 30 mm Hg of diastolic blood pressure is concerning for compartment syndrome.

○ **What incisions would you use to perform fasciotomies to the lower leg?**

Two vertical incisions 2 cm to either side of the subcutaneous border of the tibia.

○ **Through which of the above incisions would you decompress the posterior compartments?**

Usually the medial one.

○ **Which compartments are released via the lateral incision?**

Anterior and lateral compartments.

○ **What is the commonest organism associated with acute osteomyelitis?**

Staphylococcus aureus.

○ **In children which organism is commonly associated with acute osteomyelitis other than *S. aureus?***

Haemophilus influenzae. However, the incidence of this has decreased in recent years with the vaccination of children for *H. influenzae.*

● ● ● REFERENCES ● ● ●

Bosse MJ, MacKenzie EJ, Kellam J, et al. An analysis of outcomes of reconstruction or amputation of leg-threatening injuries. *N Engl J Med.* 2002;347:1924–1931.

Bosse MJ, MacKenzie EJ, Kellam JF, et al. A prospective evaluation of the clinical utility of lower extremity injury-severity scores. *J Bone Joint Surg Am.* 2001;83:3–14.

Bosse MJ, McCarthy ML, Jones AL, et al. The Lower Extremity Assessment Project (LEAP) stud. The insensate foot following severe lower extremity trauma: an indication for amputation? *J Bone Joint Surg Am.* 2005;87:2601–2608.

Ferraresi S, Garozzo D, Buffatti P. Common peroneal nerve injuries results with one-stage nerve repair and tendon transfer. *Neurosurg Rev.* 2003;26:175–179.

Hijjawi JB, Dumanian GA. The diabetic and ischemic lower extremity. In: McCarthy JG, Galiano RD, Boutros S, eds. *Current Therapy in Plastic Surgery.* 1st ed. Philadelphia, PA: Elsevier Science-Saunders; 2006.

Lindner NJ, Ramm O, Hillmann A, et al. Limb salvage and outcome of osteosarcoma. The University of Muenster experience. *Clin Orthop Relat Res.* 1999;(358):83–89.

MacKenzie EJ, Bosse MJ, Pollak AN, et al. Long-term persistence of disability following severe lower-limb trauma. results of a seven-year follow-up. *J Bone Joint Surg Am.* 2005;87:1801–1809.

MacKenzie EJ, Jones AS, Bosse MJ, et al. Health-care costs associated with amputation or reconstruction of a limb-threatening injury?. *J Bone Joint Surg Am.* 2007;89(8):1685–1692.

Millesi H. Brachial plexus injuries: management and results. In: Terzis JK, ed. *Microreconstruction of Nerve Injuries.* Philadelphia, PA: WB Saunders; 1987:243–249.

Rao S, Saltzman C, Yack HJ. Segmental foot mobility in individuals with and without diabetes and neuropathy. *Clin Biomech (Bristol, Avon).* 2007;22:464–471.

Schroeder J, Saris D, Besselaar PP, Marti RK. Comparison of the results of the Girdlestone pseudarthrosis with reimplantation of a total hip replacement. *Int Orthop.* 1998;22:215–218.

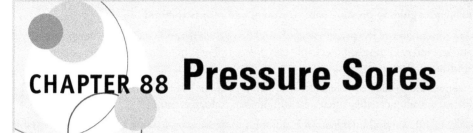

CHAPTER 88 Pressure Sores

Ryan Stehr, MD and
Robert J. Havlik, MD

○ **What is the etiology of pressure sores?**

Pressure sores arise as a result of tissue ischemia developing from pressure over a bony prominence. Pressure between the surface the patient rests on and the underlying bone may approach or exceed the patient's blood pressure, leading to tissue ischemia and/or tissue death.

○ **What are the risk factors of pressure sore development?**

Increased age, spinal cord injury, spasticity, decreased skin sensation, paraplegia, quadriplegia, prolonged immobilization, bowel or bladder incontinence. Malnutrition is not proven to be a risk factor.

○ **Where are the most common sites of pressure sores?**

The most common site is overlying the ischial tuberosity, followed by the trochanters or the sacrum.

○ **What are the stages of pressure sores?**

Revised in 2007, the National Pressure Ulcer Advisory Panel stages are the following:

Suspected deep tissue injury: Areas of purple or maroon discoloration with intact skin or blistering in the setting of excessive pressure and shear.

Stage I: Intact skin with nonblanching erythema, usually over a bony prominence.

Stage II: Partial-thickness loss of dermis.

Stage III: Full-thickness skin loss with visible subcutaneous fat, which may extend down to the deep fascia. There may be slough in the wound and undermining or tunneling.

Stage IV: Full-thickness tissue loss beyond the deep fascia with exposed bone, tendon, or muscle.

Unstageable: Excessive slough or eschar prevents accurate assessment of wound depth.

○   **What are some basic principles guiding pressure sore treatment and reconstruction?**

All contributing factors to the etiology of the pressure sore should first be addressed. For example, incontinence must be controlled or else any interventions will inevitably fail. A recent illness in the patient or loss of family support may even be contributing factors.

Stages I and II—These wounds are considered reversible, and with proper local wound care, adequate nutritional support and pressure off-loading adjuncts, they often heal without surgical intervention.

Stages III and IV—Usually require surgical intervention in addition to pressure off-loading adjuncts. All nonviable tissue should be debrided and then soft-tissue coverage should be undertaken. In the paraplegic population, spasticity should be addressed as this can cause flap breakdown by making pressure problems worse or causing shearing.

○   **What infections are commonly associated with pressure sores?**

Urinary tract infections and pneumonia. For the majority of patients with spinal cord injury and pressure sores who present with a fever, the source will be the urinary tract or the lungs. Fever is much less commonly caused by the pressure sore, as this is usually a clean, contaminated wound that is adequately draining.

○   **What laboratory tests are useful in the diagnosis of osteomyelitis in a pressure sore?**

A white blood cell count will often be elevated in osteomyelitis; however, it is nonspecific. An elevated erythrocyte sedimentation rate >120 mm/hr is much more specific for osteomyelitis.

○   **What radiologic test is most helpful in the diagnosis of osteomyelitis in a pressure sore?**

Unfortunately, there is no single radiologic test that remains the gold standard. Some authors advocate MRI, CT scan, or bone scans; however, plain film of the pelvis appears to have equivalent sensitivity.

○   **What is the gold-standard test to confirm osteomyelitis in a pressure sore?**

While laboratory and radiologic tests are often used to aid in the diagnosis of osteomyelitis, definitive diagnosis is obtained at the time of surgery with a sterile, open bone biopsy and culture to guide antibiotic therapy. Antibiotics should be held until cultures are obtained, if possible.

○   **What are the more common bacteria associated with pressure sores?**

Staphylococcus aureus, *Proteus mirabilis*, *Pseudomonas aeruginosa*, and *Bacteroides fragilis* are commonly isolated; however, the cultures are usually polymicrobial.

○   **What is appropriate treatment for osteomyelitis in pressure sores?**

Six to eight weeks of intravenous antibiotic therapy guided by antimicrobial susceptibility results from a sterile, open bone biopsy.

Two schools of thought exist on the timing of reconstruction. One recommends immediate reconstruction at the time of excision followed by IV antibiotics, while the other recommends negative pressure wound therapy until IV antibiotics are completed followed by delayed closure.

○   **What is the etiology of spasticity in paraplegics?**

Elimination of higher CNS suppression of spinal reflex arcs leading to hypertonia and hyperreflexia.

○ **What is the significance of spasticity in pressure sore management?**

It can exacerbate pressure points, place tension on wound edges, and contribute to joint or muscle contracture.

○ **What are some treatments for spasticity?**

Systemic diazepam or baclofen, intrathecal baclofen pump, phenol or alcohol, neurosurgical treatment with cordotomy or rhizotomy.

○ **What are the reconstructive options for sacral pressure sores?**

1. Gluteus maximus musculocutaneous flap.
2. Gluteal fasciocutaneous rotation flap.
3. Superior gluteal artery perforator flap.

○ **What are the reconstructive options for ischial pressure sores?**

1. Gluteus maximus musculocutaneous flap.
2. Inferior gluteal thigh fasciocutaneous flap.
3. V-Y hamstring fasciocutaneous flap with or without biceps femoris muscle.

○ **What are the reconstructive options for trochanteric pressure sores?**

1. Tensor fascia lata flap.
2. Thigh rotational flap.
3. Inferior gluteal thigh flap.

○ **What is a Girdlestone arthroplasty and when is it indicated?**

Girdlestone arthroplasty involves resection of the femoral head and a portion of the proximal femur. This is usually performed to treat septic arthritis of the hip joint. The acetabulum should also be debrided. In order to obliterate the dead space between the acetabulum and the femoral shaft, the vastus lateralis muscle flap may be used.

○ **Why do patients with spinal cord injury and denervated tissues experience poor wound healing?**

The exact etiology of delayed wound healing in patients with denervated tissues is not completely elucidated; however, current research indicates that nerve growth factor (NGF) and substance P (SP) play an important role in normal wound healing. NGF is produced by target tissues such as the skin and subcutaneous tissue and undergoes retrograde transport by sensory nerve fibers. NGF regulates the release of substance P, which then acts as a chemoattractant for neutrophils and macrophages. Additionally, substance P acts as a vasodilator and regulates a number of other inflammatory mediators produced by leukocytes. Patients with spinal cord injuries or other causes of denervated tissue have been shown to have decreased levels of substance P in their wounds. Rat models have shown improved wound healing with administration of exogenous substance P.

○ **What surgical tactics can be used to potentially decrease pressure sore recurrence?**

In selected patients with a low spinal cord injury, use of a sensate flap can be used to restore protective sensation to the injured area. This can be done for sacral sores by using tissue expansion in the lower pack. No strong evidence exists to show that this technique reduces recurrence.

○ **What nonsurgical tactics can be used to prevent future pressure sores?**

Minimize pressure over bony prominences and reconstructions by frequent turning and pressure relieving mattresses, proper hygiene, control of incontinence, aggressive management of spasticity and contracture.

● ● ● **REFERENCES** ● ● ●

Barker AR, Rosson GD, Dellon AL. "Wound healing in denervated tissue." *Ann Plast Surg.* 2006;57(3)339–342.

Bauer J, Phillips LG. MOC-PSSM CME article: pressure sores. *Plast Reconstr Surg.* 2008;121(1 suppl):1–10.

Braden BJ, Bergstrom N. Clinical utility of the Braden scale for predicting pressure sore risk. *Decubitus.* 1989;2(3):44–46, 50–51.

Di Caprio G, Serra-Mestre JM, Ziccardi P, et al. Expanded flaps in surgical treatment of pressure sores: our experience for 25 years. *Ann Plast Surg.* 2014;75:552–555.

Evans GR, Lewis VL Jr, Manson PN, Loomis M, Vander Kolk CA. Hip joint communication with pressure sore: the refractory wound and the role of girdlestone arthroplasty. *Plast Reconstr Surg.* 1993;91(2):288–294.

Larson DL, Gilstrap J, Carrera GF. Is there a reliable and cost efficient way to diagnose osteomyelitis in the pressure sore patient?. *Presented at AAPS Meeting.* 2010.

Levi B, Rees R. Diagnosis and management of pressure ulcers. *Clin Plast Surg.* 2007;34:735–748.

Lewis VL Jr, Bailey MH, Pulawski G, Kind G, Bashioum RW, Hendrix RW. The diagnosis of osteomyelitis in patients with pressure sores. *Plast Reconstr Surg.* 1988;81(2):229–232.

National Pressure Ulcer Advisory Panel. Retrieved December 18, 2009, from www.npuap.org

Neves RI, Kahler SH, Banducci DR, Manders EK. Tissue expansion of sensate skin for pressure sores. *Ann Plast Surg.* 1992;29(5): 433–437.

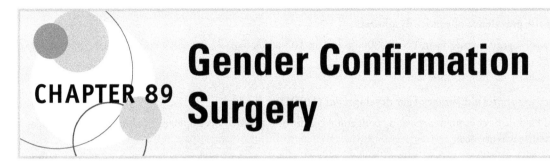

CHAPTER 89

Gender Confirmation Surgery

Nicholas Kim, MD and
Loren S. Schechter, MD, FACS

○ **What is gender identity?**

One's basic sense of self as a man or woman.

○ **What is gender dysphoria?**

A term introduced by Fisk in 1973, gender dysphoria refers to distress resulting from conflicting gender identity and sex of assignment. It has replaced the term Gender Identity Disorder in the Diagnostic and Statistical Manual of Mental Disorders-5th edition (DSM-5), which was implemented in 2014. This revision of the DSM-4's Gender Identity Disorder was intended to avoid the stigmatizing effect of the previous diagnostic term without jeopardizing access to effective treatment options.

○ **What are the diagnostic criteria for gender dysphoria according to the DSM-5?**

There must be marked difference between the individual's expressed gender and the gender others would assign him or her. This must continue for at least 6 months. The critical element is the presence of clinically significant impairment in social, occupational, or other important areas of functioning.

○ **What is transsexualism?**

A term coined by Magnus Hirschfield in 1923, a transsexual is an individual who desires to live permanently in the social role of the opposite gender, and wants to undergo sex reassignment. In 1994, the DSM-4 committee replaced the diagnostic term Transsexualism with Gender Identity Disorder, which has since been replaced by Gender Dysphoria. The International Classification of Diseases-10 (ICD-10) continues to use Transsexualism as a diagnostic term under the heading of Gender Identity Disorders.

○ **What are the diagnostic criteria for transsexualism according to the ICD-10?**

There are three criteria: (1) the desire to live and be accepted as a member of the opposite sex; (2) the transsexual identity has been present persistently for at least 2 years; and (3) the disorder is not a symptom or another mental disorder or a chromosomal abnormality.

○ **What is the prevalence of gender dysphoria?**

The DSM-5 reports a range from 1 in 20,000 up to 1 in 10,000 biological men and a range from 1 in 50,000 up to 1 in 30,000 biological women.

○ **Is gender dysphoria a disorder of sex development (DSD)?**

No, DSD is a distinct entity representing congenital conditions in which development of chromosomal, gonadal, or anatomic sex is atypical.

○ **What are the Standards of Care for the Health of Transsexual?**

Previously known as the Harry Benjamin International Gender Dysphoria Association Guidelines for Diagnosis and Treatment, the Standards of Care is a publication of the World Professional Association for Transgender Health (WPATH). It is intended to provide flexible clinical guidelines to meet the diverse health care needs of individuals with gender dysphoria. The most current set, Version 7, was published in 2011.

○ **What are the mechanisms of feminization through hormone therapy?**

Feminization is achieved by two mechanisms: androgen suppression using medications such as spironolactone or finasteride, and induction of female characteristics using estrogen.

○ **What are the effects of feminization hormone therapy?**

Within the first 6 months there is redistribution of fat, decreased muscle mass, softening of the skin, and decreased libido. Breast growth may be expected after 3 to 6 months of therapy and may continue for over 2 years.

○ **What are the effects of masculinization hormone therapy?**

Testosterone therapy results in increased muscle mass, decreased fat mass, increased facial hair and acne, male pattern baldness, and increased libido. In female-to-male individuals, testosterone therapy results in clitoromegaly, temporary or permanent decreased fertility, deepened voice, vaginal atrophy, and cessation of menses.

○ **Why use the term "Gender Confirmation Surgery" as opposed to "Sex Change" or "Gender Reassignment Surgery"?**

The latter two phrases suggest that a person is making a choice to switch genders. Gender confirmation surgery should be seen as a therapeutic tool to enable a person to feel comfortable as their gendered self.

○ **What are the anatomic differences between the male and female chest that are relevant in top surgery?**

The male chest is wider than the female chest, and the male pectoral muscle is usually more developed. The male areola is smaller than the female areola, and the distance between the nipple and inframammary crease is shorter in males.

○ **What are the methods of top surgery performed for female-to-male individuals?**

A subcutaneous mastectomy with varying incisions (and possible free nipple graft) is performed. The technique depends upon on skin elasticity, breast volume, and breast ptosis. The double-incision technique (inframammary crease with free nipple-areolar graft) is the most commonly performed procedure. Other incisions, such as periareolar and short vertical incisions, may also be performed.

○ **What is breast binding?**

Breast binding is a practice commonly performed by female-to-male individuals in order to flatten the breasts. This may lead to a loss of skin elasticity, thereby necessitating skin removal at the time of chest wall contouring surgery.

○ **What are the most common types of breast surgery performed for male-to-female individuals?**

Breast augmentation is most often performed through an inframammary crease incision. Transaxillary or periareolar incisions may also be performed, and the use of shaped implants is gaining popularity.

○ **What are the surgical options for sexual reassignment surgery (SRS) or vaginoplasty in male-to-female individuals?**

There are three options: (1) penile disassembly and inversion vaginoplasty; (2) intestinal transplantation; and (3) nongenital flaps.

○ **What are the typical components of vaginoplasty?**

They include: (1) formation of a neovagina using penile and scrotal (or sigmoid colon in the case of intestinal vaginoplasty); (2) formation of a neoclitoris, typically formed from the dorsal glans penis; (3) shortening of urethra; and (4) formation of labia minora and majora.

○ **What are the potential complications of vaginoplasty?**

There is risk of rectal injury, which, when recognized intraoperatively, should be repaired in two layers and drained. The use of diverting colostomy may be required in the case of rectovaginal fistula. Additional complications include, but are not limited to vaginal stenosis, lack of sensation, delayed wound healing, venous thromboembolism, and urethral injury.

○ **What are the long-term care instructions following vaginoplasty?**

Annual speculum exam and digital prostate exam are performed. Routine vaginal dilation by the patient is required in order to prevent vaginal stenosis. Frequency of vaginal dilation may be reduced with sexual intercourse. Intermittent intravaginal washing (douching) is performed once or twice weekly using dilute povidone-iodine solution or mild soap.

○ **What are the advantages of intestinal transplantation?**

The ability to create a vascularized neovagina with a moist lining. This may lessen the need for postoperative vaginal dilation as well as the need for lubrication during intercourse.

○ **What are the drawbacks of intestinal transplantation?**

The need for an intra-abdominal operation with a bowel anastomosis, possibility of diversion colitis in the defunctionalized sigmoid colon, risk of GI malignancy, and small amounts of postcoital bleeding as a result of friable colonic mucosa.

○ **Does estrogen hormone therapy present a perioperative risk?**

Yes. Estrogen hormone therapy should be discontinued approximately 2 weeks prior to surgery to reduce the risk of venous thromboembolism.

○   **What are the surgical options for bottom surgery or genital surgery in female-to-male individuals?**

The options are metoidioplasty versus pedicled/free flap phalloplasty. Both phalloplasty and metoidioplasty procedures may be combined with vaginectomy and scrotoplasty. Hysterectomy and oophorectomy are typically performed prior to phalloplasty or metoidioplasty. Staged placement of testicular implants and penile prostheses may also be performed

○   **What is metoidioplasty?**

Metoidioplasty involves lengthening of the hormonally hypertrophied clitoris by release of the suspensory ligament and resection of the ventral chordae. Lengthening of the female urethra may be performed with the aid of labia minora vaginal musculomucosal flaps.

○   **What are the most common complications associated with metoidioplasty?**

Urethral fistula and strictures.

○   **What are the flap options for phalloplasty?**

The three most commonly used flaps are: (1) radial forearm flap; (2) anterolateral thigh flap; and (3) latissimus dorsi myocutaneous flap. The radial forearm flap provides a sensate flap that is amenable to the tube-in-a-tube design, but leaves a noticeable donor site. The bulk of the anterolateral thigh flap prohibits tubularization, and the latissimus flap lacks sensation.

○   **What is an option for vascular anastomoses and nerve coaptations?**

The radial artery is typically anastomosed end-to-side to the common or superficial femoral artery, and the cephalic vein anastomosed end-to-end to the greater saphenous vein. Additional venous anastomoses between the basilic and median cubital veins to the superficial inferior epigastric and superficial circumflex iliac veins may also be performed. The medial and lateral antebrachial cutaneous nerves may be coapted to the ilioinguinal nerve and dorsal clitoral nerve for protective sensation and erogenous sensation, respectively.

○   **Does the WPATH Standards of Care recommend a referral from a mental health professional for other surgeries?**

No. Other surgeries such as facial feminization surgery, facial masculinization surgery, reduction thyroid chondroplasty, voice surgery, etc. do not require a referral according to the Standards of Care. However, mental health professionals can play an important role in assisting transgender individuals in making a fully informed decision about the timing and implications of such procedures.

○   **What are the characteristic differences between a masculine and feminine forehead?**

When compared to a masculine forehead, the feminine forehead is shorter and has a more continuous, convex curvature. The masculine forehead has more pronounced supraorbital bossing due to larger frontal sinuses. The female eyebrow is located above the supraorbital rim and has more of an arched appearance, whereas the male eyebrow typically sits at the supraorbital rim.

○   **What are the characteristic differences between a masculine and feminine nose?**

The feminine nose is overall smaller than the masculine nose. The masculine nose is associated with a more acute nasofrontal angle. In addition, the nasolabial angle is more obtuse in the feminine nose due to an upturning nasal tip.

○ **What are the characteristic differences between a masculine and feminine mandible?**

The masculine mandible has a more acute angle and greater lateral flaring due to a thicker masseter muscle. This results in lower face fullness when compared to the narrower, and more tapered, feminine lower face. The feminine chin is smaller in both the vertical and horizontal dimensions, resulting in a narrower and more pointed appearance.

○ **What are the surgical techniques for facial feminization?**

The techniques include: (1) supraorbital burring or frontal osteotomy with set back; (2) brow lift; (3) anterior hairline advancement or hair transplantation; (4) feminizing rhinoplasty; (5) mandibular angle reduction; and (6) reduction genioplasty.

○ **What are the surgical techniques for facial masculinization?**

The techniques include: (1) forehead augmentation; (2) mandibular angle implant augmentation; and (3) implant or sliding genioplasty.

○ **What is reduction thyroid chondroplasty?**

An outpatient procedure performed either open or endoscopically to lessen the appearance of the "Adam's apple" or prominent thyroid cartilage.

○ **What is voice surgery?**

Various techniques designed to shorten the vocal cords, increase vocal cord tension, or reduce the vibrating vocal cord mass in order to raise vocal pitch. Estrogen hormone therapy does not commonly affect vocal pitch, and this may result in residual stigma of masculinity.

● ● ● REFERENCES ● ● ●

Coleman E, Bockting W, Botzer M, et al. Standards of care for the health of transsexual, transgender, and gender-nonconforming people, version 7. *Intl J Transgend*. 2012;13(4):165–232.

Hage JJ. Metaidioplasty: an alternative phalloplasty technique in transsexuals. *Plast Reconstr Surg*. 1996;97:161–167.

Kwun Kim S, Hoon Park J, Cheol Lee K, et al. Long-term results in patients after rectosigmoid vaginoplasty. *Plast Reconstr Surg*. 2003;112(1):143–151.

Monstrey S, Selvaggi G, Ceulemans P, et al. Chest-wall contouring surgery in female-to-male transsexuals: a new algorithm. *Plast Reconstr Surg*. 2008. 121(3):849–859.

Ousterhout DK. Dr. Paul Tessier and facial skeletal masculinization. *Ann Plast Surg*. 2011;67(6):S10–S15.

Ousterhout DK. Feminization of the forehead: contour changing to improve female aesthetics. *Plast Reconstr Surg*. 1987;79(5):701–713.

Schechter LS. Surgery of gender identity disorder. In: Song DH, Neligan PC. *Plastic Surgery. Trunk and Lower Extremity*. 3rd ed. Volume 4. Philadelphia, PA: Elsevier Health Sciences; 2012.

Selvaggi G, Ceulemans P, De Cuypere G, et al. Gender identity disorder: general overview and surgical treatment for vaginoplasty in male-to-female transsexuals. *Plast Reconstr Surg*. 2005;116(6):135e–145e.

Selvaggi G, Monstrey S, Hoebeke P, et al. Donor-site morbidity of the radial forearm free flap after 125 phalloplasties in gender identity disorder. *Plast Reconstr Surg*. 2006;118(5):1171–1177.

CHAPTER 90
Infiltration and Extravasation Injuries

Jenna Cusic, MD and
Patrick Hettinger, MD

• • • DEFINITIONS • • •

○ **What is the difference between an extravasation and an infiltration?**

- Extravasation
  - Leakage of a vesicant (most common definition).
  - Administration of a harsh solution that causes vein damage leading to rupture.
- Infiltration
  - Leakage of an irritant (most common definition).
  - Administration of a solution outside a vein into surrounding tissues.

○ **What is a vesicant?**

- Agent that is inherently toxic, which may cause blistering, sloughing, or deep tissue damage.
- They have a wide range of necrotic potential.
- Examples include, calcium solutions, potassium solutions, radiographic contrast, sodium bicarbonate, vasoconstrictor agents, doxorubicin, fluorescein, mitomycin-C, vinblastine, and vincristine.

○ **What is an irritant?**

- Agent that is not directly toxic, which may cause an inflammatory reaction with erythema, warmth, and tenderness.
- Examples include, albumin, blood products, asparginase, bleomycin, cyclophosphamide, methotrexate, cisplatin, fluorouracil, and valium.

○ **What is a nonirritant?**

Agent that is nontoxic and rarely produces an acute reaction.

○ **Can an irritant produce the same symptoms as a vesicant?**

• Any agent in high enough concentration or volume may become an irritant or vesicant.

• A vesicant may not always produce necrotic tissue changes depending on the volume, concentration, or infusion rate.

• • • EPIDEMIOLOGY, RISK FACTORS, AND COMPLICATIONS • • •

○ **What is the incidence of extravasation?**

• Many go unreported, thereby the true incidence is difficult to ascertain.

• Extravasation injury has been generally reported at 0.1% to 6%, yet has been documented up to 22% of cytotoxic administrations.

○ **Which agents may cause an extravasation/infiltration injury?**

Maintenance fluids, electrolytes, blood products, chemotherapeutic agents, vasopressors, antibiotics, anesthetic agents, other medications, TPN, and contrast agents.

○ **What are the risk factors for extravasation/infiltration?**

• Unable to communicate pain—infants or elderly, nonverbal or cognitive impairment, ICU, under anesthesia.

• Decreased sensation—neuropathy (diabetic or chemotherapy side effects).

• Comorbidities—peripheral vascular disease, Raynaud phenomenon, and diabetes.

• Vessels and their flow—lymphedema, obstructed vena cava, venous hypertension; chemotherapy patients have fragile, mobile veins.

• Procedure technique—multiple attempts, large gauge or metal needles, bolus or high flow injections.

• Agents—vesicants, high osmolarity, extremes of pH, and vasoconstrictive agents.

○ **What complications may ensue from extravasation/infiltration?**

• Pain, scarring (aesthetically displeasing and functional impairment), functional loss (consider character of surrounding tissue such as thickness of skin, as well as underlying structures such as neurovascular structures or tendons/joints), soft-tissue loss, infection, compartment syndrome, further operations, and amputations.

• Delay in oncological treatment if receiving chemotherapy or radiation.

• Longer hospital stays and increased costs.

• • • PREVENTION • • •

○ **What strategies can be used for prevention?**

Check IV site on an hourly basis and recognize high-risk patients; optimize veins (hot towels, nitroglycerin); use the smallest needle appropriate in a larger vein; avoid multiple perforations to the same vein (second attempt made more proximal), unnecessary dressings, extremities with lymphedema, infusion under pressure; use large or central veins for resuscitative efforts; and maximally dilute chemotherapy agents.

• • • PATHOPHYSIOLOGY • • •

○ **What are the pathophysiologic mechanisms of extravasation/infiltration?**
- Infusion of the agent.
  - Leakage around the cannulation site of infusion directly into the surrounding tissues.
    - Occlusion of distal flow due to pressure from extravasated fluid into interstitial space or local irritation, including phlebitis, vasoconstriction or thrombosis → increases intraluminal pressure → leakage of agent.
  - Infusion with high pressure or large volumes increases extracellular hydrostatic pressure → venous compression → further extravasation/infiltration → arterial compromise.
    - May lead to compartment syndrome.
    - Increased height from which fluid travels into the vein leads to increased pressure; the higher the IV fluid bag, the higher the potential pressure of infusion.
    - Pressure (mm Hg) = $0.7418 \times$ height of fluid column (cm) $- 6.109$
- Agent properties.
  - Osmotic damage, ischemic damage, direct cellular toxicity, and bacterial colonization.

○ **How may osmolarity induce damage to tissues?**
- Hypertonic solutions, TPN, contrast media, antibiotics, and cations in ionized form.
- Pulls fluid from intracellular to extracellular → dehydration and death of cells, disruption of transport mechanisms, and increased interstitial fluid and pressure leading to compartment syndrome.
- Calcium and potassium salts can cause cell death by cellular fluid overload.

○ **How may ischemic damage be induced from extravasation?**
- Vasopressor agents lead to vasoconstriction → lack of tissue perfusion.
  - α-adrenergic agonists–epinephrine, norepinephrine, dopamine, and phenylephrine.
    - Duration of effect has more impact that concentration.
  - V1 agonists–vasopressin.
- Cation solutions cause prolonged depolarization → contraction of vascular smooth muscle → lack of tissue perfusion.

○ **How may cells be directly damaged through extravasation?**
- Ions can form salts and precipitate proteins, killing cells.
- DNA-binding agents cause an ongoing lethal cycle.
  - Kill the cells, releasing agent into surrounding tissue → agent is taken up by another cell → kill the cells, releasing agent into tissue, etc.
- Agents with extremes of pH may be caustic to endothelial tissue.
- Direct local damage by agent or its vehicle.

○ **How does extravasation affect tissues via bacteria?**
Open wounds may become colonized and can increase extent of wound and impair healing.

• • • PRESENTATION • • •

○ **What are the signs and symptoms of extravasation/infiltration?**

- Patient report or physical examination—pain, swelling, erythema or discoloration, induration, and blistering.

- Character of infusion—change in rate (usually slows with increased resistance), lack of blood return.

○ **What are the grades of extravasation/infiltration by clinical examination?**

Grade 1	Blanched skin. Edema <1 inch in any direction. Cool to touch. With or without pain.
Grade 2	Same as above in addition to • Edema 1 to 6 inches in any direction.
Grade 3	Same as above in addition to • Blanched, translucent skin. • Gross edema >6 inches in any direction. • Mild to moderate pain. • Possible numbness.
Grade 4	Same as above in addition to • Tight, leaking, discolored/bruised, and swollen skin. • Deep pitting edema. • Circulatory impairment. • Moderate to severe pain. • All extravasations.

Grading should be assigned by most severe clinical indicator of injury.

○ **What details of extravasation/infiltration are important to obtain?**

- Agent, as this will guide treatment and administration of potential antidotes.
  - Vesicant versus irritant; DNA-binding versus non–DNA-binding vesicant.
- Concentration.
- Volume administered and force of infusion.
- Timing of infusion
  - Antidotes have limited time intervals to be administered; necrosis interval (see below text)

• • • TREATMENT • • •

○ **What are the immediate interventions?**

- Stop the infusion, leave the catheter in place and aspirate any available fluid.
- Elevate the extremity/area.
- Obtain the details of extravasation/infiltration.

○ **What are the definitive interventions?**

- Warm or cold compresses.
- Administration of hyaluronidase if indicated (see below).
- Steroid creams—evidence is controversial, but considered to decrease inflammation.
- Administer antidotes if available.
  - Phentolamine within 12 hours after extravasation of α-adrenergic agents; may also provide some benefit with other vasoconstrictive agents like vasopressin.
  - Derazoxane within 6 hours after extravasation of anthracyclines (doxorubicin).
- Normal saline infusion techniques to dilute agent.
  - Gault technique and variants (see below).
- Surgical intervention if warranted.
  - Consider the necrosis interval, and the timing and severity of extravasation.
- Rehabilitation.

○ **Should a warm or cold compress be used?**

Depends if a "dilute and disperse" or "localize and neutralize" effect is indicated.

○ **What is the effect of a warm compress?**

- Vasodilation, which increases local blood flow and dilutes and disperses the agent.
- Used in conjunction with hyaluronidase.
  - TPN, mannitol, calcium, potassium, phenytoin, and contrast media.

○ **Are there instances when a warm compress should not be used?**

- Yes, as it could increase the area of toxicity by dispersing the agent.
- Do not use with DNA-binding vesicants.

○ **What is the effect of a cold compress?**

- Vasoconstriction, which decreases inflammation and keeps the agent localized.
- Can decrease cellular uptake of the agent.
  - Used for DNA-binding vesicants; may be used for contrast media (may also use warm pack).
  - Generally acceptable for chemotherapeutic agents except non–DNA-binding vesicants.

○ **Are there instances where cold compresses should not be used?**

- Yes, vinca alkaloids (type of non–DNA-binding vesicant) as this may increase tissue ulceration.
  - Vincristine, vinblastine.

○ **How does hyaluronidase assist with treatment?**

Reversibly breaks down hyaluronic acid (dominant GAG in connective tissue) → decreases viscosity → increases tissue permeability → absorption and dispersal of agent.

○ **When should hyaluronidase be injected?**

• Within 1 hour of extravasation.

• May be used for vinca alkaloids, calcium, potassium, hypertonic glucose, TPN, and mannitol, among other agents.

• Avoid with vasoconstrictive agents, DNA-binding vesicants, controversial in contrast media.

○ **Which conditions may predispose resistance to hyaluronidase?**

• Large doses of corticosteroids, salicylates, estrogens, and antihistamines.

• Elderly may be less responsive due to their skin inelasticity.

○ **What is the "Gault technique"?**

• Saline flushout of the extravasated/infiltrated area.

  • Hyaluronidase is infiltrated, stab incisions around periphery of affected area are made and normal saline is flushed through a blunt ended cannula in 20 to 50 cc aliquots, up to 500 mL total.

  • Fluid returned can be analyzed for extravasated/infiltrated agent.

  • Area may also be liposuctioned.

• Variations of liposuction and normal saline clysis have been shown in a number of studies to result in improved rates of ulceration and soft tissue damage, as well as preserved function, even in cytotoxic extravasations.

○ **What is the necrosis interval?**

• Time from extravasation to point of irreversible tissue damage.

• Early surgical intervention within this time frame may prevent necrosis.

  • Vasopressor agents: 4 to 6 hours.

  • Radiographic contrast agents: 6 hours.

  • Chemotherapeutic agents: 72 hours.

○ **What determines "wait and see" approach versus "early surgical intervention"?**

• May generally observe a mild or moderate injury consisting of an irritant or a small volume, low concentration vesicant, with no blistering or necrosis.

• Consider early surgical intervention with severe injuries, including vesicant extravasations, large volumes, tissue necrosis, or within the necrosis interval of vasopressors, contrast media, or chemotherapeutic agents.

  • On examination, the amount of tissue damage is often underestimated.

  • Early surgical intervention within 72 hours of severe injuries or within the necrosis interval of respective agents can improve outcomes.

○ **How are vasopressors deleterious to tissues?**

• Vasoconstriction leads to tissue ischemia.

  • α-adrenergic receptors (epinephrine, norepinephrine, phenylephrine, and dopamine) or V1 receptors (vasopressin).

• Generally acidic, causing local tissue toxicity.

○ **How may vasopressor extravasation injury present?**

Blanching, swelling, erythematous or purple discoloration, bullae and eventually an eschar or gangrene.

○ **What are early interventions for vasopressor extravasations?**

- Do not place a cold pack (already vasoconstricted) or give hyaluronidase (can extend ischemic area).
- Phentolamine—competitive α-receptor antagonist → vasodilation.
  - Antidote for α-agonist agents, and may also indirectly improve vasopressin extravasation.
  - May see partial reversal of ischemia within 7 to 10 minutes.
  - Inject into subcutaneous area within 12 hours.
- Terbutaline–β_2-agonist → vasodilation.
  - Second-line agent.
  - Use with caution in underlying cardiac disease, as it may induce arrhythmias or myocardial infarction in at-risk populations.
- Topical nitroglycerin–increases cGMP → vasodilation.
- Stellate ganglion block–blocks sympathetic input, decreasing vasoconstriction.

○ **What are the early interventions for mannitol?**

- Warm compresses, hyaluronidase.
  - Hyperosmolarity can cause extreme edema, potentially leading to compartment syndrome; dispersion and dilution of the agent will assist in decreasing its effect.

○ **What are the early interventions for TPN?**

- Warm or cold compresses have been proposed; hyaluronidase may also be used.
  - TPN is hyperosmotic and acidic.

○ **Is calcium gluconate or calcium chloride more detrimental?**

- Calcium chloride's osmolarity is 2,040 mOsm/L and it dissociates more extensively with a higher risk of precipitation, whereas calcium gluconate's osmolarity is 669 mOsm/L.
  - Absolute calcium content may be the strongest predictor of tissue necrosis due to direct protein precipitation and vasoconstriction.
- Calcium may cause ischemic necrosis from prolonged depolarization or may precipitate proteins and cause cellular toxicity.

○ **How may calcium extravasation present?**

- Early—erythema and pain progressing to eschar formation and eventually necrosis, but may take weeks to develop.
- Late—calcinosis cutis.

○ **What is calcinosis cutis?**

Extravasation of calcium, leading to soft tissue calcification through formation of hydroxyapatite; forms subcutaneous white to yellow plaques that are visible in radiographs.

○ **What are the possible interventions for calcium extravasation?**

- Hyaluronidase.
- Sodium thiosulfate—forms calcium thiosulfate which has a higher solubility.
- Surgical resection.

○ **What is "purple glove syndrome"?**

- Phenytoin related soft-tissue injury.
  - Phenytoin is hyperosmolar and alkalotic, and may form precipitates leading to thrombosis.
- Three phases:
  - Pain and purple/blue discoloration distal to venous access site.
  - Glove-like circumferential erythema with edema.
  - Bullae formation, skin necrosis, and possible compartment syndrome.
    - One-third of patients progress to this phase.

○ **What are the potential treatments for phenytoin extravasation?**

- Warm compresses, hyaluronidase.
- May prevent injury with a lower rate of infusion.
- Surgical intervention.

○ **What are examples of chemotherapeutic DNA-binding and non–DNA-binding agents?**

- DNA-binding
  - Anthracyclines—doxorubicin, daunorubicin, epirubicin, and idarubicin.
  - Alkylating agents—mechlorethamine.
  - Other—mitomycin.
- Non–DNA-binding
  - Vinca alkaloids—vincristine, vinblastine.
  - Taxanes—paclitaxel.

○ **Why do DNA-binding vesicants have the potential to be so detrimental?**

- They form a vicious cycle of cell death → agent is released and taken up by another cell → cell death → agent is released, etc.
- May present early to late with ongoing and extensive tissue damage.

○ **What is the "recall effect"?**

Reactivation of skin toxicity with administration of chemotherapy or radiation at a remote site.

○ **How do doxorubicin extravasations present?**

- Progressive, central necrosis with raised, erythematous, and painful edges.
- These injuries heal slower as they contain chronic fibroblast disorganization; they show a delayed presence of myofibroblasts.

○ **Can doxorubicin cause local irritation?**

Doxorubicin infusion may cause a local "flare" which usually subsides within 1 to 2 hours.

○ **What are the initial treatments for doxorubicin extravasation?**

- Cold compresses, as this is a DNA-binding agent and should be localized, not dispersed, to avoid extending the area of injury.
- Dexrazoxane is the first-line antidote, but needs to be administered within 6 hours.
  - Free radical scavenger inhibits topoisomerase II.
  - Side effects: transient transaminitis, slight myelosuppression.
- Dimethyl sulfoxide (DMSO) may also be used.
  - Neutralizes free radicals, may cause vasodilation.

○ **If surgical intervention is required, what may be used to assess that doxorubicin laden tissue is removed?**

UV light causes doxorubicin tissue to glow reddish/orange.

○ **If surgical intervention is required, what may be used to assess that contrast media laden tissue is removed?**

Obtain x-ray imaging, which will reveal location of contrast media if it remains in tissues.

⦿ ⦿ ⦿ REFERENCES ⦿ ⦿ ⦿

Al-Benna S, O'Boyle C, Holley J. Extravasation injuries in adults. *ISRN Dermatol.* 2013:856541.

Ball R, Henao J. Ibinson JW, Metro DG. Peripheral intravenous catheter infiltration: anesthesia providers do not adhere to their own ideas of best practice. *J Clin Anesth.* 2013;25:115–120.

Boulanger J, Ducharme A, Dufour A, et al. Management of the extravasation of anti-neoplastic agents. *Support Care Cancer.* 2015; 23(5):1459–1471.

Erickson BA, Yap RL, Pazona JF, Hartigan BJ, Smith ND. Mannitol extravasation during partial nephrectomy leading to forearm compartment syndrome. *Int Braz J Urol.* 2007;33(1):68–71; discussion 71.

Gault DT. Extravasation injuries. *Br J Plast Surg.* 1993;46:91–96.

Hahn JC, Shafritz AB. Chemotherapy extravasation injuries. *J Hand Surg Am.* 2012;37:360–362.

Hannon MG, Lee SK. Extravasation injuries. *J Hand Surg Am.* 2011;36:2060–2065.

Khan MS, Holmes JD. Reducing the morbidity from extravasation injuries. *Ann Plast Surg.* 2002;48:628–632.

Kumar RJ, Pegg SP, Kimble RM. Management of extravasation injuries. *ANZ J. Surg.* 2001;71:285–289.

Larson D. Treatment of tissue extravasation by antitumor agents. *Cancer.* 1982;49:1796–1799.

Le A, Patel S. Extravasation of noncytotoxic drugs: a review of the literature. *Ann Pharmacother.* 2014;48(7):870–886.

Loth T, Eversmann W. Extravasation injuries in the upper extremity. *Clin Orthop Relat Res.* 1991;272:248–254.

Napoli P, Corradino B, Badalamenti G, et al. Surgical treatment of extravasation injuries. *J Surg Oncol.* 2005;91:264–268.

Reynolds P, MacLaren R, Mueller S, Fish DN, Kiser TH. Management of extravasation injuries: a focused evaluation of noncytotoxic medications. *Pharmacotherapy.* 2014;34(6):617–632.

Rhys-Davies NC, Stotter AT. The Rhys-Davies exsanguinator. *Ann R Coll Surg Engl.* 1985;67:193–195.

Rudolph R, Larson DL. Etiology and treatment of chemotherapeutic agent extravasation injuries: a review. *J Clin Oncol.* 1987;7(5): 1116–1126.

Schaverien MV, Evison D, McCulley SJ. Management of large volume CT contrast medium extravasation injury: technical refinement and literature review. *J Plast Reconstr Aesthet Surg.* 2008;61:562–565.

Tofani BF, Rineair SA, Gosdin CH, et al. Quality improvement project to reduce infiltration and extravasation events in a pediatric hospital. *J Pediatr Nurs.* 2012;27:682–689.

Tsai YS, Cheng SM, Ng SP, et al. Squeeze maneuver: an easy way to manage radiological contrast-medium extravasation. *Acta Radiol.* 2007;48:605–607.

Tsavaris NB, Karagiaouris P, Tzannou I, et al. Conservative approach to the treatment of chemotherapy-induced extravasation. *J Dermatol Surg Oncol.* 1990;16:519–522.

Tsavaris NB, Komitsopoulou P, Karagiaouris P, et al. Prevention of tissue necrosis due to accidental extravasation of cytostatic drugs by a conservative approach. *Cancer Chemother Pharmacol.* 1992;30:330–333.

Upton J, Mullliken JB, Murray JE. Major intravenous extravasation injuries. *Am J Surg.* 1979;137:497–506.

Section VIII GENERAL TOPICS

CHAPTER 91 Basic Statistical Methods

Pieter G.L. Koolen, MD

• • • DESCRIPTIVE STATISTICS • • •

○ **Why use descriptive statistics?**

- To describe the basic characteristics of a data set.
- To identify patterns in your data set.
- To generate hypotheses.

○ **What are common measures of central tendency?**

- Mean.
- Median.
- Mode.

○ **What is the mean?**

The statistical average.

○ **How is the mean estimated?**

To estimate the mean, sum up all the values and divide the sum by the number of values.

○ **What is the median?**

The exact "middle" value.

○ **How is the median determined?**

Sort the data from the lowest to the highest value and find the value in the middle. If there is an even number of data points, average the two values in the middle.

○ **When the data are highly skewed, which measure of central tendency is preferred?**

The median because the mean is sensitive to outliers or data points that are very different than most others.

○ **What is the most frequently occurring score in a set of scores?**

The mode.

○ **Measures of dispersion include?**

• Range.

• Standard deviation.

• Standard error.

○ **What does the standard deviation describe?**

• How spread out the values are in a data set, OR

• How closely the values of a data set cluster around the mean value.

○ **What is the standard error?**

The standard error refers to the likelihood that the mean and standard deviation of a specific sample of participants reflect the mean and standard deviation of the full population of potential participants. It is computed by dividing the standard deviation by the square root of the sample size (n).

○ **What is the range?**

The distance between the minimum value and maximum value.

○ **What is the interquartile range?**

The distance between the 25th and 75th percentiles.

• • • TYPES OF VARIABLES • • •

○ **What is a categorical variable?**

A variable made of categories that cannot be quantified (e.g., blood type, gender, and pregnant/not pregnant).

○ **What kind of statistical analysis is appropriate for categorical variables?**

Nonparametric statistics.

○ **What is a continuous variable?**

A variable that gives a score for each subject in a sample and can take on any value on a measurement scale (e.g., blood pressure and cholesterol).

○ **What kind of statistical analysis is appropriate for continuous variables?**

Parametric statistics.

○ **What is an ordinal variable?**

An ordinal variable is a variable that is recorded on an interval scale from highest to lowest but does not involve use of the numerical relationship between numbers (e.g., having patients rate their level of pain on a scale from 1 to 10).

○ **What kind of statistical analysis is appropriate for ordinal variables?**

Technically, nonparametric statistics are most appropriate for ordinal variables, but researchers often use parametric statistics.

○ **What is the difference between parametric and nonparametric tests?**

Parametric tests assume that the data are <u>normally</u> distributed and nonparametric tests are typically more stringent because they are based on the assumption of <u>nonnormal</u> distribution.

Examples of parametric tests and the nonparametric equivalent

Parametric Test	*Nonparametric Test*
Ratio or interval data	Ordinal or nominal
Two-sample unpaired *t*-test	Mann–Whitney *U*-test *or* Wilcoxon rank-sum test
One-sample matched pairs *t*-test	Wilcoxon matched pairs test
One-way ANOVA (*F*-test)	Kruskal–Wallis analysis of variance by ranks
One-way repeated-measures ANOVA	Friedman ANOVA test
Chi-square	Fisher exact test
Pearson *r*—product moment correlation coefficient	Spearman rank correlation coefficient

• • • INFERENTIAL STATISTICS • • •

○ **The probability that any particular outcome would have occurred by chance is known as?**

<u>The *P* value</u>: the probability of the observed result or something more extreme under the null hypothesis.

○ **What is a confidence interval?**

A range of values around the sample mean within which a researcher can be certain (typically 95% certain) contains the true mean of the population.

• • • PARAMETRIC TESTS • • •

○ **What types of analysis can you use when both variables are continuous?**

• Regression.

• Correlation.

○ **What does regression analysis mean?**

Whether you can predict the value of one variable (the dependent variable) from the value of another variable (the independent variable) (e.g., predicting a patient's cholesterol level from the number of years he or she has been smoking).

○ **What is the statistic for a regression called?**

R^2.

○ **What does a B or β mean when it is reported with regression results?**

That is the value by which the independent variable must be multiplied to determine the value of the dependent variable.

Note: most journals now require researchers to report the 95% confidence interval around the B or β.

○ **What is a correlation?**

Examining whether two variables are positively or negatively related to each other (e.g., weight and height).

○ **What is the statistic for a correlation called?**

r.

○ **What is the range for r?**

+1 to −1.

○ **What does a +1 r-value mean?**

Two variables are perfectly positively related to each other (as one increases so does the other).

○ **What does a −1 r-value mean?**

Two variables are perfectly inversely related to each other (as one increases the other decreases).

○ **What is a partial correlation?**

It is essentially a correlation you can run with three values. It involves correlating two values to each other, while accounting for the correlation each value has with a third value (e.g., removing the correlation with age while still examining a correlation between height and weight).

○ **What type of analysis can you use when one variable is categorical and the other variable is continuous?**

- *t*-tests.
- analysis of variance (ANOVA).

○ **What does a *t*-test involve?**

Examining whether two groups of participants significantly differ on a variable (e.g., comparing findings between a control group and an experimental group).

○ **What does an ANOVA involve?**

Examining whether two or more groups significantly differ on a variable. You can use this when you have more than one experimental group.

○ **What is an omnibus *F*-test?**

This tells you whether there is an overall difference between your groups.

○ **How can you compare multiple groups to each other within an ANOVA?**

- Planned contrasts.

- Posthoc tests (e.g., Bonferroni and Tukey).

○ **What tests do you use when you want to compare only one or two of your groups to each other?**

Planned contrasts (e.g., compare experimental group 1 to the control group and experimental group 2 to the control group, but not experimental groups 1 and 2 to each other).

○ **What tests do you use when you want to compare all of your groups to each other?**

Posthoc tests (e.g., compare the control group with both experimental groups and the experimental groups to each other).

• • • NONPARAMETRIC TESTS • • •

○ **When is logistic regression appropriate?**

When you want to predict a dichotomous variable from a continuous variable (e.g., predicting whether someone is male or female from knowing their weight).

○ **When is a Wilcoxon signed-ranks test appropriate?**

This test functions as a *t*-test for ordinal variables (e.g., examining whether the control group and the experimental group differ in their pain ratings).

○ **To determine if a difference exists between two different groups, which statistical test is most appropriate?**

Mann–Whitney *U*-test.

○ **What are the characteristics of the Mann–Whitney *U*-test?**

- Used to determine if a difference exists between two different groups.

- Equivalent to the two-sample *t*-test.

- Nonparametric test.

○ **The Wilcoxon rank-sum test is equivalent to which other statistical test?**

- The Mann–Whitney *U*-test.

- Used to test differences between two conditions and different subjects in each condition.

○ **What is an appropriate test to determine the relationship between two categorical variables?**

Pearson chi-square test.

○ **What does a Pearson chi-square test involve?**

It is a hypothesis test which may be performed on contingency tables and is used to discover if there is a relationship between two categorical variables (e.g., being female and having breast cancer).

● ● ● TYPES OF ERROR ● ● ●

○ **The probability of falsely rejecting the null hypothesis is what type of error?**

Type I error.

○ **When a researcher concludes that there is a difference between two conditions when there is no difference, the researcher is making what type of error?**

Type I error.

○ **What is a Type II error?**

Probability of failing to reject the null hypothesis when it is true, and the researcher concludes there is no difference between two conditions when there is a real difference.

○ **What is a null hypothesis?**

That there is no real difference between two groups (or treatments).

○ **What is the purpose of the binomial test?**

Used to compare two dichotomous variables to each other and if you want to know if the proportion of individuals falling into each category has resulted from chance.

○ **What is the term that refers to the statistical likelihood that a researcher will find a significant effect that exists based on the sample size and number of variables?**

Power.

○ **What determines how many degrees of freedom you have for a particular test?**

The number of participants and the number of variables in your analyses.

● ● ● EVIDENCE-BASED MEDICINE ● ● ●

○ **What is evidence-based medicine?**

Clinical decision making based on the integration of research, clinical expertise, and patient needs.

○ **How many different levels of evidence are there?**

Five.

○ **What is Level I type of evidence?**

The highest quality of evidence (e.g., systematic reviews or randomized controlled trials).

○ **What is Level II type of evidence?**

Evidence gathered from a lesser quality randomized clinical trial (e.g., high attrition rates, improper randomization of subjects, or nonrandomization of subjects) or a cohort study or systematic review of such studies.

○ **What is Level III type of evidence?**

Evidence gathered from a well-designed quasi-experimental study (e.g., case–control study or systematic review of such studies).

○ **What is Level IV type of evidence?**

Evidence gathered from well-designed nonexperimental study (e.g., descriptive studies and case series).

○ **What is Level V type of evidence?**

Evidence gathered from expert opinion, case reports, and clinical examples. This is the weakest level of evidence.

● ● ● ASSESSMENT OF DIAGNOSTIC STUDIES ● ● ●

○ **What is sensitivity?**

The probability that a patient <u>with</u> a disease will have a <u>positive</u> test result.

○ **What is specificity?**

The probability that a patient <u>without</u> a disease will have a <u>negative</u> test result.

○ **What is the positive predictive value (PPV)?**

The probability that a patient with a <u>positive</u> test result <u>has</u> the disease. The more specific a test, the higher is its PPV.

○ **What is the negative predictive value (NPV)?**

The probability that a patient with a <u>negative</u> test result <u>does not have</u> the disease. The more sensitive a test, the higher its NPV.

● ● ● BIAS IN STUDY DESIGN ● ● ●

○ **What is a selection bias?**

When participants or samples are selected that differ from other groups in additional determinants of outcome. The sample obtained is not representative of the population intended to be analyzed.

○ **What is a confounding bias?**

The differential effect of unknown or uncontrolled factors on study groups.

○ **What is a measurement/information bias?**

A systematic error in the measurement of the outcome.

○ **What is a recall bias?**

A difference between two groups caused by the inaccuracy of retrospective recollections retrieved.

○ **What is a lead time bias?**

Results when comparing two screening tests and the new or experimental test identify the disease earlier than the traditional test, thus giving the impression of prolonged survival.

● ● ● **REFERENCES** ● ● ●

Field A. *Discovering Statistics Using SPSS*. Los Angeles, CA: Sage; 2009.

Garrett-Mater E. *Basic Biostatistics for Clinicians: How to Use and Interpret Statistics*. Available online at: http://people.musc.edu/~elg26/talks/BasicBiostatisticsforClinicians.pdf.

Greenhalgh T. Statistics for the non-statistician I: different types of data need different statistical tests. *BMJ*. 1997;315:364–366.

Greenhalgh T. Statistics for the non-statistician II: "Significant" relations and their pitfalls. *BMJ*. 1997;315:422–425.

Rich NC. Levels of Evidence. *J Womens Health Phys Ther*. 2005;29:2.

Sackett DL, Strauss SE, Richardson WS, et al. *Evidence-Based Medicine: How to Practice and Teach EBM*. Philadelphia, PA: Churchill-Livingstone; 2000.

Sackett DL, Rosenberg WM, Gray JA, Haynes RB, Richardson WS. Evidence based medicine: what it is and what it isn't. *BMJ*. 1996;312:71–72.

Siegel S. *Nonparametric Statistics for the Behavioral Sciences*. New York, NY: McGraw-Hill; 1956.

Song JW, Hass A, Chung KC. Applications of statistical tests in hand surgery. *J Hand Surg Am*. 2009;34(10):1872–1881.

Witte RS. *Statistics*. 4th ed. Fort Worth, TX: Harcourt Brace; 1993.

CHAPTER 92 Special Topics in General Surgery

Erez Dayan, MD and
Emily M. Clarke-Pearson, MD, MEd

• • • HEMATOLOGY/BLOOD PRODUCTS • • •

○ **Name common supplements that should be discontinued to avoid increased bleeding risk.**

Ginko biloba, garlic, ginseng, omega-3, vitamin E, chondroitin, and saw palmetto.

○ **How should one manage a Jehovah's Witness patient with a low preoperative Hgb?**

First evaluate the patient for cause: iron deficiency (i.e., possible GI malignancy), renal dysfunction, or folate/B12 deficiency. Once these causes of anemia are ruled out, the patient should be started on oral iron and recombinant erythropoietin.

○ **What are the indications for RBC transfusion?**

Evidence of active bleeding/hemorrhagic shock or generally Hgb <7 (Hgb <8 in patients with acute coronary syndromes). Previous guidelines to initiate transfusion for Hgb 10/Hct 30 have shown no benefit.

○ **What is the most common acquired hypercoagulable disorder?**

Smoking. Other common acquired causes: oral contraceptive pills, obesity, cancer, and antiphospholipid syndrome.

○ **Three days after starting warfarin on a patient skin begins sloughing skin off their arms and legs. What is the most likely cause?**

Warfarin induced skin necrosis may result if warfarin is started without first starting heparin. Protein C and S have shorter half-lives and decrease before the other vitamin-k dependent factors when warfarin is initiated. This leads to hypercoagulable state and skin necrosis. Treatment is heparin.

○ **How do you treat a hemophiliac joint?**

Do not aspirate. Elevate, range of motion exercises, and ice.

○ **What is the most common location of a deep vein thrombosis?**

Calf. However, iliofemoral DVTs are most likely to cause a pulmonary embolus. Left leg is twice as likely as right because the left iliac vein is compressed by the right iliac artery.

● ● ● FLUIDS/ELECTROLYTES/NUTRITION ● ● ●

○ **What are the indications for total parental nutrition (TPN)?**

Enteral nutrition is always preferred over parenteral nutrition. TPN may be the only option for patients who require total bowel rest or do not have a functional GI tract (i.e., bowel obstruction, radiation enteritis, and congenital GI anomalies).

○ **What does TPN formula usually consist of?**

Water (30–40 mL/kg/day), protein (20% calories), fat (30% calories), dextrose (50% calories), trace minerals, vitamins, and electrolytes.

○ **A patient presents for an elective procedure 3 months after thyroidectomy. What should you be cautious of?**

A common cause of hypocalcemia is iatrogenic injury. Check for signs of hypocalcemia (perioral tingling/numbness, Chvostek's sign, Trousseau's sign, and prolonged QT on EKG). You may need to correct Mg before being able to correct Ca.

○ **How can you assess a patient's preoperative nutritional status?**

Albumin ($t^{1/2}$ 18 days), transferrin ($t^{1/2}$ 8 days), and prealbumin ($t^{1/2}$ 2 days) are all useful indicators of nutritional status. Albumin <2.5 and/or >20% weight loss in 6 months are strong risk factors for morbidity/mortality.

○ **What is a respiratory quotient (RQ)?**

RQ is a measurement of energy expenditure (ratio of CO_2 produced to O_2 consumed). RQ is important for patients who are ventilator dependent. RQ >1 (lipogenesis) indicates high carbohydrate and CO_2 buildup. Conversely, RQ <0.7 suggests fat oxidation (starvation) and carbohydrates should be increased.

○ **What is the benefit of D51/2NS maintenance IV fluid?**

5% dextrose stimulates insulin release, amino acid uptake, and protein synthesis. When given at 125 cc/hr it provides 150 g glucose/day.

● ● ● ONCOLOGY ● ● ●

○ **What is radiation enteritis?**

GI toxicity may result when the radiation field includes GI structures (thorax, abdomen, or pelvis). Effects include early toxicity (i.e., diarrhea and nausea) and late toxicity (i.e., ulceration and stricture). Combining chemotherapy with radiation increases the risk of radiation enteritis.

○ **What is the difference between a core needle biopsy (CNBx) and fine needle aspiration (FNA)?**

CNBx gives architecture, FNA gives cytology.

○ **Is higher energy radiation worse or better for the skin?**

Better, maximal ionizing potential is not reached until deeper structures.

○ **In which cases is it appropriate to resect a normal organ to prevent cancer?**

(1) Colon (familial adenomatous polyposis), (2) Breast (BRCA I/II with strong family history), and (3) Thyroid (Ret protoncogene or MENIN gene with strong family history).

○ **What are the guidelines for biopsy of an extremity sarcoma?**

Excisional biopsy for lesions <4 cm and longitudinal incisional biopsy if >4 cm. The incisional biopsy is oriented longitudinally so that the scar can be easily resected after re-excision for margins.

• • • THORACIC • • •

○ **What anatomy is relevant to thoracic outlet syndrome?**

The thoracic outlet is the space between the clavicle and the first rib. The subclavian vein runs anterior to the anterior scalene, the subclavian artery and brachial plexus run between the middle/anterior scalenes. Patients can experience neurogenic, venous, or arterial manifestations of compression in this region.

○ **What is a Pancoast tumor?**

Superior pulmonary sulcus tumor. Invasion of the sympathetic chain leads to Horner's syndrome (ptosis, miosis, and anhydrosis) or ulnar nerve symptoms (weakness of intrinsic hand muscles and pain/paresthesia of 4th and 5th digits).

○ **What are the key features of chylothorax and its treatment?**

The thoracic duct runs along the right side of the chest and crosses to the left side at T4–5 in order to drain into the left subclavian vein. Chylothorax is often due to iatrogenic injury of the thoracic duct. Management usually is conservative at first (chest tube, octreotide, and low fat diet). Surgical ligation can be performed if conservative measures fail.

○ **What is the best way to measure alveolar ventilation?**

$PaCO_2$ is the only blood gas measurement that gives you the relationship of alveolar ventilation to CO_2 production.

• • • HEAD AND NECK • • •

○ **Massive bleeding 1 week after tracheostomy creation is most likely:**

Tracheoinnominate artery fistula. First obtain bedside control of hemorrhage by overinflating the cuff or placing your finger through the tracheostomy site to compress the innominate artery against the sternum. Urgent median sternotomy in OR and then either ligate the innominate artery, bypass, or place interposition graft.

○ **In a trauma patient, what are different ways to treat elevated intracranial pressure (ICP)?**

(1) Sedation/paralysis, (2) elevated head of bed, (3) relative hyperventilation (CO_2 30–35), (4) keep serum Na 140–150 (may need hypertonic saline), (5) Mannitol, and (6) ventriculostomy with CSF drainage or burr hole/craniotomy.

○ **What is Cushing's triad?**

(1) Hypertension, (2) bradycardia, and (3) slow respiratory rate. All three of these findings in a patient with head injury suggest impending herniation.

● ● ● **TRANSPLANT** ● ● ●

○ **Describe the different types of rejection?**

Type of Rejection	Time	Cause
Hyperacute	Minutes to hours	Preformed antibodies against donor tissue
Acute	Days to weeks	T cells mediated against foreign MHC
Chronic	Months to years	T cell mediated against foreign MHC "looking like" self MHC

○ **Name the two most common posttransplant malignancies.**

(1) Skin Ca (SSC #1) and (2) posttransplant lymphoproliferative disorder.

○ **What is the mechanism of steroid use in transplant?**

Steroids inhibit macrophages and genes for cytokine synthesis (IL-1 and IL-6).

● ● ● **ANESTHESIA/AIRWAY MANAGEMENT** ● ● ●

○ **What is Rapid Sequence intubation (RSI)?**

RSI allows for rapid control of the airway but using a fast acting induction agent and paralytic. RSI is often used in emergency airway management or in patients that are high risk for aspiration (i.e., bowel obstruction, pregnancy, and recent oral intake).

○ **How do you perform an open cricothyroidotomy?**

Cricothyroidotomy is the last resort when an emergent airway is needed. A 1-cm vertical incision is made between the inferior aspect of the thyroid cartilage and the superior aspect of the cricoid ring down to depth of laryngeal structures. Then a horizontal incision is made near the inferior edge of the cricothyroid membrane (to avoid superior cricothyroid vessels), then dilate and place an endotracheal/tracheostomy tube.

○ **What are some advantages of dexmedetomidine (precedex) versus propofol?**

Dexmedetomidine is a selective α_2-agonist that provides "cooperative" sedation and analgesia without depressing the respiratory drive. Patients may be extubated while on dexmedetomidine. Propofol has a rapid on/off effect of complete sedation and does not have analgesic properties. Propofol causes respiratory depression. Side effects of both medications may include bradycardia and hypotension.

○ **How should patients on chronic steroids be managed postoperatively?**

Function of hypothalamic–pituitary–adrenal (HPA) axis and need for perioperative steroids.

• Nonsuppressed HPA axis	• Any dose of exogenous steroids for <3 wks. • <5 mg prednisone for any duration or <10 mg prednisone every other day.	• Do not require preop evaluation of HPA axis or additional steroids perioperatively.
• Suppressed HPA axis	• Prednisone >20 mg/day for >3 wks.	• Minor procedures–no steroids. • Moderate procedures–25 mg hydrocortisone q8h × 24 hrs. • Major procedure–100 mg IV hydrocortisone before induction, 50 mg q8h × 24 hrs, taper down.

Patients with intermediate HPA suppression require biochemical evaluation to determine severity of suppression.

○ **What is malignant hyperthermia and how is it treated?**

Malignant hyperthermia is a life-threatening hypermetabolic state that occurs when susceptible patients are exposed to volatile anesthetics or succinylcholine. Clinical presentation includes masseter muscle rigidity, hypercarbia, fever, tachycardia, acidosis, and hyperkalemia. Treatment: (1) discontinue trigger agents, (2) oxygenate/ventilate, (3) dantrolene, (4) monitor and treat hyperkalemia, and (5) supportive care.

○ **Name some of the physiologic changes that occur in the elderly population that must be considered perioperatively?**

Cardiovascular: decreased cardiac contractility and stroke volume.

GU: impaired ability to concentrate urine. Reduced creatinine function (nl creatinine ≠ nl renal function)

Respiratory: decreased response to hypoxia and hypercapnia, decreased vital lung capacity, and increased residual volume.

Wound healing: longer rate of collagen turnover and reduced inflammatory response.

● ● ● TRAUMA AND CRITICAL CARE ● ● ●

○ **What are the trauma zones of the neck?**

Zone 1—clavicle to cricoid; explore if symptomatic or significant finding (workup: angio, bronch, EGD, and swallow study).

Zone 2—cricoid to angle of mandible; explore all if penetrating platysma.

Zone 3—angle of mandible to skull base; explore if symptomatic or significant finding (workup: angio and laryngoscopy).

○ **What are common fractures from an upright fall?**

Calcaneus, lumbar spine, and wrist/forearm.

○ **What are proven methods to decrease surgical site infections?**

Preop use clippers to remove hair (not shave), smoking cessation, and appropriate skin prep.

Abx within 1 hour of incision and discontinuation within 24 hours.

Maintain blood glucose control (80–120 in diabetic patients).

Keep PaO$_2$ high during operation.

Keep patient warm (Bair hugger best method).

Intraoperatively obliterate dead space, sterile dressing for 24 to 48 hours, and ensure hemostasis.

○ **What are the advantages and disadvantages of different central line access (i.e., subclavian, internal jugular, and femoral)?**

Type	Advantages	Disadvantages
• Internal Jugular	• Less risk of pneumothorax. • Bleeding controlled by direct pressure.	• Not good for prolonged access. • Risk for carotid injury.
• Subclavian	• Easier landmarks in obese patient. • Can be performed while airway being established.	• Increased risk of pneumothorax. • Difficult to hold pressure with bleeding.
• Femoral	• Quick access away from chest and airway. • No need for trendelenburg position.	• More likely to get infected. • Risk of iliofemoral thrombosis.

○ **Describe the hemodynamic findings of hemorrhagic, septic, cardiogenic, and neurogenic shock.**

	CVP/PCWP	Cardiac Index	Systemic Vascular Resistance	SvO$_2$
Hemorrhagic	⇓	⇓	⇑	⇓
Septic	⇑	⇑	⇓	⇑
Cardiogenic	⇓	⇓	⇑	⇓
Neurogenic	⇑	⇓	⇓	⇑

○ **What is needed to diagnose necrotizing fasciitis?**

Necrotizing fasciitis is a clinical diagnosis (sepsis, erythema, edema, crepitus, blisters, pain out of proportion, and drainage). Patients should be taken to the OR for fascial/ muscle debridement immediately and broad-spectrum antibiotics should be started until organisms are isolated.

○ **What is the most important prognostic indicator of the Glasgow coma scale (GCS)?**

Motor score. GCS includes assessment of motor function (1–6), verbal function (1–5), and eye function (1–4). The lowest score is 3 and highest is 15. Intubated patients are given a verbal score of 1T.

○ **What are indications for an ICP monitor?**

GCS <8, suspected elevated ICP from CT scan findings, and inability to follow neurologic examination (i.e., sedated/paralyzed patient). Patients with GCS <14 require CT scan and GCS <10 need intubation.

○ **What diagnostic tests should be performed on a patient with posterior knee dislocation?**

Posterior knee dislocations are highly associated with popliteal injuries. Perform extremity vascular examination and ankle-brachial index. If normal, admit for serial vascular examinations. If any abnormalities found, proceed to OR for angiogram.

○ **What is the treatment for venous air embolus?**

Supportive care (mechanical ventilation, pressors, and volume), immediately place in left lateral decubitus position with head down. In contrast, patients with arterial embolism should be placed flat. In severely unstable patients, one may attempt to aspirate air (limited benefit).

○ **What are commonly used ventilator settings?**

Assist control—full preset breath given in coordination with patient's inspiratory effort. Independent spontaneous breathing is not allowed.

Synchronous intermittent mandatory ventilation—preset breaths given in coordination with patient's inspiratory effort. Spontaneous breathing is allowed.

Pressure support—decreases work of breathing for spontaneously breathing patient. Patient effort determines volume and rate.

○ **When should enterocutaneous fistula resection be considered?**

Enterocutaneous fistulas are associated with inflammation and dense adhesions, making early surgery risky. If the fistula has failed to resolve after ~6 weeks of nonoperative management it will likely need surgery.

○ **Name some commonly used eponyms for the examination of the acute abdomen?**

Eponym	*Location*	*Pain Suggests*
• McBurny's point	• 1/3 the distance from ASIS to umbilicus.	• Appendicitis.
• Rovsing's sign	• Palpation of left lower quadrant causes pain in right lower quadrant.	• Appendicitis.
• Murphy's sign	• Palpation of subcostal right upper quadrant when patient breathes in.	• Cholecystitis.
• Carnett's sign	• Abdominal pain increases when patient tenses abdominal wall muscles.	• Abdominal wall etiology vs. abdominal cavity (i.e., rectus sheath hematoma vs. diverticulitis).
• Markle's sign	• Exceptional abdominal tenderness elicited by shaking bed or foot.	• Peritonitis.
• Blumberg's sign	• Abdominal wall is compressed slowly and then rapidly released (rebound).	• Peritonitis.

○ **What is the most common cause of abdominal pain in patients <50 years old? How about >50 years old?**

<50 years old—acute appendicitis, >50 years old—cholecystitis.

• • • VASCULAR • • •

○ **What are the absolute indications for an IVC filter?**

Presence of DVT or PE with: (1) contraindication to anticoagulation (i.e., head trauma and retroperitoneal hematoma), (2) recurrent PE despite anticoagulation, and (3) anticoagulation related complication.

○ **What happens if you ligate the carotid artery?**

20% of patients will have stroke.

○ **What are three risk factors for venous thrombosis?**

Virchow's triad: (1) stasis, (2) endothelial injury, and (3) hypercoagulability.

○ **Name differences between unfractionated heparin (UFH) and low–molecular-weight heparin (LMWH)?**

LMWH (i.e., lovenox) has a much smaller risk of heparin induced thrombocytopenia (HITT) and does not require PTT monitoring. Unlike LMWH, UFH can be reversed with protamine.

○ **What is the most common peripheral aneurysm?**

Popliteal artery. Must screen for other aneurysms (50% incidence).

○ **What is the most common visceral aneurysm?**

Splenic artery. Repair for patients who are symptomatic and women who are pregnant or of childbearing age.

○ **What is the treatment for lower extremity claudication?**

Conservative therapy first: ASA, smoking cessation, and exercise until painful to improve collateral flow.

○ **What are the best tests to diagnose osteomyelitis?**

Needle bone biopsy is the best diagnostic test. Tagged WBC scan has the highest sensitivity but is not specific (may be falsely positive with surrounding inflammation).

○ **What are the indications for angiogram in extremity trauma?**

Angiogram should be performed for soft signs of vascular injury (i.e., ABI <0.9, unequal pulses, large stable hematoma, and injury near a major artery). For major signs of vascular injury (i.e., active hemorrhage, pulse deficit, expanding hematoma, and distal ischemia) go to OR.

● ● ● **REFERENCES** ● ● ●

Albertos R, Caralt B, Rello J. Ventilator-associated pneumonia management in critical illness. *Curr Opin Gastroenterol.* 2011;27(2): 160–166.

Barrack RL. Current guidelines for total joint VTE prophylaxis: dawn of a new day. *J Bone Joint Surg Br.* 2012;94(11 Suppl A):3–7.

Barrera LM, Perel P, Ker K, Cirocchi R, Farinella E, Morales Uribe CH. Thromboprophylaxis for trauma patients. *Cochrane Database Syst Rev.* 2013;3:CD008303.

Bisbe Vives E, Basora Macaya M. Algorithm for treating preoperative anemia. *Rev Esp Anestesiol Reanim.* 2015;62 Suppl 1:27–34.

Burgess CA, Dale OT, Almeyda R, Corbridge RJ. An evidence based review of the assessment and management of penetrating neck trauma. *Clin Otolaryngol.* 2012;37(1):44–52.

Chandrashekar S, Kantharaj A. Legal and ethical issues in safe blood transfusion. *Indian J Anaesth.* 2014;58(5):558–564.

Curley GF, Shehata N, Mazer CD, Hare GM, Friedrich JO. Transfusion triggers for guiding RBC transfusion for cardiovascular surgery: a systematic review and meta-analysis*. *Crit Care Med.* 2014;42(12):2611–2624.

da Silva Fink J, Daniel de Mello P, Daniel de Mello E. Subjective global assessment of nutritional status - a systematic review of the literature. *Clin Nutr.* 2015;34(5):785–792.

Goodnough LT, Levy JH, Murphy MF. Concepts of blood transfusion in adults. *Lancet.* 2013;381(9880):1845–1854.

Kuhn JE, Lebus VG, Bible JE. Thoracic outlet syndrome. *J Am Acad Orthop Surg.* 2015;23(4):222–232.

Lawson T Ralph C. Perioperative Jehovah's Witnesses: a review. *Br J Anaesth.* 2015;115(5):676–687.

Mahmoodie M, Sanei B, Moazeni-Bistgani M, Namgar M. Penetrating neck trauma: review of 192 cases. *Arch Trauma Res.* 2012;1(1): 14–18.

Ricci Z, Iacoella C, Cogo P. Fluid management in critically ill pediatric patients with congenital heart disease. *Minerva Pediatr.* 2011;63(5):399–410.

Schulz RJ, Bischoff SC, Koletzko B; Working group for developing the guidelines for parenteral nutrition of The German Association for Nutritional Medicine. Gastroenterology - Guidelines on Parenteral Nutrition, Chapter 15. *Ger Med Sci.* 2009;7:Doc13.

Shah A, Stanworth SJ, McKechnie S. Evidence and triggers for the transfusion of blood and blood products. *Anaesthesia.* 2015;70 Suppl 1:10–9, e3–e5.

CHAPTER 93 High-Yield Topics

Peter F. Koltz, MD and
Samuel J. Lin, MD, MBA, FACS

● ● ● BREAST AND COSMETIC ● ● ●

Breast

○ **What is the next step following reduction mammaplasty when the resection specimen contains invasive ductal carcinoma?**

Determine tumor margins; decide on completion mastectomy.

○ **What is a critical factor in deciding breast contouring following implant removal?**

Preoperative ptosis (remains unchanged following removal).

○ **What best determines performing contouring and implant removal in the same setting?**

Thickness of residual breast (minimum thickness of 4 cm required).

○ **Compared to traditional transaxillary submuscular breast augmentation, endoscopic techniques are associated with a decreased rate of what?**

Malpositioning of the implant.

○ **Breast ptosis results from elongation and laxity of what structure?**

Cooper ligaments.

○ **What is the most appropriate CPT code used for fat grafting?**

Fat grafting is reported with code 20926 (tissue grafts, other [e.g., paratenon, fat, dermis]) and includes the following: Harvest of the fat graft material by any method, closure of the donor site, processing of fat graft material, injection of fat graft into recipient site, and 90 days of routine postoperative care.

○ **Mastectomy resulting in decreased bulk in the inferior and lateral portions of the right pectoral muscle is caused by denervation of what nerve?**

Medial pectoral; C8–T1 supplies lower and lateral sternal portion of pectoralis major and pectoralis minor muscle.

○ **What does the lateral pectoral nerve supply?**

Arises from C5–6, supplies the medial portion of the pectoralis muscle.

○ **How does one assess the status of the pectoralis muscle in postmastectomy reconstruction?**

Have the patient place hands on hips and contract chest muscles.

○ **During breast augmentation, underfilling of the implants below the manufacturer's recommended minimum will most likely have what effect?**

Decreases longevity of the implant and leads to early rupture.

○ **What advantage does an extended latissimus dorsi flap have over a standard latissimus dorsi flap in the setting of breast reconstruction?**

A decreased need for adjuvant breast implantation.

○ **What mammographic finding is seen 6 to 18 months following an inferior pedicle reduction mammoplasty?**

Parenchymal redistribution, nipple elevation, calcifications, oil cysts from localized fat necrosis.

○ **Breast reduction by liposuction is most useful in breasts with what percentage of fat?**

50%.

○ **In a young patient undergoing MRM with postoperative radiation, what procedure will provide the best aesthetic reconstruction?**

Delayed reconstruction with autologous tissue.

○ **In a study comparing early and late complications in patients who underwent TRAM reconstruction followed by radiation versus radiation treatment followed by TRAM reconstruction, what were the differences?**

The early complications did not differ, but the late complications were more frequent in the group undergoing immediate reconstruction.

○ **A woman who has the *BRCA2* mutation has a lifetime incidence of what percentage of developing breast cancer?**

60%.

○ **Sharp dissection lateral to the lateral edge of the pectoralis muscle during augmentation mammaplasty may result in what complication?**

Numbness of the nipple–areola complex; the fourth and fifth anterolateral intercostal nerves provide sensation to the nipple–areola complex.

○ **What is consistently the best marking for the new nipple position during reduction mammaplasty?**

The inframammary fold.

○ **What represents the lateral border of the breast footprint?**

Anterior axillary fold.

○ **Sensation to the nipple–areolar complex is derived from what?**

Anterolateral branches of the third through fifth intercostal nerves (primarily the fourth nerve).

○ **Define pseudoptosis of the breast.**

The nipple remains above the IMF, but the breast mass descends below the NAC.

○ **What is first-degree ptosis?**

The NAC descends to the level of the IMF.

○ **What is second-degree ptosis?**

The nipple is located beneath the IMF, but is not the lowest point of the breast.

○ **In polymastia, where are accessory mammary structure most commonly found?**

The axilla.

○ **What supplies sensation to the upper breast?**

Cervical branches from the third and fourth.

○ **The medial and inferior breast?**

Branches from the anterior cutaneous branches.

○ **What is the most common cause of asymmetric enlargement of a breast over a year with a palpable mass in a teenage girl?**

Fibroadenoma; treat with excision.

○ **What is the first treatment for nipple cyanosis following breast reduction?**

Releasing the sutures surrounding the NAC and return to the OR.

○ **What are the criteria for free nipple grafting?**

Reduction amount greater than 1,500 g, nipple transposition length greater than 25 cm, and a history of smoking or diabetes.

○ **What affects the quality of mammography with breast implants?**

Implant position, capsular contracture, native breast volume.

○ **What common medications may cause gynecomastia?**

Tagamet, Digoxin, Minocycline, spironolactone.

○ **What are key elements of the Lejour reduction mammaplasty?**

Central vertical gland excision and excision of skin in one direction, upper pedicle, more difficult to determine resection end point.

○ **What is considered the best reconstructive option for the breast as a secondary procedure following mastectomy and irradiation?**

TRAM reconstruction; implant reconstruction associated with increased capsular contraction rate with prior irradiation.

○ **What condition has an increased risk of hypercoaguability and must be considered in free flap reconstruction?**

Systemic lupus erythematosus (SLE).

○ **What is the next appropriate step for a woman preceding breast augmentation with milky discharge and regular menstrual cycles?**

Obtaining a serum prolactin level to rule out a pituitary lesion; thyroid function studies, medication history (e.g., tricyclic antidepressants).

○ **What is the most frequent complication following periareolar mastopexy?**

Areolar widening.

○ **What defines a tuberous breast?**

Constricted appearance of breast; unilateral narrowing of the breast; narrow breast diameter, superior displacement of the IMF; areola enlarged; breast hypoplasia.

○ **How is a tuberous breast treated?**

Augmentation mammaplasty with IMF adjustment, radial scoring of the breast glandular tissue, areola reduction.

○ **What is the rate of additional procedures following breast implant augmentation?**

25% of patients requiring additional procedure within 13 years.

○ **What is the rate of deflation after implant augmentation?**

1% annually.

○ **What is the approximate rate of capsular contraction?**

20% to 25%.

○ **What portion of breast parenchyma is affected after implant augmentation?**

Estimated 5%, not entirely seen on mammography.

○ **What nerve supplies the nipple–areola complex?**

The lateral branch of the fourth intercostal nerves.

○ **What factors are increased in smokers who undergo free TRAM breast reconstruction?**

Necrosis of the mastectomy skin, abdominal skin, and hernia rates.

○ **What factors are not increased with smokers undergoing free TRAM breast reconstruction?**

Vessel thrombosis, fat necrosis, flap loss, or wound infection.

○ **What are the grades of gynecomastia?**

I: mild enlargement without redundant skin.

IIA: moderate enlargement without redundant skin.

IIB: moderate enlargement with skin redundancy.

III: marked enlargement with significant redundant skin.

○ **What are the methods of treating gynecomastia?**

Suction lipectomy, excising a concentric circle of skin, amputation with free nipple grafting, glandular resection with liposuction.

○ **What are the general indications for delayed mastopexy following implant explantation?**

Marked ptosis requiring nipple elevation of greater than 4 cm, breast mound less than 4 cm, smoking history.

○ **What is the procedure that should be done for grade II breast ptosis?**

For repositioning of the nipple–areola complex of 2 to 4 cm, a Wise pattern mastopexy may be performed.

○ **What procedure is recommended for pseudoptosis?**

Wedge excision from the inframammary fold.

○ **What is the most appropriate next step for a smoker having undergone implant explantation with marked ptosis and less than 4 cm of breast thickness?**

Delayed mastopexy for 3 months at minimum.

○ **What patients are appropriate candidates for nipple sparing mastectomy?**

Tumor size of 3 cm or less, at least 2 cm from the nipple, not multicentric, and those with clinically negative nodes.

○ **After bilateral TRAM elevation, what supplies the umbilicus primarily?**

Ligamentum teres.

○ **To minimize hernia recurrence following abdominal-based autologous reconstruction, where is the optimal position to place mesh to minimize recurrence?**

Between rectus muscle and posterior rectus sheath.

○ **What are the venous thromboembolism guidelines based on Caprini score (risk assessment model)?**

Patients undergoing major plastic and reconstructive operative procedures performed during general anesthesia that last longer than 60 minutes should receive VTE prevention. For patients with Caprini score of 3 to 6, the use of postoperative low–molecular-weight heparin (LMWH) or unfractionated heparin (UH) should be considered. For patients with Caprini score of 3 or more, use of mechanical prophylaxis throughout the duration of chemical prophylaxis for nonambulatory patients should be considered. For patients with Caprini score of 7 or more, the use of extended LMWH postoperative prophylaxis should be strongly considered.

○ **What is the greatest source of dissatisfaction following breast reduction?**

Noticeable scarring.

○ **Following reduction mammaplasty, what is the percentage of being able to breast-feed?**

30%.

○ **What is the best radiologic study to assess for silicone breast implant rupture? What is the linguine sign?**

MRI. The linguine sign is a finding on MRI of multiple curvilinear low–signal-intensity lines within the high–signal-intensity silicone gel signifying implant rupture.

○ **Patient presents 6 weeks after breast reduction with a firm, painless mass in the breast. Diagnosis?**

Fat necrosis.

○ **Define the following chest wall abnormalities:**

Anterior thoracic hypoplasia	Anterior chest wall depression, posteriorly displaced ribs, ipsilateral breast hypoplasia, superiorly displaced nipple complex.
Pectus excavatum	Most common deformity. Results in concave anterior chest wall, typically the lower third of the sternum. Normal breasts.
Pectus carinatum	Sternum and ribs are displaced anteriorly. Normal breasts.
Poland syndrome	Unilateral anomaly of varying severity consisting of absent sternal head of pectoralis, hypoplasia of breast/nipple, ipsilateral upper extremity anomalies, +/− chest wall abnormalities.
Sternal cleft	Rare congenital anomaly in which the sternum fails to fuse in the midline. Normal breasts.

○ **What findings are seen in Poland syndrome?**

Pectoralis muscle sternal head hypoplasia, hypoplasia/aplasia of the breast, ipsilateral hand anomalies; males and females equally affected; chest wall anomalies.

○ **What is the initial management of gynecomastia in puberty in the absence of other abnormalities?**

Observation and follow-up in 12 months.

○ **How old do you have to be to get cosmetic silicone breast augmentation?**

The FDA has approved silicone gel breast implants for women aged 22 and older. Younger patients get saline implants.

○ **What is the proper shape and location of the male nipple–areola complex?**

Oval in shape and located at the fourth to fifth intercostal spaces.

○ **True/False: Size of the implant in breast augmentation influences postoperative nipple sensation.**

True.

○ **What is the downside to using a textured silicone implant over a smooth silicone implant?**

Increased rate of rippling.

○ **True/False: Textured implants have a higher rate of capsular contracture than smooth implants?**

False, they have slightly less.

○ **What nerves may be injured during transaxillary breast augmentation?**

Intercostobrachial and medial brachial cutaneous nerves providing sensation to the medial aspect of the upper arm.

○ **What is the lifetime risk of breast cancer in a male with the *BRCA2* gene mutation? Female with *BRCA1* mutation? Female with *BRCA2* mutation?**

7% in males, in females, 85% *BRCA1*, 60% *BRCA2*.

○ **What is a phyllodes tumor? How is it treated?**

Tumors from the periductal stromal cells of the breast. They are typically fast growing but 90% are benign. Management is local excision and close annual surveillance.

Nose

○ **How is a "hanging" columella treated?**

Trimming of the caudal margin of the septum and medial crura of the lower lateral cartilage.

○ **What is the best flap to use for a defect of the lateral nasal ala?**

Nasolabial flap, superiorly based.

○ **What should be used for a defect of the lateral nasal wall above the ala?**

Cheek advancement flap.

○ **A defect of the caudal third of the nose centrally?**

Frontonasal flap.

○ **What skin characteristics negatively affect results after rhinoplasty?**
Thick skin with large sebaceous glands; skin envelope does not conform easily.

○ **What are the three zones of injury occurring in a nasal fracture?**
Upper vault (nasal bones, ethmoid, vomer, cephalic septal border); middle vault (upper lateral cartilages, septum, maxilla); lower vault (alar cartilages, inferior septum).

○ **What is the limit at which airway resistance increases in the internal nasal valve?**
Less than 10 to 12 degrees.

○ **What defines the internal nasal valve area?**
The caudal margin of the upper lateral cartilage, septum, nasal floor, and anterior edge of inferior turbinate.

○ **Secondary healing of what part of the nose is least likely to provide an acceptable cosmetic result?**
The nasal tip.

○ **What techniques have important roles in providing tip projection in addition to tip grafting?**
Suturing of the medial crura, placing a strut graft between the medial crura.

○ **What effect occurs with resection of the lateral and medial crura and the nasal spine?**
Decrease of tip projection.

○ **What effect does a complete transfixion incision have?**
Decreases projection secondary to weakening of nasal support.

○ **True/False: The evaluation of the nasal airway should include the nasal dorsum.**
False.

○ **In a patient with a negative Cottle maneuver, what procedure is likely to improve the nasal airway?**
Lateral strut graft of the crus.

○ **What comprises the external nasal valve?**
Columella, ala, nasal sill.

○ **What comprises the internal nasal valve?**
Area of the angle between the upper lateral cartilage and septum.

○ **How is vestibular stenosis treated?**
An alar base flap.

○ **What factors lead to a saddle nose deformity?**

Excessive dorsal or septal resection, nasal bone comminution during infracture, or a fracture of the perpendicular ethmoid plate.

○ **What supplies sensation to the nasal radix?**

The supratrochlear and infratrochlear nerves.

○ **What supplies sensation to the nasal tip?**

External nasal branch of the anterior ethmoidal nerve; emerges from nasal bone and lateral nasal cartilage.

○ **What part of the nose is innervated by the infraorbital nerve?**

Lower lateral half and skin of the columella.

○ **What is supplied by the infratrochlear nerve?**

Superior portion of the nasal side wall and skin over the radix.

○ **Where is a 1-cm defect on the nose most amenable to healing by secondary intention?**

Area of the medial canthus, glabella, nasolabial fold, and philtrum.

○ **What is the blood supply to the nasal tip during an open rhinoplasty?**

Lateral nasal artery that arises from the angular artery.

○ **What artery is divided during open rhinoplasty?**

The columellar branch of the superior labial artery.

○ **What vessels from the internal carotid artery supply the nasal skin?**

Dorsal nasal artery, external branch of the ethmoidal artery.

○ **What defect is a dorsal nasal flap typically used for?**

A defect of the nasal tip up to 2 cm.

○ **What is the polybeak deformity following rhinoplasty due to?**

Excessive reduction of the tip particularly in the setting of poor nasal tip projection.

○ **What is the treatment for alar collapse with inspiration and a pinched nasal tip?**

Grafting of the nasal tip with cartilage.

○ **What are the causes of a saddle nose deformity after rhinoplasty?**

Overresection of the septum, separation of the cartilaginous septum from the vomer, collapse of the vertical component of the L-strut.

○ **What causes the inverted V deformity after rhinoplasty?**

Collapse of the upper lateral cartilage.

○ **What causes the open-roof deformity after rhinoplasty?**

Failure of the nasal bones to come together in the midline after osteotomies.

○ **What causes a stair-step deformity after rhinoplasty?**

An osteotomy that is too high on the nasal process and not flush with the maxilla resulting in a visible and palpable deformity.

○ **How do you correct the inverted V deformity after rhinoplasty?**

Spreader grafts correct the collapse of the internal nasal valve.

○ **What is the advantage of partial submucous resection of the inferior turbinate over turbinate ablation?**

Decreased incidence of atrophic rhinitis.

○ **How do you treat a collapsed external nasal valve?**

Alar batten grafts.

Ear

○ **What is the Antia–Buch flap used for?**

Lesions located on the lateral rim; tissue used from postauricular skin to reconstruct the helical margin.

○ **Where on the avulsed pinna is anastomosis of the arteries most appropriate?**

The posterior surface; larger arteries enter the pinna on the posterior surface.

○ **Treatment of an auricular hematoma by needle aspiration is likely to result in what?**

Seroma.

○ **A 6-year-old boy with an obtuse concha-mastoid angle with a normal antihelical fold is best treated by what technique?**

Setback of the concha using concha-mastoid sutures.

○ **What are common causes of prominent ears?**

Enlarged conchal bowl, obtuse concha-mastoid angle, loss of the antihelical fold.

○ **How is ear prominence corrected from loss of the antihelical fold?**

Abrading or scoring the antihelix and placing Mustarde sutures between the conchal and scaphoid eminence.

○ **True/False: Microtia and inner ear abnormalities may be closely related.**

False.

○ **What is orbital auricular vertebral syndrome otherwise known as?**

Goldenhar syndrome (associated with microtia, cervical spine abnormalities, mandibular hypoplasia, preauricular pits/sinuses, hemifacial microsomia).

○ **What develops from the first three hillocks of the ear during development?**

First three hillocks are from the first arch; tragus, helical root, superior helix.

○ **What develops from the second three hillocks of the ear?**

Antitragus, antihelix, inferior helix and lobule; from the second branchial arch.

○ **What is the treatment principle of cryptotia?**

Detaching the superior auricle from the temporal area and placing a skin graft in the retroauricular area.

○ **How is Stahl ear treated?**

Advancing the third crus of the antihelix.

○ **Placing sutures from the concha to the mastoid bowl and rasping the anterior surface of the antihelix has been described for what condition?**

Correction of prominent ears.

○ **How is the constricted ear treated?**

Partially detaching the helix from the scapha and suturing the helix.

○ **What is the treatment for an auricular implant (porous polyethylene) covered with a temporoparietal fascial flap with subsequent exposure of the implant?**

Dressing changes and secondary wound healing for at least 6 months.

○ **What principle guides the Mustarde otoplasty approach?**

Using mattress sutures to bend the antihelix.

○ **What is the Stenstrom technique?**

Using an otoabrader to bend the anterior antihelical surface.

○ **What is the Graham and Gault otoplasty technique?**

Endoscopic scoring and suture of the cartilage posteriorly.

○ **What is the Luckett procedure?**

Excision of a crescent-shaped piece of skin/cartilage.

○ **What is the Furnas technique?**

Sutures spanning the concha to the mastoid.

○ **What are the common descriptive findings in the prominent ear?**

Conchal valgus, cranioauricular angle greater than 40 degrees, antihelical underfolding; widened conchoscaphal angle (greater than 90 degrees).

○ **What are general options for correcting the prominent ear?**

Concha to scapha sutures, concha to mastoid sutures, scoring the cartilage anteriorly, conchal resection, postauricular skin resection.

○ **What is the optimal timing for microtia surgery in a child?**

At 6 to 7 years of age, the ear is practically fully developed by age 7.

○ **What is the ear canal typically created in microtia with respect to auricular reconstruction?**

Typically following the creation of the auricle.

○ **What is the initial management of the neonate with prominent ears?**

Molding with tape and splinting.

○ **How long do maternal estrogens remain in the neonate?**

6 months, which allows for shaping of auricular cartilage.

○ **What is the Stahl ear deformity?**

A third crus, antihelical flattening, scaphoid fossa deformity.

○ **What is the constricted ear?**

Helical and scaphal hooding.

○ **What is seen in cryptotia?**

Upper pole of the ear is buried beneath skin; absence of superior auriculocephalic sulcus missing.

○ **What nerve supplies sensation to the superior cranial surface of the ear?**

Lesser occipital nerve.

○ **What nerve supplies sensation to the skin of the anterosuperior EAC?**

Lesser occipital nerve.

○ **What areas are supplied by the great auricular nerve?**

Inferior half of the lateral ear and inferior portion of the cranial surface of the ear.

○ **What area is supplied by the auriculotemporal nerve?**

Sensation to the anterosuperior surface of the external ear.

○ **What does Arnold nerve supply?**

Sensation to the concha and posterior EAC.

○ **At what trimester does maldevelopment occur and microtia result?**

First trimester between 4.5 and 10 weeks.

○ **What is the treatment for a complete upper auricular defect from a burn several years ago?**

Rib cartilage framework for the upper ear with temporoparietal fascia flap and skin graft.

○ **What is the likely cause of recurrent prominence of ears following otoplasty at 7 months?**

Suture failure at the antihelical fold.

Eye

○ **What is the treatment for chronic ectropion and excessive scleral show after a chemical burn?**

Full-thickness skin grafting.

○ **What is the mechanism of involutional ectropion?**

Laxity of the lower lid from the lower lid retractors becoming disinserted from the tarsal plate.

○ **What is the treatment for involutional ectropion?**

Lateral canthoplasty, lateral wedge excision, or excising of a full-thickness wedge from the lateral canthal region.

○ **What structure does the common canaliculus enter the lacrimal sac posterior to?**

The medial canthal tendon.

○ **What muscle is most commonly injured in blepharoplasty?**

Superior oblique; clinically may see tilting of head, and depression of chin.

○ **What is the procedure required for a patient who exhibits a Jones I test without dye and a Jones II test with dye in the tear sac?**

Dacryocystorhinostomy.

○ **How is a Jones I test performed?**

Instill 2% fluorescein dye into the conjunctival fornices; recovery of dye indicates a normal lacrimal system (or positive result); a negative result necessitates a Jones II test.

○ **How is a Jones II test performed?**

Dilation of the punta is performed first; fluid passing into the nose indicates that obstruction of the nasolacrimal duct is cleared.

○ **A negative Jones I and a positive Jones II test indicate what?**

Blockage of the nasolacrimal duct system.

○ **What procedure will address lower eyelid skin laxity with 2 mm of scleral show bilaterally?**

Lower lid blepharoplasty with lateral canthopexy.

○ **Following lower lid blepharoplasty, a woman exhibiting scleral show, round, sad-looking eyes, photophobia, epiphora, what has anatomically occurred?**

Scarring between the orbital septum and the capsulopalpebral fascia, resulting in lower lid retraction (without lid eversion); other causes include lateral canthal tendon laxity, midface descent.

○ **What is the eyelid function in patients with Bell palsy?**

Ectropion from dysfunction of the orbicularis muscle; inability to close the eye.

○ **What characterizes aponeurotic ptosis?**

Good levator function; elevation of eyelid crease, ability to visualize shadow of iris with eyelid closure (positive Nesi sign), or translucent upper eyelid.

○ **What may be done to improve excess scleral show and slowed retraction of a "snap-back" test following blepharoplasty?**

Lateral canthopexy.

○ **How is a patient treated with 3.5 mm of ptosis and 10-mm levator function?**

Resuturing of the levator aponeurosis.

○ **What are the classifications of ptosis?**

Neurogenic, myogenic, mechanical, aponeurotic.

○ **When is eyebrow suspension used for ptosis treatment?**

Poor levator function (less than 4 mm) and greater than 3 mm of ptosis.

○ **When is the Fasanella–Servat procedure used?**

Good levator function and minimal ptosis (less than 2 mm).

○ **What procedure is used for levator function between 4- and 10-mm and 3-mm ptosis?**

Levator resection.

○ **What is the treatment of 4-mm ptosis and 2-mm levator function in a 5-year-old child?**

Frontalis suspension.

○ **What is associated with inadvertent blepharoptosis—Botox injection of the corrugator or lateral orbicularis?**

The corrugator.

○ **Transcutaneous lower lid blepharoplasty is associated with what undesired finding most commonly?**

Malpositioned lower eyelids.

○ **What may be done for asymmetrical lower eyelids following blepharoplasty?**

Conservative (taping, Frost stitches) treatment first; surgery for failed conservative treatment (tarsal strip, wedge tarsectomy).

○ **What percentage of patients undergoing orbital floor fracture repair through a preseptal transconjunctival approach develop ectropion?**

Close to 0%.

○ **What clinical findings are seen in levator aponeurosis dehiscence?**

Ptosis, elevated supratarsal crease, thinning of upper eyelid skin.

○ **What is typically done for levator aponeurosis dehiscence?**

Levator advancement.

○ **What is a likely cause of chronic lower lid deformity following ORIF of the orbital floor?**

Posterior lamella shortening; posterior lamella (capsulopalpebral fascia) comprising tarsus, lower lid retractors, conjunctiva.

○ **What is done for nasolacrimal duct obstruction?**

Dacryocystorhinostomy.

○ **What predisposing factors cause patients to have dry eye syndrome after blepharoplasty?**

Exophthalmos, scleral show, lower lid hypotonia, maxillary hypoplasia.

○ **What is blepharochalasis?**

Recurrent episodes of painless edema of the eyelids; unclear etiology; caused by elastic tissue deficiency; leading to "baggy" appearance of lids.

○ **What is dermatochalasis?**

Excess eyelid skin.

○ **What is the blepharophimosis syndrome?**

Genetic condition; telecanthus, ptosis, upper eyelid phimosis.

○ **What is the most common form of acquired ptosis?**

Involutional; results from thinning of the levator aponeurosis; good levator function, elevated eyelid creases.

○ **What characterizes blepharophimosis syndrome?**

Type I: large epicanthal folds, epicanthus inversus, horizontal shortening of the eyelids, marked ptosis.

Type II: telecanthus, epicanthal fold absence, bilateral ptosis, no levator function, shortened eyelids.

Type III: missing epicanthal folds, telecanthus, antimongoloid slant; telecanthus.

○ **What treatment is done for blepharophimosis?**

Epicanthal fold repair, levator resection, medial canthoplasty, eyelid suspension.

○ **What defines normal levator function?**

Greater than 10 mm of excursion.

○ **What degree of ptosis is the Fasanella–Servat procedure performed for?**

Mild ptosis.

○ **What is given for ptosis seen in Horner syndrome?**

Phenylephrine eye drops.

○ **What is the treatment of choice 14 days after blepharoplasty in a patient with lagophthalmos?**

Corneal lubrication.

○ **What structure are the upper eyelid fat pads immediately posterior to?**

The orbital septum; the fat pads sit just anterior to the levator aponeurosis.

○ **In the lower lids the fat pads are located just anterior to what structure?**

The inferior retractors.

○ **What separates the medial and middle fat pads in the lower lid?**

The inferior oblique.

○ **What is an epiblepharon?**

A congenital anomaly in which a fold of skin lies across the upper or lower lid margin. In the lower eyelid it causes a turning inward of the eyelashes.

○ **What is senile ptosis?**

Most common cause of ptosis in elderly patients, the result of dehiscence of the levator aponeurosis. The supratarsal crease is elevated on examination.

○ **How do you measure the prominence of the globe in relation to the orbit?**

Distance from anterior border of globe to most anterior aspect of the lateral orbital rim. Enophthalmos is <14 mm, exophthalmos is >18 mm.

○ **What happens to the lacrimal drainage system on eyelid closure?**

Lacrimal puncta are closed, the lacrimal diaphragm is compressed, the lacrimal sac opens.

○ **What is the appropriate amount of pretarsal eyelid show?**

2 to 5 mm.

○ **What is symblepharon?**

Pathologic adhesion of the palpebral conjunctiva to the bulbar conjunctiva, usually related to thermal injury.

○ **What is chemosis?**

Edema of the bulbar conjunctiva.

○ **What is a chalazion?**

A cyst on the eyelid caused by inflammation from a blocked meibomian gland.

○ **What is a hordeolum?**

Also known as a sty, it is an infection of the sebaceous glands at the base of the eyelashes. Unlike a chalazion, these are acute, painful and usually do not resolve without intervention.

○ **What is the function of the inferior oblique muscle? Superior oblique muscle?**

Inferior oblique: abducts, elevates, laterally rotates; superior oblique: abducts, depresses, medially rotates.

○ **What is the most commonly injured muscle during blepharoplasty?**

Inferior oblique muscle. Presents as diplopia with upward gaze.

○ **What muscle acts as the primary depressor of the lateral eyebrow?**

Orbicularis oculi muscle.

Face

○ **What type of genioplasty should be performed in a patient with sagittal deficiency and vertical excess with class I occlusion?**

Jumping genioplasty.

○ **Where should the brow peak in a female patient undergoing browlifting?**

At the lateral limbus to lateral canthal area.

○ **What branch of the facial nerve is injured most frequently during face lift?**

Buccal.

○ **What effect do corticosteroids have on edema and ecchymosis following rhytidectomy?**

No change in both instances.

○ **Compared with primary rhytidectomy, distortion of the hairline is more or less frequent in secondary rhytidectomy?**

More likely to occur; if the same incisions are used, recession of the temporal hairline, obliteration of sideburn hair, and alopecia may occur.

○ **Are the risks of hematoma, hypertrophic scarring, and skin slough higher in the setting of secondary rhytidectomy?**

Typically not.

○ **What adverse effect is lessened by endoscopic browlifting as opposed to conventional coronal browlifting?**

Scalp sensibility changes.

○ **In a patient with microgenia who has both bony deficiencies in the anteroposterior and vertical dimensions, what is the most appropriate treatment?**

Osseous genioplasty.

○ **How well does chin implantation correct vertical deficiency of the chin?**

It only corrects anteroposterior dimension.

○ **Transverse rhytids along the root of the nose are from which muscle group?**

Procerus (originates from upper lateral cartilage inserting into skin/glabella).

○ **What is the origin/insertion of the corrugator?**

Originate along periosteum/medial orbital rim inserting into dermis of upper eyelid.

○ **Following a face lift, an inability to raise the upper lip on one side is due to what complication?**

Injury to the buccal branch of the facial nerve (innervates levator labii oris).

○ **What does injury to the cervical branch of the facial nerve manifest as?**

Platysmal weakening, or an asymmetric smile.

○ **What must be evaluated first during a consult for chin implantation?**

The patient's occlusion.

○ **Fullness of the lateral orbit noted during browlift may be due to what structure?**

A ptotic lacrimal gland.

○ **What is the treatment of a ptotic lacrimal gland?**

Suspension of the gland, not resection.

○ **What approach is used for browlift in a 60-year-old woman with a high hairline with brow descent under the level of the supraorbital rim?**

Open browlift through a hairline incision.

○ **What may cause resorption of the malar fat pad following rhytidectomy?**

Disruption of the branches of the angular artery; significant in malar fat pad advancement greater than 2 cm.

○ **What is the treatment for bone resorption following chin implantation with chin asymmetry?**

Implant removal, bone graft, and sliding genioplasty.

○ **What is the treatment of an obtuse cervicomental angle, marked fat pads in anterior neck, subcutaneous banding, and loose redundant skin in the neck?**

Removal of cervical fat and platysmaplasty.

○ **What is the relation of the temporal branch of the facial nerve to the superficial temporal fascia above the zygomatic arch?**

Deep to the superficial temporal fascia.

○ **What is the most frequent rhytidectomy complication?**

Hematoma (0.3–8.1%).

○ **What are risk factors for hematoma following rhytidectomy?**

Male patients and hypertension.

○ **What vascular supply are the temporal scalp flap and Washio flap based on?**

Posterior temporal branch of the superficial temporal artery.

○ **What does the deep branch of the supraorbital nerve innervate?**

Central frontoparietal scalp.

○ **What does the superficial branch of the supraorbital nerve innervate?**

Central forehead and hairline.

○ **What supplies sensation to the temporal forehead?**

V2 and V3.

○ **What supplies sensation to the temporal scalp?**

The occipital nerve.

○ **What is the most worrisome component of a secondary rhytidectomy regarding postoperative complications?**

Hairline distortion.

○ **How does the vascular supply of the skin flap compare in a secondary rhytidectomy?**

Usually good or better due to the delay factor following the primary procedure; skin slough is less frequent.

○ **What is the mechanism of outward pseudoherniation of the buccal fat pad?**
Buccopharyngeal membrane attenuation.

○ **What is the natural progression of Bell palsy?**
85% have recovery spontaneously within 3 weeks.

○ **What is the description of the mandible in Pierre Robin sequence?**
Retrognathia; normal mandibular dimensions.

○ **What defines microgenia?**
Maldevelopment of the mental symphysis.

○ **What is the likely cause of increased show of the lower incisors following genioplasty?**
Inadequate repair of the mentalis muscle on closure; lower lip drifts downward with healing.

○ **What muscle supplies blood to the anterior bony segment following a horizontal genioplasty?**
The anterior digastric.

○ **What are the zones of the malar region?**
Zone I: First third of the zygomatic arch and malar bone.
Zone II: Middle third of the zygomatic arch.
Zone III: Paranasal.
Zone IV: Posterior third of the zygomatic arch.
Zone V: Submalar region.

○ **What is the largest zone?**
Zone I.

○ **Which malar zones are rarely augmented in aesthetic surgery?**
Zone III and zone IV.

○ **What is the appearance with zone V malar augmentation?**
Midface fullness, rounded appearance of the cheeks.

○ **What is the management of an anterior platysmal band?**
Plication in the midline.

○ **What is the most important factor in facial reanimation following trauma?**
Length of time between injury and reconstruction; facial muscles are viable for 2 years following paralysis; after 2 years, free muscle transfer is required.

○ **What is the appropriate amount of tooth show in repose?**

2-mm upper incisor show (may be 4 mm in women). Lower incisors should not show in repose.

○ **What is the most commonly injured nerve during rhytidectomy?**

Great auricular nerve.

○ **What is the MACS lift?**

Minimal access cranial suspension. A short scar rhytidectomy technique in which the SMAS is purse-string sutured to the deep temporal fascia above the zygomatic arch using a vertical vector.

Body Contouring

○ **When do serum lidocaine concentrations peak postoperatively?**

Approximately 12 hours.

○ **How do you increase graft survival in autologous fat grafting?**

Maximize surface area contact between fat graft and vascularized bed. Minimize the amount of fat injected per pass.

○ **What is the safe dose of lidocaine when used in tumescent solution for liposuction?**

35 mg/kg.

○ **What diagnosis should be considered with disorientation after massive weight loss surgery?**

Wernicke–Korsakoff encephalopathy from thiamine deficiency, which can be present from malnutrition of massive weight loss. Treat with intravenous thiamine.

○ **What cosmetic procedure is associated with the highest incidence of venous thromboembolic events (VTE)?**

Abdominoplasty.

○ **What is the most common complication of brachioplasty?**

Hypertrophic scarring in as many as 40% of patients.

○ **Numbness of the anterolateral thigh after abdominoplasty is due to what complication?**

Injury to the lateral femoral cutaneous nerve (becomes superficial 10 cm below the anterior superior iliac spine).

○ **What is the course of the lateral femoral cutaneous nerve?**

Arises from L2–3, passes 1 cm medial to the ASIS, superficial to the sartorius, and branches anteriorly and posteriorly.

○ **What does the genitofemoral nerve innervate?**

Sensation to skin of scrotum, mons pubis, labia, and over the superior portion of the femoral triangle.

○ **What does the iliohypogastric supply?**

Sensation to the skin of the lateral buttocks and abdomen above the pubis.

○ **What does the ilioinguinal nerve supply?**

Sensation to the superomedial thigh and scrotum or mons pubis.

○ **The obturator nerve?**

Skin of the medial and lower thigh.

○ **With tumescence during suction lipectomy, what percentage of total blood loss is to be expected of the total aspirate?**

1%.

○ **The wet technique?**

This technique utilizes 300 mL of fluid per region—25% blood in the aspirate.

○ **Complications from smoking arise in what percentage of patients undergoing abdominoplasty?**

50%.

○ **In addition to contour irregularities, UAL is likely to cause what complication more frequently than SAL?**

Thermal injury.

○ **A 1:1 infiltrate to aspirate ratio during liposuction indicates which technique?**

Superwet.

○ **What defines tumescent technique during liposuction?**

2 to 3 cc wetting solution/1 cc of aspirate.

○ **What is the wet technique?**

Injecting 100 to 300 cc of wetting solution per area regardless of the amount of aspirate removed.

○ **What specific technique has been shown to decrease the recurrence rate in thigh lifts?**

Superficial fascial system suspension; anchoring skin flap to Colles fascia.

○ **What is the most likely cause of death following liposuction?**

Thromboembolism; followed by abdominal wall perforation, anesthetic complication, infection.

○ **In a patient returning several days after liposuction with clear gray fluid from incisions, erythema, and early sepsis, what is the most appropriate management?**

Surgical debridement of involved tissues. Necrotizing fasciitis is a rapidly progressive soft-tissue infection that occurs in 0.4 per 100,000 patients following liposuction.

○ **What is the most frequent chronic complication following brachioplasty?**

Scar widening.

○ **What surrounding nerves are at risk during abdominoplasty?**

Ilioinguinal, iliohypogastric, and intercostals.

○ **What procedure is appropriate for a 33-year-old patient who has lost 140 lb after a gastric bypass?**

Lower body lift.

○ **What procedure is appropriate for a 40-year-old patient with good skin tone and muscle tone with a localized area of excess fat?**

Suction lipectomy.

○ **Is the umbilicus altered in mini abdominoplasty?**

No.

○ **What area of the incision is most at risk for necrosis after abdominoplasty?**

Area of the suprapubic region; lower midline flap is most at risk for ischemia.

○ **Skin laxity of the arms following massive weight loss is due to laxity of what structure?**

The clavipectoral fascia.

○ **What is the most frequent complication of abdominoplasty combined with liposuction?**

Seroma formation.

○ **What normally supplies the umbilical skin?**

Vessels from the deep inferior epigastric arteries, ligamentum teres, and the medial umbilical ligament.

○ **What is the likely cause of a supraumbilical bulge after abdominoplasty?**

Not placating the rectus muscle.

Skin/Lasers

○ **What type of basal cell carcinoma (BCC) requires additional excision by Mohs technique?**

Morpheaform; also known as sclerosing BCC.

○ **True/False: Suction lipectomy may be an effective procedure for the management of axillary hyperhidrosis, HIV-associated lipodystrophy, lymphedema, and Madelung disease.**

True.

○ **What is Madelung disease?**

Benign symmetric lipomatosis; diffuse growth of nonencapsulated lipomas, in neck, shoulders, posterior trunk.

○ **What nerve is typically involved in Frey syndrome?**

Auriculotemporal nerve, a branch of V.

○ **What is the nerve of Jacobson?**

The tympanic branch of IX, which provides sensation to the tympanic cavity.

○ **What is the mechanism of greater dermal injury with the CO₂ laser as compared with the Er:YAG laser?**

The Er:YAG laser has an affinity for water that is 10× greater; also, the pulse rate is shorter than that of the CO_2 laser.

○ **A painful vesicular rash in the days following CO₂ laser treatment of facial rhytids is best treated by what method?**

Acyclovir (prophylactic treatment is important).

○ **Is isotretinoin used for premedicating laser patients?**

No; Accutane is contraindicated.

○ **What is the most common complication following 30% TCA peeling?**

Hyperpigmentation.

○ **What complication is associated with phenol peeling?**

Cardiac arrhythmias.

○ **With laser treatments?**

HSV reactivation.

○ **What agent is typically used in rejuvenating fine facial rhytids?**

TCA (15–35%).

○ **What patients should Botox not be injected into?**

Egg/albumin sensitivity.

○ **What agents are administered before dermabrasion to prevent hyperpigmentation?**

Hydroquinones.

○ **Is tretinoin or isotretinoin used for skin preparation before dermabrasion?**

Tretinoin; isotretinoin (Accutane) is contraindicated for 1 year before laser or dermabrasion due to risk of scarring and delayed healing.

○ **What is the mechanism of Botox?**

Prevents acetylcholine uptake.

○ **What is the latency period and duration of effect of Botox?**

Onset beginning 3 to 7 days and lasting for 4 to 6 months.

○ **What is pachydermoperiostosis?**

Genetic syndrome resulting in enlarged hands, feet, eyelids, and toes.

○ **What is the mechanism of retinoids in regard to the skin?**

Decreased activity of metalloproteases from AP1 transcription inhibition.

○ **What is the mechanism of tretinoin?**

Thinning the stratum corneum, epidermal thickening, atypia reversal, increased collagen synthesis.

○ **What is the mechanism of topical vitamin C?**

Decreased free radical effects of UVB and increased collagen production.

○ **What is the mechanism of alpha hydroxy acids?**

Increased desquamation from decreased corneocyte adhesion.

○ **What is the mechanism of hydroquinones?**

Block conversion of dopamine to melanin; blocking tyrosinase.

○ **What level of dermis is dermabrasion performed at?**

Down to the upper third of the dermis.

○ **What treatment is recommended for ice-pick acne scars?**
Excision.

○ **What skin layer are hair follicles found at?**

The subcutaneous level.

○ **What treatment relieves burning and itching associated with keloids?**

Intralesional injection of steroid.

○ **What lasers are used for blue-green tattoos?**

Q-switched Nd:YAG and alexandrite lasers.

○ **What colors is the Nd:YAG laser used for?**

Red, brown, and orange.

○ **What is the Q-switched ruby laser used for?**

Tattoos with purple and violet pigments.

○ **What are features of Gorlin syndrome?**
Nevoid BCC syndrome; AD; multiple BCCs; mandibular cysts; intracranial calcifications.

○ **The stratification of Fitzpatrick skin types is important for what?**
Risk of pigmentary changes following chemical peeling.

○ **What Fitzpatrick skin types are at risk for pigmentary changes after chemical peel?**
4, 5, and 6.

○ **What physiologic changes with collagen are seen with application of tretinoin for periorbital rhytids?**
Increased type III collagen over 6 to 12 months; up to 80% increase in collagen.

○ **What changes are seen in the skin with tretinoin therapy?**
Thickened dermis; skin elasticity improves.

○ **What is the best treatment for multiple actinic keratoses of the face?**
Topical 5-fluorouracil (5-FU) treatment.

○ **What is the most common infection following facial laser resurfacing?**
Reactivation of latent herpes simplex virus. Treat with antivirals (e.g., acyclovir).

○ **What is the difference between botulinum toxin type A (BOTOX Cosmetic) and botulinum toxin type B (Myobloc)?**
Lower pH results in greater pain with injection, shorter duration of action, quicker onset of action, greater diffusion area.

○ **What test should be performed prior to the use of bovine collagen fillers?**
Skin test to assess for allergic reaction.

● ● ● **CRANIOFACIAL** ● ● ●

○ **What is the only facial muscle to compress the cheek?**
Buccinator.

○ **True/False: The metopic suture usually fuses before 1 year of age?**
True.

○ **What common medication can contribute to osteonecrosis of the mandible?**
Bisphosphonate therapy, often used to treat osteoporosis and as chemotherapy to treat bone metastases.

○ **A patient with a prior cleft lip and palate undergoes Le Fort I advancement for maxillary hypoplasia, what postoperative complication is he or she at higher risk for?**

Velopharyngeal incompetence.

○ **Patient with partial tongue numbness after third molar removal. Diagnosis?**

Injury to the lingual nerve, which provides sensation to the anterior two-thirds of the tongue.

○ **What is the sensory nerve supply to the tongue?**

Lingual nerve: general sensation to anterior two-thirds. Chorda tympani (CN VII): taste to anterior two-thirds. Glossopharyngeal nerve: taste and sensation to posterior one-third.

○ **How do you treat a small salivary leak presenting 10 days after pharyngeal reconstruction?**

Conservatively with local wound care.

○ **What is the "coup de sabre" deformity?**

Frontal linear scleroderma, an acquired condition presenting as a linear band of atrophy and a furrow in the skin on the frontal or frontoparietal scalp.

○ **What imaging study should be obtained on patients with progressive hemifacial atrophy (Parry–Romberg syndrome)?**

Brain MRI.

○ **Progressive hemifacial atrophy follows the distribution of branches of what nerve?**

Trigeminal nerve (CN V).

○ **A mother and first child have a cleft lip and palate, what is the risk that the next child will have the deformity?**

14%.

○ **What is the ideal free flap for a hemiglossectomy defect?**

Radial forearm free flap.

○ **Where should the medial canthus be reattached in relation to the lacrimal fossa?**

Posterior and superior to the posterior crest of the lacrimal fossa.

○ **What is the treatment for proptosis, increased intraocular pressure, and decreased visual acuity after trauma?**

Lateral canthotomy and cantholysis (within 90 minutes!).

○ **In Bell palsy, paralysis of what structure results in hypersensitivity to sound? Changes in taste?**

Stapedius muscle dampens sound. Chorda tympani provides taste to anterior two-thirds of tongue.

○ **What nerve innervates the tensor tympani and tensor veli palatine muscles?**

Trigeminal nerve.

○ **What nerve innervates the levator palatine muscle?**

Vagus nerve.

○ **What is the initial treatment of cutaneous angiosarcoma?**

Surgical excision with wide margins.

○ **What type of bone graft can result in overgrowth when used in the pediatric temporomandibular joint reconstruction?**

Rib graft due to the presence of a cartilaginous cap.

○ **What joint type best describes the temporomandibular joint?**

Hinge-sliding (ginglymoarthrodial).

○ **What is Cobb syndrome?**

A rare congenital disorder characterized by visible skin lesions with underlying spinal angiomas or AVMs.

○ **What is nevus flammeus neonatorum?**

A lesion that is present at birth, usually in the upper face and posterior neck, but disappears or fades by 1 year of age.

○ **What is the most appropriate flap for nasal lining in a large full-thickness nasal sidewall defect? What is the blood supply?**

Mucoperichondrial flap; anterior ethmoidal artery.

○ **Which tooth root is longest?**

Canine, approximately 30 mm.

○ **In treatment of oral cancer, how do you decide whether to do a marginal mandibulectomy or a segmental mandibulectomy?**

If the tumor abuts the mandible, marginal mandibulectomy (removal of the alveolar process) is an option. If the tumor invades bone, segmental mandibulectomy is indicated.

○ **At what point during ear reconstruction should a bone-anchored hearing aid be placed?**

After completion of ear reconstruction because it is placed in the mastoid region that may be used during ear reconstruction.

○ **What is Möbius syndrome?**

Congenital disorder characterized by facial weakness combined with abnormal ocular abduction (weakness of CN VI and CN VII). Limb abnormalities are also common.

○ **A teenager presents with a facial mass that has been gradually enlarging since birth, MRI shows a high vascular flow. Diagnosis?**

Arteriovenous malformation.

○ **What is the diagnosis in a patient with a clicking sensation on jaw opening?**

Subluxation of the articular disk of the TMJ joint.

○ **What is a thyroglossal duct cyst?**

A remnant of the thyroglossal duct that forms anywhere along the course of the embryologic migration of the thyroid gland from the base of the tongue to the anterior midline neck.

○ **What is the most common congenital nasal mass?**

Dermoid cyst.

○ **A pediatric patient presents with a midline nasal mass, what is the next step?**

Imaging study to rule out intracranial communication, which is often suggested by broadening of the nasal root or increased intercanthal distance.

○ **What is a pilomatrixoma?**

A rare, benign superficial skin neoplasm originating from the hair matrix cells.

○ **What is the most appropriate surgical approach to a patient with a defect compromising 75% of the central upper lip?**

Bilateral Karapandzic flaps with a central Abbe flap.

○ **A free gracilis transfer is planned for facial reanimation, the vector of pull should mimic which muscle of facial expression?**

Zygomaticus major.

○ **What is the lifetime risk of a malignant peripheral nerve sheath tumor in patients with neurofibromatosis type 1?**

Approximately 10%, usually arising from a pre-existing neurofibroma.

○ **After a facial nerve laceration, how long can the distal end of the nerve be successfully stimulated?**

Approximately 72 hours, after which the neurotransmitter stores are depleted.

○ **What is a branchial cleft fistula?**

Embryologic remnant of the cleft between the second and third branchial arches, usually located at the anterior border of the lower sternocleidomastoid muscle.

○ **What nerve is at risk when excising a branchial cleft fistula?**

Hypoglossal nerve (CN XII). The fistula follows the carotid sheath superiorly and crosses the hypoglossal nerve.

○ **What is the treatment for osteoradionecrosis of the mandible associated with a pathologic fracture?**
Segmental resection and free tissue transfer.

○ **What is the landmark for mental nerve block?**
The mandibular second premolar.

○ **What is the landmark to locate the opening of Stensen duct?**
The maxillary second molar.

○ **What is the landmark for the location of the inferior alveolar nerve?**
The sigmoid notch.

○ **What findings are consistent with vertical maxillary excess (long face syndrome)?**
Gummy smile, long obtuse nasolabial angle, class II angle classification, obtuse nasolabial angle, lip incompetence, show of upper incisors with lips in repose; mentalis muscle strain.

○ **What is appearance of the chin in vertical excess syndrome?**
Chin is retruded; mandible appears retrognathic.

○ **What defines a "gummy" smile?**
Greater than 4 mm of incisor show at rest and greater than 2 mm with active movement.

○ **What is the lip-to-tooth relationship in long face syndrome?**
Lip-to-tooth relationship greater than 3 mm.

○ **What differentiates mandibular deficiency from vertical maxillary excess?**
SNB angle decreased with mandibular deficiency.

○ **What are the characteristics of mandibular excess?**
Wide lower third of face, prominent lower lip, anterior crossbite, class III angle classification, increased SNB angle.

○ **What are the characteristics of vertical maxillary deficiency (short face syndrome)?**
Decreased facial height, absence of maxillary show with edentulous look, protruding chin, wide alar bases, class III angle, normal or greater SNB.

○ **In patients younger than 2 years, when should mandibular distraction osteogenesis be performed?**
When there is tongue-based airway compromise secondary to mandibular hypoplasia that pulls the mandible forward relieving airway obstruction.

○ **Why should children younger than 2 years with only selected congenital hypoplasia or aplasia of only selected portions of the mandible not undergo distraction osteogenesis?**
Risk for permanent dental injury in patients who do not have airway compromise.

○ **How reliably does distraction osteogenesis improve patients with laryngomalacia or tracheomalacia?**

It will not reliably improve airway obstruction.

○ **At what time is distraction osteogenesis initiated in patients with hemifacial microsomia?**

Older than 1 year.

○ **What is the treatment of patients with an acute open lock deformity of the mandible?**

Attempted closed reduction under sedation in the ED.

○ **What is the deformity in open lock deformity?**

Condyle slips into position anterior to the articular eminence.

○ **What is the treatment of a teenaged girl with RA and mandibular retrusion and anterior open bite?**

Maxillary impaction (to close the open-bite deformity), advancement genioplasty.

○ **A 35-year-old man sustains nasal trauma resulting in a localized purplish mass on the left side of the septum—what is the next step in management?**

Immediate incision and drainage of the septal mass.

○ **What is a long-term sequelae of septal hematoma?**

Septal perforation leading to saddle nose deformity.

○ **Application of an arch bar to the maxillary alveolus requires anesthesia of which nerves?**

Nasopalatine and anterior superior alveolar.

○ **What nerve trunk does the nasopalatine nerve originate from?**

V2.

○ **Which nerve provides sensation to the posterior palate?**

Greater palatine nerve.

○ **Following resection of a pleomorphic adenoma, a recurrent multinodular tumor requires what type of therapy next?**

XRT.

○ **In patients sustaining bilateral parasymphysial fractures, which muscle exerts a distractive force on the anterior fracture segment?**

The geniohyoid.

○ **What is the function of the geniohyoid muscle?**

To depress and retract the mandible.

○ **What is the function of the posterior belly of the digastric muscle?**

Elevates the hyoid, has only a secondary effect on the anterior mandible.

○ **Which Tessier cleft has displacement of the medial canthus of the eyelid?**

No. 3 cleft is characteristic of having a medially displaced medial canthus; also referred to as a naso-ocular cleft (inferomedial wall is absent); nose is shortened, colobomas, NLD obstruction.

○ **What are the characteristics of a No. 1 cleft?**

Just lateral to midline, begins at Cupid bow and passes through dome of nostril; notching of alar dome; nasal bone may be absent; septum unaffected; hypertelorism and encephalocele may be associated.

○ **A No. 4 cleft?**

Passes between the piriform aperture and infraorbital foramen, begins lateral to Cupid bow and philtrum, passes lateral to the nasal ala onto cheek, terminates in lower eyelid, medial canthal tendon unaffected.

○ **A No. 5 cleft?**

Begins behind canine and extends through maxillary sinus to orbital floor; colobomas of lateral lower lids and clefting of upper lip medial to oral commissure associated.

○ **Which cleft is the incomplete form of Treacher Collins syndrome?**

No. 6; passes inferior and lateral to the oral commissure, toward angle of mandible; colobomas of lateral lower eyelids; downward slant of palpebral fissures.

○ **Which is the most common atypical cleft?**

No. 7; 1 per 3,000 births; absent zygomatic arch.

○ **Where does a No. 8 cleft extend?**

From lateral commissure of palpebral fissure to temporal region; colobomas of lower eyelids also seen.

○ **Which cleft is the supraorbital extension of the No. 5 cleft?**

No. 9.

○ **A patient sustaining a frontal sinus fracture in an MVA with CSF rhinorrhea and displacement of anterior/posterior sinus walls and injured nasofrontal ducts requires what operation?**

Cranialization of the frontal sinus in conjunction with neurosurgery.

○ **What are the steps in cranialization?**

Bifrontal craniotomy to repair dura, removal of posterior wall of frontal sinus and associated mucosa; occlusion of nasofrontal duct with a pericranial flap or fat; burring down sharp edges; allowing the brain to expand into this new potential space.

○ **Frontal sinus exenteration involves what?**

Removal of the anterior table of the frontal sinus only.

○ **What is involved in frontal sinus obliteration?**

Removing all the mucosa within the frontal sinus; allowing the nasofrontal duct to occlude.

○ **Which muscles produce side-to-side grinding motions of the mandible?**

Medial and lateral pterygoid; rotation occurs around the vertical axis of the contralateral condyle.

○ **What is the origin/insertion of the medial pterygoid? How does it function?**

Originates from the medial surface of the lateral pterygoid plate and tuberosity of maxilla and inserts into the medial surface of the mandibular angle/ramus; elevates and pulls mandible medially.

○ **What is the origin/insertion of the lateral pterygoid? Its function?**

Originates from the lateral surface of the lateral pterygoid plate (inferior head) and infratemporal surface of the greater wing of the sphenoid (superior head) and inserts into the mandibular condylar neck (inferior head) and articular disk of TMJ (superior head); protrudes the mandible forward and opens mouth.

○ **Simultaneous action of all four pterygoid muscles results in what motion of the mandible?**

Protrusion of the mandible.

○ **Where does the masseter originate/insert?**

Originates from zygomatic arch; inserts onto ramus.

○ **Where does the temporalis muscle insert?**

Originates from the temporal fossa and attaches to the coronoid process of the mandible; primarily elevates mandible, but also can retract mandible.

○ **Following a bilateral cleft lip repair, tightness of the upper lip with a wide hypoplastic philtrum with the absence of muscle competence and redundant lower lip may be treated with what kind of flap?**

Abbe flap (to create a functional philtrum in patients with tightness of the upper lip following cleft lip repair).

○ **What are the dimensions of a reconstructed philtrum in the adult?**

No wider than 10 mm and no longer than 15 mm.

○ **What is the incidence of concomitant cervical spine injury with a mandibular fracture?**

10%.

○ **In a patient with VPI with central velopharyngeal closure and poor lateral wall motion, what procedure is indicated?**

Sphincter pharyngoplasty.

○ **What muscle is transposed in sphincter pharyngoplasty?**

Palatopharyngeus (incorporated into the posterior pharyngeal wall to create a sphincter).

○ **When is a pharyngeal flap indicated?**

Correction of deficits of the central palate with good lateral wall motion; the levator veli palatini is used as well in the palate for attachment of the posterior wall flap.

○ **Where is the tensor veli palatini muscle located relative to the levator veli palatini?**

The TVP is anterior to the LVP.

○ **Where are the palatoglossus muscles located—in the anterior or posterior tonsillar pillar?**

Anterior.

○ **A neonate with a 1.5-cm reddish mass adjacent to the nasal root with overlying telangiectasias that is firm, not compressible and nonpulsatile is most likely what type of mass?**

Glioma (rarely with bony defects, intracranial connections).

○ **What embryonic tissue derives nasal dermoids?**

Mesoderm and ectoderm (hair follicles, sebaceous glands, smooth muscle).

○ **What external nasal lesions transilluminate and are compressible?**

Encephaloceles (external, or sincipital) are soft, bluish, compressible, and pulsatile lesions that transilluminate; Furstenberg sign.

○ **What nerve innervates the oral commissures bilaterally?**

Buccal nerve, a branch of V3.

○ **What causes a 10-month-old boy to tilt his head to the right who also has an uncorrected left coronal synostosis?**

Paresis of the ipsilateral superior oblique muscle (foreshortening of the orbital roof on the affected side; relative paresis of superior oblique occurs).

○ **In surgically correcting the patient with NOE fracture, what is the most appropriate management of the lacrimal system?**

Observation; generally low incidence of duct injury in patients undergoing ORIF without overlying lacerations.

○ **How does one evaluate persistent epiphora following surgery for an NOE fracture?**

Dacryocystography; followed by a DCR if required for treatment.

○ **What muscle courses around the pterygoid hamulus?**

The tensor veli palatini.

○ **Where does the levator veli palatini run relative to the hamulus?**

It passes posterior to the hamulus creating a muscular sling.

○ **A complete unilateral cleft lip is associated with what type of movement of the ala?**

Lateral, inferior, and posterior (the piriform rim is also deficient, which also supports the ala).

○ **Treacher Collins syndrome involves which Tessier cleft(s)?**

No. 6, 7, and 8 clefts.

○ **What is the class occlusion seen in Treacher Collins?**

Class II.

○ **What are the characteristics of the maxilla, palate, and mandible in Treacher Collins?**

Maxilla protrudes, palatal plane is moved upward and posteriorly; micrognathia, decreased length of the ramus and body; hypoplastic or absent condyle; cleft in the inferolateral orbital floor also occurs; hypoplastic zygoma, maxilla, and mandible.

○ **What type of synostosis is seen in Crouzon?**

Bilateral coronal synostosis (acrocephalosyndactyly) forehead and superior orbital rim retrusion, proptosis, midface hypoplasia.

○ **What type of occlusion is seen in Crouzon?**

Angle type III.

○ **What abnormalities are seen in Goldenhar?**

Oculoauriculovertebral dysplasia; subset of hemifacial microsomia, epibulbar dermoids and scapula/spine anomalies seen; may be bilateral; resemble a No. 7 cleft; mandibular hypoplasia.

○ **What is Romberg syndrome?**

Progressive hemifacial atrophy, appears initially as cutaneous pigmentation and progresses to destruction of facial soft tissues and skeleton.

○ **What are the zones of distraction osteogenesis?**

Fibrous zone (central region of the distraction gap); transitional zone (adjacent to the fibrous zone, contains fibrous tissue undergoing ossification); zone of remodeling bone (surrounded by zone of mature bone).

○ **What nerve supplies sensation to the buccal mucosa?**

The trigeminal nerve (V).

○ **What are the clinical findings of a unilateral condylar fracture?**

Upward cant of mandible to the fractured side, early contact of molars on ipsilateral side; contralateral lateral open bite.

○ **What are the clinical findings of a bilateral condylar fracture?**

Anterior open-bite secondary to loss of posterior vertical height.

○ **What is the malocclusion seen in a 6-year-old who has undergone a unilateral cleft lip/palate previously with an unrepaired alveolar cleft?**

Posterior crossbite (an unrepaired alveolar cleft causes maxillary arch collapse, the arch will be deficient in the A-P, transverse, and vertical directions.

○ **What is the clinical appearance of a posterior crossbite?**

Lower dentition is labial to the upper dentition.

○ **What is the definition of Angle class I?**

The mesiobuccal cusp of the first maxillary molar sits in the buccal groove of the first mandibular molar.

○ **Define overbite and overjet.**

Overbite describes the distance between the mandibular and maxillary incisors in the vertical plane; overjet describes the distance between the incisors in the horizontal plane.

○ **What direction does the central mandibular segment move in a patient sustaining bilateral vertically and horizontally unfavorable fractures adjacent to the canine roots?**

Downward and posterior (actions of the digastric and geniohyoid/genioglossus).

○ **What points of fixation are required in patients with zygomaticomaxillary complex fractures?**

Z-F suture, inferior orbital rim, and zygomaticomaxillary buttress.

○ **What is the most common type of nonsyndromic single-suture craniosynostosis?**

Sagittal (50% of patients with single-suture fusions); elongated skull with frontal/occipital bossing.

○ **What is turribrachycephaly?**

Shortened, wide skull with increased vertical height at top of skull; from bilateral coronal synostosis.

○ **How common is lambdoid suture fusion?**

Extremely rare, in 1% to 2% in patients with craniosynostosis.

○ **What is trigonocephaly?**

Metopic suture fusion; leaves a prominent midline ridge in forehead; occurs in 10% of all single-suture fusions; triangularly shaped forehead.

○ **How often does single-suture squamosal synostosis occur?**

Isolated fusion does not occur.

○ **What areas are affected in auriculotemporal nerve paresis during superficial parotidectomy?**

Numbness of tragus, EAC, tympanum, and temporal skin; fibers also go to the parotid gland as secretomotor fibers and articular fibers to the TMJ.

○ **What branch is the auriculotemporal nerve from?**

V3, mandibular division of V.

○ **What nerve innervates the concha? The antihelix?**

Auricular branch of X.

○ **What areas are supplied by the great auricular nerve? The lesser occipital nerve?**

Both these nerves are derived from C2 to C3; the areas supplied are the helix and lobule.

○ **What procedure is most appropriate for a 15 year old with Apert in need of 25 mm of midface advancement?**

Le Fort III with distraction osteogenesis for advancement; distraction osteogenesis preferred over bone grafting for greater than 10 mm.

○ **In an infant with hemifacial microsomia, should macrostomia or deficiencies of the mandibular ramus/body be corrected first?**

Macrostomia; hemifacial microsomia associated with first and second branchial arch anomalies and Tessier No. 7 cleft.

○ **What nerve passes through the foramen ovale?**

V3.

○ **Where does V1 pass through?**

The superior orbital fissure.

○ **What nerve passes through the foramen rotundum?**

V2.

○ **What is the most likely diagnosis of a patient with a painless mass at the angle of the mandible for the past 10 years with a biopsy showing luminal ductal cells mixed with sheets of myoepithelial cells?**

A pleomorphic adenoma; most common benign tumor of the parotid; contains two populations of cells (epithelial and mesenchymal cells).

○ **How does a myoepithelioma of the parotid differ from a pleomorphic adenoma?**

More rare, affects parotid or palate, histologically similar but also shows spindle cells.

○ **What parotid tumor has a characteristic of being bilateral?**

Warthin's (papillary cystadenoma lymphomatosum); male smokers; 10% multicentric, 10% bilateral.

○ **What structures arise from the lateral nasal processes?**

The nasal ala.

○ **What structures arise from the medial nasal processes?**

The columella, nasal tip, philtrum, and premaxilla; this occurs during the sixth week of gestation.

○ **What structures arise from the frontonasal processes?**

The bridge and root of the nose.

○ **Which muscle of mastication pulls the mandible upward, medially, and forward?**

The medial pterygoid.

○ **What is the origin/insertion of the anterior digastric muscle? The posterior digastric?**

Originates from the inside lower border of the symphysis and attaches to the lateral corner of the hyoid bone. Posterior belly extends between the hyoid and mastoid.

○ **How does the digastric function in distracting the mandible in the setting of a fracture?**

The digastric pulls the anterior mandibular fragments posteroinferiorly.

○ **What is the function of the mylohyoid?**

Elevates the tongue.

○ **Abnormalities of the corpus callosum is most frequently associated with premature fusion of which cranial suture?**

The metopic suture (trigonocephaly); also associated with higher incidence of developmental delay.

○ **What is the most appropriate initial step in evaluating an infant in respiratory distress with retrogenia and glossoptosis?**

Prone positioning; Pierre Robin sequence occurs with a 50% incidence of high-arched clefts of the soft palate; hard palate clefting also occurs in some patients.

○ **What are alternative treatments if prone positioning does not help the neonate with Pierre Robin sequence?**

Lip–tongue adhesion, tracheostomy, mandibular distraction osteogenesis.

○ **What cranial suture has the greatest incidence of synostosis associated with mutations in the loci for FGF receptors?**

Coronal; in both unilateral and bilateral.

○ **What bony segments are moved together in a Le Fort I osteotomy?**

The entire alveolar process of the maxilla, vault of the palate, pterygoid processes.

○ **What bony segments are included in a Le Fort II?**

A central maxillary segment is undisturbed; also included are portions of the medial orbital walls, orbital floor, and nasofrontal junction.

○ **The external auditory canal develops from which embryologic structure?**

First branchial groove.

○ **Which hillocks does the first branchial arch give rise to?**

The first three hillocks.

○ **What cranial nerve innervates the temporalis muscle?**

V3.

○ **An anterior chamber hemorrhage of the eye is known as what?**

A hyphema.

○ **What defines subconjunctival hemorrhage?**

Bleeding occurring in the bulbar or palpebral conjunctiva; from extravasation of conjunctival capillaries.

○ **What is the most common complication of a sagittal split osteotomy?**

Loss of lower lip sensibility.

○ **Craniofacial microsomia is the most common major craniofacial anomaly—how is it transmitted?**

It does not demonstrate genetic transmission—likely an intrauterine event; for example, hematoma.

○ **How are Apert and Crouzon patients differentiated clinically?**

Apert's patients have severe syndactyly of the middle three digits of the hands and feet; Crouzon patients have normal extremities; both have craniosynostosis, exorbitism, and midface retrusion.

○ **How is Treacher Collins transmitted?**

Autosomal dominant.

○ **What are clinical characteristics of Treacher Collins?**

Facial clefting, antimongoloid slant, colobomas, absence of eyelashes on medial portion of the lower eyelid, preauricular displacement of hair, micrognathia, malar/mandibular defects.

○ **What is the maximum bony defect (in mm) that will not require bone grafting?**

5 mm.

○ **What structures pass through the superior orbital fissure?**

III, IV, V_1, VI, sympathetic nerve fibers.

○ **What is the superior orbital fissure syndrome?**

Fractures that extend to the superior orbital fissure and orbital roof; vision is not affected.

○ **What is orbital apex syndrome?**

Injury to the optic nerve from extension of the fracture into the optic canal; loss of vision.

○ **Prominence of the ear is caused by effacement of what part of the ear?**

Superior crus of the antihelix; conchoscaphal angle is greater than 90 degrees; helix is greater than 12 to 15 mm from the temporal skin.

○ **Prominence of the middle portion of the ear is caused by hypertrophy of what structure?**

Concha cavum; here the concha cavum has a depth of more than 1.5 cm.

○ **What soft-tissue change is most likely seen following Le Fort I advancement?**

Increased nasolabial angle, widened alar base; shortened upper lip, increased incisor show.

○ **How is upper lip shortening prevented during Le Fort I advancement?**

V-Y advancement during closure.

○ **Regarding the chin, lower facial height, labiomental fold, and sagittal deficiency, alloplastic chin augmentation is best recommended in what setting?**

Symmetric chin, normal lower facial height, shallow labiomental fold, minimal sagittal deficiency.

○ **How is velocardiofacial syndrome diagnosed?**

FISH analysis; for deletion of 22q11.2.

○ **What are the components of velocardiofacial syndrome?**

AD; VPI, developmental delay, upward slanting of palpebral fissures, prominent nose with broad nasal root, aberrant carotid arteries; submucous cleft.

○ **Define Angle class I.**

The mesiobuccal cusp of the first maxillary molar fits into the buccal groove of the first mandibular molar.

○ **Define Angle class II, division 1.**

The mesiobuccal cusp of the first maxillary molar is anterior to the buccal groove of the first mandibular molar; division 1: lateral incisors angled labially.

○ **Define Angle class II, division 2.**

Same previous Angle class II but the lateral incisors are angled lingually; retrognathic on appearance.

○ **What are operative indications for TMJ pathology?**

Internal derangement associated with neoplasia, trauma.

○ **What are surgical options for internal derangement?**

Intracapsular repositioning of the disk, excision of the disk, temporalis fascia flap placement.

○ **A decreased SNA and normal SNB indicate what process of the maxilla?**

Maxillary retrusion.

○ **What are normal values of SNA and SNB?**

SNA 82 degrees; SNB 80 degrees.

○ **Normally how much incisor show appears at rest?**

2 to 3 mm.

○ **What muscle causes the medial displacement of the condyle following a fracture?**

Lateral pterygoid.

○ **What is the sequence of repair in a patient with midface fractures and bilateral condylar neck fractures?**

ORIF of condylar neck fractures followed by midface fractures.

○ **What is the most common cause of an open-bite deformity following Le Fort I and bilateral sagittal split osteotomy in a patient?**

Centric relation not equaling centric occlusion, or having the condyles not seated properly in each respective glenoid fossa.

○ **What population of patients does progressive condyle resorption occur in?**

Young women; a late cause of open-bite deformity causing shortening of the condyle and clockwise rotation of the mandible.

○ **What defines vertical maxillary deficiency?**

Decrease in vertical height, absence of maxillary incisor show, short/flat upper lip, protrusive chin, acute mandibular plane.

○ **During pediatric distraction osteogenesis, what techniques optimize bone formation?**

Lower-energy corticotomy (minimizing central medullary bone trauma); less than 5 mm of intraoperative immediate distraction; stable fixator placement.

○ **What passes through the stylomastoid foramen?**

The facial nerve and stylomastoid artery.

○ **What passes through the jugular foramen?**

IX, X, XI, and the internal jugular vein.

○ **What passes through foramen ovale?**

V3 and accessory meningeal artery.

○ **How is scaphocephaly treated?**

Cranial vault remodeling with barrel staving.

○ **What is scaphocephaly?**

Premature closure of the sagittal suture; skull is long, narrow, and characteristically keel shaped.

○ **What procedures are done for unicoronal and bicoronal synostosis?**

Bilateral frontal craniotomy and bilateral fronto-orbital advancement.

○ **The buccal nerve is a branch of which nerve?**

V3; arises from surface of the buccinator. Supplies sensation to medial cheek.

○ **What is the dorsal nasal nerve a branch of?**

Nasociliary nerve, V1.

○ **What is the sensory territory of the infratrochlear nerve?**

The nasal root and medial eyelid.

○ **What is the zygomaticofacial nerve a branch of?**

V2; supplies zygomatic skin and upper portion of central cheek.

○ **What symptoms define Pierre Robin sequence?**

Micrognathia, glossoptosis, respiratory distress, and cleft palate.

○ **What is the initial management of a neonate with Pierre Robin?**

Prone positioning; evaluation of the lower airway for synchronous anomalies; later, other interventions include distraction osteogenesis, tongue–lip adhesion, tracheotomy.

○ **What are symptoms of Binder syndrome?**

Nasomaxillary hypoplasia, low/flat nasal tip, absent nasal spine; Angle class III malocclusion.

○ **What is Klippel–Feil syndrome?**

Shortened neck, low posterior hairline, hearing loss, cleft palate, facial abnormalities; fusion of cervical spine.

○ **What is Shprintzen syndrome?**

Otherwise known as velocardiofacial syndrome; most common syndrome seen in cleft lip/palate; thymus/parathyroid glands absent; cardiac anomalies, velopharyngeal dysfunction.

○ **What is van der Woude syndrome?**

Cleft lip/palate, LOWER lip pits (from accessory saliva glands); extremity anomalies.

○ **Does the medial or lateral pterygoid elevate the mandible?**
The medial.

○ **What action does the digastric muscle have on the mandible following a fracture?**

Pulls anterior mandibular segment posteriorly and inferiorly.

○ **What is the action of the lateral pterygoid in unilateral subcondylar fractures?**

The ipsilateral condylar head is pulled anteriorly and medially; the contralateral lateral pterygoid continues to protrude the mandible, thus deviating the jaw to the fracture side.

○ **In patients with subcondylar fractures, what is the most appropriate duration of maxillomandibular fixation (MMF)?**

4 weeks.

○ **Embryologically, what arises from the frontonasal process?**

The nasal bridge and root.

○ **What arises from the medial nasal processes?**

Columella, tip, philtrum, premaxilla.

○ **What arises from the lateral nasal processes?**

The alae.

○ **Which branchial arch gives rise to the stylopharyngeus muscle?**

The third.

○ **What muscles are derived from the first branchial arch?**

Muscles of chewing, anterior digastric, mylohyoid, tensor tympani.

○ **What is the most appropriate next step for treatment of a naso-orbital-ethmoid fracture?**

ORIF and bone grafting.

○ **What muscle travels around the hamulus in the mouth?**

The tensor veli palatini.

○ **What bone does the hamulus arise from?**

The medial pterygoid plate.

○ **A 5-month-old child with anterior displacement of the right ear and zygoma and right side of the forehead with flattening of the right side of the occiput has what process?**

Right-sided posterior deformational plagiocephaly.

○ **What are the most common causes of synostotic plagiocephaly?**

Unilateral coronal and lambdoidal craniosynostosis.

○ **How frequent is deformational plagiocephaly?**

1 per 70 infants.

○ **What findings are seen in posterior deformational plagiocephaly?**

Unilateral; parallelogram-shaped head; ipsilateral flattening of the occiput with anterior displacement of ipsilateral ear.

○ **What findings are seen in bilateral deformational plagiocephaly?**

Flattening of the occipital area, mastoid bulging bilaterally, biparietal eminence bossing.

○ **What is seen in lambdoidal craniosynostosis?**

Ipsilateral occipital flattening with lambdoid suture ridging (from fusion of the suture); INFERIOR displacement of the ear.

○ **What shape is the skull in lambdoidal craniosynostosis?**

Trapezoid-like.

○ **On the basis of radiographic CT findings, what are operative indications for an orbital blowout fracture?**

Orbital floor defect greater than 2 cm, low vertical height of the globe, coexisting other facial fractures.

○ **What are clinical indications for operative intervention in orbital blowout fractures?**

Symptomatic diplopia, positive forced duction testing, failed resolution of extraocular muscle entrapment after 1 week.

○ **Does the supraorbital artery derive its blood supply from the internal or external system? The supratrochlear artery?**

Both are branches of the ophthalmic artery, which branches from the internal carotid artery.

○ **What is an important consideration when deciding whether to use an external or internal distraction device following a Le Fort III?**

Using an external device allows for in-office removal, saving an operative procedure for the patient.

○ **Nerve injury during osseous genioplasty most likely results in what symptom?**

Numbness of the lower lip (mental nerve).

○ **In a teenaged boy with Angle class III, 12 mm of negative overjet, and normal SNB angle, what procedure is most appropriate for maxillary advancement?**

Distraction osteogenesis of the maxilla; Le Fort I single-stage advancement of more than 10 mm is considered unpredictable.

○ **What is the procedure of choice in a patient to advance the maxilla who has had cleft lip/palate repair and pharyngeal flap with a 14-mm negative overjet?**

Maxillary distraction osteogenesis.

○ **What environmental exposure has been linked to squamous cell carcinoma of the maxillary sinus?**
Nickel.

○ **What is the most useful component to anatomically reduce in a ZMC fracture?**
The lateral orbital wall, alternatively, the sphenoid wing can be also used.

○ **Where does the levator palpebrae superioris originate from?**
The lesser wing of the sphenoid.

○ **Where do the superior oblique and rectus muscles originate from?**
The annulus tendineus communis.

○ **What structure does the inferior oblique arise from?**
The maxilla.

○ **Gustatory sweating following parotid surgery is due to malfunction of what nerve?**
Auriculotemporal.

○ **What is the mechanism of Frey syndrome?**
Aberrant connections between postganglionic parasympathetic fibers from the otic ganglion and postganglionic sympathetic fibers to sweat glands.

○ **What effect does Botox have on Frey syndrome?**
Intracutaneous administration blocks acetylcholine transmission and may improve symptoms for up to a year.

○ **What structure does the stapes derive from?**
The second branchial arch.

○ **A melanoma with a Clark level of IV and Breslow thickness of 2.8 mm with an in-transit metastasis has what stage?**
Stage III (T4, N0).

○ **How is vertical maxillary excess and a retruded chin treated?**
Typically by Le Fort I with maxillary impaction and genioplasty.

○ **What is the appearance of the nose in vertical maxillary excess typically?**
Alar base constriction and an obtuse nasolabial angle.

○ **What are other signs of vertical maxillary excess?**
Lip incompetence, incisor show, mentalis strain.

○ **Where does the nasolacrimal duct drain into the nasal cavity?**
Inferior meatus.

○ **What structures drain into the middle meatus?**
The frontal, anterior ethmoid, and maxillary sinuses.

○ **What areas of the mandible are fractured most commonly?**
The angle and body.

○ **What is most appropriate initial therapy for a child with an enlarging hemangioma of the eyelid?**
Oral steroids 2 to 3 mg/kg per day (low dose); surgical management if steroids are unsuccessful.

○ **What structure is incised during a preseptal transconjunctival approach to the orbital floor?**
The capsulopalpebral fascia.

○ **What nerve supplies the superior helix of the auricle?**
The auriculotemporal nerve (CN V).

○ **What nerves provide sensation to the ear?**
Auriculotemporal branch (V), VII, Jacobson nerve (IX), Arnold nerve (X), lesser occipital nerve (C2), great auricular nerve (C2,3).

○ **What system controls pupillary constriction?**
Parasympathetics of the eye; travel with CN III and the inferior oblique.

○ **What clinical finding is seen in direct trauma to the optic nerve?**
Afferent pupillary defect (Marcus Gunn pupil).

○ **What muscle of the tongue is supplied by CN X?**
The palatoglossus.

○ **What is the appearance of the palpebral fissure following zygomatic fractures?**
Downward cant due to pulling of Whitnall ligament inferiorly.

○ **What finding during facial fracture causes rounding of the palpebral fissure?**
Lateral canthal ligament detachment or comminuted frontal process of the zygoma.

○ **What structures travel through the superior orbital fissure?**
V1, III, IV, and VI.

○ **What branches off CN V1?**
The frontal, nasociliary, and lacrimal nerves.

○ **What syndrome has brachycephaly, hypertelorism, bregmatic prominence, maxillary hypoplasia, and bony syndactyly of toes and hands?**

Apert.

○ **Members of a family with frontal recession, maxillary retrusion, proptosis, and exorbitism without extremity anomalies have what syndrome?**

Crouzon.

○ **What findings are seen in Carpenter syndrome?**

Brachydactyly, syndactyly, polydactyly, cardiac disease, obesity, GU anomalies; AR.

○ **What is seen in Nager syndrome?**

Acrofacial dysostosis; AR; cleft palate, orbital, zygomatic, maxillo-mandibular hypoplasia, preaxial hypoplasia or agenesis; auricular defects, mental retardation; syndactyly of the second web space.

○ **What is seen in Pfeiffer syndrome?**

Synostosis, acrocephalosyndactyly, broad thumbs, midface hypoplasia.

○ **What procedure is done for horizontal deficiency and vertical excess of the chin?**

Jumping genioplasty.

○ **What embryologic anomaly is responsible for primary cleft palate?**

Failed lateral and median palatine process fusion.

○ **What causes secondary cleft palate?**

Failed lateral palatine process fusion to each other and the nasal septum.

○ **What causes cleft lip?**

Fusion of the medial nasal prominence and maxillary prominence.

○ **What causes macrostomia?**

Failed fusion of the maxillary and mandibular prominences.

○ **In a maxillary advancement for 1 cm of negative overjet, what primary factor is the most significant risk for VPI?**

Midface hypoplasia due to cleft palate repair (higher risk than other craniofacial syndromes such as microsomia or Crouzon).

○ **What is the most common Tessier facial cleft?**

No. 7 (macrostomia, zygomatic arch absence).

○ **Which Tessier cleft includes the same position as a unilateral cleft lip?**

No. 3; also extends to affect nasal ala and medial canthus.

○ **What is the appropriate management of Romberg hemifacial atrophy?**

Parascapular flap; deepithelialized and placed under skin flap.

○ **What is the most common cause of late enophthalmos following ORIF of an orbital floor and zygomatic arch fracture?**

Inadequate reduction.

○ **Where does a frontonasal encephalocele communicate intracranially?**

Foramen cecum.

○ **What is the metachronous incidence of squamous cell carcinoma in a patient who continues to smoke?**

40%; those who stop tobacco have an incidence of 6%.

○ **What is the normal latency period in mandibular distraction in a 6-year-old child?**

1 week.

○ **What are the symptoms of TMJ internal derangement?**

Anterior excursion of the meniscus with posterior and superior positioning of the condyle; jaw clicking; preauricular pain.

○ **What is the relationship of the condyle during an acute TMJ dislocation?**

Anterior excursion of the condyle past the eminence.

○ **What is the safest landmark for identifying the facial nerve during parotid surgery?**

Using the tympanomastoid suture line.

○ **Following a Le Fort I, what provides vascularity to the maxillary segment?**

The ascending pharyngeal artery and ascending palatine artery (of the facial artery).

○ **What does the greater palatine artery supply?**

Palate and roof of mouth.

○ **What does the lesser palatine artery supply?**

Soft palate and palatine tonsils.

○ **What is cryptotia?**

Absence of the superior auriculocephalic sulcus; upper pole is buried beneath the scalp.

○ **What normally supplies blood to the maxilla?**

Internal maxillary artery by descending palatine, posterior superior alveolar, and infraorbital arteries.

○ **What is cup ear?**

Hooding of the scapha and helix and antihelical flattening.

○ **What is lop ear?**

Auricular protrusion and superior helical folding.

○ **What are the characteristics of mandibular prognathism?**

Angle class III, lower facial third prominence.

○ **What are the characteristics of mandibular retrognathism?**

Anterior teeth protrusion, lip incompetence, deep labiomental crease.

○ **What treatment should be undertaken for an anterior frontal sinus fracture with a nondisplaced posterior wall fracture and patency of the nasofrontal duct?**

Repair of the anterior wall alone.

○ **What approach is undertaken if the nasofrontal duct is obstructed?**

Obliteration of the frontal sinus.

○ **What situation necessitates cranialization?**

Comminution of the posterior wall; concomitant CSF leak.

○ **What clinical symptoms define superior orbital fissure syndrome?**

Fracture affecting III, IV, V1, and VI; extraocular muscle paralysis, levator palpebrae weakness, numbness of the forehead, eyebrow, upper eyelid.

○ **What is orbital apex syndrome?**

Superior orbital fissure syndrome with blindness (from optic nerve involvement).

○ **When do the permanent canine teeth erupt?**

Between 10 and 11 years of age.

○ **When do the permanent first molars erupt?**

Between 6 and 7 years of age.

○ **What nerve is the cause of Frey syndrome?**

Aberrant regeneration of the auriculotemporal nerve.

○ **What is the mechanism of Frey syndrome?**

Aberrant regeneration of the auriculotemporal nerve to sweat glands; test with Minor starch-iodine test.

○ **What is the treatment of Frey syndrome?**

Tympanic neurectomy, topical glycopyrrolate, and/or Prantal (diphemanil methylsulfate) to control gustatory sweating.

○ **Where does the great auricular nerve travel within the neck?**

Exists on top of the SCM, 9 cm from the caudal EAC and 6.5 cm inferior to the tragus.

○ **What type of mandible fracture is seen in a patient with chin deviation to the left, upward mandibular cant to the left, and right-sided open-bite deformity?**

Left condylar fracture; also with loss of posterior ramus height on left, chin deviated to left due to right lateral pterygoid.

○ **What growth factor has been associated with craniosynostosis in the animal model?**

TGF-beta in the posterior frontal suture line.

○ **When does the anterior fontanelle close?**

24 months.

○ **When does the posterior fontanelle close?**

2 months.

○ **What is the treatment for bilateral subcondylar fractures?**

ORIF through preauricular incisions.

○ **What is the most common craniofacial anomaly?**

Hemifacial microsomia.

○ **Fractures of what part of the mandible are most significant for growth in the child?**

Fractures of the condyle.

○ **What are late complications of frontal sinus fractures?**

Orbital abscess, mucocele, osteomyelitis.

○ **What are complications of frontal sinus fractures occurring within the first few weeks?**

Meningitis, mucocele, frontal sinusitis.

○ **What does the first branchial groove develop into?**

The EAC.

○ **What is the most common site of squamous cell carcinoma of the paranasal sinuses?**

The maxillary sinus (chronic exposure to nickel and wood working materials).

○ **What is most common cause of TMJ ankylosis?**

Trauma.

○ **What permanent tooth erupts first?**

The first molar (6–7 years of age).

○ **What are the commonly used cranial base planes?**

Frankfort horizontal, basion-nasion, sella-nasion.

○ **What are the common maxillary planes used?**

Axis of the maxillary incisor, nasion to A point, occlusal, and palatal.

○ **What bones form the lateral orbital wall?**

Zygoma, greater wing of the sphenoid.

○ **What bones form the orbit?**

Greater wing of sphenoid, lacrimal, palatine, maxilla, ethmoid, frontal, lesser wing of the sphenoid.

○ **What structures drain into the middle meatus?**

The anterior ethmoid, maxillary, and frontal sinuses.

○ **What drains into the inferior meatus?**

The nasolacrimal duct.

○ **What is the primary action of the superior oblique?**

Depression; also abduction and intorsion; innervated by the trochlear nerve.

○ **What is the percentage of coexisting spine injuries with panfacial MVC trauma?**

10%.

○ **What muscle is used in sphincter pharyngoplasty for reconstruction?**

Palatopharyngeus.

○ **What is the blood supply to the sternocleidomastoid muscle?**

Occipital, superior thyroid, and thyrocervical trunk.

○ **What metal on CT scan exhibits the greatest amount of scatter?**

Stainless steel; titanium and vitallium have the least scatter.

○ **What suture line is broken in Le Fort III but not monobloc advancement?**

Frontozygomatic suture and nasofrontal junction.

○ **What muscles are important for closure of the velum?**

Levator veli palatini, uvulus, palatopharyngeus, and superior pharyngeal constrictors (NOT the tensor veli palatini).

○ **What is the mechanism of velopharyngeal insufficiency with the levator veli palatini in cleft palate?**

The levator inserts on the posterior hard palate; repair reproduces the sling required for closure.

○ **What is the role of the tensor veli palatini?**

Tenses the soft palate; important for eustachian tube function.

○ **What attaches to Whitnall tubercle?**

Lateral rectus fascial extension, lateral check ligament, lateral levator aponeurosis horn, and lateral palpebral ligaments.

○ **What is the suspensor ligament of Lockwood composed of?**

Fascia from the inferior rectus and inferior oblique.

○ **What is the most frequent site of mandible fractures?**

Angle (35%), parasymphysial region (24%), and body (18%).

○ **What mandible fracture location is most commonly associated with anterior open bite?**

Subcondylar/condylar.

○ **What premature fusion causes brachycephaly?**

Bilateral coronal synostosis, cranial vault is shortening in A-P dimension, frontal skull is flat and wide.

○ **What is lambdoid synostosis known as?**

Occipital or posterior plagiocephaly; oblique and posterior flattening.

○ **What is the condition present with a normal SNA and decreased SNB?**

Mandibular retrusion.

○ **What is the Landes angle?**

Frankfort horizontal and N-A plane; normal value 88 degrees.

○ **What is the likely cause of a gradual bony enlargement of the left fronto-orbital region in a 9-year-old child?**

Fibrous dysplasia.

○ **What is McCune Albright syndrome?**

Polyostotic fibrous dysplasia, hyperthyroidism, abnormal pigmentation, sexual precocity.

○ **In a patient with mandibular prognathism and maxillary hypoplasia, what is the required treatment?**

Le Fort I with sagittal split osteotomy.

○ **What is the likely cause of enophthalmos after trauma?**

Bony orbital volume increase.

○ **What is the next course of treatment following a Le Fort I with a unilateral posterior open-bite deformity?**

Removal of hardware and disimpaction of the maxillary fracture.

○ **What is Binder syndrome?**

Midface hypoplasia, flat nasal dorsum, retracted columella, anterior nasal spine absence; Angle class III occlusion.

○ **What do the first three hillocks give rise to?**

The tragus, root of the helix, and superior helix.

○ **What do the second three hillocks give rise to?**

The antihelix, antitragus, and lobule.

○ **What does Meckel cartilage form?**

Malleus, incus, mandible, sphenomandibular ligament.

○ **What does Reichert cartilage form?**

Stapes, styloid process, stylohyoid ligament, lesser cornu of the hyoid, part of the hyoid body.

○ **What is the first structure to be released during treatment of a retrobulbar hematoma?**

The lateral canthal tendon.

○ **Where is Tenon capsule located?**

It covers the globe and extraocular muscles; lower portion constitutes Lockwood ligament.

○ **What is the study of choice in patients with painless jaw clicking after trauma?**

MRI to rule out internal derangement.

○ **What Tessier cleft is associated with macrostomia?**

No. 7.

○ **Which cleft is associated with absence of the zygomatic arch?**

Also No. 7.

○ **What is the likelihood of malignant transformation in acinic cell carcinoma of the parotid?**
Infrequent, bilateral, or multicentric lesion.

○ **What is the most common malignant tumor of the parotid?**
Mucoepidermoid carcinoma.

○ **What is the layer underneath which is used for the Gillies approach to a zygomatic arch fracture?**
Deep layer of the deep temporal fascia.

○ **What is the mechanism of action of the TMJ during the last portion of jaw opening?**
Upper joint space translation.

○ **What is the sequence of events in TMJ opening?**
Rotation (condyle in lower joint space), rotation/translation, translation within the joint (condyle in upper joint space).

○ **What innervates the tensor veli palatini?**
Cranial nerve V.

○ **What innervates the levator veli palatini?**
The superior laryngeal branch of CN X.

○ **What innervates the stylopharyngeus?**
CN IX.

○ **What innervates the palatopharyngeus?**
CN X.

○ **What supplies vascularity to the trapezius flap?**
The transverse cervical artery, secondary source occipital artery, type II muscle flap.

○ **What supplies sensation to the lobule and posterior two-thirds of the ear?**
The great auricular nerve.

○ **What supplies sensation to the posterior ear and EAC?**
Arnold nerve (branch of X).

○ **What supplies sensation to the anterior superior helix and tragus?**
Auriculotemporal nerve (branch of V).

○   **What supplies sensation to the posterior auricle and concha?**

Posterior auricular nerve, lesser occipital nerve.

○   **What is the rate of distraction osteogenesis in the pediatric mandible?**

1 mm/day.

○   **What process causes the changing of recipient mesenchymal cells into osteoprogenitor cells from BMP stimulation?**

Osteoinduction.

○   **What is osteoconduction?**

Bone ingrowth into grafted material.

○   **What structures should be inspected following nasal trauma regarding septal deviation?**

Septal cartilage, perpendicular plate of the ethmoid, vomer.

○   **What is the first-line treatment for nasopharyngeal carcinoma?**

Radiation therapy.

○   **What is the likely response to a 2-cm squamous cell carcinoma of the lower lip to radiotherapy?**

90% complete response.

○   **What permanent teeth have the longest roots?**

The cuspids (canines); 27 mm height.

○   **What bone mainly comprises the medial orbital wall?**

Ethmoid bone.

○   **The lingual nerve is a branch of what nerve?**

The mandibular branch of CN V.

○   **What are the main branches of the mandibular division of CN V?**

Lingual nerve, inferior alveolar nerve, long buccal branch, mental nerve, auriculotemporal branch.

○   **What does the auriculotemporal nerve innervate?**

Sensation to the anterior auricle, temporal region, and portion of EAC and TMJ.

○   **What are the main branches of the maxillary division of CN V?**

Infraorbital nerve, nasopalatine nerve, posterosuperior alveolar nerve, posterosuperior nasal nerve.

○ **What structure is the likely cause of ectropion following an orbital floor fracture reduction through a subciliary incision?**
Scarring of the orbital septum.

○ **What structure is avoided when making an incision into the first lower eyelid crease during an orbital floor fracture case?**
This incision preserves the innervation of the pretarsal portion of the orbicularis oculi; normal lid tone is preserved.

○ **The mental nerve located in relation to what tooth of the mandible?**
The second bicuspid.

○ **Where is Stensen duct located relative the maxillary teeth?**
Opposite the second molar.

○ **What muscle contributes to medial displacement of the condyle following a fracture?**
Lateral pterygoid.

○ **The Frankfort horizontal passes through which points?**
The porion and orbitale.

○ **What is the treatment for a unilateral nondisplaced coronoid fracture?**
Short-term mandibulomaxillary fixation.

○ **What is the treatment for a mandibular osteogenic sarcoma?**
Wide excision, followed by radiation/chemotherapy.

○ **Where do the most minor salivary gland tumors arise in the mouth?**
The palate.

○ **What is the histological subtype of most minor salivary gland tumors?**
Adenoid cystic carcinoma.

○ **In an edentulous patient, what can be used for MMF?**
Intraoral splints that are custom made; fixed to the maxilla or mandible using wires/screws.

○ **What is advocated for first-line treatment for a chylous fistula in the neck?**
Medium chain triglyceride diet with closed drainage on suction.

○ **Which side is a chylous fistula usually associated on?**
Injury to the thoracic duct on the left.

○ **What are the physical findings associated with a unilateral cleft lip?**

Rotation of the premaxilla and outward projection; collapsed lateral maxillary segment; shortened columella, attenuation of the lower lateral cartilage; alar base rotated outward; shortened philtrum.

○ **What direction are the septum and cartilage deviated toward in a unilateral cleft lip?**

Toward the noncleft side.

• • • HAND AND EXTREMITIES • • •

○ **What is the Gustilo classification?**

Classification of open lower extremity fractures.

Type I	Low energy, soft-tissue defect <1 cm
Type II	Soft-tissue defect >1 cm with moderate soft-tissue damage
Type III	Soft-tissue defect >1 cm with extensive soft-tissue damage
IIIa	Local soft-tissue coverage possible
IIIb	Local soft-tissue coverage not possible
IIIc	Vascular injuries that require repair

○ **What management option should be considered with Gustilo IIIC injuries with an insensate foot?**

Below-knee amputation.

○ **What is lymphedema praecox? Lymphedema Tarda?**

It is the most likely form of hereditary lymphedema—typically manifests at puberty and has a chronic course. It is usually seen bilaterally. Lymphedema tarda arises in middle age by definition. It is another form of primary lymphedema.

○ **What is infantile digital fibromatosis? Treatment?**

Rapidly growing fibrous lesions appearing on the lateral or dorsal aspects of fingers of children. Pathology shows intracytoplasmic inclusion bodies. Treatment is wide excision.

○ **What is the initial management of lymphedema?**

Elevation and compression, also consider intermittent pneumatic compression therapy.

○ **At what age should thumb reconstruction be performed in the complete absence of the thumb?**

1 year of age.

○ **What structures need to be divided with release of the ulnar tunnel?**

Pisohamate ligament, volar carpal ligament.

○ **What is Osborne ligament?**

The band of fascia bridging between the two heads of the FCU and the medial epicondyle, a common site of ulnar nerve compression.

○ **What nerve may be injured with harvest of the lateral gastrocnemius flap?**

Common peroneal nerve (approximately 8%).

○ **How can you distinguish a preganglionic from a postganglionic nerve injury?**

Preganglionic lesions are associated with nerve root avulsions and are not reconstructable by nerve repair or nerve grafts. Sensory nerve conduction is intact but with the absence of somatosensory-evoked potentials.

○ **A manual laborer presents with avulsion amputation of the index finger, what is the best treatment?**

Revision amputation.

○ **What is the initial management of epithelioid sarcoma?**

Preoperative radiation.

○ **A patient presents with delayed rupture of a flexor tendon repair, what is the best treatment option?**

Staged tendon reconstruction with initial placement of Hunter rods.

○ **Patient presents after mastectomy and radiation for breast cancer with ipsilateral hand swelling, numbness, and generalized weakness without pain, what is the diagnosis?**

Radiation-induced plexopathy, most common in the C5–6 distribution.

○ **What is the femoral triangle? What is its importance in medial thigh lift?**

The femoral triangle is formed by the inguinal ligament, the sartorius muscle, and the adductor longus muscle. Avoiding the lymphatics in this area during thigh lift reduces seroma rate.

○ **What is melanonychia?**

Benign pigmented streaks in the nail plate, commonly seen in African Americans.

○ **What is the initial management of a pigmented lesion under the nail?**

Shave biopsy (full-thickness biopsy is unnecessarily morbid).

○ **A patient has burn scar over half of his nail bed and requests cosmetic improvement, what is the best treatment?**

Excision of scar, eponychial flap, and nail bed graft from a toe.

○ **What is the Wassel classification of duplicated thumb? Which is most common?**

I: bifid distal phalanx; II: duplicated distal phalanx; III: bifid proximal phalanx; IV: duplicated proximal phalanx; V: bifid metacarpal; VI: duplicated metacarpal; VII: triphalangism.

*Type IV is most common.

○ **An FDP tendon ruptures with a large piece of bone, the tendon will get caught on what structure?**

A4 pulley.

○ **Polydactyly falls under what category of congenital anomalies?**

Duplication.

○ **Syndactyly falls under what category of congenital anomalies?**

Failure of differentiation.

○ **What are the innervations of the flexor pollicis brevis muscle?**

Deep head: ulnar nerve; superficial head: median nerve.

○ **What nerve transfer can restore intrinsic function after high ulnar nerve injury?**

Anterior interosseous nerve to the pronator quadratus transferred to the ulnar motor branch.

○ **What is the reverse cross-finger flap?**

The flap transfers only the subcutaneous tissue of the dorsum of the donor finger to the recipient finger providing an adequate bed for skin grafting.

○ **What is a DISI deformity in the wrist?**

Dorsal intercalated segmental instability (DISI) is when the scaphoid and lunate are dissociated from an injury to the scapholunate ligament (indicated by widened scapholunate interval). The lunate goes into dorsiflexion and the scaphoid goes into volar flexion.

○ **In Klippel–Trenaunay syndrome (KTS), what are the major health risks?**

DVT, pulmonary embolism.

○ **At the level of the wrist, where are the motor fibers of the median nerve in relation to the sensory fibers?**

Volar and radial.

○ **What is the Blauth classification of hypoplastic thumb?**

I	Minor generalized hypoplasia
II	Absence of thenar muscles, first webspace narrowing, ulnar collateral ligament insufficiency
III	Extrinsic muscle abnormalities, skeletal deficiency (A: stable CMC; B: unstable CMC)
IV	Pouce flottant of floating thumb (rudimentary thumb)
V	Absent thumb

○ **What is the main arterial supply to the reverse sural flap?**

The flap is based on the sural artery via perforators from the peroneal artery. The main perforator arises approximately 5 cm superior to the malleolus.

○ **A patient can still flex her DIP joint after cutting her FDP, why?**

Preservation of the vincula.

○ **A patient can still extend the DIP joint after cutting the extensor tendon at the middle phalanx, why?**

Oblique retinacular ligament.

○ **On nerve conduction studies, what is the significance of increased latency?**

Latency measures the time for nerve conduction, nerve compression, and subsequent demyelination result in increased latency.

○ **On EMG, what changes signify denervation?**

Fibrillations and positive sharp waves.

○ **True/False: Biodegradable materials are preferable for use as spacers in CMC arthroplasty?**

True.

○ **What is the most important structure providing stabilization to the CMC joint?**

Dorsal ligament complex.

○ **What is the management of perilunate dislocations?**

Open reduction and internal fixation.

○ **What is the treatment for loss of the thumb at the level of the MCP joint?**

Toe-to-thumb transfer.

○ **True/False: At the level of the wrist, the FDS tendons of the index and small fingers are dorsal to the long and ring fingers.**

True.

○ **What tendon transfer is most appropriate in a child with spastic cerebral palsy with mental retardation and a clenched fist with ulnar palmar maceration?**

FDS to FDP; this will lengthen and weaken the finger flexors; may also arthrodese wrist rather than transferring to wrist extensors.

○ **When is texture discrimination appropriate for children with CP?**

Age 2 to 3 years.

○ **Trauma to the dorsalis pedis artery in the lower leg is most likely associated with what neuropraxia?**

Decreased deep peroneal nerve function; first webspace decreased sensation.

○ **What innervates the dorsal aspect of the foot?**

Superficial peroneal nerve.

○ **What innervates the lateral foot?**

Sural nerve.

○ **Medial?**

Saphenous nerve.

○ **Which of these nerves travels with an artery?**

Deep peroneal nerve.

○ **What innervates the plantar surface?**

Tibial nerve; travels with PT.

○ **What is the immediate treatment for hydrofluoric acid burns?**

Calcium gluconate gel application (prevention of hypocalcemia, hypomagnesemia, hyperkalemia).

○ **What is given for phenol burns?**

Mineral oil.

○ **What is given for creosol burns?**

Polyethylene glycol.

○ **What is the most common primary benign tumor of the hand?**

Enchondroma (benign cartilaginous tumor).

○ **What signifies pain in the absence of fracture with enchondroma?**

Malignant degeneration.

○ **What is the radiographic finding in enchondroma?**

Scalloped, lytic lesion within the medullary canal.

○ **What is Ollier disease?**

Multiple enchondromatosis.

○ **What is Maffucci syndrome?**

Multiple enchondromas with subcutaneous hemangiomas.

○ **How often do chondromyxoid fibromas occur in the upper extremity?**

Rarely.

○ **How often do giant cell tumors occur in the distal upper extremity?**

Only 2% to 5% in hand; radius is the third most commonly affected site.

○ **How often do osteoid osteomas cause pain?**

Frequently, at night, give NSAIDs.

○ **What defines the midpalmar space?**

Flexor tendons, metacarpal bone and interosseous fascia, septum from the third metacarpal to FDP, superficial aponeurosis (deep to the flexor tendon to fascia over second/third volar interossei and third/fourth metacarpals).

○ **What is the thenar space?**

Radial to vertical septum between the third MC and FDP of long finger; extends to radial edge of abductor pollicis brevis.

○ **What tendons are ruptured most commonly in RA?**

EPL (treat with ECRL transfer) and EDQ.

○ **How do extensor tendon ruptures progress in the RA patient?**

Ulnar to radial progression (Vaughn–Jackson progression); EDQ then EDC to small, ring, then long fingers.

○ **What is a Mannerfelt lesion?**

Rupture of FPL over a scaphoid spur (flexor ruptures far less frequently, usually affecting radial digits).

○ **What prevents closed reduction of the little finger in a volar dislocation of the PIP joint?**

Extensor tendon; when condyle has pushed through the extensor tendon and acts as sling.

○ **What is more common—volar or dorsal dislocations of the PIP?**

Dorsal.

○ **What may prevent dorsal dislocations of the PIP from adequate closed reduction?**

Volar plate and flexor tendons, though rarely.

○ **What is the most common primary blood supply to the great toe in toe-to-thumb transfer?**

First dorsal metatarsal artery from DP; may travel dorsal or plantar to interosseous muscle.

○ **What hand tumor has an affinity for immunosuppressed patients?**

Keratoacanthoma (thought to be a variant of SCCa); appears as red papule, expands rapidly over several weeks.

○ **What is the likelihood for future siblings to be affected with constriction band syndrome?**

No genetic transmission; fourth most common congenital hand anomaly.

○ **What are the three most common congenital hand anomalies?**

Polydactyly, syndactyly, and trigger thumb.

○ **What other anomalies are seen with amniotic band syndrome?**

Club foot, cleft lip/palate, craniofacial defects, hemangioma, meningocele.

○ **What is the most appropriate treatment for radial nerve palsy after a humeral ORIF 6 months later?**

Tendon transfers.

○ **What transfers are performed for radial nerve palsy?**

Pronator teres to ECRB for wrist extension.

○ **What transfers are performed for finger extension?**

FCR, FCU, FDS(3, 4) to EDC.

○ **What transfers are performed for thumb extension?**

PL or FCR to EPL.

○ **What is the best option for reconstruction of volar skin of the index when dorsal skin of the long finger is not available?**

Thenar flap (for tips of index/long fingers); these fingers flex easily into the thenar crease.

○ **What option is there for ring and small finger volar skin defects?**

Hypothenar flaps.

○ **What procedure may be used for volar pad defects of the thumb?**

Moberg flap; volar advancement flap; composed completely of palmar thumb skin.

○ **With an SLAC wrist what procedure is most appropriate in a dockworker?**

SLAC wrist, with DISI and radioscaphoid arthrosis, is best treated with scaphoid excision and four-corner arthrodesis (lunate, capitate, hamate, triquetrum) in a dockworker.

○ **How is SLAC wrist classified?**

Stage I: radioscaphoid

Stage II: radial midcarpal

Stage III: ulnar midcarpal

Stage IV: pancarpal

○ **What structure defines the growth and differentiation of the new limb during embryologic development?**

Apical ectodermal ridge (which arises from the Wolffian ridge, protruding from the main trunk).

○ **What structure defines anterior–posterior morphology of the limb?**

Zone of polarizing activity.

○ **When do the upper extremities begin to develop?**

At 4 weeks; by the fifth week, the hand is recognizable; the apical ectodermal ridge becomes flattened; hand appears initially as paddle.

○ **When are the fingernails identifiable?**

At the 17th week of gestation.

○ **What is the first step in a patient with a 2-cm gap in the ulnar nerve following trauma?**

Ulnar nerve transposition (provides up to 4 cm of length; 2 cm of length at distal forearm and wrist).

○ **PIP contractures in fifth finger Dupuytren is most likely caused by what structures?**

Central, lateral, and spiral cords.

○ **What other fascial structures may contribute to flexion contractures?**

Grayson, Cleland, lateral digital sheath, natatory ligament, pretendinous and spiral bands, superficial transverse ligament.

○ **What does the central cord arise from?**

The pretendinous band.

○ **What is the lateral cord from?**

Central digital sheath.

○ **What is the spiral cord composed of?**

Pretendinous and spiral bands, lateral digital sheath, and Grayson ligament.

○ **Contraction of the spiral cord has what effect on the neurovascular bundle?**

Medial and superficial displacement of the bundle.

○ **What causes contracture of the MP joint?**

Action from the pretendinous cord (which does not contribute to PIP contracture).

○ **What does the natatory cord cause?**

Adduction contractures of the digits (passes transversely across palm at level of webspaces).

○ **What is the most common organism causing septic arthritis of the hand/wrist?**

Staphylococcus aureus. Streptococcus is next.

○ **What organism will likely be cultured from a human bite wound?**

Eikenella corrodens.

○ **What is the best option for a distal third defect following trauma with exposed bone?**

Fasciocutaneous flap.

○ **What defects will a gastrocnemius flap cover in the leg?**

Upper, some middle third of the leg defects.

○ **How is onychomycosis treated?**

6 weeks of terbinafine or itraconazole.

○ **Is terbinafine associated with any side effects?**

Stevens–Johnson, neutropenia, hepatic failure.

○ **What is lumbrical plus deformity?**

Extension of the PIP on attempting to make a fist (occurs following repair; secondary to release of FDP of index).

○ **How is lumbrical plus treated?**

Division of the lumbrical (with attempted flexion lumbrical exerts tension through lateral band).

○ **When is transfer of the interosseous muscle performed?**

Correction of rheumatoid ulnar drift.

○ **What is the acceptable limit of before surgical correction is necessary in a pediatric patient with camptodactyly?**

30 degrees of extension of the PIP.

○ **How are minimal extension deficits corrected in camptodactyly?**

Transfer lumbrical tendon into central slip.

○ **How are extension deficits greater than 30 degrees treated?**

Release of abnormal lumbrical and superficialis tendons; release of accessory collateral ligaments to volar plate; FTSG.

○ **What is the Zancolli lasso procedure?**

Portions of FDS brought through A2 pulley; for the correction of ulnar palsy digital clawing.

O **What are Kanavel signs?**

Fusiform swelling, partial flexed posturing of finger, tenderness over flexor tendon sheath, pain with passive extension; open and irrigate flexor sheath.

O **Where are the incisions made for flexor tenosynovitis?**

Palm incision to inspect proximal A1 pulley and distal incision to visualize A4, A5 at minimum.

O **What is the best postoperative dressing for an infant following simple complete syndactyly release of the third webspace?**

Long arm cast.

O **What zone of flexor tendon repair is associated with the best prognosis?**

Zone 5.

O **Which finger has the most lacerations of the nail bed?**

The long finger.

O **How are nail bed lacerations classified?**

Simple, stellate, crush, amputated, avulsion.

O **Following a ring avulsion replantation failure, what is the next step in management?**

Ray amputation with most or all of the metacarpal.

O **What is the Littler flap?**

A neurovascular island flap based on the digital nerve/vascular bundle of long or ring.

O **What is the Shaw flap?**

Superficial inferior epigastric artery (SIEA) flap; can be used for coverage of hand/forearm.

O **Where are the landmarks of the SIEA?**

Intersection of inguinal ligament and femoral artery; travels superiorly and laterally toward anterior axilla.

O **What is the arterial supply of the groin flap?**

SCIA.

O **What are landmarks for the SCIA?**

Originates from femoral artery, travels parallel to inguinal ligament, 1 cm deep to the ligament.

O **What is the best treatment of trapeziometacarpal DJD in factory worker?**

Arthrodesis.

○ **When is reconstruction of the palmar (oblique) ligament performed?**

Situations of prearthritic instability with pain of CMC joint.

○ **How are lunate dislocations classified?**

Midcarpal lunocapitate, complete lunate, and perilunate.

○ **How is a complete lunate injury differentiated from a perilunate injury?**

Presence of radiolunate joint dislocation concurrently.

○ **What other bony structures are involved in greater arc injury?**

High-energy trauma; radial styloid, scaphoid, capitate, hamate, triquetrum, ulnar styloid fractures.

○ **What structures are involved in lesser arc injury?**

SL, LT, lunocapitate intervals.

○ **What is a collar button abscess?**

Pus communicating from volar webspace to dorsal hand by palmar fascia or lumbrical canal.

○ **What is a characteristic finding of a collar button abscess?**

Finger abduction.

○ **Where is Parona space?**

Between pronator quadratus and FDP tendons; communicates with radial and ulnar palmar bursa and midpalmar space.

○ **What area of swelling is associated with Parona space infection?**

Volar wrist proximal to distal flexion crease.

○ **How is the scaphoid vascularized?**

Perforators enter distally and supply most proximal part last; high risk of avascular necrosis of proximal pole fractures.

○ **What nerve is typically decompressed during Volkmann contracture reconstruction with a muscle free flap?**

Median nerve at all points of compression.

○ **What forearm muscles are affected most often in compartment syndrome?**

FPL, FDP; in severe cases, FDS, FCU, FCR.

○ **What areas of compression are important in decompressing the median nerve?**

Lacertus fibrosus, two heads of pronator teres, proximal arch of FDS, carpal canal; ligament of Struthers (band between supracondylar humeral process and medial epicondyle).

O   **Does Volkmann's ischemic contracture involve the anterior interosseous nerve?**

No.

O   **What is ectrodactyly?**

Partial or total absence of fingers suggesting central hand deficiency.

O   **What is typical central hand deficiency?**

Absence of third ray; usually bilateral, cleft lip/palate, congenital heart disease, syndactyly and foot involvement common.

O   **What is camptodactyly?**

Nontraumatic flexion deformity of PIP; usually bilateral; involves small finger.

O   **What is hypothenar hammer syndrome?**

Ulnar artery thrombosis; symptoms include pain, paresthesia, temperature decrease, numbness of ulnar digits.

O   **What is the treatment of a neuroma in continuity in the extremity?**

Neuroma excision and nerve grafting (e.g., with sural nerve).

O   **What influences the success of a replanted digit?**

Most importantly, mechanism of injury (crush, avulsion lower success rates); cooling of amputated part improves success.

O   **What differentiates complex and simple syndactyly?**

Complex: skin and bones are fused.

O   **When do infants with syndactyly undergo release?**

Typically by 18 months.

O   **What is the best diagnostic study for a high-flow vascular malformation in the extremity?**

MRA.

O   **What symptoms accompany ulnar nerve compression at Guyon canal?**

Weakness of grip, limited abduction/adduction of fingers, difficulty in crossing fingers, decreased sensation over ulnar-sided digits.

O   **What is the significance of dorsoulnar sensation of the hand?**

Sensation to this area is supplied by ulnar nerve fibers arising 6 cm PROXIMAL to Guyon canal.

O   **What are the most common sites of compression of the ulnar nerve?**

Band of Osborne (cubital tunnel), Guyon canal, arcade of Struthers (thin aponeurotic band from medial triceps head to medial intermuscular septum), origin of the FCU.

○ **What describes the arcade of Struthers?**

Fascial bands extending from the medial intermuscular septum that can compress the ulnar nerve.

○ **What is another name for the deep branch of the radial nerve?**

Posterior interosseous nerve.

○ **What are compression sites of the radial nerve?**

Arcade of Frohse (band over supinator), vascular leash of Henry (radial recurrent vessels that cross the nerve), ECRB, proximal supinator, distal supinator.

○ **What is the most appropriate treatment for split nail deformity?**

Full-thickness nail grafting from the toe; injured nail bed does not carry growth of new nail plate.

○ **What are the likely anatomic causes of failed closed reduction of a dorsal dislocation of the MP joint of the index finger?**

Lumbrical muscle, volar plate, FDP.

○ **What is the mechanism of failed closed reduction in this case?**

MC head protrudes volar between lumbrical and flexor tendons; volar plate is folded within the joint.

○ **What are symptoms of complex regional pain syndrome (CRPS) I?**

Otherwise known as RSD; pain, stiffness, vasomotor instability; hyperhidrosis, osteoporosis may occur.

○ **How is RSD diagnosed?**

Stellate ganglion blocks; thermography has also been used.

○ **How is CRPS characterized?**

Chronic pain that persists in the absence of ongoing cellular damage and is characterized by autonomic dysfunction, trophic changes, and impaired function. This contributes to or creates one or more of the following: clinically significant osteopenia, delayed bony healing or nonunion, joint stiffness, tendon adhesions, arthrofibrosis, pseudo-Dupuytren palmar fibrosis, swelling, and atrophy.

○ **What is the incidence of CRPS?**

5.5 to 26.2 per 100,000 person-years, and the prevalence is reported as 20.7 per 100,000 person-years. Women are more frequently affected than men, with a ratio of 3:1 to 4:1; the upper extremity is involved more frequently than the lower extremity; and fracture is the most common causative event. Incidence of CRPS after distal radius fracture has been reported to be between 22% and 39%.

○ **What drug is associated with a decreased incidence of CRPS?**

Ascorbic acid.

○ **What is causalgia?**

Otherwise known as CRPS II; persistent pain following trauma with a known nerve injury.

○ **What is most appropriate treatment following transverse nonhealing fractures of the fourth and fifth metacarpal shafts?**

Open reduction, miniplate fixation.

○ **What is the most common mode of inheritance in typical cleft hand?**

Autosomal dominant.

○ **What are the characteristics of typical cleft hand?**

V-shaped cleft, absence of central digit, syndactyly of ulnar-sided digits; associated with syndromes (EEC: ectrodactyly, ectodermal dysplasia, cleft lip/palate); cleft foot.

○ **What are the characteristics of atypical cleft hand?**

U-shaped hand that is broad; sometimes termed symbrachydactyly.

○ **What is the common cause of swan neck deformities in rheumatoid arthritis?**

Intrinsic tendon tightness.

○ **What procedures are recommended for swan neck deformities?**

MP arthroplasty, intrinsic releases, centralizing extrinsic extensor tendons; Zancolli-FDS reconstruction.

○ **What muscle harvested with a distally based posterior interosseous flap will maintain blood supply of the ulna?**

Muscle to the EPL.

○ **What fascial structures normally surround the neurovascular bundle in the finger?**

Cleland, Grayson ligaments, lateral digital sheet, retrovascular band.

○ **Where do EDC ruptures occur in RA?**

At the level of distal ulna; must differentiate from extensor subluxation.

○ **Can FDS ruptures cause swan neck deformities in RA?**

Yes, less commonly.

○ **What is Cleland ligament?**

Fascial structure lying deep and dorsal to neurovascular bundle; originates from side of phalanges and travels obliquely to skin.

○ **What is Grayson ligament?**

Superficial to neurovascular bundle; arises from tendon sheath and goes to the skin; travel volar to the neurovascular bundle; thought to be involved in Dupuytren's.

○ **What is the lateral digital sheath?**

Composed of superficial fascia on both sides of the phalanges; fibers from the natatory ligament and spiral band contribute as well.

○ **What is the most appropriate time for correction of syndactyly?**

12 to 18 months for third webspace; earlier for first or fourth webspace syndactyly.

○ **What defines complete syndactyly?**

Inclusion of the entire webspace.

○ **What supplies the sartorius muscle flap?**

The superficial circumflex iliac (SCIA) and superficial femoral arteries.

○ **What potential flaps are supplied by the lateral circumflex femoral artery?**

Rectus femoris, TFL, vastus lateralis.

○ **What is a pincer nail deformity?**

Otherwise known as trumpet nail deformity; excess transverse nail curvature; pinching of the soft tissue of the fingertip.

○ **How is trumpet nail deformity treated?**

Lateral nail matrix elevation and dermal grafting.

○ **In neonatal brachial plexus palsy, complete recovery is likely if activity is seen in the deltoid and biceps by what week?**

Week 8.

○ **What is Dupuytren diathesis?**

An early, aggressive form of Dupuytren involving knuckles, plantar fascia, and Peyronie disease.

○ **What digits are involved in Dupuytren disease? In Dupuytren diathesis?**

In Dupuytren the ulnar digits; in diathesis the radial digits.

○ **What distinguishes the location of Heberden and Bouchard nodes?**

Both seen in OA; Heberden affect the DIP; Bouchard affect the PIP.

○ **What response is sometimes seen following surgery for Dupuytren disease?**

A flare response (type of localized RSD).

○ **What is hypothenar hammer syndrome?**

Trauma to hand causing crushing of the ulnar artery at Guyon canal resulting in a true aneurysm sending emboli to the digits.

○ **What upper extremity findings are seen in thoracic outlet syndrome?**

Sensorimotor findings in C8–T1; numbness in fingers (particularly small finger); test with Roos, Adson tests.

○ **What patient population is Buerger disease seen in?**

Middle-aged smokers.

○ **What incision is used for compartment syndrome of the hand in releasing the adductor pollicis and interossei?**

Dorsal incision over the second metacarpal.

○ **What compartments are released in a hand compartment syndrome?**

Four dorsal, three volar interossei, adductor pollicis, and thenar/hypothenar eminences.

○ **What incisions are made for releasing all of the hand compartments?**

All dorsal incisions over the second and fourth metacarpals; ulnar fifth metacarpal, radial first metacarpal.

○ **What is the best means of reducing a dorsal dislocation of the MP joint of the index?**

Wrist flexion with placing pressure distally and volarly; traction places the volar plate more dorsally preventing the MP joint from being reducible and tightens lumbricals and flexor tendons.

○ **What is the likely cause of point tenderness of the base of the nail that is sensitive to cold and painful on palpation?**

Glomus tumor; bright lesion on T2 MRI.

○ **What are the two most common tumors of the hand?**

Ganglions, followed by giant cell tumors.

○ **Where are giant cell tumors usually found?**

Palmar surfaces of the wrist and hand.

○ **What is Vaughn–Jackson progression?**

Extensor tendon rupture from ulnar to radial-sided digits.

○ **What is caput ulna?**

Prominence and dorsal subluxation of the ulna causing tendon ruptures.

○ **What is done for extensor tendon ruptures in RA?**

Transfer to radial extensors; centralized over MP joints.

○ **What comprises tendon transfers for radial nerve palsy?**

Pronator teres to ECRB, FCU to EDC, palmaris longus to EPL.

○ **What is done in the Boyes sublimis transfer?**

FDS(3) transferred to the EDC(3,4,5); FDS(4) to EIP and EPL; and FCR to adductor longus and EPB.

○ **What is seen on radiographs of the hand in scleroderma?**

Calcium deposits in the soft tissue; treat with calcium channel antagonists, NSAIDs, penicillamine.

○ **What is clinically seen in the hands in hypoparathyroidism?**

Carotenemia on the palms and soles.

○ **What is pronator syndrome?**

Compression proximally of the median nerve; sensory symptoms in the median nerve distribution; decreased palm sensation.

○ **What maneuvers reproduce pronator syndrome?**

Elbow flexion with elbow in pronation, resisted elbow flexion, resisted pronation with wrist flexion.

○ **What are compression points of the median nerve?**

The supracondylar process and ligament of Struthers (from supracondylar humeral process and medial epicondyle, lacertus fibrosis (fascia of aponeurosis from biceps tendon to flexor mass), pronator teres, FDS arch.

○ **What is anterior interosseous syndrome?**

Pain in proximal forearm; weakness/paralysis of FDP of index and long, FPL, and pronator quadratus.

○ **Where is the anterior interosseous nerve compressed potentially?**

Deep head of the pronator teres, FDS(4) tendinous origin, origin of FCU, accessory FPL, palmaris profundus.

○ **What is cubital tunnel syndrome?**

Compression of the ulnar nerve at the elbow; pain over proximal forearm; weakness of FDP of ring and small and first dorsal interosseous and abductor digiti minimi; numbness/tingling of ring/small fingers; sensory deficit of ring/small.

○ **What is posterior interosseous syndrome?**

Motor deficits without sensory deficits; weakness of wrist/thumb/thumb abduction/digit extensors; radial deviation of the wrist (ECRL innervated proximally); initially weakness and pain in forearm.

○ **What likely is the site of compression of the posterior interosseous nerve?**

Arcade of Frohse.

○ **Where do most patients have compression with radial tunnel syndrome?**

At the arcade of Frohse (band over deep radial nerve entering supinator); also vascular leash, ECRB tendon.

○ **What is the primary symptom seen in radial tunnel?**

Pain rather than numbness or weakness over the mobile wad with extension, resisted supination, or passive flexion/pronation of the wrist.

○ **What motor or sensory loss is seen with radial tunnel syndrome?**

None.

○ **What is the most appropriate step for avascular necrosis of the proximal pole of the scaphoid following ORIF?**

Bone pedicle flap; based on perforators from neighboring extensor compartments.

○ **What percentage of nondisplaced scaphoid fractures heal by casting alone?**

90%.

○ **What is the incidence of complete healing in scaphoid fractures displaced by more than 1 mm?**

55% have nonunion; 50% have eventual avascular necrosis.

○ **What is Kienböck disease?**

Avascular necrosis of the lunate.

○ **What most likely prevents closed reduction in PIP dislocations?**

FDP tendon (flexion causes entrapment of the proximal phalangeal condyles); volar plate also is a potential cause of failed reduction.

○ **What is the treatment for extrinsic tendon tightness of the PIP following an old burn injury?**

Central slip release.

○ **What is the treatment for intrinsic tendon tightness?**

Release of the lateral bands.

○ **What is the sequence of replantation for a five-finger amputation?**

Thumb, followed by long or ring, with index least in order of importance.

○ **What is the sequence of reconstructing the structures of an amputated digit?**

First bone/tendon, then vein/artery, then nerves last.

○ **What position on the metacarpal is most appropriate for an index to long finger transposition?**

At the level of the metacarpal base.

○ **What is the likely effect on power grip and key pinch following a ray resection of the index finger?**

20% decrease; loss of supination strength.

○ **What is the treatment for an acute scapholunate tear?**

Open repair through a dorsal incision; Blatt capsulodesis further secures the repair.

○ **What are Mayfield classification of perilunate instability patterns?**

I: SL instability or tearing of SL and volar radioscaphoid ligaments

II: dislocation of the capitate

III: LT separation

IV: lunate dislocation

○ **What encompasses greater arc injuries in the setting of perilunate dislocations?**

Fractures of the radial styloid, capitate, triquetrum, ulnar styloid.

○ **When is scaphoidectomy recommended?**

In scaphoid nonunion advanced collapse; progressive chronic arthritis in conjunction with a proximal row carpectomy or four corner arthrodesis.

○ **What artery courses through the triangular space?**

The circumflex scapular.

○ **What are the boundaries of the triangular space?**

The long head of the triceps, teres major and teres minor.

○ **Where is the quadrangular space in relation to the triangular space?**

Immediately lateral.

○ **What comprises the quadrangular space?**

Surgical humeral neck, lateral head of the triceps, teres major, teres minor.

○ **What passes through the quadrangular space?**

The axillary nerve and posterior humeral circumflex artery.

○ **What is the period of immobilization for a nondisplaced scaphoid waist fracture?**

10 to 14 weeks in a thumb spica cast.

○ **What is the lumbrical plus deformity?**

Occurs following transection of the FDP tendon; in flexion, the lumbrical through the radial lateral band causes paradoxical PIP extension.

○ **What is the treatment of lumbrical plus deformity?**

Division of the lumbrical tendon or releasing the radial lateral band.

○ **What flexor tendon ruptures are seen most frequently in RA?**

FPL and FDP of the index because of bony spurs over the distal scaphoid.

○ **What is intersection syndrome?**

Second dorsal compartment tenosynovitis; near intersection of first and second extensor compartments; pain and swelling 4 cm proximal to wrist; proximal to Lister tubercle.

○ **What is Wartenberg syndrome?**

Compression of the dorsal sensory branch of the radial nerve between the brachioradialis and ECRL tendons; pain, numbness of dorsoradial wrist following wearing a bracelet.

○ **What length of bone is provided by the fibula free flap?**

More than 20 cm.

○ **What procedure may be done for a 1.5-cm diameter defect of the volar distal thumb?**

Moberg flap (palmar advancement flap).

○ **What is the most appropriate treatment for a full-thickness burn of the forearm?**

Early tangential excision to punctate bleeding and coverage with split-thickness skin grafts.

○ **What joints are affected in osteoarthritis of the thumb?**

CMC, STT, radiocarpal joints; initially, there is volar beak ligament failure.

○ **What are felons?**

Infections of the pulp space usually caused by *S. aureus*.

○ **What is the mechanism in congenital clasp thumb?**

Absence of the EPB and/or EPL; MP flexion and thumb adduction.

○ **Where does the first dorsal metacarpal artery travel in relation to the first dorsal interosseous muscle?**

Within the fascia of the muscle; communicates with perforators from the superficial arch near the MP joint.

○ **What is a Stener lesion?**

Palpable mass on the ulnar metacarpal head; composed of adductor pollicis fascia interposed between torn ulnar collateral ligament and MP joint of thumb.

○ **What muscle may cause carpal tunnel syndrome in a heavy laborer?**

Lumbrical. The lumbrical inserts into radial sagittal band and aids in extension of the interphalangeal joints as well as flexion of MP joints.

○ **What is the appropriate treatment of a chronic paronychia of the finger?**

Usually due to *Candida*; if topical/oral antifungals are not successful, eponychial marsupialization.

○ **What are the associated syndromes of radial club hand?**

VATER, Holt-Oram, Fanconi anemia, TAR syndrome (thrombocytopenia-absent radius syndrome).

○ **What test is performed to detect Fanconi anemia?**

Mitomycin testing to prevent pancytopenia complications.

○ **What structures are involved in Dupuytren contractures of the PIP joint?**

Central, lateral, retrovascular, and spiral cord (pretendinous band, vertical band, spiral band, Grayson ligaments, lateral digital sheath contribute to the spiral cord).

○ **What are the subtypes of the thumb-in-palm deformity in cerebral palsy?**

Type I: simple adduction contracture.

Type II: type I with MP flexion deformity.

Type III: adduction with hyperextension deformity and/or MP instability.

Type IV: type I with FPL spasticity.

○ **What level of amputation should be done for a subungual melanoma?**

At the DIP joint.

○ **What manipulations of the upper extremity will increase median and ulnar nerve length during repair?**

Shoulder abduction and elbow flexion.

○ **What is the best treatment for a 30-year-old steelworker with CMC arthritis?**

Trapeziometacarpal arthrodesis.

○ **What are the characteristics of juvenile RA?**

Exhibit wrist flexion with loss of wrist extension; carpal bone and metacarpals are deviated ulnarly, loss of IP flexion, loss of MP flexion, and radial deviation of MP joints.

○ **How common are tendon ruptures seen in juvenile RA?**

Rare.

○ **In adult RA, what direction does the carpus tend toward?**

Radial deviation and supination.

○ **What is the guiding principle in zone II flexor tendon repairs to ensure greatest motion?**

Immediate early active flexion to prevent adhesions.

○ **What spatial relation does the ulnar motor group have with respect to the sensory group in the wrist?**

Ulnar and dorsal to the sensory group; at Guyon's the motor fascicles become dorsal and radial.

○ **What is the treatment for a type IV mallet injury?**

Closed reduction and pin fixation; 30% of the articular surface of the phalanx has been avulsed.

○ **What is the treatment for a type I mallet injury?**

Stack splinting; immobilizes DIP joint in extension.

○ **What is the quadriga effect?**

Excessive distal pull by one FDP tendon; leaves other digits with decreased flexion.

○ **What is the treatment for a CMC dislocation of the thumb?**

Closed reduction by axial traction and pronation with application of pressure to the metacarpal base and pinning.

○ **What is normal total active motion for an index finger?**

90 (MP) + 110 (PIP) + 70 (DIP) = 270 degrees.

○ **What is the appropriate treatment for the third MP joint of a piano player with severe OA?**

Silicone implant arthroplasty.

○ **What is the best way to correct a supination defect in a quadriplegic?**

Redirection of the biceps tendon through the interosseous membrane.

○ **What is a Moberg flap used for?**

Volar defects of the thumb; two arteries and two nerves are included; may be advanced 1 to 1.5 cm.

○ **What are common causes of the lumbrical plus deformity?**

Distal amputations, lengthy FDP interposition grafts; excessive profundus lengthening procedures.

○ **What is the local muscle flap used for antecubital fossa wounds?**

Brachioradialis flap; based on the radial recurrent artery.

○ **What is the lateral arm flap based on?**

Perforating branches of the profunda brachii artery.

○ **What nerve palsy is occasionally seen in tourniquet usage during hand surgery?**

Radial nerve palsy.

○ **What is arthrogryposis?**

Multiple joint contractures seen at birth.

○ **What is Madelung deformity?**

Radial shortening, palmar subluxation of the carpus, ulnar head prominence; slowed growth of the ulnar distal radius.

○ **What is the treatment of most Salter fractures?**

Closed reduction with pin fixation.

○ **What is the first step in managing an above-elbow amputation 5 hours later?**

Arterial shunting.

○ **What is a longitudinally bracketed epiphysis?**

Causes angular deformity of the finger; longitudinal growth is delayed on one side while the other side of the phalanx grows normally; associated with delta phalanx.

○ **What is Secrétan disorder?**

Peritendinous fibrosis following minor work-related trauma; may be associated with lymphedema.

○ **Where do the perforators arise to supply the osteocutaneous radial forearm flap?**

Between the brachioradialis and flexor carpi radialis.

○ **What is the appearance of an enchondroma on plain films?**

Radiolucent neoplasm; thinning and expansion of the bony cortex.

○ **What is the risk of multiple enchondromas?**

Degeneration to chondrosarcomas.

○ **Following a Gustilo IIIB injury, what pulse lavage agent is likely to preserve cellular function while cleaning the wound?**

1% surgical soap.

○ **What is the earliest clinical sign of upper extremity compartment syndrome?**

Worsening pain with passive muscle stretching.

○ **What organism is associated with medicinal leech therapy during antibiotic prophylaxis?**

Aeromonas hydrophila.

○ **What sensation is detected by Pacinian corpuscles?**

Vibration.

○ **What skin component detects burning pain?**

Free endings of C fibers.

○ **What detects moving two-point discrimination?**

Meissner corpuscles.

○ **What detects static two-point discrimination?**
Merkel cells.

○ **What webspace is most frequently affected in syndactyly?**
The third webspace.

○ **What is the inheritance of syndactyly?**
Sporadic.

○ **What is Carpenter syndrome?**
Simple syndactyly, brachydactyly, broad thumbs, craniosynostosis.

○ **What is Pfeiffer syndrome?**
Partial syndactyly, broad thumbs, midface hypoplasia.

○ **What is a traumatic boutonniere deformity?**
Central slip disruption at the PIP joint with volar migration of the lateral bands; PIP flexion causes DIP extension.

○ **What causes PIP contractures in Dupuytren?**
Central cord most likely cause contractures; lateral and spiral cords can also cause contractures.

○ **What is the clinical finding of a natatory cord?**
Loss of finger abduction.

○ **What cord causes contractures of the DIP joint?**
The retrovascular cord; dorsal to the neurovascular bundle and palmar to Cleland ligament.

○ **What contractures do pretendinous cords cause?**
MP contractures.

○ **What can be used for coverage for a dorsal exposed IP joint of the thumb?**
Kite flap.

○ **What is the kite flap based on?**
First or second dorsal metacarpal artery; dorsal skin of the respective proximal phalanx is taken with the flap; superficial radial sensory nerve branch may be used for sensation.

○ **Where is the origin of the first dorsal metacarpal artery located?**
Just proximal to the bifurcation of the dorsal radial artery into the princeps pollicis and deep palmar arch.

○ **What congenital deformity is seen with a delta phalanx?**
Clinodactyly.

○ **What causes camptodactyly?**

Skin deficit, volar plate shortening, central slip deficiency, shortening of the sublimis tendon.

○ **What is the most frequent finding in late Volkmann contractures?**

Flexor muscle fibrosis.

○ **In what population of patients do Volkmann contractures occur?**

Children who have supracondylar fractures (brachial artery compromise).

○ **What nerve is most commonly involved in Volkmann contracture?**

Median nerve neuropathy most common.

○ **What is the typical clinical appearance of the hand in Volkmann contracture?**

Wrist flexion, flexion/adduction of the thumb, MP extension, PIP/DIP flexion.

○ **What characterizes intrinsic plus deformities?**

Intrinsic muscle contracture; MP flexion, PIP extension.

○ **What is a Stener lesion?**

The ulnar collateral ligament of the thumb MP joint tears and retracts proximally; the adductor aponeurosis intercedes the space and prevents healing.

○ **What treatment is done for a Stener lesion?**

Open reduction, internal fixation.

○ **What is the treatment principle behind patients with RA regarding order of progression?**

Proximal to distal sequence (i.e., elbow arthroplasty before wrist arthrodesis before MP joint arthroplasties).

○ **What diagnosis should be considered with rapid onset of psoriatic arthritis or Reiter syndrome (arthritis, conjunctivitis, uveitis)?**

HIV infection.

○ **What forearm muscles lie the deepest when considering sequelae of compartment syndrome?**

The FDP and FPL.

○ **What are known as the superficial flexors of the forearm?**

FDS, FCR, FCU, pronator teres.

○ **What are the deep extensors?**

EPL, EPB, APL, EIP.

○ **What are the superficial extensors?**

Brachioradialis, ECRL, ECRB, EDC, ECU.

○ **What are the more aggressive subtypes of BCC?**
Infiltrative, ulcerative, sclerosing, morpheaform.

○ **For a subungual melanoma of the thumb, what is the most appropriate level of amputation?**
The diaphysis of the proximal phalanx.

○ **What prevents a Clark level from being assigned in subungual melanomas?**
Absence of subcutaneous tissue in the nail bed.

○ **What maneuvers are done to preserve webspace and function following a proximal phalanx amputation of the thumb?**
Z-plasty, first dorsal interosseous tendon detachment, more proximally reattaching the adductor pollicis.

○ **What structures may be released to improve PIP motion following a severe pilon fracture?**
Collateral ligaments, volar plate, capsule, check rein ligaments; capsulectomy to improve finger motion.

○ **What borders the lunula of the nail bed?**
Sterile matrix distally and germinal matrix proximally.

○ **What percentage of people do not have a plantaris muscle on one side?**
15%.

○ **What clinical finding may be seen with a glomus tumor of the nail bed?**
Blue discoloration of the nail bed and distal phalanx erosion.

○ **Where are giant cell tumors of the hand found?**
Palmar wrists, hands, fingers.

○ **Where are mucous cysts typically located in the hand?**
They are ganglions of the DIP joint; Heberden nodes associated.

○ **What study is typically done for evaluating osteomyelitis of the calcaneus?**
MRI.

○ **What procedure may be done for osteomyelitis of the proximal phalanx of the thumb following EPL repair?**
Decortication and removal of all affected bone; IV antibiotics.

○ **What is next appropriate step for a 2-year-old child with a functional thumb but adactyly of the other digits at the level of the MP joint?**
Second toe-to-hand transfer.

○ **What is Kienböck disease?**

Avascular necrosis of the lunate.

○ **What is the end-stage result of scapholunate dissociation?**

SLAC wrist.

○ **What does the lunate appear like with perilunate dislocation?**

Triangular on A-P.

○ **What are the characteristics of scleroderma of the hand?**

Joint stiffness, "shiny" edema of the hands; may also be associated with dysphagia.

○ **What components form CREST syndrome?**

Calcinosis, Raynaud's, esophageal dysfunction, sclerodactyly, telangiectasias.

○ **A laceration over the MP joint of the thumb is likely in what extensor zone?**

V; EPL likely injured.

○ **What is the role of the intrinsics in thumb extension?**

Able to extend thumb IP joint to a neutral position.

○ **What is the treatment for a volar dislocation of the PIP joint with middle phalanx volarly subluxed?**

Lateral band and central slip repair; classically described as irreducible by closed means.

○ **What structures are injured in a volar dislocation of the PIP joint?**

Volar plate, collateral ligament, accessory collateral ligament; may attempt reduction by flexing the MP and PIP joints.

○ **What is the treatment for unstable dorsal dislocations of the PIP joint?**

Volar plate arthroplasty.

○ **What are the borders of the anatomic snuffbox?**

Volar (APL and EPB) and dorsal border (EPL).

○ **How does C7 nerve compression present?**

Weakness in the muscles supplied by the radial nerve (including triceps) and muscles in median nerve distribution (pronator teres, FCR, FDS, FPL).

○ **What is the next step in treating gangrene of the distal tip in a patient with severe peripheral vasculitis?**

Venous bypass; amputation only as a last resort.

○ **What tendon transfer may be done for severe carpal tunnel syndrome with difficulty opposing the thumb in all positions?**

Palmaris longus (Camitz) to aid the abductor pollicis longus; this is an abductorplasty.

○ **What is done for a pit viper bite to the hand?**

Fasciotomy, IV antibiotics, antivenin.

○ **What is the recommended treatment for asymptomatic pediatric carpal ganglions?**

Observation and splinting.

○ **What does the Bunnell opponensplasty involve?**

Transfer of the ring FDS.

○ **What does a Huber opponensplasty involve?**

Abductor digiti minimi.

○ **A Phalen–Miller?**

Transfer of the ECU tendon.

○ **A Burkhalter opponensplasty?**

Transfer of the EIP tendon.

○ **What is the treatment principle of the ulna in radial club hand surgery?**

Centralization of the ulna.

○ **What is the status of the thumb in type IV radial club hand?**

Absence of the thumb with the absence of the radius; scaphoid and trapezium usually absent; index pollicization may be performed.

○ **What other common syndromes are associated with radial club hand?**

VATER, Holt-Oram, TAR.

○ **What is a flag flap used for?**

Defects of the proximal or MP joints of the digits; not used for the thumb.

○ **Following a distal radius fracture ORIF, thumb pain and numbness may be due to what?**

Acute carpal tunnel syndrome; release the carpal tunnel.

○ **What procedure may be done for severe ischemic peripheral vascular disease before amputation?**

Distal venous arterialization bypass.

○ **What is the mechanism of a boutonniere deformity of the PIP joint?**

Extensor mechanism (central slip, transverse and oblique retinacular ligaments, lateral bands) becomes imbalanced; central slip injured.

○ **What is the management for a stage I boutonniere deformity?**

Splinting the PIP joint at 0 degrees.

○ **What is the likely cause of recurrent paronychia?**

Candida albicans.

○ **What do radiographs show in giant cell tumors of the hand?**

Radiolucent expansile lesions of the epiphysis; multifocal tumor.

○ **What nerve graft may be used for a 2.7-cm defect of a digital nerve?**

Terminal branch of the posterior interosseous nerve.

○ **Where is the posterior interosseous nerve located?**

Deep to the extensors at the wrist; lies in the floor of the fourth compartment radially; ulnar and deep to the EPL.

○ **What findings on radiographs are seen in pantrapezial arthritis?**

CMC and STT joint narrowing and arthritic changes.

○ **What is the length of advancement that is able to be accomplished using a Moberg flap?**

1.5 cm.

○ **What prevents being able to use a Moberg-type advancement flap in the digits?**

The digits do not have a dual arterial supply like the thumb.

○ **What are the earliest carpal bones visible on radiographs?**

The capitate and hamate; appositional growth occurs in the carpal bones.

○ **What is the last carpal bone to be seen on x-ray?**

The pisiform, at 6.5 years.

○ **What nonoperative management exists for Dupuytren?**

Collagenase, cortisone, skeletal traction, extension splinting.

○ **What is a thenar flap used for?**

Coverage of defects of the index and middle finger tips.

● ● ● COMPREHENSIVE ● ● ●

○ **Which is essential to have in the operative suite according to the Guidelines for Office-Based Anesthesia?**

Materials and equipment necessary to provide anesthesia, recovery ministration, cardiopulmonary resuscitation, and provisions for potential emergencies. This includes: suctioning apparatus, appropriately sized airway equipment, including laryngoscope blades, means of positive-pressure ventilation, intravenous equipment, pharmacologic antagonists, basic resuscitative medications, and defibrillator equipment.

○ **What effect might garlic supplements have on surgery?**

Increased risk of bleeding.

○ **When does the physician–patient relationship begin?**

It begins when a doctor has any professional contact with a patient (not necessarily in person).

○ **If you excise a lesion and perform an adjacent tissue transfer closure at the same time, can you code for both?**

No, code only for the flap closure.

○ **What is the most common genetic mutation increasing risk of VTE?**

Factor V Leiden (activated protein C resistance) present in 3% to 7% of the Caucasian population.

○ **What is the genetic transmission of male pattern alopecia?**

X-linked autosomal inheritance.

○ **What is the result of increased 5-alpha reductase activity?**

Alopecia.

○ **Regarding hair growth phases, what characterizes male pattern alopecia?**

Lengthened telogen phase; shortened anagen phase.

○ **What growth phase of hair is active growth in?**

The anagen phase; lasts 3 years.

○ **What is the pattern of hair growth following hair transplant?**

1 month of hair growth, loss of hair, and normal growth following 3 months; 6 months required for permanent hair growth into area.

○ **What is the most appropriate procedure for a patient with Hamilton class VI alopecia?**

Scalp reduction; followed by recreating the anterior hairline.

○ **What period of time should be told to the smoking patient undergoing surgery?**

Discontinue smoking 4 to 8 weeks before surgery and 4 weeks after surgery.

○ **Reanimation of the lower face 3 years following Bell palsy with resultant good eye coverage is best treated in what manner?**

Neurotized free muscle transfer using cross-facial grafts; facial muscle atrophy occurs after 18 months of absent innervation.

○ **What initiates the process of epithelial migration in healing incisions?**

The loss of contact inhibition between cells.

○ **In the setting of an electrical injury to an extremity, what concerning diagnosis should be ruled out? How is it treated?**

Suspect compartment syndrome. Treat with fasciotomy.

○ **What is the most common worldwide cause of secondary (i.e., acquired) lymphedema?**

Filariasis, infestation of lymph nodes by the parasite *Wuchereria bancrofti*. Other causes are prior surgery, radiation, infection, and tumor invasion.

○ **What is Charles procedure?**

A classic procedure used to treat lower extremity lymphedema consisting of excision of skin down to fascia and immediate autografting using the excised skin. Rarely used.

○ **Which anesthetic induction agent should be avoided in the setting of significant burns?**

Succinylcholine, which can cause hyperkalemia because of massive release of potassium from skeletal muscle.

○ **How large of an abdominal wall fascial defect can be closed with a component separation technique?**

Epigastric region: 10 cm, mid abdomen: 20 cm, low abdomen: 6 cm.

○ **What factors increase complication rates of hydroxyapatite use in cranioplasty?**

Radiation, pediatric patients, defects in the frontal region, defects greater than 25 cm^2.

○ **What are the classic features of BCC?**

Shiny, pearly nodule; telangiectasias; nonhealing ulcer.

○ **What is the preferred treatment modality for BCC of the face?**

Mohs micrographic surgery.

○ **What is the Mathes and Nahai flap classification? Name two muscles of each type.**

I	One dominant pedicle (gastrocnemius, rectus femoris, tensor fascia lata)
II	One dominant pedicle and one minor pedicle (gracilis, trapezius, vastus lateralis)
III	Two dominant pedicles (rectus abdominus, gluteus maximus, serratus)
IV	Multiple segmental pedicles (sartorius, tibialis anterior)
V	One dominant pedicle and minor segmental (pectoralis major, latissimus)

○ **What is the preferred flap for mid-thoracic spinal defects?**

Latissimus dorsi flap.

○ **What is Apligraf?**

A biomaterial containing two types of cells: cultured foreskin-derived human keratinocytes and fibroblasts on a matrix of bovine collagen. Used for difficult wounds.

○ **What is Biobrane?**

A biomaterial consisting of silicone film with embedded nylon fabric coated with porcine collagen.

○ **What is Integra?**

A bilayer membrane system for skin replacement. It consists of a porous matrix layer of bovine collagen and glycosaminoglycans covered by a thin layer of silicone. Aids in the development of a granulation bed for skin grafting difficult wounds.

○ **What is AlloDerm?**

Acellular dermal matrix derived from human cadaveric donors without epidermal and cellular components.

○ **What is Surgisis?**

A biosynthetic matrix consisting of collagen and other proteins derived from porcine small intestine.

○ **What is the most common bacteria in cat bite infections?**

Pasteurella species.

○ **What is antibiotic prophylaxis for cat bites?**

Amoxicillin-clavulanate (penicillin allergy: moxifloxacin or ciprofloxacin/clindamycin).

○ **What is the treatment for doxorubicin extravasation?**

Topical dimethyl sulfoxide.

○ **What is the biochemical mechanism of vitamin C deficiency (scurvy)?**

Vitamin C is essential for cross-linking collagen through the hydroxylation of proline and lysine.

○ **What are the pathologic characteristics of radiated skin?**

Decreased acute inflammatory response, decreased fibroblast proliferation, decreased neutrophil function, decreased tissue oxygenation, increased vessel thrombosis.

○ **What is the blood supply to the lateral arm flap? Reverse lateral arm flap?**

Posterior radial collateral artery. Radial recurrent artery.

○ **How do you reverse epinephrine-induced vasoconstriction?**

Injection of phentolamine.

○ **In cases of accidental digital self-injection of epinephrine with an EpiPen, what is the appropriate management?**

Observation. There have been no documented cases of digital necrosis following injection, and observation is indicated. Vasoconstriction lasts 90 minutes and resolves on its own.

○ **What is the best measure of fluid status in burn patients?**

Urine output, ideally 0.5 mL/kg/hr in adults.

○ **What is the most important factor in the development of decubitus ulcers?**

Prolonged pressure above end-capillary pressure (32 mm Hg).

○ **What is the treatment for eyelid ectropion secondary to burns?**

Release and grafting.

○ **What is the most common adverse outcome after labioplasty?**

Incomplete correction.

○ **What should be suspected when thrombotic events occur after heparin therapy?**

Heparin-induced thrombocytopenia (HIT), check the platelet count first.

○ **What is a dermatofibroma?**

Benign skin lesion presenting as a small (<1 cm), firm, symmetric, and regular-appearing nodule. Occurs anywhere on the body, but most commonly anterior thighs and legs. Treat with excision if bothersome or uncertain diagnosis.

○ **What is the Fitzpatrick sign?**

Skin dimples downward with lateral compression of a skin lesion. This finding is associated with dermatofibromas.

○ **What is the most carcinogenic component of sunlight?**

Ultraviolet B (290–320-nm wavelength), which is more carcinogenic than ultraviolet A (320–400-nm wavelength).

○ **What dermal structure is implicated in hidradenitis suppurativa?**

Apocrine sweat glands.

○ **HIV-positive male with painful, erythematous vesicles on the fingertip. Diagnosis? Treatment?**

Herpes simplex infection. Diagnose with Tzanck smear showing giant cells or intranuclear inclusions. Treat with antiviral such as acyclovir.

○ **What is the transmission rate following an HIV needle stick?**

0.3%.

○ **What is the risk reduction of using AZT within 2 hours following an HIV needle stick?**

80%.

○ **What is the initial treatment of frostbite?**

Rapid rewarming in a water bath (104–108°F). Avoid radiant heat source.

○ **What medications can be useful in the initial management of frostbite?**

NSAIDs (i.e., ibuprofen) provide antiprostaglandin activity that can limit secondary damage.

○ **What is the vascular risk of microsurgery in the sickle cell patient?**

Sludging leading to compromised flap perfusion.

○ **What is the mechanism of action of topical imiquimod?**

Often used for actinic keratoses and nonmelanoma skin cancers, imiquimod is thought to act by stimulating host cytokine production and induction of tumor apoptosis.

○ **What is the mechanism of action of topical 5-FU?**

Direct inhibition of DNA synthesis.

○ **What are the characteristics of body dysmorphic disorder (BDD)?**

Excessive preoccupation with a perceived physical flaw that causes significant distress and behavioral impairment. Cosmetic surgery unlikely to benefit BDD.

○ **What are the three most common pathogens of burn wound infections?**

MRSA, *Pseudomonas, Klebsiella.*

○ **The area between which two muscle layers of the abdominal wall is preserved in a component separation?**

Internal oblique and transversus abdominis (contains intercostals nerves and vessels).

○ **What type of anticoagulation has been proven to increase microsurgical anastomotic patency rate? What type of suture technique?**

No form of anticoagulation or suture technique has been consistently proven superior in improving patency rates or free flap survival.

○ **90% of all thrombotic complications in microsurgery occur in what time period?**

First 24 hours.

○ **What is the most appropriate initial treatment of calcinosis cutis in CREST syndrome?**

Debridement of calcific deposits.

○ **Which abdominal flap used in breast reconstruction has the greatest functional morbidity? The lowest morbidity?**

Greatest: bilateral pedicled TRAM flap. Lowest: SIEA free flap.

○ **When is vascular compromise most likely to occur following free flap reconstruction?**

1 to 2 days.

○ **A patient has a Mohs defect on the nasal sidewall subunit. What is the appropriate flap for a defect 10 to 15 mm? Greater than 15 mm?**

Bilobed flap. Paramedian forehead flap.

○ **What is xeroderma pigmentosum (XP)?**

Autosomal recessive defect resulting in abnormal DNA repair mechanism. Patients are prone to skin malignancies from UV exposure. Treatment is avoidance of sun exposure.

○ **A portion of what muscle may need to be taken with an ALT flap?**

Vastus lateralis.

○ **For each flap, name the arterial supply.**

ALT	Descending branch of the lateral femoral circumflex
Gracilis	Medial femoral circumflex
Tensor fascia lata	Ascending branch of the lateral femoral circumflex

○ **What is the adverse effect of nicotine on wound healing?**

Microvascular vasoconstriction.

○ **What is cutis laxa?**

A rare disorder in which abnormal elastin fibers cause hypoblastic skin. The skin of these patients does not spring back when stretched. There is an increased risk of hernia formation.

○ **What is Ehlers–Danlos syndrome?**

Also known as cutis hyperelastica, it is characterized by skin and joint laxity due to an inherited defect in collagen. Results in greater incidence of wound complications, hernia formation, and wide and thin scars.

○ **What is the recurrence rate of keloids following simple excision?**
At least 55% and reported even higher.

○ **What is the most likely result of axillary silicone granulomas following breast augmentation?**
They are a known tissue response to the presence of foreign material and should be resected when present.

○ **What is the optimal treatment for carbonaceous material embedded in the face?**
ND:YAG laser treatment (also used for road asphalt, amateur tattoo ink).

○ **What artery does the saphenous artery arise from?**
Descending genicular artery.

○ **What does the superficial femoral artery become at the knee?**
Popliteal artery.

○ **What does the lateral circumflex femoral artery arise from?**
The profunda femoris artery.

○ **What medication is most appropriate to treat heterotopic ossification?**
Etidronate.

○ **How often may heterotopic ossification occur in spinal cord injury patients?**
40%.

○ **What agent most readily decreases the depth of a phenol peel?**
Liquid soap.

○ **What effects do antibiotic ointment and taping have on phenol peel?**
Increasing the depth.

○ **What is the most appropriate treatment for a patient exhibiting a dark bluish discoloration of a TRAM flap following free TRAM reconstruction with signs of venous congestion?**
Operative intervention.

○ **What clinical appearance characterizes the end point of dermabrasion at the level of the superficial reticular dermis?**
Confluent bleeding with a coarse tissue background.

○ **When does reepithelialization begin following dermabrasion?**
7 to 10 days.

○ **What clinical appearance occurs with dermabrasion to the superficial papillary dermis?**

Sparse punctate bleeding.

○ **What theoretical gain in length is achieved with a Z-plasty angle of 60 degrees?**

75%.

Z-plasty	Length Gain (%)
30	25
45	50
60	75
75	100

○ **What is the mechanism of Botox?**

Inhibition of acetylcholine release at the neuromuscular junction.

○ **What age group characterizes keratoacanthomas?**

Men older than 50 years.

○ **What clinical appearance describes keratoacanthomas?**

Umbilicated center with a keratin plug.

○ **Where do cylindromas form?**

They are found firm, fleshy tumors of the scalp, rarely solitary.

○ **What cutaneous lesion is characteristically found on the lower extremities of young adults?**

Dermatofibroma (fibrous popular lesion).

○ **Where do syringomas form?**

In females during adolescence occurring only on the lower eyelids.

○ **For the treatment of a sacral pressure sore, what is the highest level at which bony debridement may be done without entering the dural space?**

S2–3.

○ **At what level does the conus medullaris lie?**

L2.

○ **What organisms are typically isolated in patients with hidradenitis?**

S. aureus and *Streptococcus viridans*.

O **Which sweat glands are affected in hidradenitis?**

The apocrine sweat glands.

O **Lesions around the nostrils that are culture negative but demonstrate noncaseating granulomas are indicative of what likely process?**

Sarcoidosis.

O **What systemic process is lupus pernio associated with?**

Sarcoidosis.

O **What is the appropriate treatment of sarcoidosis?**

Intralesional steroids, oral hydroxychloroquine, or methotrexate.

O **What is rhinosporidiosis?**

A chronic fungal condition of the nose caused by *Rhinosporidium seeberi* bacteria; cultures may be negative.

O **What is Apligraf composed of?**

Bilayer of neonatal epidermal keratinocytes and dermal fibroblasts within a matrix of bovine collagen.

O **What is AlloDerm composed of?**

Lyophilized cellular cadaveric dermis.

O **What is Biobrane composed of?**

Nylon and silicone fabric coated with porcine collagen.

O **Integra?**

Dermal matrix of bovine collagen and shark-derived chondroitin sulfate covered by bilayer of silastic epidermis; silicone layer is removed and skin graft is placed on underlying dermal matrix.

O **TransCyte?**

Neonatal dermal fibroblasts cultured onto a thin membrane of silicone bonded to nylon mesh and bovine collagen.

O **What are the common characteristics of von Hippel–Lindau disease?**

Hemangiomas affecting the retina and hemangioblastomas of the cerebellum/visceral organs; seizures/mental retardation.

O **What are the common characteristics of Klippel–Trenaunay syndrome?**

Port-wine stain (usually over one extremity) and overlying venous/lymphatic malformations; limb hemihypertrophy (usually the leg).

○ **What is Parkes–Weber syndrome?**

Similar to Klippel–Trenaunay syndrome but distinguished by the presence of A-V fistulas; also hypertrophy of upper extremity.

○ **What is Osler–Weber–Rendu syndrome?**

Hereditary hemorrhagic telangiectasia; AD; multiple ecstatic vessels; epistaxis, hematuria, hematemesis.

○ **What is Sturge–Weber syndrome?**

Port-wine stain in distribution of V1 and V2; may be associated with seizures, intracranial calcifications, hemiparesis, glaucoma; leptomeningeal venous malformations.

○ **What blood level is increased in calciphylaxis?**

Parathyroid hormone; protein C is decreased.

○ **What surgical interventions may be beneficial in patients with calciphylaxis?**

Debridement, skin grafting, subtotal thyroidectomy.

○ **What finding is more likely to occur in patients undergoing with the Erbium:YAG laser than with the CO_2 laser?**

Transudative wound.

○ **What laser currently is felt to be the treatment of choice for ablative resurfacing of the skin?**

Er:YAG laser (absorbs water within the epidermis a minimum of 10 times more efficiently than the CO_2 laser); photomechanical rather than photothermal process.

○ **How frequent is permanent hypopigmentation with Er:YAG versus CO_2?**

Less than 5% with Er:YAG and as much as 40% in CO_2.

○ **What physiologic changes occur in acute burn injury?**

Decreased cardiac output, decreased plasma volume, increased systemic vascular resistance, decreased capillary pressure.

○ **What characterizes the anagen and telogen phases in male pattern alopecia?**

Decreased anagen (active phase of hair follicle), increased telogen phase (resting phase).

○ **Follicles changing from terminal to villous fibers are seen in what process?**

Male pattern alopecia.

○ **How is the Parkland formula administered?**

Lactated Ringer solution (4 mL/kg/% TBSA [second and third degree only]) administered during the first 24 hours. The first half administered during the first 8 hours and the second half administered during the remaining 16 hours.

○ **What distinguishes the long duration of bupivacaine compared to lidocaine?**
Protein binding.

○ **What factor determines the potency of a local anesthetic?**
Lipid solubility—higher solubility leads to higher potency.

○ **Local anesthetics with a higher pKa have what characteristic onset of action?**
Slower onset of action.

○ **What pigmented nevus is classified as a hamartoma?**
Becker nevus (has epidermal and dermal elements); males more frequently involved; brown patches on upper trunk; hypertrichosis; underlying smooth muscle hamartoma present.

○ **Where are acral nevi typically located?**
Palmar or plantar surfaces (typically junctional or compound).

○ **What terms also describe a dysplastic nevus?**
Clark nevus, atypical nevus, or atypical mole (precursor to malignant melanoma).

○ **What is a Sutton nevus?**
Otherwise known as a halo nevus; central melanocytic nevus surrounded by halo of hypopigmented skin.

○ **What patients do Spitz nevi form in?**
In children; benign proliferation of melanocytes on face, trunk, or extremities; characterized by irregular growth phase; difficult to distinguish from malignant melanoma.

○ **What is the most likely adverse effect from topical silver sulfadiazine?**
Neutropenia.

○ **What adverse effect occurs with silver nitrate?**
Hyponatremia; penetrates tissue poorly.

○ **Sulfamylon (mafenide acetate)?**
Metabolic acidosis and pain; excellent penetration of burn eschar.

○ **What type of vascular malformation changes in size with body position?**
Venous malformation, due to its compressibility and propensity to fill with blood.

○ **What characterizes the bone adjacent to lymphatic malformations?**
Bony overgrowth.

○ **What is the first-line intervention for a large, symptomatic, macrocystic, lymphatic malformations? What about arteriovenous malformations?**

Sclerotherapy (e.g., doxycycline) for lymphatic malformations, emolization for AVMs.

○ **How often will squamous cell carcinoma develop in actinic keratoses?**

20%.

○ **What is Bowen disease?**

Intraepithelial squamous cell carcinoma; solitary lesions with red discoloration; potentially caused by UV, arsenic, viral infections, chronic trauma.

○ **Why do keratoacanthomas require excision?**

Keratoacanthomas grow rapidly over weeks and regress spontaneously; in rare instances progress to carcinoma; initially firm, flesh-colored then progress to dome-shaped nodules with umbilicated center with keratin plug.

○ **Where do keratoacanthomas typically occur?**

Face, neck, and dorsal aspect of arms.

○ **What defines a T3 melanoma?**

Tumor with a Breslow thickness of 1.5 to 4 mm.

○ **What laser wavelength has the greatest affinity for water?**

2,940 nm.

○ **Which laser is used for cutaneous vascular lesions?**

585-nm-pulsed dye laser.

○ **What is the double Q-switched Nd:YAG laser used for?**

Has a 1,064-nm wavelength; used for hair removal or tattoos.

○ **What is the millisecond pulsed Nd:YAG laser used for?**

Treatment of vascular lesions.

○ **What is the wavelength of the CO_2 laser?**

10,600 nm; mechanism of photothermal injury.

○ **Which cell type is predominantly involved in wound contracture?**

Fibroblast; TGF-beta may also contribute to wound contracture.

○ **What is the time frame for wound contracture?**

Begins 4 to 5 days after initial injury and continues until at least 21 days after injury.

○ **Which vascular lesion is characterized by an arteriole central vessel?**

Spider angioma (arteriolar malformation).

○ **Where do spider angiomas occur?**

On face in both children and adults. Treat with laser or electrocautery.

○ **Where are macular stains seen?**

On skin of neonates, not true vascular nevi.

○ **Are pyogenic granulomas true vascular malformations?**

No. They receive their blood from capillaries.

○ **What type of vascular malformation is a strawberry hemangioma?**

Venous malformation; do not grow commensurately with the child.

○ **Where is the most appropriate donor site for hair from the scalp?**

The occipital region (donor dominance greatest in the occipital region).

○ **How long must a person's hands be splinted following toxic epidermal necrolysis syndrome?**

These patients have skin sloughing at the dermal–epidermal junction; injury only to the level of superficial dermis; skin will heal without contracture.

○ **What are long-term complications of toxic epidermal necrolysis syndrome in the integument?**

Changes in skin pigmentation, complications involving eyes and fingernails.

○ **What is the mechanism of action of silicone sheeting in scar maturation?**

Increasing the static electronegative field inducing favorable wound effects.

○ **Has silicone sheeting been shown to decrease wound tension, affect contact inhibition, or regulate intracellular integrins?**

No.

○ **How is a 8 mm × 8 mm traumatic defect of the alar margin treated most commonly?**

Composite graft from the ear.

○ **What is the effect of skin treatment with topical tretinoin (retinoic acid)?**

Thinning of the stratum corneum, thickening of epidermis, inhibits binding of AP1 transcription factor to DNA by 70% (decreases collagenase).

○ **What is the recurrence rate of an ischial pressure sore after undergoing debridement/coverage?**

80% within 9 to 18 months.

○ **What is the advantage of using Integra for coverage of full-thickness burns?**

Allowing for use of thinner autografts; Integra revascularized in 2 to 3 weeks.

○ **What is Integra?**

Synthetic bilaminar membrane with dermal matrix of bovine collagen cross-linked with chondroitin sulfate covered by temporary silastic epidermis.

○ **What requirement is needed before injection of bovine collagen (Zyderm)?**

Test dose 4 weeks prior to injection (3%) allergic reaction.

○ **What supplies the secondary pedicle of the gracilis muscle flap?**

Superficial femoral artery/vein.

○ **What type of flap is the gracilis?**

Type II muscle flap (one dominant and one secondary pedicle); dominant pedicle is ascending branch of the medial femoral circumflex artery.

○ **What pedicle supplies the rectus femoris flap?**

Lateral femoral circumflex.

○ **What supplies the vastus lateralis?**

The lateral femoral circumflex.

○ **What is the recurrence rate of a BCC less than 2 cm following initial treatment?**

10%.

○ **Where is recurrence of BCC highest?**

In periorbital, periauricular, perinasal regions.

○ **What particular BCC is prone to recurrence?**

Morpheaform BCC.

○ **Which benign lesion has been shown to result from sun exposure?**

Lentigines (benign pigmented macules); do not fade in the absence of sun exposure.

○ **What are ephelides?**

Common pigmented freckles not related to sun exposure.

○ **What is xanthelasma?**

Multiple soft yellow orange plaques occurring around eyes as a result of deposition of lipid-laden macrophages.

○ **Name two type III muscle flaps.**

Gluteus maximus and rectus abdominis (dual dominant pedicles).

○ **What are type I muscle flaps?**

One dominant pedicle (gastrocnemius, TFL, vastus lateralis).

○ **What are type II muscle flaps?**

One dominant pedicle and secondary pedicle (gracilis, trapezius).

○ **What is a type IV muscle flap?**

Segmental blood supply (external oblique, sartorius).

○ **Type V?**

Dominant pedicle and multiple secondary segmental pedicles (latissimus, pectoralis major).

○ **What is an absolute contraindication for VAC therapy?**

Presence of exposed blood vessels.

○ **What auricular lesion is painful and is associated with the side down when the patient sleeps?**

Chondrodermatitis nodularis helices; painful erythematous nodule on helix or antihelix; treatment is excision.

○ **What are acrochordons?**

Skin tags.

○ **What is the most appropriate treatment following blepharoptosis after Botox?**

Use of alpha-adrenergic agonist eye drops; ocular decongestion (naphazoline); contract Mueller's.

○ **What are known complications of Botox?**

Diplopia, retrobulbar hemorrhage, globe perforation, lagophthalmos, photophobia, epiphora, ectropion, exposure keratitis.

○ **What are the immune responses in a 60% TBSA burn in a young healthy adult?**

Impairment of cell-mediated immunity; impairment of T lymphocyte function; suppression of circulating T cells; activation of T helper lymphocytes; decrease in Ig; marked decrease in IgG; increased IL-7.

○ **What is contained in Jessner solution?**

Resorcinol, salicylic acid, lactic acid, ethanol.

○ **What is Jessner solution often used for?**

Hyperpigmentation.

○ **What is the histopathologic examination of a proliferating hemangioma going to show?**

Increased collagenase, increased mast cells, multilaminate BM, plump endothelial cells, increased levels of circulating 17 beta-estradiol.

○ **What do the mast cells in hemangiomas produce?**

Heparin, stimulating capillary endothelial cell migration.

○ **What properties do vascular malformations exhibit in the endothelium and basement membrane?**

Flattening of endothelium, thinning of BM, normal quantity of mast cells.

○ **Following a partial-thickness burn, what antimicrobial dressing is applied to the wound without having to consider patient allergy?**

Acticoat.

○ **Do Biobrane and TransCyte have antimicrobial activity?**

No.

○ **What is the procedure of choice in an ambulatory patient with a grade IV sacral pressure sore?**

Superior gluteal artery perforator flap (unilateral).

○ **What is the mechanism of finasteride?**

Inhibition of 5-alpha reductase (which converts testosterone into dihydroxytestosterone).

○ **What is the most frequently seen problem with fat grafting?**

Undercorrection.

○ **Where is the greatest amount of "take" for a fat graft in the face?**

Along the nasolabial folds.

○ **Thromboxane B2 and prostaglandin F2a are thought to have what effect on tissues?**

Induction of microvascular thrombosis.

○ **What effects do prostaglandin I2 and E2 have?**

Antiplatelet activity, causing vasodilation.

○ **What is the ratio of type I collagen to type III in hypertrophic scars?**

2:1, normally 4:1.

○ **Where is type I collagen found?**

In 90% of the tissues (bone, tendon, skin).

○ **Where is type II found?**

Hyaline cartilage and eye tissue.

○ **Where is type III found?**

Skin, arteries, uterus, intestinal wall, fetal wound collagen; hypertrophic and immature scar can contain up to 30% type III.

○ **Where is type IV found?**

Basement membranes.

○ **What is the effect of deep mechanical massage on the skin?**

Collagen band accumulation in the middle and deep subcutaneous regions.

○ **Compare and contrast hypertrophic and keloid scars.**

Hypertrophic scars generally arise during the first few weeks following the initial scar, grow rapidly, and then regress. On the other hand, keloid scars appear later following the initial scar, and then gradually proliferate, often indefinitely. Both keloid and hypertrophic scars demonstrate increased fibroblast density. Keloid scars demonstrate increased fibroblast proliferation rates compared with hypertrophic scars. Keloid scars demonstrate a decreased ratio of type III to type I collagen. This is not observed in hypertrophic scars. Keloid scars demonstrate thicker, larger, and more randomly oriented collagen fibers compared with hypertrophic scars.

○ **What is Fitzpatrick type II skin characterized by?**

Usually burns, rarely tans.

Skin Type	Skin Color	Characteristics
I	White	Always burns, never tans
II	White	Usually burns, rarely tans
III	White	Sometimes burns, tans average
IV	White	Rarely burns, tans more than average
V	Brown	Rarely burns, tans profusely
VI	Black	Never burns, deep pigmentation

○ **What is the main concern for using autologous cartilage grafting?**

Risk of warping.

○ **During burn physiology, monoclonal antibodies limit the depth of injury in which zone?**

The zone of stasis.

○   **Going from superficial to deep, what are the zones of burn injury?**

Zone of coagulation, zone of stasis (microthrombi, neutrophil adherence, vasoconstriction), zone of hyperemia (vasodilation and vasoactive mediator release).

○   **What humoral factor has been shown to stimulate collagen-producing fibroblasts?**

TGF-beta.

○   **What factor increases the ability of cartilage to survive as a graft prior to placement?**

Proteoglycan matrix (composed of type II collagen).

○   **What is the required concentration of factor VIII before major surgery is undertaken?**

Hemophilia A requires 80% of normal factor VIII levels.

○   **What is the most likely finding following flap coverage of one ischial pressure sore?**

Development of a pressure sore on the opposite side from transfer of weight to contralateral side.

○   **What is a Marjolin ulcer?**

Malignant degeneration of a chronic wound edge to carcinoma.

○   **What are clinical findings of systemic inflammatory response syndrome?**

Body temperature lower than 96.8°F or greater than 101.5°F, pulse greater than 90, RR greater than 20, leukocyte count fewer than 4,000 or greater than 12,000.

○   **Wound sepsis occurs in what concentration of organisms per gram of tissue?**

10^5 per gram of tissue.

○   **Rhinophyma in an older male patient is best treated by what means?**

Tangential excision with healing by secondary intention.

○   **What mechanism occurs during tissue expansion of random skin flaps?**

Increased survival; secondary to delayed-type phenomenon.

○   **What is seen histologically with the dermis and epidermis during tissue expansion?**

Total collagen content increased; thinning of the dermis, thickening of the stratum spinosum (epidermis).

○   **Following a burn injury, what is the time limit after which secondary healing will lead to hypertrophic scarring?**

After 3 weeks, open wounds have a higher chance of hypertrophic scarring.

○   **How is embolization used in AVM treatment?**

Used to target the center of the AVM.

○ **What is the distal limit of the reversed sural artery flap when raising the pedicle?**

Pivot the pedicle at least 5 cm above the lateral malleolus (to decrease risk of disruption of the peroneal perforators).

○ **Where is the sural nerve located with respect to the short saphenous vein?**

The nerve is lateral to both the superficial sural artery and short saphenous vein.

○ **What have studies indicated regarding pain control in DIEP versus free TRAM breast reconstruction?**

Less use of analgesia postoperatively in DIEP flaps.

○ **What flap has greater abdominal wall morbidity?**

Free TRAM.

○ **What flap has greater fat necrosis?**

DIEP.

○ **What is likely to occur with trunk flexion following a DIEP harvest?**

Decrease in flexion strength.

○ **What are some of the standard accreditation necessities of an ambulatory facility?**

The American Association for Accreditation of Ambulatory Surgery Facilities (AAAASF) requires surgeons to be Board Certified or Board Eligible with a Board recognized by the American Board of Medical Specialties. A patient who underwent general anesthesia needs a responsible adult to supervise him/her for 12 to 24 hours. Surgeons are required to demonstrate that they hold unrestricted hospital privileges at an acute-care hospital within 30 minutes' driving time of the ambulatory facility. If pediatric patients are cared for, at least one member of the team needs to be certified in Pediatric Advance Life Support (PALS). Ambulatory care facilities are inspected every 3 years by the AAAASF.

○ **Which laser is used most frequently for treating lymphatic malformations?**

Erbium (2,910 nm).

○ **What are the alexandrite (755 nm) and diode (810 nm) lasers used for?**

Removing hair, blue/green pigments.

○ **What are the Nd:YAG (532 nm) and pulsed dye (585 nm) lasers used for?**

Small vascular lesions.

○ **What is the Nd:YAG (1,064 nm) used for?**

Tattoo pigments (blue, black); 2- to 6-mm skin penetration.

○ **What is the most appropriate treatment for a burn to the dorsum of the hand?**

Early excision and split-thickness grafting.

○ **What occurs to the bone surrounding cervical lymphatic malformations?**

Hypertrophy of the bone (typically the maxilla and mandible, causing open-bite deformity, prognathism, and malocclusion).

○ **What premalignant skin condition is associated with melanoma?**

Xeroderma pigmentosum (AR).

○ **What is the likelihood of malignancy with actinic keratoses?**

They harbor a 10% chance of developing into squamous cell carcinoma; treat actinic keratoses with 5-FU or excision.

○ **What is Bazex syndrome?**

X-linked; hypotrichosis, hypohidrosis, multiple BCC.

○ **What is the erythroplasia of Queyrat?**

Otherwise known as Bowen disease/squamous cell in situ affecting the penis.

○ **Where does the nevus sebaceous of Jadassohn occur?**

Head and neck; 10% may develop BCC.

○ **Of the more frequently known genetic collagen disorders (e.g., Ehlers–Danlos), which is a candidate for rhytidectomy?**

Cutis laxa (nonfunctioning elastase inhibitor); aneurysms and hernias prone to develop.

○ **What is the mechanism behind Ehlers–Danlos syndrome?**

Lysyl oxidase deficiency; joint hypermobility, thin skin.

○ **What is progeria?**

Hutchinson–Gilford syndrome; AR; growth retardation, cardiac disease, skin laxity, premature aging.

○ **What are the characteristics of Werner syndrome?**

Premature facial aging, short stature, alopecia, arteriosclerosis; cataracts; AR.

○ **What is Restylane composed of?**

Hyaluronic acid.

○ **What is Isolagen composed of?**

Autologous agent from human skin cells with an extracellular matrix.

○ **What does the deep inferior epigastric artery arise from?**

The external iliac.

○ **What are calcium alginate dressings most useful for during pressure sore treatment?**
Absorbing exudate; also may trap debris and microorganisms, but no inherent antimicrobial activity.

○ **What is most important for growth of a reconstructed ear in microtia repair?**
Perichondrium.

○ **Isolated orbital fractures most commonly occur in which bone?**
Maxillary.

○ **What are copper vapor lasers used for?**
Absorbed by red and brown pigment.

○ **The lateral thigh flap is supplied by what arterial supply?**
The third branch of the profunda femoris artery.

○ **Name the deep adductor muscles from superior to inferior.**
The pectineus, adductor brevis, adductor longus, adductor magnus.

○ **What supplies the gracilis?**
The medial circumflex artery.

○ **Name common examples of a type I flap.**
TFL, gastrocnemius, vastus lateralis.

○ **Name examples of a type II flap.**
Gracilis, abd digiti minimi, soleus.

○ **Name examples of a type III flap.**
Rectus abdominis, gluteus maximus serratus.

○ **Name examples of a type IV flap.**
Sartorius, extensor hallucis longus, tibialis anterior.

○ **Name examples of a type V flap.**
Latissimus dorsi, pectoralis major.

○ **What defines a giant congenital nevus?**
Larger than 20 cm in diameter, twice the size of the patient's palm.

○ **What is a range of melanoma risk in giant congenital nevi?**
4% to 8% (though controversial).

○ **What is the laser most appropriate for large capillary vascular malformations of the eyelid?**

The flashlamp pumped pulsed dye laser (585 nm).

○ **What vitamin has been shown to reverse the negative effects of steroid use?**

Vitamin A counteracts the negative effect on wound healing by restoring monocytic activity.

○ **What are the effects of smoking on free TRAM breast reconstruction regarding fat necrosis and vessel thrombosis?**

Generally not believed to increase the rate of fat necrosis or vessel necrosis; however, hernia, mastectomy skin flap, and abdominal skin flap necrosis may occur at increased rates.

○ **Preoperative delay of smoking for what period of time is recommended before surgery?**

4 weeks.

○ **What factors are associated with nonmelanocytic skin malignancy?**

Frequency of lifetime sunburns, sun exposure during adolescence/childhood, exposure at irregular intervals.

○ **What is the relationship of depth of sunburn and development of skin malignancy?**

No association.

○ **What is the type of UV radiation emitted by tanning beds?**

UVA.

○ **What are proposed mechanisms of dextran?**

Decreased factor VIII and von Willebrand factor, increased electronegativity, modification of fibrin, volume expansion, inhibits alpha-2 antiplasmin.

○ **What is the most appropriate duration of MMF for treatment of minimally displaced bilateral subcondylar fractures of the mandible?**

4 weeks.

○ **What are general characteristics of vascular malformations?**

Present at birth, do not regress, grow with child.

○ **What are general characteristics of hemangiomas?**

True neoplasms; develop by 1 year and then may regress spontaneously.

○ **What findings are seen with Klippel–Feil syndrome?**

Short neck, lower posterior hairline, cervical vertebral fusion.

○ **What is seen with Maffucci syndrome?**

Multiple enchondromas (mostly in hand) and venous malformations; deformities of fingers and toes; chondrosarcoma risk.

○ **What bone substitute has the capacity for osteoconduction and osseointegration?**
Hydroxyapatite.

○ **What is osteoconduction?**
The ability of a material to encourage bone to grow toward and along its surface.

○ **What is osseointegration?**
The direct chemical bonding of an alloplast to the surface of bone without an intervening layer of fibrous tissue.

○ **What are common characteristics of venous malformations?**
Dark lesions that become enlarged with dependency and change with position.

○ **What treatments are advocated for venous malformation?**
Laser treatment and wedge resection if small enough, sclerotherapy and excision for larger lesions.

○ **What protein has been implicated in breast capsule formation?**
Fibrinogen.

○ **What is cutis aplasia?**
Absence of the skin and scalp at birth; also may include the bone.

○ **What is the treatment for cutis aplasia?**
Maintaining a clean, moist wound environment; silver sulfadiazine dressing changes.

○ **What muscle is the gracilis immediately posterior to during harvest?**
Adductor longus.

○ **What muscle is posterior to the gracilis?**
Adductor magnus.

○ **What relative levels of ATP are typically found in keloid and hypertrophic scars?**
Increased.

○ **What is the general rule in using a groin flap regarding the vascularity of the SCIA artery?**
The SCIA and superficial inferior epigastric arteries have separate origins in 40% of the time; the SCIA is from the common femoral artery and travels parallel to the inguinal ligament 2 to 3 cm inferior to the ligament.

○ **What is the Parkland formula?**
4 mL/kg/% TBSA burned given within the first 24 hours; half is given within the first 8 hours and the remainder given over 16 hours.

○ **What margins are required for the treatment of Merkel cell carcinoma in the head and neck?**

Wide 3-cm margins with primary neck dissection. The standard of management is surgical excision combined with radiation therapy. Radiation therapy decreases local recurrence rates. Node-negative patients with no distant metastasis treated with surgery and radiation have 5-year survival rates of approximately 90%.

○ **When should a delay procedure be performed for a pedicled TRAM?**

In patients with risk factors for flap loss: obesity, smokers, prior radiation, or large breast volume needed.

○ **What is the treatment of a hydrofluoric acid burn?**

Administration of 10% calcium gluconate gel and local injection.

○ **What is used for phosphorus burns?**

Copper sulfate irrigation.

○ **What is used for phenol burns?**

Polyethylene glycol or vegetable oil.

○ **What is the most common adverse effect with AlloDerm lip augmentation?**

Resorption of the graft.

○ **Why should halo nevi be excised?**

Melanoma similarity; melanomas can develop in an incomplete halo; the pigmentary change or "halo" surrounding the nevus (leukoderma) not painful usually.

○ **What is the likely process seen with brown recluse spider bite treatment (dapsone)?**

Hemolysis; there is no antivenin.

○ **What is the most effective means of detecting silicone implant rupture?**

MRI; one report stated 13.4 years as the mean age; one report stated half of patients with implants 7 to 10 years with rupture or hemorrhage on MRI.

○ **What is Muir–Torre syndrome?**

AD; multiple cutaneous malignancies (BCC, SCCa, keratoacanthomas) as well as malignancies of colon, bladder, ovary, and kidneys.

○ **What is Proteus syndrome?**

Partial gigantism of the extremities; hemifacial hemihypertrophy, macrocephaly; subcutaneous lipomas; vascular anomalies (capillary, lymphatic, venous malformations).

○ **What forms of BCC are prone to recurrence?**

Sclerosing and morpheaform types.

○ **What area of the face is at increased risk for fat embolism and blindness during fat injection?**
The glabellar region; ophthalmic artery communicates with this region.

○ **What is the likely physiologic change seen in vitamin C deficiency?**
Decreased hydroxylation of lysine and proline; decreased collagen cross-linking.

○ **What are physiologic effects seen with vitamin A deficiency?**
Decreased fibronectin production and monocyte activation.

○ **What are the physiologic changes seen with a large second/third-degree burn?**
Decreased leukocyte function, T helper lymphocyte production and immunoglobulins decreased, complement activation and T suppressor lymphocytes are increased; circulating complement decreased; decreased B lymphocyte activity.

○ **How resistant are cultured epithelial autografts to infection?**
Low resistance; 100 to 1,000 colonies per cm^3 are required for infection.

○ **How resistant are STSGs to infection?**
10^4 to 10^5 colonies per cm^3 for infection.

○ **What fraction of hemangiomas are noted in the first month?**
4/5.

○ **How frequent are cutaneous horns associated with malignancy?**
May contain malignant cells; 20% seen with premalignant conditions.

○ **What is the best placement of AlloDerm for lip augmentation?**
Submucosally along the dry/wet vermilion border.

○ **Where are Spitz nevi located in children?**
The head and neck region; in adults, these are found on the extremities.

○ **What is a Hutchinson freckle?**
Otherwise known as lentigo maligna melanoma; only located within epidermal layers; invasive melanoma occurring 5% to 30%.

○ **What substance has been shown to reverse premalignant skin conditions?**
Retinoids (topical application).

○ **What arteries supply the gastrocnemius muscle flap?**
Medial and lateral sural arteries.

○ **What is the treatment of scorpion stings?**

Observation and cold compresses in adults usually; in children hospitalization with monitoring for arrhythmias, muscle spasms, airway control.

○ **What is the mechanism of cellular growth in hemangiomas?**

Hyperplasia.

○ **What characterizes amateur tattoos?**

Irregular placement of dye in the superficial dermis; small pigment particles (professional tattoos are of larger pigment sizes).

○ **What is the most frequent cause of infectious secondary lymphedema?**

W. bancrofti.

○ **What is Kasabach–Merritt syndrome?**

Marked thrombocytopenia with single or multiple hemangiomas; treat with embolization, compression, interferon, steroids, or radiation.

○ **What distinguishes ester and amide local anesthetics?**

Amides have an "I" in the prefix before the "caine" (e.g., bupivacaine, lidocaine, mepivacaine); amides are more stable and cause fewer allergic reactions.

○ **What are the phases of wound healing and the predominant cells in each phase?**

Inflammation (PMNs, macrophages; first week); proliferative (fibroblasts; 1 to 5 weeks); maturation (cross-linking of collagen; 5 weeks to 2 years).

○ **In a 3-year-old child with an oral commissure electrical burn, what is the length of time required for splinting?**

6 months to prevent microstomia.

○ **What free flap provides bone as well as a sensate skin paddle for the floor of the mouth?**

Lateral arm; radial collateral artery and posterior brachial cutaneous nerve (C5–6).

○ **What topographic portion of the humerus is used in the lateral arm flap?**

The posterolateral portion.

○ **What is the blood supply of the parascapular flap?**

The circumflex scapular artery.

○ **What characterizes the toxin of the black widow spider?**

Neurotoxin; treat with IV calcium gluconate and diazepam.

○ **What characterizes the toxin of the brown recluse spider?**
Dermonecrotic.

○ **What is Wolff law of bone grafting?**
Stress is important for survival of grafted bone.

○ **Do membranous or endochondral bone grafts last longer?**
Membranous bone grafts.

○ **What type of skin grafts grow commensurately with a child?**
Full-thickness grafts.

○ **What is the main drawback with unilaminar skin substitutes?**
Poor mechanical protection.

○ **What are advantages with unilaminar skin substitutes?**
Helpful in wound debridement, fluid absorption, decreasing bacterial count, and stimulating granulation.

○ **Bovine collagen is best injected into what skin layer?**
The dermis.

○ **What characterizes the bone formation with hydroxyapatite cement?**
Osteoconduction; peripheral ingrowth of new bone.

○ **What is the mechanism of silicone sheeting in improving scars?**
Static electronegative field increase.

○ **What is the venous drainage for the reversed radial forearm flap?**
Radial venae comitantes.

○ **What flap may be used for an ischial pressure sore and prior ligation of the profunda femoris artery on the same side?**
Gluteal thigh flap; based on the inferior gluteal artery.

○ **What is the blood supply for the rectus femoris?**
Descending branch of the lateral circumflex.

○ **What is the blood supply of the gracilis muscle?**
Ascending branch of the medial circumflex.

○ **What is the supply of the TFL?**
Ascending branch of the lateral circumflex.

○ **What is Milroy disease?**
X-linked dominant; primary lymphedema; unilateral pitting edema; normal bone growth, no hemihypertrophy.

○ **What best describes the status of the shell of a subglandular breast implant placed a decade ago?**
Loss of shell strength as compared to preimplantation.

○ **What skin lesion is found in the distribution of CN V?**
Nevus of Ota (V_1 and V_2); 80% in females.

○ **What is an ephelis?**
Pigmented freckle with normal number of melanocytes and high concentration of melanin.

○ **What areas are the nevus of Ito seen?**
In the areas of the lateral brachiocutaneous and supraclavicular nerves.

○ **Where is the nevus of Jadassohn seen?**
On the scalp and face.

○ **What is the malignant potential of the nevus of Jadassohn?**
15% develop into BCC.

○ **What is the treatment of a hemangioma of the upper lid that is obstructing the visual axis?**
Excision; amblyopia may develop in as short as 1 week.

○ **What is the percentage of hair growth if two-thirds of the hair shaft is transplanted?**
Growth in 30% of the time; hair bulb is not required for growth.

○ **What head and neck free flap allows the greatest movement of skin in relation to the bone?**
The scapular free flap.

○ **What supplies vascularity to the inferior pole of the scapula?**
Angular branch of the thoracodorsal artery.

○ **Skin grafts of what type are used for dorsal burn contractures of the hand?**
Full thickness.

○ **What population of people have Merkel cell carcinoma?**
Most frequently seen in the head and neck region of elderly women.

○ **What area of the body is most frequently affected by sebaceous carcinoma?**

Eyelid; meibomian gland.

○ **For what defects of the scalp is tissue expansion most appropriate?**

Greater than 15%.

○ **Can rhytidectomy be performed in a patient with pseudoxanthoma elasticum?**

Disorder of premature skin laxity, calcium deposition within the elastic fibers; yes, rhytidectomy may be performed.

○ **What bony landmarks are used for locating the superior gluteal artery?**

A third of the way down starting from the PSIS along a line drawn from the PSIS to the trochanter.

○ **What is the most common cause of death in paraplegics with pressure sores?**

Renal failure due to amyloid disease.

○ **What effect on epithelialization does isotretinoin have?**

Decreases epithelialization; otherwise known as Accutane; thinning of the stratum corneum.

○ **What retinoid is often used as a pretreatment for chemical peeling and laser?**

Tretinoin.

○ **What supplies motor innervation to the gracilis?**

Anterior branch of the obturator nerve; travels between the adductor longus and adductor brevis.

○ **What nerve supplies the rectus femoris?**

Femoral nerve.

○ **What supplies motor innervation to the TFL?**

Inferior branch of the superior gluteal nerve.

○ **The erythroplasia of Queyrat has squamous cell carcinoma affecting what site?**

The penis; part of Bowen disease; 15% of Bowen disease becomes invasive SCCa.

○ **What is the treatment of rhinocerebral mucormycosis?**

Emergent debridement of the sinuses and orbital exenteration.

○ **Where are keloids likely to form?**

Face, cheek, ear, shoulder, upper arm, anterior chest.

○ **What is the best treatment for a 1-cm skin defect of the upper eyelid in a 75-year-old woman?**

Skin graft from the contralateral side.

○ **What skin cream provides protection against UVA (long and short wave) and UVB?**

Zinc oxide.

○ **SPF rating is limited by what fact?**

It only rates UVB protection, not UVA.

○ **What microbe is associated with leech therapy?**

A. hydrophila; treat with Bactrim or fluoroquinolones.

○ **What happens to glucose concentration after a burn injury?**

Increases; glucose should not be added to the resuscitation fluids.

○ **What happens to cardiac output after a burn injury?**

Decreases; decreased plasma volume, increased SVR.

○ **A purple "cobblestone" lesion in an adult is likely what type of vascular malformation?**

A capillary malformation; usually in distribution of the VI and VII nerves.

○ **What is the Branham sign?**

Decreased heart rate after compression of an AVM (causing a baroreceptor response).

○ **What histologic change is seen with tretinoin use?**

Compact stratum corneum that causes smoothing of the skin; increase in hyaluronic acid, increase in epidermal thickness, increase in dermal mucin, decrease in melanin production.

○ **What adverse effects are seen with tretinoin use?**

Retin-A has been associated with erythema, crusting, and sun-sensitivity.

○ **What type of antibodies are formed in a reaction to bovine collagen?**

IgG antibodies; 3% of all patients may have a reaction.

○ **What is the collagen makeup of Zyderm?**

95% type I and 5% type II.

○ **What characteristic of full-thickness skin grafts has the most effect on inhibiting wound contraction?**

The fraction of grafted dermis.

○ **What dressings are typically used for burns of the ear?**

Mafenide acetate dressing changes; in preventing suppurative chondritis.

○ **What is the average time for maturation (time from application to removal of silicone layer) of Integra with simple gauze dressings only?**

3 weeks.

○ **During wound healing, collagen synthesis and breakdown reach a steady state at what time?**

21 days.

○ **What is an appropriate method of reconstructing the scalp following a 35% burn wound?**

Tissue expansion.

○ **What has a higher rate of infection when applied to the donor site of a skin graft—Duoderm or Biobrane?**

Biobrane.

○ **What is the best choice of flap for a 1.7-cm defect of the columella?**

Nasolabial flap.

● ● ● **REFERENCES** ● ● ●

Ablove RH, Howell RM. The physiology and technique of skin grafting. *Hand Clin.* 1997;13:163–173.

Abrahams JJ, Eklund JA. Diagnostic radiology of the cranial base. *Clin Plast Surg.* 1995;22:373–405.

Achauer BM, Adair SR. Acute and reconstructive management of the burned eyelid. *Clin Plast Surg.* 2000a;27:87–96, vi.

Achauer BM, et al. Burn reconstruction. In: Achauer BM, Eriksson E, Guyuron B, et al., eds. *Plastic Surgery: Indications, Operations, and Outcomes.* Vol 1. St Louis, MO: Mosby-Year Book; 2000b:431–432.

Achauer BM, Applebaum R, Vander Kam VM. Electrical burn injury of the upper extremity. *Br J Plast Surg.* 1994;47:331–340.

Achauer BM, et al. Vascular lesions. *Clin Plast Surg.* 1982;69:412–420.

Achauer BM. Reconstructing the burned face. *Clin Plast Surg.* 1992;19:623–636.

Achauer BM. Scalp. In: *Burn Reconstruction.* New York, NY: Thieme Medical Publishers; 1991:13–22.

Achauer BM. The burned hand. In: Green DP, Hotchkiss RN, Pederson WC, eds. *Operative Hand Surgery.* Vol 2. 4th ed. New York, NY: Churchill Livingstone; 1999:2045–2060.

Acland RD. The free iliac flap: a lateral modification of the free groin flap. *Plast Reconstr Surg.* 1979;64:30–36.

Adams WP Jr, Robinson JB Jr, Rohrich RJ. Lipid infiltration as a possible biologic cause of silicone gel breast implant aging. *Plast Reconstr Surg.* 1998;101:64–68.

Adams WP Jr. Discussion—the role of plastic surgery in congenital cutis laxa: a 10-year follow-up. *Plast Reconstr Surg.* 1999;104:1179.

Adams WP, Bengston BP, Glicksman CA, et al. Decision and management algorithms to address patient and food and drug administration concerns regarding breast augmentation and implants. *Plast Reconstr Surg.* 2004;114(5):1252–1257.

Adamson GJ, et al. Amputations. In: Achauer BM, Eriksson E, Guyuron B, et al., eds. *Plastic Surgery: Indications, Operations, and Outcomes.* Vol 4. St Louis, MO: Mosby-Year Book; 2000:1831–1843.

Adamson JE, Horton CE, Crawford HH. The growth pattern of the external ear. *Plast Reconstr Surg.* 1965;36:466–470.

Adani R, Busa R, Bathia A, Caroli A. The "kite flap" for dorsal thumb reconstruction. *Acta Chir Plast.* 1995;37:63–66.

Adcock D, Paulsen S, Davis S, Nanney L, Shack RB. Analysis of cutaneous and systemic effects of Endermologie in the porcine model. *Aesthetic Surg J.* 1998;18:414–420.

Adcock D, Paulsen S, Jabour K, Davis S, Nanney LB, Shack RB. Analysis of the effect of deep massage in the porcine model. *Plast Reconstr Surg*. 2001;108:233–240.

Afifi AM, Mahboub TA, Losee JE, Smith DM, Khalil HH. The reverse sural flap: modifications to improve efficacy in foot and ankle reconstruction. *Ann Plast Surg*. 2008;61(4):430–436.

Agur AM, et al. The neck. In: Gardner JN, ed. *Grant's Atlas of Anatomy*. Vol 7. 9th ed. Baltimore, MD: Williams & Wilkins; 1995: 556–557.

Akin S, Ozgenel Y, Ozcan M. Osteocutaneous posterior interosseous flap for reconstruction of the metacarpal bone and soft-tissue defects in the hand. *Plast Reconstr Surg*. 2002;109:982–987.

Al-Attar A, Mess S, Thomassen JM, Kauffman CL, Davison SP. Keloid pathogenesis and treatment. *Plast Reconstr Surg*. 2006;117(1): 286–300.

Aldrete JA, Johnson DA. Evaluation of intracutaneous testing for investigation of allergy to local anesthetic agents. *Anesth Analg*. 1970;49:173–183.

Alexander CS. Craniofacial anomalies and principles of their correction. In: Georgiade GS, Riefkohl R, Levin LS, eds. *Textbook of Maxillofacial and Reconstructive Surgery*. 3rd ed. Baltimore, MD: Williams & Wilkins; 1997:273–296.

Allcroft RA, Friedman CD, Quatela VC. Cartilage grafts for head and neck augmentation and reconstruction. *Otolaryngol Clin North Am*. 1994;27:69–80.

Allen RJ, Treece P. Deep inferior epigastric perforator flap for breast reconstruction. *Ann Plast Surg*. 1994;32:32–38.

Allison GR. Anatomy of the auricle. *Clin Plast Surg*. 1990;17:209–212.

Allison GR, Rappaport I. Prevention of Frey's syndrome with superficial musculoaponeurotic system interpretation. *Am J Surg*. 1993;166:407–410.

Almeida MF, da Costa PR, Okawa RY. Reverse-flow island sural flap. *Plast Reconstr Surg*. 2002;109:583–591.

Alster TS. Cutaneous resurfacing with CO_2 and erbium:YAG lasers: preoperative, intraoperative, and postoperative complications. *Plast Reconstr Surg*. 1999;103:619–634.

Alster TS. Q-switched alexandrite laser treatment (755 nm) of professional and amateur tattoos. *J Am Acad Dermatol*. 1995;33:69–73.

Alster TS, ed. *Manual of Cutaneous Laser Techniques*. Philadelphia, PA: Lippincott Williams & Wilkins; 2000:33–51, 119–134.

Alster TS, Lupton JR. An overview of cutaneous laser resurfacing. *Clin Plast Surg*. 2001;28:37–52.

Alster TS, Lupton JR. Erbium: YAG cutaneous laser resurfacing. *Dermatol Clin*. 2001;19:453–466.

Alster TS, Lupton JR. Treatment of complications of laser skin resurfacing. *Arch Facial Plast Surg*. 2000;2(4):279–284.

Alster TS, West TB. Treatment of scars: a review. *Ann Plast Surg*. 1997;39:418–432.

Alter BP. Arm anomalies and bone marrow failure may go hand in hand. *J Hand Surg Am*. 1992;17:566–571.

Alter G. Aesthetic genital surgery. In: Mathes SJ, Hentz VR, eds. *Plastic Surgery*. 2nd ed. Philadelphia, PA: WB Saunders; 2005:404–408.

Alvi A, et al. Malignant tumors of the salivary glands. In: Myers EN, Suen JY, eds. *Cancer of the Head and Neck*. Philadelphia, PA: WB Saunders; 1996:525–527.

Amadio PC, et al. Fractures of the carpal bones. In: Green DP, Hotchkiss RN, Pederson WC, eds. *Operative Hand Surgery*. Vol 1. 4th ed. New York, NY: Churchill Livingstone; 1999:809–864.

Amadio PC, Mackinnon SE, Merritt WH, Brody GS, Terzis JK. Reflex sympathetic dystrophy syndrome: consensus report of an ad hoc committee of the American Association of Hand Surgery on the definition of reflex sympathetic dystrophy syndrome. *Plast Reconstr Surg*. 1991;87:371–375.

American Association for Accreditation of Ambulatory Surgery Facilities, Inc. Regular Standards and Checklist for Accreditation of Ambulatory Surgery Facilities. Version 13, August 2011. Available at http://www.aaaasfsurveyors.org/asf_web/PDF%20FILES/ASC%20Standards%20and%20Checklist%20Version%2013.pdf; accessed 25 March, 2013.

American Association for Accreditation of Ambulatory Surgery Facilities, Inc. Procedural Standards and Checklist for Accreditation of Ambulatory Surgery Facilities. Published August 2011. Available at www.aaaasf.org.

American Joint Committee on Cancer. *Manual for Staging of Cancer*. 4th ed. Philadelphia, PA: JB Lippincott; 1992.

American Medical Association. *CPT 2014 Professional Edition*. Chicago, IL: American Medical Association; 2013.

American Medical Association. *Current Procedural Terminology 2009: Professional Edition*. Chicago, IL: Prentice Hall; 2008.

American Medical Association. *Guides to the Evaluation of Permanent Impairment*. 4th ed. Chicago, IL: American Medical Association; 1995:18–20.

American Society of Anesthesiologists Task Force on Sedation and Analgesia by Non-Anesthesiologists. Practice guidelines for sedation and analgesia by non-anesthesiologists. *Anesthesiology*. 2002;96(4):1004–1017.

American Society of Anesthesiologists. Guidelines for office-based anesthesia. 2004.

Aminoff M. Nervous system. In: Tierney LM Jr, McPhee SJ, Papadakis MA, eds. *Medical Diagnosis and Treatment.* 38th ed. Stamford, CT: Appleton & Lange; 1999:932.

Anderson JE, ed. *Grant's Atlas of Anatomy.* 8th ed. Baltimore, MD: Williams & Wilkins; 1983.

Anderson RL, Dixon RS. Aponeurotic ptosis surgery. *Arch Ophthalmol.* 1979;97:1123–1128.

Andreason TJ, Green SD, Childers BJ. Massive infectious soft tissue injury: diagnosis and management of necrotizing fasciitis and purpura fulminans. *Plast Reconstr Surg.* 2001;107:1025–1034.

Angel MF. Beneficial effects of staphage lysate in treatment of chronic recurrent hidradenitis suppurativa. *Surg Forum.* 1987;38:111.

Angelides AC. Ganglions of the hand and wrist. In: Green DP, Hotchkiss RN, Pederson WC, eds. *Operative Hand Surgery.* Vol 2. 4th ed. New York, NY: Churchill Livingstone; 1999:2171–2183.

Angrigiani C, Grilli D, Dominikow D, Zancolli EA. Posterior interosseous reverse forearm flap: experience with 80 consecutive cases. *Plast Reconstr Surg.* 1993;92:285–293.

Anthony JP, Mathes SJ, Alpert BS. The muscle flap in the treatment of chronic lower extremity osteomyelitis: results in patients over 5 years after treatment. *Plast Reconstr Surg.* 1991;88:311–318.

Anthony JP, Mathes SJ. Update on chronic osteomyelitis. *Clin Plast Surg.* 1991;18:515–523.

Antia NH, Buch VI. Chondrocutaneous advancement flap for the marginal defect of the ear. *Plast Reconstr Surg.* 1967;39:472–477.

Antonyshyn O. Principles in management of facial injuries. In: Georgiade GS, Riefkohl R, Levin LS, eds. *Textbook of Maxillofacial and Reconstructive Surgery.* 3rd ed. Baltimore, MD: Williams & Wilkins; 1997:339–350.

Anvar BA, Evans BC, Evans GR. Lip reconstruction. *Plast Reconstr Surg.* 2007;120(4):57e–64e.

Apesos J, Muntzing MG 2nd. Autologen. *Clin Plast Surg.* 2000;27:507–513.

Apfelberg DB, Manchester GH. Decorative and traumatic tattoo biophysics and removal. *Clin Plast Surg.* 1987;14(2):243–251.

Arca E, Taştan HB, Akar A, Kurumlu Z, Gür AR. An open, randomized, comparative study of oral fluconazole, itraconazole and terbinafine therapy in onychomycosis. *J Dermatol Treatment.* 2002;13:3–9.

Arey LB, ed. *Developmental Anatomy.* 26th ed. Philadelphia, PA: WB Saunders; 1970.

Argenta LC, Marks MW, Pasyk KA. Advances in tissue expansion. *Clin Plast Surg.* 1985;12:159–171.

Argenta LC, VanderKolk C, Friedman RJ, Marks M. Refinements in reconstruction of congenital breast deformities. *Plast Reconstr Surg.* 1985;76:73–82.

Argenta LC, Morykwas MJ. Vacuum-assisted closure: a new method for wound control and treatment: clinical experience. *Ann Plast Surg.* 1997;38:563–577.

Ariyan S, et al. Radiation effects: biologic and surgical considerations. In: McCarthy JG, ed. *Plastic Surgery.* Vol 1. Philadelphia, PA: WB Saunders; 1990:831.

Ariyan S. Sternocleidomastoid muscle and musculocutaneous flap. In: Strauch B, Vasconez LO, Hall-Findlay EJ, eds. *Grabb's Encyclopedia of Flaps.* Vol 1. Boston, MA: Little Brown & Co; 1990:485–491.

Armstrong MB, Villalobos RE, Leppink DM. Free-tissue transfer for lower-extremity reconstruction in the immunosuppressed diabetic transplant recipient. *J Reconstr Microsurg.* 1997;13:1–5.

Arnaud E, Meneses P, Lajeunie E, Thorne JA, Marchac D, Renier D. Postoperative mental and morphological outcome for nonsyndromic brachycephaly. *Plast Reconstr Surg.* 2002;110:6–12.

Arnold J. Pursuing the perfect strip: harvesting donor strips with minimal hair transection. *Internat J Aesthet Restorative Surg.* 1995;3:148–153.

Arnold M, Barbul A. Nutrition and wound healing. *Plast Reconstr Surg.* 2006;117(7 Suppl):42S–58S.

Aronson J, Shen X. Experimental healing of distraction osteogenesis comparing metaphyseal with diaphyseal sites. *Clin Orthop Relat Res.* 1994;(301):25–30.

Aronson J. Experimental and clinical experience with distraction osteogenesis. *Cleft Palate Craniofac J.* 1994;31:473–482.

Aronson J, Harrison B, Boyd CM, Cannon DJ, Lubansky HJ. Mechanical induction of osteogenesis: the importance of pin rigidity. *J Ped Orthop.* 1988;8:396–401.

Aronson J. Principles of distraction osteogenesis: the orthopedic experience. In: McCarthy JG, ed. *Distraction of the Craniofacial Skeleton.* New York, NY: Springer-Verlag; 1999:55–56.

Arturson MG. The pathophysiology of severe thermal injury. *J Burn Care Rehabil.* 1985;6:129–146.

Ash MM, et al. Clinical occlusion. In: Ash MM, Ramfjord S, eds. *Occlusion.* 4th ed. Philadelphia, PA: WB Saunders; 1995:50–62.

Apesos J, Muntzing MG 2nd. Autologen. *Clin Plast Surg.* 2000;27:507–513.

Athanasian EA, Wold LE, Amadio PC. Giant cell tumors of the bones of the hand. *J Hand Surg Am.* 1997;22:91–98.

Athanasian EA. Bone and soft tissue tumors. In: Green DP, Hotchkiss RN, Pederson WC, eds. *Operative Hand Surgery.* Vol 3. 4th ed. New York, NY: Churchill Livingstone; 1999:2223–2253.

Atiyeh BS, Hashim HA, El-Douaihy Y, Kayle DI. Perinipple round-block technique for correction of tuberous/tubular breast deformities. *Aesthetic Plast Surg.* 1998;22:284–288.

Attinger C, Cooper P. Soft tissue reconstruction for calcaneal fractures or osteomyelitis. *Ortho Clin North Am.* 2001;32:135–170.

Ausprunk DH, Folkman J. Migration and proliferation of endothelial cells in preformed and newly formed blood vessels during tumor angiogenesis. *Microvasc Res.* 1977;14:53–65.

Austad ED. Breast implant-related silicone granulomas: the literature and litigation. *Plast Reconstr Surg.* 2002;109:1724–1730.

Ayliffe P, et al. Nasoethmoid fractures. In: Booth PW, Schendel SA, Hausamen JE, eds. *Maxillofacial Surgery.* Vol 1. London, UK: Churchill Livingstone; 1999:141–159.

Back SM. Two new cutaneous flaps: the medial and lateral thigh flaps. *Plast Reconstr Surg.* 1983;71:354–365.

Bafaqeeh SA, Al-Qattan MM. Simultaneous open rhinoplasty and alar base excision: is there a problem with the blood supply of the nasal tip and columellar skin? *Plast Reconstr Surg.* 2000;105:344–347.

Bahr W, Bagambisa FB, Schlegel G, Schilli W. Comparison of transcutaneous incisions used for exposure of the infraorbital rim and orbital floor: a retrospective study. *Plast Reconstr Surg.* 1992;90:585–591.

Bailey AJ, Bazin S, Sims TJ, Le Lous M, Nicoletis C, Delaunay A. Characteristics of the collagen of human hypertrophic and normal scars. *Biochem Biophys Acta.* 1975;405:412–421.

Baird WL, et al. Maxillofacial trauma. In: Jurkiewicz JM, Krizek TJ, Mathes SJ, et al., eds. *Plastic Surgery: Principles and Practice.* Vol 1. Philadelphia, PA: Mosby-Year Book; 1990:231–270.

Baker DC, Conley J. Avoiding facial nerve injuries in rhytidectomy. Anatomical variations and pitfalls. *Plast Reconstr Surg.* 1979;64:781–795.

Baker DC, Strauss RB. The physiologic treatment of nasal obstruction. *Clin Plast Surg.* 1977;4:121–130.

Baker DC. Complications of cervicofacial rhytidectomy. *Clin Plast Surg.* 1983;10:543–562.

Baker DC. Facial paralysis. In: McCarthy JG, ed. *Plastic Surgery.* Vol 3. Philadelphia, PA: WB Saunders; 1990:2237–2319.

Baker JL Jr. A practical guide to ultrasound-assisted lipoplasty. *Clin Plast Surg.* 1999;26:363–368.

Baker S. Orthognathic Surgery. In: Thorne CH, Chung KC, Gosain AK, et al., eds. *Grabb and Smith's Plastic Surgery.* 7th ed. Philadelphia, PA: Lippincott Williams & Wilkins; 2013:252.

Baker TJ, et al. Chemical peeling and dermabrasion: injectable collagen. In: McCarthy JG, ed. *Plastic Surgery.* Vol 1. Philadelphia, PA: WB Saunders; 1990:781–784.

Baker TJ, Stuzin JM, Baker TM, eds. *Facial Skin Resurfacing.* St Louis, MO: Quality Medical Publishing; 1998.

Baker TM. Dermabrasion. As a complement to aesthetic surgery. *Clin Plast Surg.* 1998;25:81–88.

Balakrishnan A, Bailey CM. Lymphangioma of the tongue: a review of pathogenesis, treatment, and the use of surface laser photocoagulation. *J Otolaryngol Otol.* 1991;105:924–929.

Bang H, Kojima T, Hayashi H. Palmar advancement flap with the V-Y closure for thumb tip injuries. *J Hand Surg Am.* 1992;17:933–944.

Banks ND, Redett RJ, Mofid MZ, Manson PN. Cutis laxa: clinical experience and outcomes. *Plast Reconstr Surg.* 2003; 111(7):2434–2442.

Bannister LH. Alimentary system. In: Bannister LH, Berry MM, Collins P, et al., eds. *Gray's Anatomy.* New York, NY: Churchill Livingstone; 1995: 1683–1812.

Bannister LH, Berry MM, Williams PL, eds. *Gray's Anatomy: The Anatomical Basis of Medicine and Surgery.* 38th ed. New York, NY: Churchill Livingstone; 1995:1392–1395.

Baran NK, Horton CE. Growth of skin grafts, flaps, and scars in young minipigs. *Plast Reconstr Surg.* 1972;50:487–496.

Barber HD, et al. Mandibular fractures. In: Fonseca RJ, Walker RV, eds. *Oral and Maxillofacial Trauma.* Vol 1. 2nd ed. Philadelphia, PA: WB Saunders; 1997:473–489.

Barfred T. The hypogastric (Shaw) skin flap. In: Strauch B, Vasconex LO, eds. *Grabb's Encyclopedia of Flaps.* Boston, MA: Little Brown & Co; 1990:1101–1104.

Barker JR, Haws MJ, Brown RE, Kucan JO, Moore WD. Magnetic resonance imaging of severe frostbite injuries. *Ann Plast Surg.* 1997;38:275–279.

Barnett MP. Labial incompetence: a marker for progressive bone resorption in Silastic chin augmentation. *Plast Reconstr Surg.* 1997;100:553–554.

Barnhill RL. Malignant melanoma, dysplastic nevi, and Spitz tumors: histologic classification and characteristics. *Clin Plast Surg.* 2000;27:331–360.

Barnsley GP, Sigurdson LJ, Barnsley SE. Textured surface breast implants in the prevention of capsular contracture among breast augmentation patients: a meta-analysis of randomized controlled trials. *Plast Reconstr Surg.* 2006;117(7):2182–2190.

Barnum M, Mastey RD, Weiss AP, Akelman E. Radial tunnel syndrome. *Hand Clin.* 1996;12:679–689.

Barrera A. Micrograft and minigraft megasession hair transplantation results after a single session. *Plast Reconstr Surg.* 1997;100: 1524–1530.

Barrera A. The use of micrografts and minigrafts for the treatment of burn alopecia. *Plast Reconstr Surg.* 1999;103:581–584.

Barrie KA, Tomak SL, Cholewicki J, Wolfe SW. The role of multiple strands and locking sutures on gap formation of flexor tendon repairs during cylindrical loading. *J Hand Surg Am.* 2000;25:714–720.

Bartlett SP, et al. Craniosynostosis syndromes. In: Aston SJ, Beasley RW, Thorne CH, eds. *Grabb & Smith's Plastic Surgery.* 5th ed. Philadelphia, PA: Lippincott-Raven; 1997:295–304, 325–326.

Bartlett SP, et al. Mandibulofacial dysostosis. In: Lin KY, Ogle RC, Jane JA, eds. *Craniofacial Surgery: Science and Surgical Technique.* Philadelphia, PA: WB Saunders; 2002:288.

Bartlett SP, Lin KY, Grossman R, Katowitz J. The surgical management of orbitofacial dermoids in the pediatric patient. *Plast Reconstr Surg.* 1993;91:1208–1215.

Barton FE Jr, et al. Acquired deformities of the nose. In: McCarthy JG, ed. *Plastic Surgery.* Vol 3. Philadelphia, PA: 1990:1924–2008.

Barton FE Jr. Aesthetic aspects of nasal reconstruction. *Clin Plast Surg.* 1988;15:155–166.

Barton FE, et al. Direct fixation of the malar pad. In: Menick FJ, ed. *Facial Aesthetic Surgery.* Philadelphia, PA: WB Saunders; 1997: 329–355.

Barton FE. Rhytidectomy and the nasolabial fold. *Plast Reconstr Surg.* 1992;90:601–607.

Bass LS. Understanding laser–tissue interactions helps predict clinical effects (letter). *Plast Reconstr Surg.* 1995;95:607–608.

Bassett CA. Clinical implications of cell function in bone grafting. *Clin Orthop Relat Res.* 1972;87:49–59.

Bauer BS, et al. Congenital deformities of the ear. In: Bentz, ed. *Pediatric Plastic Surgery.* Stamford, CT: Appleton & Lange; 1998:359.

Baum Ra, et al. Multicenter trial to evaluate vascular magnetic resonance angiography of the lower extremity. *JAMA.* 1995;274:875–880.

Baumann A, Ewers R. Use of preseptal transconjunctival approach in orbit reconstruction surgery. *J Oral Maxillofac Surg.* 2001;59: 287–291.

Baylis HI, et al. Complications of lower blepharoplasty. In: Putterman AM, ed. *Cosmetic Oculoplastic Surgery.* 2nd ed. Philadelphia, PA: WB Saunders; 1993:356–363.

Bays RA. Surgery for internal derangement. In: Bays RA, Quinn PD, eds. *Oral and Maxillofacial Surgery.* Philadelphia, PA: WB Saunders; 2000:275–300.

Beahrs OH, et al. *Manual for Staging of Cancer—American Joint Committee on Cancer.* 3rd ed. Philadelphia, PA: JB Lippincott; 1988:27–32.

Becker GD, Adams LA, Levin BC. Nonsurgical repair of perinasal skin defects. *Plast Reconstr Surg.* 1991;88:768–776.

Bednar MS, Weiland AJ, Light TR. Osteoid osteoma of the upper extremity. *Hand Clin.* 1995;11:211–221.

Beekman WH, van Straalen WR, Hage JJ, Taets van Amerongen AH, Mulder JW. Imaging signs and radiologists' jargon of ruptured breast implants. *Plast Reconstr Surg.* 1998;102:1281–1289.

Beekman WH, Feitz R, Hage JJ, Mulder JW. Life span of silicone gel-filled mammary prostheses. *Plast Reconstr Surg.* 1997;100: 1723–1726.

Beer GM, Kompatscher P. A new technique for the treatment of lacrimal gland prolapse in blepharoplasty. *Aesthet Plast Surg.* 1994;18:65–69.

Beimer E, Stock W. Total thumb reconstruction: a one-stage reconstruction using an osteocutaneous forearm flap. *Br J Plast Surg.* 1983;36:52–55.

Bell ML. Scalp reduction. *Clin Plast Surg.* 1982;9:269–278.

Berde CB, et al. Local anesthetics. In: *Anesthesia.* 5th ed. New York, NY: Churchill Livingstone; 2000:516.

Berdoll MS, et al. *Toxic Shock Syndrome.* Boston, MA: CRC Press; 1991:33–45.

Berger RA, et al. Arthroplasty in the hand and wrist. In: Green DP, Hotchkiss RN, Pederson WC, eds. *Operative Hand Surgery.* Vol 1. 4th ed. New York, NY: Churchill Livingstone; 1999:147–191.

Berger RA. A method of defining palpable landmarks for the ligament-splitting dorsal wrist capsulotomy. *J Hand Surg Am.* 2007; 32(8):1291–1295.

Bergman RA, et al. *Compendium of Human Anatomic Variation.* 1998:12–27.

Berkovitz BKB, Moxham BJ. The face. In: Berkovitz BKB, Moxham BJ, eds. *Head and Neck Anatomy: A Clinical Reference.* London, UK: Informa Healthcare; 2002:108–113.

Berman B, Flores F. The treatment of hypertrophic scars and keloids. *Eur J Dermatol.* 1998;8:591–595.

Bernard SL. Reconstruction of the burned nose and ear. *Clin Plast Surg.* 2000;27:97–112.

Bessette RW, et al. Temporomandibular joint dysfunction. In: Aston SJ, Beasley RW, Thorne CH, eds. *Grabb & Smith's Plastic Surgery.* 5th ed. Philadelphia, PA: Lippincott-Raven; 1997:345.

Bettinger PC, Linscheid RL, Berger RA, Cooney WP 3rd, An KN. An anatomic study of the stabilizing ligaments of the trapezium and trapeziometacarpal joint. *J Hand Surg Am.* 1999;24(4):786–798.

Betts NJ, et al. Soft tissue changes associated with orthognathic surgery. In: *Modern Practice in Orthognathic and Reconstructive Surgery.* Philadelphia, PA: WB Saunders; 1992:2170–2209.

Bhandari M, Adili A, Schemitsch EH. The efficacy of low-pressure lavage with different irrigating solutions to remove adherent bacteria from bone. *J Bone Joint Surg Am.* 2001;83:412–419.

Bhandari PS. Total ear reconstruction in post burn deformity. *Burns.* 1998;24:661–670.

Bhawan J, Olsen E, Lufrano L, Thorne EG, Schwab B, Gilchrest BA. Histological evaluation of the long term effects of tretinoin on photodamaged skin. *J Dermatol Sci.* 1996;11:177–182.

Bibbo C. Plantar heel reconstruction with a sensate plantar medial artery musculocutaneous pedicled island flap after wide excision of melanoma. *J Foot Ankle Surg.* 2012;51(4):504–508.

Binder WJ. Submalar augmentation. An alternative to face lift surgery. *Arch Otolaryngol Head Neck Surg.* 1981;115:797–802.

Bishop AT, et al. Flexor mechanism reconstruction and rehabilitation. In: Peimer CA, ed. *Surgery of the Hand and Upper Extremity.* Vol 2. New York, NY: McGraw-Hill; 1996:1139.

Bite U, Jackson IT, Forbes GS, Gehring DG. Orbital volume measurements in enophthalmos using three-dimensional CT imaging. *Plast Reconstr Surg.* 1985;75:502–508.

Blackburn WD Jr, Grotting JC, Everson MP. Lack of evidence of systemic inflammatory rheumatic disorders in symptomatic women with breast implants. *Plast Reconstr Surg.* 1997;99:1054–1060.

Blackman JR. Spider bites. *J Am Board Fam Pract.* 1995;8:288–294.

Blaisdell FW, Lim RC Jr, Hall AD, Thomas AN. Revascularization of severely ischemic extremities with an arteriovenous fistula. *Am J Surg.* 1966;112:166–174.

Blatt G, et al. Scapholunate injuries. In: Lichtman DM, Alexander AH, eds. *The Wrist and Its Disorders.* Philadelphia PA: WB Saunders; 1997:268–306.

Blondeel PN, Hijjawi J, Depypere H, Roche N, Van Landuyt K. Shaping the breast in aesthetic and reconstructive breast surgery: an easy three-step principle. *Plast Reconstr Surg.* 2009;123(2):455–462.

Blondeel PN. Refinements in free flap breast reconstruction: the free bilateral deep inferior epigastric perforator flap anastomosed to the internal mammary artery. *Br J Plast Surg.* 1997;50:322.

Blondeel PN. The sensate free superior gluteal artery perforator (S-GAP) flap: a valuable alternative in autologous breast reconstruction. *Br J Plast Surg.* 1999; 52:185–193.

Boles DS, Schmidt CC. Pyogenic flexor tenosynovitis. *Hand Clin.* 1998;14:567–578.

Boon LM, MacDonald DM, Mulliken JB. Complications of systemic corticosteroid therapy for problematic hemangioma. *Plast Reconstr Surg.* 1999;104:1616–1623.

Bosker FS, Cytryn AS, Putterman AM, Marschall MA. Postoperative mydriasis after repair of orbital floor fracture. *Am J Ophthalmol.* 1993;115:372–375.

Bostwick J 3rd, ed. *Plastic and Reconstructive Breast Surgery.* St Louis, MO: Quality Medical Publishing; 1990.

Botte MJ, et al. Compartment syndrome and Volkmann's contracture. In: Peimer CA, ed. *Surgery of the Hand and Upper Extremity.* Vol 2. New York, NY: McGraw-Hill; 1996:1539–1558.

Botte MJ, Keenan MA, Gelberman RH. Volkmann's ischemic contracture of the upper extremity. *Hand Clin.* 1998;14:483–497.

Boussen H, et al. Chemotherapy of metastatic and/or recurrent undifferentiated nasopharyngeal carcinoma with cisplatin, bleomycin, and fluorouracil. *J Clin Oncol.* 1991;9:1675–1681.

Boutin RD, Brossmann J, Sartoris DJ, Reilly D, Resnick D. Update on imaging of orthopedic infections. *Orthop Clin North Am.* 1998;29:41–66.

Bove A, Chiarini S, D'Andrea V, Di Matteo FM, Lanzi G, De Antoni E. Facial nerve palsy: which flap? Microsurgical, anatomical, and functional considerations. *Microsurgery.* 1998;18:286–289.

Bovet JL, Nassif TM, Guimberteau JC, Baudet J. The vastus lateralis musculocutaneous flap in the repair of trochanteric pressure sores: technique and indications. *Plast Reconstr Surg.* 1982;69:830–834.

Bowers WH, et al. Treatment of chronic disorders of the distal radioulnar joint. In: Lichtman DM, ed. *The Wrist and Its Disorders.* 2nd ed. Philadelphia, PA: WB Saunders; 1997:438.

Bowers WH. The distal radioulnar joint. In: Green DP, Hotchkiss RN, Pederson WC, eds. *Operative Hand Surgery*. Vol 1. 4th ed. New York, NY: Churchill Livingstone; 1999:1019–1021.

Boyd J, et al. Lip cancer. In: Medina JE, et al., eds. *Clinical Practice Guidelines for the Diagnosis and Management of Cancer of the Head and Neck*. American Society for Head and Neck Surgeons; 1996:17–25.

Boyd JB, Mulliken JB, Kaban LB, Upton J 3rd, Murray JE. Skeletal changes associated with vascular malformations. *Plast Reconstr Surg*. 1984;74:789–797.

Boyer MI, Gelberman RH. Complications of the operative treatment of Dupuytren's disease. *Hand Clin*. 1999;15:161–166.

Boyer MI, Mih AD. Microvascular surgery in the reconstruction of congenital hand anomalies. *Hand Clin*. 1998;14:135–142.

Boyes JH, ed. *Bunnell's Surgery of the Hand*. 5th ed. Philadelphia, PA: JB Lippincott; 1970:653.

Bradley PJ. Tumors of the salivary gland. In: Jones AS, Phillips DE, Hilgers FJ, eds. *Diseases of the Head and Neck, Nose and Throat*. London, UK: Arnold; 1998:329–346.

Brashear A, Gordon MF, Elovic E, et al. Intramuscular injection of botulinum toxin for treatment of wrist and finger spasticity after a stroke. *N Engl J Med*. 2002;347:395–400.

Braunstein GD, Glassman HA. Gynecomastia. *Curr Ther Endocrinol Metab*. 1997;6:401–404.

Braunstein GD. Clinical practice. Gynecomastia. *NEnglJMed*. 2007;357(12):1229–1237.

Braunwald E, et al. *Harrison's Principles of Internal Medicine*. Vol 2. 15th ed. New York, NY: McGraw-Hill; 2001:2036–2037.

Bray PW, Bell RS, Bowen CV, Davis A, O'Sullivan B. Limb salvage surgery and adjuvant radiotherapy for soft tissue sarcomas of the forearm and hand. *J Hand Surg Am*. 1997;22(3):495–503.

Brcic A. Primary tangential excision for hand burns. *Hand Clin*. 1990;6:211–219.

Brent B. Reconstruction of the auricle. In: McCarthy JG, ed. *Plastic Surgery*. Vol 3. Philadelphia, PA: WB Saunders; 1990;2094–2152.

Brent B. Repair and grafting of cartilage in perichondrium. In: McCarthy JG, ed. *Plastic Surgery*. Vol 1. Philadelphia, PA: WB Saunders; 1990:559–582.

Brent B. Technical advances in ear reconstruction with autogenous rib cartilage grafts: personal experience with 1200 cases. *Plast Reconstr Surg*. 1999;104:319–334.

Brink RR. Management of true ptosis of the breast. *Plast Reconstr Surg*. 1993;91:657–662.

Britton EN, et al. Acute flexor tendon injury: repair and rehabilitation. In: Peimer CA, ed. *Surgery of the Hand and Upper Extremity*. Vol 1. New York, NY: McGraw-Hill; 1996:1113–1132.

Brody GA, Maloney WJ, Hentz VR. Digital replantation applying the leech Hirudo medicinalis. *Clin Orthop Relat Res*. 1989;(245):133–137.

Brody GS. On the safety of breast implants. *Plast Reconstr Surg*. 1997;100:1309–1313.

Brody GS. Silicone technology for the plastic surgeon. *Clin Plast Surg*. 1988;15:517–520.

Brody HJ. Complications of chemical resurfacing. *Dermatol Clin*. 2001;19:427–438.

Brody HJ. Update on chemical peels. *Adv Dermatol*. 1992;7:275–288.

Broughton G 2nd, Crosby MA, Coleman J, Rohrich RJ. Use of herbal supplements and vitamins in plastic surgery: a practical review. *Plast Reconstr Surg*. 2007;119(3):48e–66e.

Broughton G 2nd, Janis JE, Attinger CE. Wound healing: an overview. *Plast Reconstr Surg*. 2006; 117(7 Suppl):1e-S–32e-S.

Brown EZ. Skin grafts. In: Green DP, ed. *Operative Hand Surgery*. Vol 2. 3rd ed. New York, NY: Churchill Livingstone; 1993:1711–1740.

Brown EZ. Skin grafts. In: Green DP, Hotchkiss RN, Pederson WC, eds. *Operative Hand Surgery*. Vol 2. 4th ed. New York, NY: Churchill Livingstone; 1999:1759–1782.

Brown MD, Weinberg M, Chong N, Levine R, Holowaty E. A cohort study of breast cancer risk in breast reduction patients. *Plast Reconstr Surg*. 1999;103:1674–1681.

Brushart TM. Nerve repair and grafting. In: Green DP, Hotchkiss RN, Pederson WC, eds. *Operative Hand Surgery*. Vol 2. 4th ed. New York, NY: Churchill Livingstone; 1999:1381–1403.

Brushart TM. Peripheral nerve biology. In: *Hand Surgery Update*. Englewood: American Society for Surgery of the Hand. 1994;1:20–21.

Brzozowski D, Niessen M, Evans HB, Hurst LN. Breast-feeding after inferior pedicle reduction mammaplasty. *Plast Reconstr Surg*. 2000;105:530–534.

Bucky LP, Vedder NB, Hong HZ, et al. Reduction of burn injury by inhibiting CD18-mediated leukocyte adherence in rabbits. *Plast Reconstr Surg*. 1994;93:1473–1480.

Budny PJ, Fix RJ. Salvage of prosthetic grafts and joints in the lower extremity. *Clin Plast Surg*. 1991;18:583–591.

Bui DT, Cordeiro PG, Hu QY, Disa JJ, Pusic A, Mehrara BJ. Free flap reexploration: indications, treatment, and outcomes in 1193 free flaps. *Plast Reconstr Surg.* 2007;119(7):2092–2100.

Bujia J, Wilmes E, Hammer C, Kastenbauer E. Class II antigenicity of human cartilage: relevance to the use of homologous cartilage grafts for reconstructive surgery. *Ann Plast Surg.* 1991;26:541–543.

Burch JM, et al. Trauma. In: Schwartz SI, ed. *Principles of Surgery.* New York, NY: McGraw-Hill; 1999:212–213.

Burge P. Closed cast treatment of scaphoid fractures. *Hand Clin.* 2001;17:541–551.

Burget GC, Menick FJ. Nasal reconstruction: seeking a fourth dimension. *Plast Reconstr Surg.* 1986;78:145–157.

Burget GC, Menick FJ. Nasal support and lining: the marriage of beauty and blood supply. *Plast Reconstr Surg.* 1989;84(2):189–202.

Burget GC. *Aesthetic Reconstruction of the Nose.* St Louis, MO: CV Mosby; 1992.

Burget GC. Aesthetic reconstruction of the tip of the nose. *Dermatol Surg.* 1995;21:419–429.

Burget GC. Aesthetic restoration of the nose. *Clin Plast Surg.* 1985;12:463–480.

Burggasser G, Happak W, Gruber H, Freilinger G. The temporalis: blood supply and innervation. *Plast Reconstr Surg.* 2002;109:1862–1869.

Burkhart CG, et al. Calciphylaxis: a case report and review of the literature. *Wounds.* 1999;11:58–61.

Burns AJ, et al. Cutaneous vascular anomalies, hemangiomas, and malformations. In: Georgiade GS, Riefkohl R, Levin LS, eds. *Textbook of Plastic, Maxillofacial and Reconstructive Surgery.* 3rd ed. Baltimore, MD: Williams & Wilkins; 1997:178–197.

Burstein FD, Cohen SR, Hudgins R, Boydston W, Simms C. The use of hydroxyapatite cement in secondary craniofacial reconstruction. *Plast Reconstr Surg.* 1999;104:1270–1275.

Burt JD, Byrd HS. Cleft lip: unilateral primary deformities. *Plast Reconstr Surg.* 2000;105:1043–1055.

Burton RI, et al. Extensor tendons—late reconstruction. In: Green DP, Hotchkiss RN, Pederson WC, eds. *Operative Hand Surgery.* Vol 2. 4th ed. New York, NY: Churchill Livingstone; 1999:1988–2021.

Burwell RG. Osteogenesis in cancellous bone grafts: considered in terms of its cellular changes, basic mechanisms, and the perspective of growth control and its possible aberrations. *Clin Orthop Relat Res.* 1965;40:35–47.

Byrd HS, Andochick SE. The deep temporal lift: a multiplanar, lateral brow, temporal, and upper face lift. *Plast Reconstr Surg.* 1996;97:928–937.

Caballero E, Frykberg RG. Diabetic foot infections. *J Foot Ankle Surg.* 1998;37:248–251.

Calkins ER. Nosocomial infections in hand surgery. *Hand Clin.* 1998;14:531–545.

Callan JP, Bickers DR, Moy RL. Actinic keratoses. *J Am Acad Dermatol.* 1997;36:650–653.

Calloway DM, Anton MA, Jacobs JS. Changing concepts and controversies in the management of mandibular fractures. *Clin Plast Surg.* 1992;19:59–69.

Campion D. Electrodiagnostic testing in hand surgery. *J Hand Surg Am.* 1996;21:947–956.

Canady KW. Evaluation of nasal obstruction in rhinoplasty. *Plast Reconstr Surg.* 1994;94:555–559.

Caouette-Laberge L, Guay N, Bortoluzzi P, Belleville C. Otoplasty: anterior scoring technique and results in 500 cases. *Plast Reconstr Surg.* 2000;105:504–515.

Cardenas-Camarena L, Andino-Ulloa R, Mora RC, Fajardo-Barajas D. Laboratory and histopathologic comparative study of internal ultrasound-assisted lipoplasty and tumescent lipoplasty. *Plast Reconstr Surg.* 2002;110:1158–1164.

Cardenas-Camarena L, González LE. Large-volume liposuction and extensive abdominoplasty: a feasible alternative for improving body shape. *Plast Reconstr Surg.* 1998;102:1698–1707.

Cardo DM, Culver DH, Ciesielski CA, et al. A case–control study of HIV seroconversion in health care workers after percutaneous exposure. Centers for Disease Control and Prevention Needlestick Surveillance Group. *N Engl J Med.* 1997;337:1485–1490.

Carels RA, Janse M, Klaver PS, de Vries I, Kager PA, Overbosch D. Acute management of patients bitten by poisonous snakes. *Ned Tijdschr Geneeskd.* 1998;142:2773–2777.

Carlotti AE Jr, Aschaffenburg PH, Schendel SA. Facial changes associated with surgical advancement of the lip and maxilla. *J Oral Maxillofac Surg.* 1986;44:593–596.

Carlson GW. Oncologic and reconstructive principles. In: Achauer BM, Eriksson E, Guyuron B, et al., eds. *Plastic Surgery: Indications, Operations, and Outcomes.* Vol 3. St Louis, MO: Mosby-Year Book; 2000:1067–1092.

Carlton JM, et al. Skin grafts and pedicle flaps. In: Peimer CA, ed. *Surgery of the Hand and Upper Extremity.* Vol 2. New York, NY: McGraw-Hill; 1996:1819–1844.

Carraway JH, et al. Reoperative blepharoplasty. In: Grotting JC, ed. *Reoperative Aesthetic & Reconstructive Surgery.* St Louis, MO: Quality Medical Publishing; 1995:205–244.

Carraway JH, Mellow CG. The prevention and treatment of lower lid ectropium following blepharoplasty. *Plast Reconstr Surg.* 1990;85:971–981.

Carraway JH. Reconstruction of the eyelids and correction of ptosis of the eyelid. In: Aston SJ, Beasley RW, Thorne CH, eds. *Grabb & Smith's Plastic Surgery.* 5th ed. Philadelphia, PA: Lippincott-Raven; 1997:529–544.

Carroll RE. Squamous cell carcinoma of the nail bed. *J Hand Surg Am.* 1976;1:92–97.

Cassidy C, et al. Tendon dysfunction in systemic arthritis. In: Peimer CA, ed. *Surgery of the Hand and Upper Extremity.* Vol 2. New York, NY: McGraw-Hill; 1996:1645–1676.

Cassileth LB, Bartlett SP, Glat PM, et al. Clinical characteristics of patients with unicoronal synostosis and mutations of fibroblast growth factor receptor 3: a preliminary report. *Plast Reconstr Surg.* 2001;108:1849–1854.

Casson P, Colen S. Dysplastic and congenital nevi. *Clin Plast Surg.* 1993;20:105–113.

Casson PR, et al. Tumors of the maxilla. In: McCarthy JG, ed. *Plastic Surgery.* Vol 5. Philadelphia, PA: WB Saunders; 1990:33317–33335.

Centers for Disease Control and Prevention (CDC). Availability of new rabies vaccine for human use. *MMWR Morb Mortal Wkly Rep.* 1998;47:12, 19.

Centers for Disease Control and Prevention (CDC). Human rabies—Virginia, 1998. *MMWR Morb Mortal Wkly Rep.* 1999;48:95–97.

Chalmers RL, Smock E, Geh JL. Experience of Integra in cancer reconstructive surgery. *J Plast Reconstr Aesthet Surg.* 2010;63(12):2081–2090.

Chan SW, et al. Rehabilitation of hand injuries. In: Cohen M, ed. *Mastery of Plastic and Reconstructive Surgery.* Vol 3. Boston, MA: Little Brown & Co; 1994:1745–1763.

Chang C, Nelson JS, Achauer BM. Q-switched ruby laser treatment of oculodermal melanosis (nevus of ota). *Plast Reconstr Surg.* 1996;98:784–790.

Chang D, Youssef A, Cha S, Reece GP. Autologous breast reconstruction with the extended latissimus dorsi flap. *Plast Reconstr Surg.* 2002;110:751–759.

Chang DW, et al. Effect of smoking on complications in patients undergoing free TRAM flap breast reconstruction. *Plast Reconstr Surg.* 1996;12:467.

Chang WT, Meals RA. Two-stage flexor tendon reconstruction. In: Chung KC, ed. *Operative Techniques: Hand and Wrist Surgery.* Philadelphia, PA: WB Saunders; 2007:545–564.

Chao KS, Perez CA, Brady LW, eds. *Radiation Oncology: Management Decisions.* Philadelphia, PA: Lippincott-Raven; 1999:221–234.

Chaplin D, Pulkki T, Saarimaa A, Vainio K. Wrist and finger deformities in juvenile rheumatoid arthritis. *Acta Rheumatoid Scand.* 1969;15:206–223.

Chen CT, Robinson JB Jr, Rohrich RJ, Ansari M. The blood supply of the reverse temporalis muscle flap: anatomic study and clinical applications. *Plast Reconstr Surg.* 1999;103:1181–1188.

Chen KT, Mardini S, Chuang DC, et al. Timing of presentation of the first signs of vascular compromise dictates the salvage outcome of free flap transfers. *Plast Reconstr Surg.* 2007;120(1):187–195.

Chen YR, Noordhoff MS. Treatment of craniomaxillofacial fibrous dysplasia: how early and how extensive? *Plast Reconstr Surg.* 1990;86:835–842.

Cheng JT, Perkins SW, Hamilton MM. Collagen and injectable fillers. *Otolaryngol Clin North Am.* 2002;35:73–85.

Chidyllo SA, Jacobs JS. Applications of dental splints in regard to the modern techniques of rigid fixation. *J Craniofac Surg.* 1994;5:136–141.

Childers BJ, Goldwyn RM, Ramos D, Chaffey J, Harris JR. Long-term results of irradiation for basal cell carcinoma of the skin of the nose. *Plast Reconstr Surg.* 1994;93:1169–1173.

Chin M, et al. Distraction of the midface. In: McCarthy JG, ed. *Distraction of the Craniofacial Skeleton.* New York, NY: Springer-Verlag; 1999:349–377.

Chin M, Toth BA. Le Fort III advancement with gradual distraction using internal devices. *Plast Reconstr Surg.* 1997;100:819–832.

Chiu DT, et al. Repair and grafting of dermis, fat, and fascia. In: McCarthy, ed. *Plastic Surgery.* Vol 1. Philadelphia, PA: WB Saunders; 1990:519–520.

Choe KS, Stucki-McCormick SU. Chin augmentation. *Facial Plast Surg.* 2000;16:45–54.

Choi DJ, Alomari AI, Chaudry G, Orbach DB. Neurointerventional management of low-flow vascular malformations of the head and neck. *Neuroimag Clin North Am.* 2009;19(2):199–218.

Choi KY, Yang JD, Chung HY, Cho BC. Current concepts in the mandibular condyle fracture management part I: overview of condylar fracture. *Arch Plast Surg.* 2012;39(4):291–300.

Choi M, Rabb H, Arnaout MA, Ehrlich HP. Preventing the infiltration of leukocytes by monoclonal antibodies blocks the development of progressive ischemia in rat burns. *Plast Reconstr Surg.* 1995;96:1177–1185.

Choi PD, Nath R, Mackinnon SE. Iatrogenic injury to the ilioinguinal and iliohypogastric nerves in the groin: a case report, diagnosis, and management. *Ann Plast Surg.* 1996;37:60–65.

Chowdry S, Seidenstricker L, Cooney DS, Hazani R, Wilhelmi BJ. Do not use epinephrine in digital blocks: myth or truth? Part II. A retrospective review of 1111 cases. *Plast Reconstr Surg.* 2010;126(6):2031–2034.

Chuinard RS, Boyes JH, Stark HH, Ashworth CR. Tendon transfers for radial nerve palsy: use of superficialis tendons for digital extension. *J Hand Surg Am.* 1978;3:560–570.

Chung KC, Greenfield ML, Walters M. Decision-analysis methodology in the work-up of women with suspected silicone breast implant rupture. *Plast Reconstr Surg.* 1998;102:689–695.

Chung KC, Wei FC. An outcome study of thumb reconstruction using microvascular toe transfer. *J Hand Surg Am.* 2000; 25(4):651–658.

Cioffi WG, Burleson DG, Pruitt BA Jr. Leukocyte responses to injury. *Arch Surg.* 1993;128:1260–1267.

Cioffi WG. What's new in surgery: burns and metabolism. *J Am Coll Surg.* 2001;192:241–254.

Clark CP 3rd. New directions in skin care. *Clin Plast Surg.* 2001;28:745–750.

Clark CP 3rd. Office-based skin care and superficial peels: the scientific rationale. *Plast Reconstr Surg.* 1999;104:854–864.

Clark HM, Curtis CG. An approach to obstetrical brachial plexus injuries. *Hand Clin.* 1995;11:563–580.

Clayman MA, Clayman LZ. Use of AlloDerm as a barrier to treat chronic Frey's syndrome. *Otolaryngol Head Neck Surg.* 2001;124:687.

Cleaver JE. Cancer in xeroderma pigmentosum and related disorders of DNA repair. *Nat Rev Cancer.* 2005;5(7):564–573.

Clemente CD, ed. *Gray's Anatomy of the Human Body.* 30th ed. Philadelphia, PA: Lea & Febiger; 1985.

Clemente CD. *Anatomy: A Regional Atlas of the Human Body.* 2nd ed. Baltimore, MD: Urban & Schwarzenberg; 1981.

Clemente CD. *Anatomy: A Regional Atlas of the Human Body.* 4th ed. Baltimore, MD: Williams & Wilkins; 1997:435–576, 730, 735–736, 739, 748–750, 782, 845, 859, 866, 872, 888, 895, 896.

Cody DT, et al. Neoplasms of the nasal cavity. In: Cummings CW, Frederickson JM, Harker LA, et al., eds. *Otolaryngology Head and Neck Surgery.* Vol 2. 3rd ed. St Louis, MO: Mosby-Year Book; 1998:883–901.

Coffey MJ, Rahman MF, Thirkannad SM. Pediatric ganglion cysts of the hand and wrist: an epidemiologic analysis. *Hand (N Y).* 2008;3(4):359–362.

Cohen M, ed. *Mastery of Plastic and Reconstructive Surgery.* Vol 3. Boston, MA: Little Brown & Co; 1994:1997.

Cohen SR. Midface distraction. *Sem Orthod.* 1999;5:52–58.

Cohen SR, Holmes RE, Amis P, Fichtner H. Internal craniofacial distraction with biodegradable devices: early stabilization and protected bone regeneration. *J Craniofac Surg.* 2000;11:354–366.

Cohen SR, et al. Midface distraction. In: Samchukov ML, Cope JB, Cherkashin AM, eds. *Craniofacial Distraction Osteogenesis.* St Louis, MO: Mosby-Year Book; 2001:520–530.

Cohen SR. Genioplasty. In: Achauer BM, Eriksson E, Guyuron B, et al., eds. *Plastic Surgery: Indications, Operations, and Outcomes.* St Louis, MO: Mosby-Year Book; 2000:2563–2582, 2683–2703.

Coker NJ, Vrabec JT. Acute paralysis of the facial nerve. In: Bailey BJ, ed. *Head and Neck Surgery—Otolaryngology.* 3rd ed. Philadelphia, PA: Lippincott Williams & Wilkins; 2001:1843–1858.

Cole JK, Engrav LH, Heimbach DM. Early excision and grafting of face and neck burns in patients over 20 years. *Plast Reconstr Surg.* 2002;109:1266–1273.

Cole P, Kaufman Y, Hollier L. Principles of facial trauma: orbital fracture management. *J Craniofac Surg.* 2009;20(1):101–104.

Coleman JJ 3rd, Sultan MR. The bipedicled osteocutaneous scapula flap: a new subscapular system free flap. *Plast Reconstr Surg.* 1991;87:682–692.

Coleman JJ 3rd. The pharynx. In: Achauer BM, Eriksson E, Guyuron B, et al., eds. *Plastic Surgery: Indications, Operations, and Outcomes.* Vol 3. St Louis, MO: Mosby-Year Book; 2000:1289–1310.

Coleman SR. Facial recontouring with lipostructure. *Clin Plast Surg.* 1997;24:347–367.

Coleman SR. Long-term survival of fat transplants: controlled demonstrations. *Aesthetic Plastic Surg.* 1995;19:421–425.

Colen SR. Pressure sores. In: McCarthy JG, ed. *Plastic Surgery.* Vol 6. Philadelphia, PA: WB Saunders; 1990:3797.

Commons GW, Halperin B, Chang CC. Large-volume liposuction: a review of 631 consecutive cases over 12 years. *Plast Reconstr Surg.* 2001;108:1753–1763.

Concannon MJ, Hurov J, eds. *Hand Pearls.* Philadelphia, PA: Hanley & Belfus; 2002:104, 141–145, 146–149.

Concannon MJ. Common hand problems. In: *Common Hand Problems in Primary Care.* Vol 8. Philadelphia, PA: Hanley & Belfus; 1999:161.

Concannon MJ. Infections of the hand. In: *Common Hand Problems in Primary Care.* Vol 7. Philadelphia, PA: Hanley & Belfus; 1999:127–132.

Connell BF, et al. Skin and SMAS flaps for facial rejuvenation. In: Achauer BM, Eriksson E, Guyuron B, et al., eds. *Plastic Surgery: Indications, Operations, and Outcomes.* St Louis, MO: Mosby-Year Book; 2000:2583–2607.

Conrad MH, Adams WP Jr. Pharmacologic optimization of microsurgery in the new millennium. *Plast Reconstr Surg.* 2001;108:2088–2096.

Constantian M. Primary rhinoplasty: basic techniques. In: Cohen M, ed. *Mastery of Plastic and Reconstructive Surgery.* Vol 2. Boston, MA: Little Brown & Co; 1994:1999–2020.

Constantian MB. The incompetent external nasal valve: pathophysiology and treatment in primary and secondary rhinoplasty. *Plast Reconstr Surg.* 1994;93:919–931.

Constantino PD, Friedman CD. Synthetic bone graft substitutes. *Otolaryngol Clin North Am.* 1994;27:1037–1074.

Cook TF, Fosko SW. Unusual cutaneous malignancies. *Semin Cutan Med Surg.* 1998;17:114–132.

Coons MS, Green SM. Boutonniere deformity. *Hand Clin.* 1995;11:387–402.

Cooper JS, Farnan NC, Asbell SO. Recursive partitioning analysis of 2105 patients treated in Radiation Therapy Oncology Group studies of head and neck cancer. *Cancer.* 1996;77:1905–1911.

Cordeiro PG, Disa JJ, Hidalgo DA, Hu QY. Reconstruction of the mandible with osseous free flaps: a 10-year experience with 150 consecutive patients. *Plast Reconstr Surg.* 1999;104:1314–1320.

Coscarella E, Vishteh AG, Spetzler RF, Seoane E, Zabramski JM. Subfascial and submuscular methods of temporal muscle dissection and their relationship to the frontal branch of the facial nerve: technical note. *J Neurosurg.* 2000;92:877–880.

Cotton VR. Module 1: the doctor–patient relationship. In: *Law and Medicine.* Hershey, PA: Law and Medicine Media; 2007.

Courtiss EH, Goldwyn RM, Anastasi GW. The fate of breast implants with infections around them. *Plast Reconstr Surg.* 1979;63:812–816.

Cowin DJ, Wright T, Cowin JA. Long-term complications of snake bites to the upper extremity. *J South Orthop Assoc.* 1998;7:205–211.

Cram AE. Split thickness skin grafts. In: Blair WF, ed. *Techniques in Hand Surgery.* Baltimore, MD: Williams & Wilkins; 1996:8–12.

Cramer SF. The melanocyte differentiation pathway in Spitz nevi. *Am J Dermatopath.* 1998;20:555–570.

Crawford F, Young P, Godfrey C. Oral treatments for toenail onychomycosis: a systematic review. *Arch Dermatol.* 2002;138:811–816.

Crawley WA, et al. Fractures of the mandible. In: Ferraro JW, ed. *Fundamentals in Maxillofacial Surgery.* New York, NY: Springer-Verlag; 1997:192–202.

Crawley WA, et al. Midface, upper face, and panfacial fractures. In: Ferraro JW, ed. *Fundamentals in Maxillofacial Surgery.* New York, NY: Springer-Verlag; 1997:203–214.

Cronin TD, et al. Deformities of the cervical region. In: McCarthy JG, ed. *Plastic Surgery.* Vol 3. Philadelphia, PA: WB Saunders; 1990:2057–2077.

Cruz MJ, Kerschner JE, Beste DJ, Conley SF. Pierre Robin sequence: secondary respiratory difficulties and intrinsic feeding abnormalities. *Laryngoscope.* 1999;109:1632–1636.

Cruz-Korchin N, Korchin L, González-Keelan C, Climent C, Morales I. Macromastia: how much of it is fat? *Plast Reconstr Surg.* 2002;109:64–68.

Cunningham BL, Lokeh A, Gutowski KA. Saline-filled breast implant safety and efficacy: a multicenter retrospective review. *Plast Reconstr Surg.* 2000;105:2143–2149.

Cutting CB, et al. Repair and grafting of bone. In: McCarthy JG, ed. *Plastic Surgery.* Vol 1. Philadelphia, PA: WB Saunders; 1990:583–629.

Czitrom AA, Keating S, Gross AE. The viability of articular cartilage in fresh osteochondral allografts after clinical transplantation. *J Bone Joint Surg Am.* 1990;72:574–581.

Dagley S, Dawes EA, Morrison GA. Inhibition of growth of aerobacter aerogenes: the mode of action of phenols, alcohol, and ethyl acetate. *J Bacteriol.* 1950;60:369–379.

Dagum AB, Best AK, Schemitsch EH, Mahoney JL, Mahomed MN, Blight KR. Salvage after severe lower-extremity trauma: are the outcomes worth the means? *Plast Reconstr Surg.* 1999; 103(4):1212–1220.

Daigeler A, Drucke D, Tatar K, et al. The pedicled gastrocnemius muscle flap: a review of 218 cases. *Plast Reconstr Surg.* 2009;123(1):250–257.

Daluiski A, Yi SE, Lyons KM. The molecular control of upper extremity development: implications for congenital hand anomalies. *J Hand Surg Am.* 2001;26:8–22.

Daniel RK, ed. *Aesthetic Plastic Surgery: Rhinoplasty.* Boston, MA: Little Brown & Co; 1993:3–39, 99, 298.

Danikas D, Kokkalis G, Vasiou K, Kyriakopoulou K. Mammographic findings following reduction mammoplasty. *Aesthetic Plast Surg.* 2001;25:283–285.

Dantzer E, Braye FM. Reconstructive surgery using an artificial dermis (Integra): results with 39 grafts. *Br J Plast Surg.* 2001;54: 659–664.

Dardour JC. Treatment of male pattern baldness and postoperative temporal baldness in men. *Clin Plast Surg.* 1991;775–790.

Davis GM, Ringler SL, Short K, Sherrick D, Bengtson BP. Reduction mammaplasty: long-term efficacy, morbidity, and patient satisfaction. *Plast Reconstr Surg.* 1995;96:1106–1110.

Davison SP, Clemens MW. Safety first: precautions for the massive weight loss patient. *Clin Plast Surg.* 2008;35(1):173–183.

Davison SP, Venturi ML, Attinger CE, Baker SB, Spear SL. Prevention of venous thromboembolism in the plastic surgery patient. *Plast Reconstr Surg.* 2004;114(3):43e–51e.

Dawson D, Hallett M, Millender L, eds. *Entrapment Neuropathies.* Boston, MA: Little Brown & Co; 1990:97–100, 136–144, 201–208.

Dayan SH, Perkins SW, Vartanian AJ, Wiesman IM. The forehead lift: endoscopic versus coronal approaches. *Aesthetic Plast Surg.* 2001;25:35–39.

De Cordier BC, de la Torre JI, Al-Hakeem MS, et al. Endoscopic forehead lift: review of technique, cases, and complications. *Plast Reconstr Surg.* 2002;110:1558–1568.

Deitch EA, Wheelahan TM, Rose MP, Clothier J, Cotter J. Hypertrophic burn scars: analysis of variables. *J Trauma.* 1983;23:895–898.

Deitch MA, Kiefhaber TR, Comisar BR, Stern PJ. Dorsal fracture dislocations of the proximal interphalangeal joint: surgical complications and long-term results. *J Hand Surg Am.* 1999;24:914–923.

Delay E, Gounot N, Bouillot A, Zlatoff P, Rivoire M. Autologous latissimus breast reconstruction: a 3-year clinical experience with 100 patients. *Plast Reconstr Surg.* 1998;102:1461–1478.

Delgado R, Maafs E, Alfeiran A, et al. Osteosarcoma of the jaw. *Head Neck.* 1994;16:246–252.

Della Rocca RC, Arthurs B, Silverstone P. Nasolacrimal disorders and their treatment. *Clin Plast Surg.* 1988;15:195–207.

Dellon AL. Peripheral nerve injuries. In: Georgiade GS, Riefkohl R, Levin LS, eds. *Textbook of Plastic, Maxillofacial and Reconstructive Surgery.* Baltimore, MD: Williams & Wilkins; 1997:1011–1013.

DeLustro F, Smith ST, Sundsmo J, Salem G, Kincaid S, Ellingsworth L. Reaction to injectable collagen: results in animal models and clinical use. *Plast Reconstr Surg.* 1987;79:581–594.

Demling RH. Burns: fluid and electrolyte management. *Crit Care Clin.* 1985;1:27–45.

Demling RH. Fluid resuscitation. In: Bostwick JA, ed. *The Art and Science of Burn Care.* Rockville, MD: Aspen Publishers; 1987.

Denkler K. A comprehensive review of epinephrine in the finger: to do or not to do. *Plast Reconstr Surg.* 2001;108(1):114–124.

Denny AD, Talisman R, Hanson PR, Recinos RF. Mandibular distraction osteogenesis in very young patients to correct airway obstruction. *Plast Reconstr Surg.* 2001;108:302–311.

deShazo RD, Nelson HS. An approach to the patient with a history of local anesthetic hypersensitivity: experience with 90 patients. *J Allergy Clin Immunol.* 1979;63:387–394.

Dhar SC, Nelson HS. The delay phenomenon: the story unfolds. *Plast Reconstr Surg.* 1999;104:2079–2091.

Diao E, Eaton RG. Total collateral ligament excision for contractures of the proximal interphalangeal joint. *J Hand Surg Am.* 1993;18:395–402.

Dillerud E. Suction lipoplasty: a report on complications, undesired results, and patient satisfaction based on 3511 procedures. *Plast Reconstr Surg.* 1991;88:239–246.

Dinehart SM, et al. Cancer of the skin. In: Myers EN, Suen JY, eds. *Cancer of the Head and Neck.* Philadelphia, PA: WB Saunders; 1996:143–159.

Dingman RO, Grabb WC. Surgical anatomy of the mandibular ramus of the facial nerve based on the dissection of 100 facial halves. *Plast Reconstr Surg.* 1962;29:266–272.

Dingman RO, et al. The clinical management of facial injuries and fractures of the facial bones. In: Converse JM, ed. *Reconstructive Plastic Surgery.* Philadelphia, PA: WB Saunders; 1977.

Dingman RO, Natvig P. *Surgery of Facial Fractures.* Philadelphia, PA: WB Saunders; 1964.

Dinner MI, Dowden RV. The tubular/tuberous breast syndrome. *Ann Plast Surg.* 1987;19:414–419.

Disa J, Alizadeh K, Smith JW, Hu Q, Cordeiro PG. Evaluation of combined sodium alginate and bio-occlusive membrane dressing in the management of split thickness donor sites. *Ann Plast Surg.* 2001;46:405–408.

Disa JJ, Chung KC, Gellad FE, Bickel KD, Wilgis EF. Efficacy of magnetic resonance angiography in the evaluation of vascular malformations of the hand. *Plast Reconstr Surg.* 1997;99:136–144.

Disa JJ, Carlton JM, Goldberg NH. Efficacy of operative cure in pressure sore patients. *Plast Reconstr Surg.* 1992;89:272–278.

Disa JJ, Cordeiro PG. Mandible reconstruction with microvascular injury. *Semin Surg Oncol.* 2000;19:226–234.

Disa JJ, Pusic AL, Hidalgo DH, Cordeiro PG. Simplifying microvascular head and neck reconstruction: a rational approach to donor site selection. *Ann Plast Surg.* 2001;47(4):385–389.

Dobyns JH, et al. Congenital hand deformities. In: Green DP, ed. *Operative Hand Surgery.* Vol 1. New York, NY: Churchill Livingstone; 1993:251–548.

Doi K, Oda T, Soo-Heong T, Nanda V. Free vascularized bone graft for nonunion of the scaphoid. *J Hand Surg Am.* 2000;25:507–519.

Dolezal J. Jessner's solution. In: Rubin MG, ed. *Manual of Chemical Peels, Superficial and Medium Depth.* Philadelphia, PA: JB Lippincott; 1992.

Dolezal RF. Fractures of the nose. In: Cohen M, ed. *Mastery of Plastic and Reconstructive Surgery.* Vol 2. Boston, MA: Little Brown & Co; 1994:1126–1135.

Dolynchuk K, Tadjalli HE, Manson PN. Orbital volumetric analysis: clinical application in orbitozygomatic complex injuries. *J Craniofac Trauma.* 1996;2:56–63.

Donald PJ, et al. Facial fractures. In: Snow JB Jr, Ballenger JJ, eds. *Ballenger's Otorhinolaryngology Head and Neck Surgery.* 16th ed. Hamilton, Ontario: BC Decker; 2003:900–950.

Donelan MB. Reconstruction of the burned hand and upper extremity. In: McCarthy JG, ed. *Plastic Surgery.* Vol 8. Philadelphia, PA: WB Saunders; 1990:5473–5476.

Dowden RV, Reisman NR. Breast implant overfill, optimal fill, and the standard of care. *Plast Reconstr Surg.* 1999;104:1185–1186.

Dowden RV, McCraw JB. The vastus lateralis muscle flap: technique and applications. *Ann Plast Surg.* 1980;4:396–404.

Dowden RV. Saline breast implant fill issues. *Clin Plast Surg.* 2002;28:445–450.

Doyle JR. Constriction ring reconstruction. In: Blair WF, ed. *Techniques in Hand Surgery.* Baltimore, MD: Williams & Wilkins; 1996:1106–1111.

Doyle JR. Extensor tendons—acute injuries. In: Green DP, Hotchkiss RN, Pederson WC, eds. *Operative Hand Surgery.* Vol 2. 4th ed. New York, NY: Churchill Livingstone; 1999:1851–1897.

Doyle JR. Sliding bone graft technique for arthrodesis of the trapeziometacarpal joint of the thumb. *J Hand Surg Am.* 1991;16:363–365.

Dray GJ, et al. Dislocations and ligament injuries in the digits. In: Green DP, ed. *Operative Hand Surgery.* 3rd ed. New York, NY: Churchill Livingstone; 1982:773–774.

Drug Facts and Comparisons 2000. St Louis, MO: Facts & Comparisons Inc; 1999:1621.

Ducic I, Shalom A, Rising W, Nagamoto K, Munster AM. Outcome of patients with toxic epidermal necrolysis syndrome revisited. *Plast Reconstr Surg.* 2002;110:768–773.

Duffy M, Friedland JA. The superficial plane rhytidectomy revisited. *Plast Reconstr Surg.* 1994;93:1392–1403.

Dufresne CR, et al. Pediatric facial trauma. In: McCarthy JG, ed. *Plastic Surgery.* Vol 2. Philadelphia, PA: WB Saunders; 1990:1142–1187.

Duguid IM. Ophthalmic injuries. In: Williams JL, ed. *Rowe and Williams' Maxillofacial Injuries.* Vol 2. 2nd ed. Edinburgh, Scotland: Churchill Livingstone; 1994:827–843.

Durham JW. Thumb metacarpophalangeal ulnar collateral ligament repair with local tissues. In: Blair WF, ed. *Techniques in Hand Surgery.* Baltimore, MD: Williams & Wilkins; 1996:533–537.

Durie BG, Katz M, Crowley J. Osteonecrosis of the jaw and bisphosphonates. *N Engl J Med.* 2005;353(1):99–102.

Dziewulski P. Burn wound healing: James Ellsworth Laing memorial essay for 1991. *Burns.* 1992;18:466–478.

Earley MJ. The arterial supply of the thumb first web space and index finger in its surgical application. *J Hand Surg Br.* 1986;11:163–170.

Eaton CJ, Lister GD. Treatment of skin and soft-tissue loss of the thumb. *Hand Clin.* 1992;8:71–97.

Echavez MI, Mangat DS. Effects of steroids on mood, edema, and ecchymosis in facial plastic surgery. *Arch Otolaryngol Head Neck Surg.* 1994;120:1137–1141.

Edgerton BW, et al. Dorsal cross-finger flaps. In: Strauch B, Vasconez LO, Hall-Findlay EJ, eds. *Grabb's Encyclopedia of Flaps.* 2nd ed. Philadelphia, PA: Lippincott-Raven; 1998.

Effron CR, Beasley RW. Compression neuropathies in the upper limb and electrophysiologic studies. In: Thorne CH, Beasley RW, Aston SJ, et al., eds. *Grabb and Smith's Plastic Surgery.* 6th ed. Philadelphia, PA: Lippincott Williams & Wilkins; 2006:830–834.

Eklund GW, Busby RC, Miller SH, Job JS. Improved imaging of the augmented breast. *Am J Radiol.* 1988;151:469–473.

El Deeb M, Wolford L, Bevis R. Complications of orthognathic surgery. *Clin Plast Surg.* 1989;16:825–840.

Eliezri YD, Sklar JA. Lymphangioma circumscriptum: review and evaluation of carbon dioxide laser vaporization. *J Dermatol Surg Oncol.* 1988;14:357–364.

Elliot LF, et al. Scalp and calvarium. In: Jurkiewicz MJ, Mathes SJ, Krizek TJ, et al., eds. *Plastic Surgery: Principles and Practice*. St Louis, MO: CV Mosby; 1990:419–440.

Ellis E 3rd, Miles BA. Fractures of the mandible: a technical perspective. *Plast Reconstr Surg*. 2007;120(7 Suppl 2):76S–89S.

Elsahy NI. Acquired ear defects. *Clin Plast Surg*. 2002;29:175–186.

Elsahy NI. Reconstruction of the ear after skin and cartilage loss. *Clin Plast Surg*. 2002;29:201–212.

Elster AD. Quadriplegia after minor trauma in the Klippel-Feil syndrome. *J Bone Joint Surg Am*. 1984;66:1473–1474.

Engstrand T. Biomaterials and biologics in craniofacial reconstruction. *J Craniofac Surg*. 2012;23(1):239–242.

Enjolras O, Riche MC, Merland JJ. Facial port-wine stains and Sturge-Weber syndrome. *Pediatrics*. 1985;76:48–51.

Enjolras O, Riche MC, Merland JJ, Escande JP. Management of alarming hemangiomas in infancy: a review of 25 cases. *Pediatrics*. 1990;85:491–498.

Erickson SJ, Johnson JE. MR imaging of the ankle and foot. *Radiol Clin North Am*. 1997;35:163–192.

Erlich P, Tarver H, Hunt TK. The effects of vitamin A and glucocorticoids upon repair and collagen synthesis. *Ann Surg*. 1973;177:222–227.

Evans GR, ed. *Operative Plastic Surgery*. New York, NY: McGraw-Hill; 2000; 166.

Evans GR, Schusterman MA, Kroll SS, et al. Reconstruction of the irradiated breast: is there a role for implants? *Plast Reconstr Surg*. 1995;96:1111–1115.

Evans GR, Dufresne CR, Manson PN. Surgical correction of pressure ulcers in an urban center: is it efficacious? *Adv Wound Care*. 1994;7:40–46.

Eversmann WW Jr. Entrapment and compression neuropathies. In: Green DP, ed. *Operative Hand Surgery*. 3rd ed. New York, NY: Churchill Livingstone; 1982:1341–1385.

Ezaki M, et al. Congenital hand deformities. In: Green DP, Hotchkiss RN, Pederson WC, eds. *Operative Hand Surgery*. Vol 1. 4th ed. New York, NY: Churchill Livingstone; 1999:325–551.

Ezaki M. Amnion disruption sequence. In: Green DP, Hotchkiss RN, Pederson WC, eds. *Operative Hand Surgery*. Vol 1. 4th ed. New York, NY: Churchill Livingstone; 1999:429–431.

Ezaki M. Syndactyly. In: Green DP, Hotchkiss RN, Pederson WC, eds. *Operative Hand Surgery*. Vol 1. 4th ed. New York, NY: Churchill Livingstone; 1999:426.

Fagien S, Brandt FS. Primary and adjunctive use of botulinum toxin type A (Botox) in facial aesthetic surgery: beyond the glabella. *Clin Plast Surg*. 2001;28:127–148.

Fagien S. Botox for the treatment of dynamic and hyperkinetic facial lines and furrows: adjunctive use in facial aesthetic surgery. *Plast Reconstr Surg*. 1999;103:701–713.

Fagien S. Extended use of botulinum toxin type A in facial aesthetic surgery. *Aesth Surg J*. 1998;18:215–219.

Fagien S. Facial soft-tissue augmentation with injectable autologous and allogeneic human tissue collagen matrix (Autologen and Dermalogen). *Plast Reconstr Surg*. 2000;105:362–375.

Failla JM. Differential diagnosis of hand pain: tendonitis, ganglia, and other syndromes. In: Peimer CA, ed. *Surgery of the Hand and Upper Extremity*. Vol 1. New York, NY: McGraw-Hill; 1996:1223–1249.

Falco NA, Upton J. Infantile digital fibromas. *J Hand Surg Am*. 1995;20(6):1014–1020.

Fara M. Anatomy and arteriography of cleft lips in stillborn children. *Plast Reconstr Surg*. 1968;42:29–36.

Fara M. The musculature of cleft lip and palate. In: McCarthy JG, ed. *Plastic Surgery*. Vol 4. Philadelphia, PA: WB Saunders; 1990:2612.

Farhadieh RD, Gianoutsos MP, Dickinson R, Walsh WR. Effect of distraction rate on biomechanical, mineralization, and histologic properties of an ovine mandible model. *Plast Reconstr Surg*. 2000;105:889–895.

Farmer KL, Goller M, Lippman SM. Prevention of nonmelanoma skin cancer: standard and investigative approaches. *Clin Plast Surg*. 1997;24:663–671.

Feinberg S, et al. Reconstruction of the temporomandibular joint with pedicled temporalis muscle flaps. In: Bell WH, ed. *Modern Practice in Orthognathic and Reconstructive Surgery*. Philadelphia, PA: WB Saunders; 1992:733.

Feinendegen DL, Baumgartner RW, Vuadens P, et al. Autologous fat injection for soft tissue augmentation in the face: a safe procedure? *Aesthetic Plast Surg*. 1998;22:163–167.

Feinstein FR, Krizek TJ. Fractures of the zygoma and zygomatic arch. In: *Surgery of Facial Bone Fractures*. New York, NY: Churchill Livingstone; 1987:136.

Feldman DL. Which dressing for split thickness skin graft donor sites? *Ann Plast Surg*. 1991;27:288–291.

Feldmann JJ. Corset platysmaplasty. *Clin Plast Surg*. 1992;19:369–382.

Feldon P, et al. Rheumatoid arthritis and other connective tissue diseases. In: Green DP, Hotchkiss RN, Pederson WC, eds. *Operative Hand Surgery*. Vol 2. 4th ed. New York, NY: Churchill Livingstone; 1999:1651–1739.

Ferlic DC. Rheumatoid flexor tenosynovitis and rupture. *Hand Clin*. 1996;12:561–572.

Fernandez DL, et al. Fractures of the distal radius. In: Green DP, Hotchkiss RN, Pederson WC, eds. *Operative Hand Surgery*. Vol 1. 4th ed. New York, NY: Churchill Livingstone; 1999:979.

Ferraro JW. Cephalometry and cephalometric analysis. In: Ferraro JW, ed. *Fundamentals in Maxillofacial Surgery*. New York, NY: Springer-Verlag; 1997a:233–245.

Ferraro JW. Local anesthesia and infiltration techniques. In: Ferraro JW, ed. *Fundamentals in Maxillofacial Surgery*. New York, NY: Springer-Verlag; 1997b:158–168.

Ferraro JW. Mandibular excess and deficiency. In: Ferraro JW, ed. *Fundamentals in Maxillofacial Surgery*. New York, NY: Springer-Verlag; 1997c:270–283.

Ferraro JW. Oral anatomy. In: Ferraro JW, ed. *Fundamentals in Maxillofacial Surgery*. New York, NY: Springer-Verlag; 1997d:127–157.

Fingeret M, et al. Jones Dye tests 1 and 2. *Atlas of Primary Eyecare Procedures*. Norwalk, CT: Appleton & Lange; 1990:120–121.

Fink JA, Akelman E. Nonmelanotic malignant skin tumors of the hand. *Hand Clin*. 1995;11:255–264.

Fink MP. The role of cytokines as mediators of the inflammatory response. In: Townsend CM Jr, ed. *Sabiston's Textbook of Surgery*. 16th ed. Philadelphia, PA: WB Saunders; 2001:41.

Fink SC, et al. Craniofacial syndromes. In: Bentz ML, ed. *Pediatric Plastic Surgery*. Vol 1. Stamford, CT: Appleton & Lange; 1998:1–43.

Finley RK 3rd, Driscoll DL, Blumenson LE, Karakousis CP. Subungual melanoma: an eighteen-year review. *Surgery*. 1994;116:96–100.

Finn MC, Glowacki J, Mulliken JB. Congenital vascular lesions: clinical application of a new classification. *J Pediatr Surg*. 1983;18:894–900.

Fischer K, Zhang F, Angel MF, Lineaweaver WC. Injuries associated with mandible fractures sustained in motor vehicle collisions. *Plast Reconstr Surg*. 2001;108:328–331.

Fitzpatrick TB. The validity and practicality of sun reactive types I-IV. *Arch Dermatol*. 1988;124:869–871.

Fix RJ, Vasconez LO. Fasciocutaneous flaps in reconstruction of the lower extremity. *Clin Plast Surg*. 1991;18:571–582.

Flatt AE. Digital artery sympathectomy. *J Hand Surg Am*. 1987;12:391–400.

Flatt AE. *The Care of Congenital Hand Anomalies*. 2nd ed. St Louis, MO: Quality Medical Publishing; 1994:292–316.

Flatt AE. *The Care of Congenital Hand Anomalies*. St Louis, MO: CV Mosby; 1977.

Flatt AE. *The Care of the Arthritic Hand*. St Louis, MO: Quality Medical Publishing; 1995.

Fleegler EJ, Zeinowicz RJ. Tumors of the perionychium. *Hand Clin*. 1990;6:113–135.

Fleegler EJ. Skin tumors. In: Green DP, Hotchkiss RN, Pederson WC, eds. *Operative Hand Surgery*. Vol 2. 4th ed. New York, NY: Churchill Livingstone; 1999:2184.

Fleisher GR. The management of bite wounds. *N Engl J Med*. 1999;340(2):138–140.

Fleming ID, Cooper J, Henson D. *AJCC Cancer Staging Manual*. 5th ed. Philadelphia, PA: Lippincott-Raven; 1997:163–170.

Floros C, Davis PK. Complications and long-term results following abdominoplasty: a retrospective study. *Br J Plast Surg*. 1991;44:190–194.

Flowers R, et al. Blepharoplasty and periorbital aesthetic surgery. In: Aston SJ, Beasley RW, Thorne CH, eds. *Grabb & Smith's Plastic Surgery*. 5th ed. Philadelphia, PA: Lippincott-Raven; 1997:617.

Flowers RS. Optimal procedure in secondary blepharoplasty. *Clin Plast Surg*. 1993;20:225–237.

Floyd WE 3rd, Troum S. Benign cartilaginous lesions of the upper extremity. *Hand Clin*. 1995;11:119–132.

Floyd WE, et al. Acute and chronic sepsis. In: Peimer CA, ed. *Surgery of the Hand and Upper Extremity*. Vol 2. New York, NY: McGraw-Hill; 1996:1731–1762.

Fodor PB. Endermologie (LPG): does it work? *Aesthetic Plast Surg*. 1997;21:68.

Ford T, Widgerow AD. Umbilical keloid: an early start. *Ann Plast Surg*. 1990;25:214–215.

Foster RD. Pressure sores. In: Mathes S, Hentz V, eds. *Plastic Surgery*. Philadelphia, PA: WB Saunders; 2006:1317–1321.

Foucher G, Khouri RK. Digital reconstruction with island flaps. *Clin Plast Surg*. 1997;24:1–32.

Foucher G, et al. Island flaps based on the first and second dorsal metacarpal artery. In: Levin E, Germann G, eds. *Local Flaps about the Hand: Atlas of the Hand Clinics*. Philadelphia, PA: WB Saunders; 1998a.

Foucher G, et al. Neurovascular skin kite flap from the index finger. In: Strauch B, Vasconez LO, Hall-Findlay EJ, eds. *Grabb's Encyclopedia of Flaps*. 2nd ed. Philadelphia, PA: Lippincott-Raven; 1998b.

Fox SA. A modified Kuhnt-Szymanowski procedure for ectropion and lateral canthoplasty. *Am J Ophthalmol*. 1966;62:533–536.

Frank DH, Vakassian L, Fisher JC, Ozkan N. Human antibody response following multiple injections of bovine collagen. *Plast Reconstr Surg.* 1991;87:1080–1088.

Freeland AE. *Hand Fractures: Repair, Reconstruction, and Rehabilitation.* New York, NY: Churchill Livingstone; 2000:14–65.

Freidrich KL, Pena-Velasco G, Olson RA. Changing trends with mandibular fractures: a review of 1,067 cases. *J Oral Maxillofac Surg.* 1992;50:586–589.

Freund RM, Nolan WB 3rd. Correlation between brow lift outcomes and aesthetic ideals for eyebrow height and shape in females. *Plast Reconstr Surg.* 1996;97:1343–1348.

Friedlaender GE. Current concepts review: bone grafts. *J Bone Joint Surg Am.* 1987;69:786.

Friedman HI, Williams T, Zamora S, al-Assaad ZA. Recurrent basal cell carcinoma in margin-positive tumors. *Ann Plast Surg.* 1997;38:232–235.

Friedman M, Levin B, Grybauskas V, et al. Malignant tumors of the major salivary glands. *Otolaryngol Clin North Am.* 1986;19: 625–636.

Friedman O. Changes associated with the aging face. *Facial Plast Surg Clin North Am.* 2005;13(3):371–380.

Friedman PM, Fogelman JP, Nouri K, Levine VJ, Ashinoff R. Comparative study of the efficacy of four topical anesthetics. *Dermatol Surg.* 1999;25:950–954.

Friedman S, Goldfien A. Breast secretions in normal women. *Am J Obstet Gynecol.* 1969;104:846–849.

Fuchs PC, Nathan PA, Myers LD. Synovial histology in carpal tunnel syndrome. *J Hand Surg Am.* 1991;16:753–758.

Fuente del Campo A, Martinez Elizondo M, Arnaud E. Treacher Collins syndrome (mandibulofacial dysostosis). *Clin Plast Surg.* 1994;21:613–623.

Fulton JE, Parastouk N. Fat grafting. *Dermatol Clin.* 2001;19:523–530.

Furnas DW. Correction of prominent ears by conchamastoid sutures. *Plast Reconstr Surg.* 1968;42:189–193.

Furnas DW. Complications of surgery of the external ear. *Clin Plast Surg.* 1990;17:305–318.

Furnas DW. External ear. In: Jurkiwqicz MJ, Krizek TJ, Mathes SJ, et al., eds. *Plastic Surgery: Principles and Practice.* St Louis, MO: CV Mosby; 1990:191–194.

Furnas DW. Otoplasty for prominent ears. *Clin Plast Surg.* 2002;29:273–288.

Furnas DW. Otoplasty for protruding ears, cryptotia, or Stahl's ear. In: Evans GR, ed. *Operative Plastic Surgery.* New York, NY: McGraw-Hill; 2000:417.

Fusco FJ. The aging face and skin: common signs and treatment. *Clin Plast Surg.* 2001;28:1–12.

Gabel GT. Nerve entrapment. In: Herndon JH, ed. *Surgical Reconstruction of the Upper Extremity.* Stamford, CT: Appleton & Lange; 1999:367–390.

Gagnon NB, Molina-Negro P. Facial reinnervation after facial paralysis: is it ever too late? *Arch Otorhinolaryngol.* 1989;246:303–307.

Gamaletsou MN, Sipsas NV, Roilides E, Walsh TJ. Rhino-orbital-cerebral mucormycosis. *Curr Infect Dis Rep.* 2012;14(4):423–434.

Garcia VF, Seyfer AE, Graeber GM. Reconstruction of congenital chest-wall deformities. *Surg Clin North Am.* 1989;69:1103–1118.

Garcia-Elias M. Carpal instabilities and dislocations. In: Green DP, Hotchkiss RN, Pederson WC, eds. *Operative Hand Surgery.* Vol 1. 4th ed. New York, NY: Churchill Livingstone; 1999:865–928.

Garfin SR, Mubarak SJ. Treatment of rattlesnake bites. *J Hand Surg Am.* 1980;5:619–621.

Garza JR, et al. Secondary deformities of the cleft lip and nose. In: Bentz ML, ed. *Pediatric Plastic Surgery.* Stamford, CT: Appleton & Lange; 1998:81.

Gasparro FP. P53 and dermatology. *Arch Dermatol.* 1998;134:1029–1032.

Gasser H. Delayed union and pseudarthrosis of the carpal navicular: treatment by compression screw osteosynthesis: a preliminary report on 20 fractures. *J Bone Joint Surg Am.* 1965;47:249–266.

Gayle LB, Lineaweaver WC, Oliva A, et al. Treatment of chronic osteomyelitis of the lower extremities with debridement and microvascular muscle transfer. *Clin Plast Surg.* 1992;19:895–903.

Georgiade NG, et al. Esthetic breast surgery. In: McCarthy JG, ed. *Plastic Surgery.* Vol 6. Philadelphia, PA: WB Saunders; 1990:3839–3896.

Georgiade S. Hypermastia and ptosis. In: Georgiade GS, Riefkohl R, Levin LS, eds. *Plastic, Maxillofacial and Reconstructive Surgery.* Baltimore, MD: Williams & Wilkins; 1997:752.

Ger E, Kupcha P, Ger D. The management of trigger thumb in children. *J Hand Surg Am.* 1991;16:944–947.

Ger R, Angus G, Scott P. Transmetatarsal amputation of the toe: an analytic study of ischemic complications. *Clin Anat.* 1999;12: 407–411.

Gerber GS. Carcinoma in situ of the penis. *J Urol.* 1994;151:829–833.

Gersoff WK, Ruwe P, Jokl P, Panjabi M. The effect of tourniquet pressure on muscle function. *Am J Sports Med.* 1989;17:123–127.

Gerwin M. Cerebral palsy. In: Green DP, Hotchkiss RN, Pederson WC, eds. *Operative Hand Surgery.* Vol 1. 4th ed. New York, NY: Churchill Livingstone; 1999:259–285.

Gherardini G, Bhatia N, Stal S. Congenital syndromes associated with nonmelanoma skin cancer. *Clin Plast Surg.* 1997;24:649–661.

Gibson T, Davis, W. B. The distortion of autologous grafts: its cause and prevention. *Br Plast Surg.* 1958;10:257–274.

Gilbert A. Long-term evaluation of brachial plexus surgery in obstetrical palsy. *Hand Clin.* 1995;11:583–594; discussion 594–595.

Gilbert DN, et al. *The Sanford Guide to Antimicrobial Therapy.* 29th ed. Sperryville, VA: Antimicrobial Therapy Inc; 1999.

Gillies H, Harrison SH. Operative correction by osteotomy of recessed malar maxillary compound in a case of oxycephaly. *Br J Plast Surg.* 1950;3:123–127.

Gilman S, Newman SW, eds. Ascending and descending pathways. In: *Manter and Gatz's Essentials of Clinical Neuroanatomy and Neurophysiology.* Philadelphia, PA: FA Davis Co; 1996.

Gilula LA. *The Traumatized Hand and Wrist: Radiographic and Anatomic Correlation.* Philadelphia, PA: WB Saunders; 1992.

Gingrass MK, Brown RE, Zook EG. The treatment of nail deformities secondary to ganglions of the distal interphalangeal joint. *J Hand SurgAm.* 1995;20:502–505.

Giovannitti JA, Bennett CR. Assessment of allergy to local anesthetics. *J Am Dent Assoc.* 1979;98:701–706.

Glat PM, et al. Distraction of the mandible: experimental studies. In: McCarthy JG, ed. *Distraction of the Craniofacial Skeleton.* New York, NY: Springer-Verlag; 1999:67–79.

Glat PM, Shapiro RL, Roses DF, Harris MN, Grossman JA. *Management considerations for melanonychia striata and melanoma of the hand. Hand Clin.* 1995;11:183–189.

Glat PM, et al. Wound healing. In: Aston SJ, Beasley RW, Thorne CH, eds. *Grabb & Smith's Plastic Surgery.* 5th ed. Philadelphia, PA: Lippincott-Raven; 1997:3–12.

Glickel SZ, et al. Dislocations and ligament injuries in the digits. In: Green DP, Hotchkiss RN, Pederson WC, eds. *Operative Hand Surgery.* Vol 1. 4th ed. New York, NY: Churchill Livingstone; 1999:772–808.

Glickel SZ. Metacarpophalangeal and interphalangeal joint injuries and instabilities. In: Peimer CA, ed. *Surgery of the Hand and Upper Extremity.* Vol 1. New York, NY: McGraw-Hill; 1996:1043–1067.

Gloviczki P, Driscoll DJ. Klippel-Trenaunay syndrome: current management. *Phlebology.* 2007;22(6):291–298.

Goitz RJ, Westkaemper JG, Tomaino MM, Sotereanos DG. Soft-tissue defects of the digits. Coverage considerations. *Hand Clin.* 1997;13:189–205.

Goldberg DP. Assessment and surgical treatment of basal cell skin cancer. *Clin Plast Surg.* 1997;24:673–686.

Goldberg NS, Rosanova MA. Periorbital hematomas. *Dermatol Clin.* 1992;10:653–661.

Goldner RD, Nunley JA. Replantation proximal to the wrist. *Hand Clin.* 1992;8:413–425.

Goldner RD, et al. Replantation. In: Green DP, Hotchkiss RN, Pederson WC, eds. *Operative Hand Surgery.* Vol 1. 4th ed. New York, NY: Churchill Livingstone; 1999:1139–1157.

Goldstein JA. Fixation principles. In: Achauer BM, Eriksson E, Guyuron B, et al., eds. *Plastic Surgery: Indications, Operations, and Outcomes.* Vol 2. St Louis, MO: Mosby-Year Book; 2000:651–655.

Goldwyn RM, Cohen MN. *The Unfavorable Result in Plastic Surgery: Avoidance and Treatment.* 3rd ed. Philadelphia, PA: Lippincott Williams & Wilkins; 2001.

Goodrich JJ, et al. *Craniofacial Anomalies: Growth and Development From a Surgical Perspective.* New York, NY: Thieme Medical Publishers; 1995.

Gorczyca DP, Gorczyca SM, Gorczyca KL. The diagnosis of silicone breast implant rupture. *Plast Reconstr Surg.* 2007;120(7 suppl 1):49S–61S.

Gordon L. Toe-to-thumb transplantation. In: Green DP, Hotchkiss RN, Pederson WC, eds. *Operative Hand Surgery.* Vol 2. 4th ed. New York, NY: Churchill Livingstone; 1999:1299–1326.

Gorlin RJ, Goltz RW. Multiple nevoid basal cell epithelioma, jaw cysts, and bifid ribs. A syndrome. *N Engl J Med.* 1960;262: 908–912.

Gorlin RJ, Cohen MM, Hennekam RC. *Syndromes of the Head and Neck.* New York, NY: Oxford University Press; 1990:740–742.

Gorney M. Sucking fat: an 18-year statistical and personal retrospective. *Plast Reconstr Surg.* 2001;107:608–613.

Gosain AK, Steele MA, McCarthy JG, Thorne CH. A prospective study of the relationship between strabismus and head posture in patients with frontal plagiocephaly. *Plast Reconstr Surg.* 1996;97:881–891.

Gosain AK, Song L, Corrao MA, Pintar FA. Biomechanical evaluation of titanium, biodegradable plate and screw, and cyanoacrylate glue fixation systems in craniofacial surgery. *Plast Reconstr Surg.* 1998;101:582–591.

Gosain AK, et al. Embryology of the head and neck. In: Aston SJ, Beasley RW, Thorne CH, eds. *Grabb & Smith's Plastic Surgery*. 5th ed. Philadelphia, PA: Lippincott-Raven; 1997:223–236.

Gosain AK, Santoro TD, Larson DL, Gingrass RP. Giant congenital nevi: a 20-year experience and an algorithm for their management. *Plast Reconstr Surg*. 2001;108:622–636.

Gosain AK, Santoro TD, Havlik RJ, Cohen SR, Holmes RE. Midface distraction following Le Fort III and monobloc osteotomies: problems and solutions. *Plast Reconstr Surg*. 2002;109:1797–1808.

Gosain AK, et al. Use of tissue glue: current status. *Perspect Plast Surg*. 2001a;15:129–145.

Gosain AK, Plastic Surgery Educational Foundation DATA Committee. Distraction osteogenesis of the craniofacial skeleton. *Plast Reconstr Surg*. 2001b;107:278–280.

Gottlieb LJ, et al. Pediatric burn reconstruction. In: Bentz ML, ed. *Pediatric Plastic Surgery*. Stamford, CT: Appleton & Lange; 1998;619–633.

Gould J. Arthroplasty of the metacarpophalangeal and interphalangeal joints of the digits and thumb. In: Peimer CA, ed. *Surgery of the Hand and Upper Extremity*. Vol 2. New York, NY: McGraw-Hill; 1996:1677–1689.

Graham GF. Cryosurgery. *Clin Plast Surg*. 1993;20:131–147.

Granick MS, et al. Salivary gland tumors. In: Aston SJ, Beasley RW, Thorne CH, eds. *Grabb & Smith's Plastic Surgery*. 5th ed. Philadelphia, PA: Lippincott-Raven; 1997:453–457.

Gray H. The respiratory system. In: Goss CM, ed. *Anatomy of the Human Body*. Philadelphia, PA: Lea & Febinger; 1973:1111–1140.

Grayson BH. Cephalometric analysis for the surgeon. *Clin Plast Surg*. 1989;16:633–644.

Grazer FM, et al. Suction-assisted lipectomy. In: Achauer BM, Eriksson E, Guyuron B, et al., eds. *Plastic Surgery Indications, Operations, and Outcomes*. St Louis, MO: Mosby-Year Book; 2000a:2859–2887.

Grazer FM, de Jong RH. Fatal outcomes from liposuction: census survey of cosmetic surgeons. *Plast Reconstr Surg*. 2000b;105:436–46; discussion 447–448.

Grazer FM. Abdominoplasty. In: McCarthy JG, ed. *Plastic Surgery*. Vol 6. Philadelphia, PA: WB Saunders; 1990a:3929–3963.

Grazer FM. Body contouring. In: McCarthy JG, ed. *Plastic Surgery*. Vol 6. Philadelphia, PA: WB Saunders; 1990b:3964.

Green DP. Carpal instability. In: Green DP, Hotchkiss RN, Pederson WC, et al., eds. *Green's Operative Hand Surgery*. 5th ed. Philadelphia, PA: Churchill Livingstone; 2005.

Green DP. Radial nerve palsy. In: Green DP, Hotchkiss RN, Pederson WC, eds. *Operative Hand Surgery*. Vol 2. 4th ed. New York, NY: Churchill Livingstone; 1999:1481–1496.

Green H. Cultured cells for the treatment of disease. *Sci Am*. 1991;265:96–102.

Green HA, Drake L. Aging, sun damage, and sunscreens. *Clin Plast Surg*. 1993;20:1–8.

Green RK, Angelats J. A full nasal skin rotation flap for closure of soft-tissue defects in the lower one-third of the nose. *Plast Reconstr Surg*. 1996;98:163–166.

Greenbaum SS. Chemical peeling, injectable collagen implants and dermabrasion. In: Aston SJ, Beasley RW, Thorne CH, eds. *Grabb & Smith's Plastic Surgery*. 5th ed. Philadelphia, PA: Lippincott-Raven; 1997:597–608.

Greenberg MF, Pollard ZF. Ocular plagiocephaly: ocular torticollis with skull and facial asymmetry. *Ophthalmology*. 2000;107:173–178; discussion 178–179.

Greene AK, Perlyn CA, Alomari AI. Management of lymphatic malformations. *Clin Plast Surg*. 2011;38(1):75–82.

Greene AK. Management of epinephrine injection injury to the digit. *Plast Reconstr Surg*. 2005 115(6):1800–1801.

Greene AK. Vascular anomalies: current overview of the field. *Clin Plast Surg*. 2011;38(1):1–5.

Greene RM, et al. Craniofacial embryology. In: Cohen M, ed. *Mastery of Plastic and Reconstructive Surgery*. Boston, MA: Little Brown & Co; 1994:459–470.

Greenwald D, Cooper B, Gottlieb L. An algorithm for early aggressive treatment of frostbite with limb salvage directed by triple-phase scanning. *Plast Reconstr Surg*. 1998;102:1069–1074.

Greenwald DP, Randolph M, May JW Jr. Mechanical analysis of explanted silicone breast implants. *Plast Reconstr Surg*. 1996;98: 269–272; discussion 273–275.

Gregory RO. Overview of lasers in plastic surgery. *Clin Plast Surg*. 2000;27:167–171.

Greider JL. Trigger thumb and finger release. In: Blair WF, ed. *Techniques in Hand Surgery*. Baltimore, MD: Williams & Wilkins; 1996; 567–573.

Greinwald JH Jr, Burke DK, Bonthius DJ, Bauman NM, Smith RJ. An update on the treatment of hemangiomas in children with interferon alfa-2a. *Arch Otolaryngol Head Neck Surg*. 1999;125:21–27.

Greuse M, Hamdi M, DeMey A. Breast sensitivity after vertical mammaplasty. *Plast Reconstr Surg*. 2001;107:970–976.

Grodstein F, Speizer FE, Hunter DJ. A prospective study of incident squamous cell carcinoma of the skin in the Nurses' Health Study. *J Natl Cancer Inst.* 1995;87:1061–1066.

Grolleau JL, Lanfrey E, Lavigne B, Chavoin JP, Costagliola M. Breast base anomalies: treatment strategy for tuberous breasts, minor deformities, and asymmetry. *Plast Reconstr Surg.* 1999;104:2040–2048.

Gross BG. Cardiac arrhythmias during phenol face peeling. *Plast Reconstr Surg.* 1984;73:590–594.

Gross MP, Apesos J. The use of leeches for treatment of venous congestion of the nipple following breast surgery. *Aesthet Plast Surg.* 1992;16:343–348.

Grossman KI. Facial scars. *Clin Plast Surg.* 2000;27:627–642.

Grossman MC, et al. Cutaneous laser surgery. In: Aston SJ, Beasley RW, Thorne CH, eds. *Grabb & Smith's Plastic Surgery.* 5th ed. Philadelphia, PA: Lippincott-Raven; 1997:205–219.

Grossman MD, Roberts DM, Barr CC. Ophthalmic aspects of orbital injury. A comprehensive diagnostic and management approach. *Clin Plast Surg.* 1992;19:71–85.

Gruss J, et al. Acute facial fractures and secondary facial deformity. In: Bell W, ed. *Modern Practice in Orthognathic and Reconstructive Surgery.* Philadelphia, PA: WB Saunders; 1992:1012–1055.

Gruss JS, Hurwitz JJ, Nik NA, Kassel EE. The pattern and incidence of nasolacrimal injury in naso-orbital-ethmoid fractures: the role of delayed assessment and dacryocystorhinostomy. *Br J Plast Surg.* 1985;38:116–121.

Guerra JJ, Bednar JM. Equipment malfunction in common hand surgical procedures: complications associated with the pneumatic tourniquet and with the application of casts and splints. *Hand Clin.* 1994;10:45–52.

Gundlach K. Fractures of the mandible. In: Cohen M, ed. *Mastery of Plastic and Reconstructive Surgery.* Vol 2. Boston, MA: Little Brown & Co; 1994:1165–1180.

Gunter JP, Antrobus SD. Aesthetic analysis of the eyebrows. *Plast Reconstr Surg.* 1997;99:1808–1816.

Gunter JP, Rohrich RJ. Correction of the pinched nasal tip with alar spreader grafts. *Plast Reconstr Surg.* 1992;90:821–829.

Gunter JP, Friedman RM. Lateral crural strut graft: technique and clinical applications in rhinoplasty. *Plast Reconstr Surg.* 1997;99: 943–952; discussion 953–955.

Gunter JP, Rohrich RJ. Management of the deviated nose. The importance of septal reconstruction. *Clin Plast Surg.* 1988;15:43–55.

Gunter JP, Rohrich RJ, Friedman RM. The classification and correction of alar-columellar discrepancies. *Plast Reconstr Surg.* 1996;97:643–648.

Gunter JP, Landecker A, Cochran CS. Frequently used grafts in rhinoplasty: nomenclature and analysis. *Plast Reconstr Surg.* 2006;118(1):14e–29e.

Guyuron B, DeLuca L. Ear projection and the posterior auricular muscle insertion. *Plast Reconstr Surg.* 1997;100:457–460.

Guyuron B, et al. Forehead rejuvenation. In: Achauer BM, Eriksson E, Guyuron B, et al., eds. *Plastic Surgery: Indications, Operations, and Outcomes.* St Louis, MO: Mosby-Year Book; 2000:2563–2582.

Guyuron B, Kadi JS. Problems following genioplasty. Diagnosis and treatment. *Clin Plast Surg.* 1997;24:507–514.

Guyuron B, Lasa CI Jr. Unpredictable growth pattern of costochondral graft. *Plast Reconstr Surg.* 1992;90(5):880–886; discussion 887–889.

Guyuron B. Blepharoplasty and ancillary procedures. In: Achauer BM, Eriksson E, Guyuron B, et al., eds. *Plastic Surgery: Indications, Operations, and Outcomes.* St Louis, MO: Mosby-Year Book; 2000:2539–2543.

Guyuron B. Combined maxillary and mandibular osteotomies. *Clin Plast Surg.* 1989;16:795–801.

Guyuron B. Genioplasty. In: Ferraro JW, ed. *Fundamentals of Maxillofacial Surgery.* New York, NY: Springer-Verlag; 1997:250–269.

Guyuron B. Nasal osteotomy and airway changes. *Plast Reconstr Surg.* 1998;102:856–860; discussion 861–863.

Guyuron B, Bokhari F, Thomas T. Secondary rhytidectomy. *Plast Reconstr Surg.* 1997;100:1281–1284.

Haagensen CD. *Disease of the Breast.* Philadelphia, PA: WB Saunders; 1971:1–28.

Habal MB, Reddi AH. *Bone Grafts and Bone Substitutes.* Philadelphia, PA: WB Saunders; 1992.

Hachulla E, Hatron PY, Janin A, Robert Y, Devulder B. [Digital arteritis, thrombosis and hypereosinophilic syndrome: an uncommon complication]. *Rev Med Interne.* 1995;16:434–436.

Hackenberg B, Lee C, Caterson EJ. Management of subcondylar mandible fractures in the adult patient. *J Craniofac Surg.* 2014;25(1): 166–171

Hackler RH, Zampieri TA. Urethral complications following ischiectomy in spinal cord patients: a urethral pressure study. *J Urol.* 1987;137:253–255.

Hagan KF, et al. Trapezius muscle and musculocutaneous flaps. In: Strauch B, Vasconez LO, Hall-Findlay EJ, eds. *Grabb's Encyclopedia of Flaps.* 2nd ed. Philadelphia, PA: Lippincott-Raven; 1998:496–511.

Haimovici H, Sprayregen S. Congenital microarteriovenous shunts. Angiographic and Doppler ultrasonographic identification. *Arch Surg.* 1986;121:1065–1070.

Hall CD, et al. The initial management of patients with facial trauma. In: Cohen M, ed. *Mastery of Plastic and Reconstructive Surgery.* Boston, MA: Little Brown & Co; 1994:1060–1068.

Hall-Findlay EJ. The three breast dimensions: analysis and effecting change. *Plast Reconstr Surg.* 2010125(6):1632–1642.

Hamdi M, Greuse M, Nemec E, Deprez C, De Mey A. Breast sensation after superior pedicle versus inferior pedicle mammaplasty: anatomical and histological evaluation. *Br J Plast Surg.* 2001;54:43–46.

Hamilton JB. Male hormone stimulation is a prerequisite and an incitant in common baldness. *Am J Anat.* 1942;71:451–481.

Hamra ST. Correcting the unfavorable outcomes following face lift surgery. *Clin Plast Surg.* 2001;28:621–638.

Handel N, et al. Factors affecting mammographic visualization of the breast after augmentation mammaplasty. *JAMA.* 1993;269: 987–988.

Hanke CW, Thomas JA, Lee WT, Jolivette DM, Rosenberg MJ. Risk assessment of polymyositis/dermatomyositis after treatment with injectable bovine collagen implants. *JAmAcad Dermatol.* 1996;34:450–454.

Hanke WC, Conner AC, Temofeew RK, Lingeman RE. Merkel cell carcinoma. *Arch Dermatol.* 1989;125:1096–1100.

Hanna EY, et al. Neoplasms of the salivary glands. In: Cummings CW, Fredrickson JM, Harker LA, et al., eds. *Otolaryngology Head & Neck Surgery.* Vol 2. 3rd ed. St Louis, MO: Mosby-Year Book; 1998:1255–1302.

Hansbrough JF, Franco ES. Skin replacements. *Clin Plast Surg.* 1998;25:407–423.

Hardesty RA, Marsh JL. Craniofacial onlay bone grafting: a prospective evaluation of graft morphology, orientation, and embryonic origin. *Plast Reconstr Surg.* 1990;85:5–14; discussion 15.

Harmon CB. Dermabrasion. *Dermatol Clin.* 2001;19:439–442, viii.

Harris AO, Levy ML, Goldberg LH, Stal S. Nonepidermal and appendageal skin tumors. *Clin Plast Surg.* 1993;20:115–130.

Harris L, Morris SF, Freiberg A. Is breast feeding possible after reduction mammaplasty?. *Plast Reconstr Surg.* 1992;89:836–839.

Harrison BJ, Mudge M, Hughes LE. Recurrence after surgical treatment of hidradenitis suppurativa. *Br Med J (Clin Res Ed).* 1987;294:487–489.

Hasegawa M, Torii S, Katoh H, Esaki S. The distally based superficial sural artery flap. *Plast Reconstr Surg.* 1994;93:1012–1020.

Haskell R. Applied surgical anatomy. In: Williams JL, ed. *Rowe and Williams' Maxillofacial Injuries.* Vol 1. 2nd ed. Edinburgh, Scotland: Churchill Livingstone; 1994:1–14.

Haug RH, et al. Management of maxillary fractures. In: Peterson LJ, ed. *Oral and Maxillofacial Surgery.* Philadelphia, PA: JB Lippincott; 469–489.

Haugh M, Helou S, Boissel JP, Cribier BJ. Terbinafine in fungal infections of the nails: a meta-analysis of randomized clinical trials. *Br J Dermatol.* 2002;147:118–121.

Hawn MT, Snyder CW, Graham LA, Gray SH, Finan KR, Vick CC. Long-term follow-up of technical outcomes for incisional hernia repair. *J Am Coll Surg.* 2010;210(5):648–655.

Haywood RM, Monk BE, Mahaffey PJ. Treatment of traumatic tattoos with the Nd:YAG laser: a series of nine cases. *Br J Plast Surg.* 1999;52:97–98.

Heaton KM, el-Naggar A, Ensign LG, Ross MI, Balch CM. Surgical management and prognostic factors in patients with subungual melanoma. *Ann Surg.* 1994;219:197–204.

Herbert TJ. Open volar repair of acute scaphoid fractures. *Hand Clin.* 2001;17:589–599, viii.

Heggers JP, et al. Cold induced injury: frostbite. In: Herndon DN, ed. *Total Burn Care.* Philadelphia, PA: WB Saunders; 1996:408–414.

Heithoff SJ, Millender LH, Nalebuff EA, Petruska AJ Jr. Median epicondylectomy for treatment of ulnar nerve compression in the elbow. *J Hand Surg Am.* 1990;15:22–29.

Helliwell TR, et al. Pathology of the head and neck. In: Jones AS, Phillips DE, Hilgers FJ, eds. *Diseases of the Head and Neck, Nose and Throat.* London, UK: Arnold; 1998:24–42.

Helm KF, Schwartz RA, Janniger CK. Juvenile melanoma (Spitz nevus). *Cutis.* 1996;58:35–39.

Hensel JM, Lehman JA Jr, Tantri MP, Parker MG, Wagner DS, Topham NS. An outcomes analysis and satisfaction survey of 199 consecutive abdominoplasties. *Ann Plast Surg.* 2001;46:357–363.

Hentz VR, Rosen JM, Xiao SJ, McGill KC, Abraham G. The nerve gap dilemma: a comparison of nerves repaired end to end under tension with nerve grafts in a primate model. *J Hand Surg Am.* 1993;18:417–425.

Herford AS, Zide MF. Reconstruction of superficial skin cancer defects of the nose. *J Oral Maxillofac Surg.* 2001;59:760–767.

Herrera FA, Lee CK, Kryger G, et al. Microsurgery in the hypercoagulable patient: a review of the literature. *J Reconstr Microsurg.* 2012;28(5):305–312.

Hester TR Jr, Douglas T, Szczerba S. Decreasing complications in lower lid and midface rejuvenation: the importance of orbital morphology, horizontal lower lid laxity, history of previous surgery, and minimizing trauma to the orbital septum: a critical review of 269 consecutive cases. *Plast Reconstr Surg.* 2009;123(3):1037–1049.

Hester TR Jr, Bostwick J 3rd. Poland's syndrome: correction with latissimus muscle transposition. *Plast Reconstr Surg.* 1982;69:226–233.

Hewitt RG. Manifestations of human immunodeficiency virus infection in the upper extremity. In: Peimer CA, ed. *Surgery of the Hand and Upper Extremity.* Vol. 1. New York, NY: McGraw-Hill; 1996:1787–1796.

Hidalgo DA, Elliot LF, Palumbo S, Casas L, Hammond D. Current trends in breast reduction. *Plast Reconstr Surg.* 1999;104:806–815; quiz 816; discussion 817–818.

Higgins JP, Orlando GS, Blondeel PN. Ischial pressure sore reconstruction using an inferior gluteal artery perforator (IGAP) flap. *Br J Plast Surg.* 2002;55:83–85.

Hilburn JW. General principles and use of electrodiagnostic studies in carpal and cubital tunnel syndromes. With special, attention to pitfalls and interpretation. *Hand Clin.* 1996;12:205–221.

Hinder F, et al. Pathophysiology of the systemic inflammatory response syndrome. In: Herndon DN, ed. *Total Burn Care.* Philadelphia, PA: WB Saunders; 1996:207–216.

Hinterberger JW, Kintzi HE. Phentolamine reversal of epinephrine-induced digital vasospasm. How to save an ischemic finger. *Arch Fam Med.* 1994;3(2):193–195.

Hirshowitz B, Lindenbaum E, Har-Shai Y, Feitelberg L, Tendler M, Katz D. Static-electric field induction by a silicone cushion for the treatment of hypertrophic scars. *Plast Reconstr Surg.* 1998;101:1173–1183.

Hobar PC, et al. Cleft palate repair and velopharyngeal insufficiency. In: Aston SJ, Beasley RW, Thorne CH, eds. *Grabb & Smith's Plastic Surgery.* 5th ed. Philadelphia, PA: Lippincott-Raven; 1997:263.

Hochman M. Reconstruction of midfacial and anterior skull base defects. *Otolaryngol Clin N Am.* 1995;28:1269–1277.

Hoffer MM. Cerebral palsy. In: Green DP, ed. *Operative Hand Surgery.* 3rd ed. New York, NY: Churchill Livingstone; 1982:215–223.

Hojer J, Personne M, Hultén P, Ludwigs U. Topical treatments for hydrofluoric acid burns: a blind controlled experimental study. *J Toxicol Clin Toxicol.* 2002;40:861–866.

Holder LE, Merine DS, Yang A. Nuclear medicine, contrast angiography, and magnetic resonance imaging for evaluating vascular problems in the hand. *Hand Clin.* 1993;9:85–113.

Hollander JE, Singer AJ, Valentine SM, Shofer FS. Risk factors for infection in patients with traumatic lacerations. *Acad Emerg Med.* 2001;8:716–720.

Hollinshead WH, ed. *Anatomy for Surgeons.* Philadelphia, PA: Harper & Row; 1982:93–155, 285, 307.

Hollinshead WH, et al. Head and neck anatomy. In: *Textbook of Anatomy.* 4th ed. Philadelphia, PA: Harper & Row; 1985:895–899.

Holmes RE. Alloplastic implants. In: McCarthy JG, ed. *Plastic Surgery.* Philadelphia, PA: WB Saunders; 1990; 1:698–731.

Holt JE, Holt GR. Reconstruction of the lacrimal drainage system. *Arch Otolaryngol.* 1984;110:211–220.

Honig SF. Incidence, trends, and the epidemiology of breast cancer. In: Spear SL, ed. *Surgery of the Breast: Principles and Art.* Philadelphia, PA: Lippincott-Raven; 1998:3–21.

Hopkins R. Mandibular fractures: treatment by closed reduction and indirect skeletal fixation. In: Williams JL, ed. *Rowe and Williams' Maxillofacial Injuries.* Vol 1. 2nd ed. Edinburgh, Scotland: Churchill Livingstone; 1994:283–285.

Horn MA, Cimino V, Angelats J. Modified autogenous latissimus breast reconstruction and the box top nipple. *Plast Reconstr Surg.* 2000;106:763–768.

Horton CE, Carraway JH, Potenza AD. Treatment of a lacrimal bulge in blepharoplasty by repositioning the gland. *Plast Reconstr Surg.* 1978;61:701–702.

Horton JB, Reece EM, Broughton G 2nd, Janis JE, Thornton JF, Rohrich RJ, . Patient safety in the office-based setting. *Plast Reconstr Surg.* 2006;117(4):61e–80e.

Hotchkiss RN. Elbow contracture. In: Green DP, et al., eds. *Operative Hand Surgery.* Vol 1. New York, NY: Churchill Livingstone; 1999:668–669, 679–681.

House F. Disorders of the thumb in cerebral palsy, stroke, and tetraplegia. In: Strickland JW, ed. *The Thumb.* New York, NY: Churchill Livingstone; 1994.

Howard BK, Beran SJ, Kenkel JM, Krueger J, Rohrich RJ. The effects of ultrasonic energy on peripheral nerves: implications for ultrasound-assisted liposuction. *Plast Reconstr Surg.* 1999;103:984–989.

Howard BK, Rohrich RJ. Understanding the nasal airway: principles and practice. *Plast Reconstr Surg.* 2002;109:1128–1146; quiz 1145–1146.

Howard PS, Oslin BD, Moore JR. Endoscopic transaxillary submuscular augmentation mammaplasty with textured saline breast implants. *Ann Plast Surg.* 1996;37:12–17.

Howard PS. The role of endoscopy and implant texture in transaxillary submuscular breast augmentation. *Ann Plast Surg.* 1999;42: 245–248.

Hoyen HA, Lacey SH, Graham TJ. Atypical hand infections. *Hand Clin.* 1998;14:613–634, ix.

Huang AB, Schweitzer ME, Hume E, Batte WG. Osteomyelitis of the pelvis/hips in paralyzed patients: accuracy and clinical utility of MRI. *J Comput Assist Tomogr.* 1998;22:437–443.

Huang MH, Gruss JS, Clarren SK, et al. The differential diagnosis of posterior plagiocephaly: true lambdoid synostosis versus potential molding. *Plast Reconstr Surg.* 1996;98:765–774; discussion 775–776.

Huber GF. Modern management of Merkel cell carcinoma. *Curr Opin Otolaryngol Head Neck Surg.* 2014;22(2):109–115.

Hudson DA. Some thoughts on choosing a Z-plasty: the Z made simple. *Plast Reconstr Surg.* 2000;106:665–671.

Huger WE Jr. The anatomic rationale for abdominal lipectomy. *Am Surg.* 1979;45:612–617.

Hurst L, et al. Dupuytren's disease. In: Peimer CA, ed. *Surgery of the Hand and Upper Extremity.* Vol 2. New York, NY: McGraw-Hill; 1996:1601–1615.

Hurst LC, Badalamente MA. Nonoperative treatment of Dupuytren's disease. *Hand Clin.* 1999;15:97–107, vii.

Hurwitz S, ed. *Clinical Pediatric Dermatology: A Textbook of Skin Disorders of Childhood and Adolescence.* Philadelphia, PA: WB Saunders; 1993:208–290.

Hwang K, You SH, Sohn IA. Analysis of orbital bone fractures: a 12-year study of 391 patients. *J Craniofac Surg.* 2009;20(4):1218–1223.

Hyakusoku H, Tonegawa H, Fumiiri M. Heel coverage with a T-shaped distally based sural island fasciocutaneous flap. *Plast Reconstr Surg.* 1994;93:872–876.

Hyman J, Disa JJ, Cordiero PG, Mehrara BJ. Management of salivary fistulas after microvascular head and neck reconstruction. *Ann Plast Surg.* 2006;57(3):270–273; discussion 274.

Hynes D, et al. Compression neuropathies: radial. In: Peimer CA, ed. *Surgery of the Hand and Upper Extremity.* Vol 2. New York, NY: McGraw-Hill; 1996:1291–1305.

Hynes DE. Neurovascular pedicle and advancement flaps for palmar thumb defects. *Hand Clin.* 1997;13:207–216.

Hynes W. Pharyngoplasty by muscle transplantation. *Br J Plast Surg.* 1950;3:128–135.

Idler RS, Steichen JB. Complications of replantation surgery. *Hand Clin.* 1992;8:427–451.

Ilizarov GA. The tension–stress effect on the genesis and growth of tissues: part I The influence of stability of fixation and soft-tissue preservation. *Clin Orthop Relat Res.* 1989;(238):249–281.

Imbriglia JE. Four-corner arthrodesis. In: Blair WF, ed. *Techniques in Hand Surgery.* Baltimore, MD; Williams & Wilkins; 1996a: 865–871.

Imbriglia JE, et al. Radial nerve reconstruction. In: Peimer CA, ed. *Surgery of the Hand and Upper Extremity.* Vol 2. New York, NY: McGraw-Hill; 1996b:1361–1397.

Incaudo G, Schatz M, Patterson R, Rosenberg M, Yamamoto F, Hamburger RN. Administration of local anesthetics to patients with a history of prior adverse reaction. *J Allergy Clin Immunol.* 1978;61:339–345.

Inigo F, Ysunza A, Rojo P, Trigos I. Recovery of facial palsy after crossed facial nerve grafts. *Br J Plast Surg.* 1994;47:312–317.

Itoh Y, Arai K. The deep inferior epigastric artery free skin flap: anatomic study and clinical application. *Plast Reconstr Surg.* 1993;91:853–853; discussion 864.

Iverson RE, Lynch DJ; American Society of Plastic Surgeons Committee on Patient Safety. Practice advisory on liposuction. *Plast Reconstr Surg.* 2004;113(5):1478–1490; discussion 1491–1495.

Jackson DM. [The diagnosis of the depth of burning]. *Br J Surg.* 1953;40:588–596.

Jackson GL, Ballantyne AJ. Role of parotidectomy for skin cancer of the head and neck. *Am J Surg.* 1981;142:464–469.

Jackson IT, Carreño R, Potparic Z, Hussain K. Hemangiomas, vascular malformations, and lymphovenous malformations: classification and methods of treatment. *Plast Reconstr Surg.* 1993;91:1216–1230.

Jackson IT, et al. Orthognathic surgery. In: *Atlas of Craniomaxillofacial Surgery.* St Louis, MO: CV Mosby; 1982:83.

Jackson IT, et al. Tumors of the craniofacial skeleton, including the jaws. In: McCarthy JG, ed. *Plastic Surgery.* Vol 5. Philadelphia, PA: WB Saunders; 1990:3336–3411.

Jackson IT. Anatomy of the buccal fat pad and its clinical significance. *Plast Reconstr Surg.* 1999;103:2059–2060; discussion 2061–2063.

Jackson IT. Intraoral tumors and cervical lymphadenectomy. In: Aston SJ, Beasley RW, Thorne CH, eds. *Grabb & Smith's Plastic Surgery.* 5th ed. Philadelphia, PA: Lippincott-Raven; 1997:439–452.

Jackson IT. Sphincter pharyngoplasty. *Clin Plast Surg.* 1985;12:711–717.

Jackson LE, Koch RJ. Controversies in the management of inferior turbinate hypertrophy: a comprehensive review. *Plast Reconstr Surg.* 1999;103:300–312.

Jackson T. Intraoral tumors and cervical lymphadenectomy. In: Aston SJ, Beasley RW, Thorne CH, eds. *Grabb & Smith's Plastic Surgery.* 5th ed. Philadelphia, PA: Lippincott-Raven; 1997:439–452.

Jacobovicz J, Lee C, Trabulsy PP. Endoscopic repair of mandibular subcondylar fractures. *Plast Reconstr Surg.* 1998;101:437–441.

Jacobs JS, et al. The application of dental splints in regard to modern techniques of rigid fixation. In: Ferraro JW, ed. *Fundamentals of Maxillofacial Surgery.* New York, NY: Springer-Verlag; 1996a:327–333.

Jacobs JS, et al. Traumatic deformities and reconstruction of the temporomandibular joint. In: Ferraro JW, ed. *Fundamentals of Maxillofacial Surgery.* New York, NY: Springer-Verlag; 1996b:307–320.

Janevicius R. CPT corner: Breast reconstruction coding continues to evolve. *Plastic Surgery News.* 2013:16–17.

Janevicius R. CPT corner: Coding fat grafting procedures is straightforward. *Plastic Surgery News.* 2009.

Janfaza P, et al. Oral cavity. In: Janfaza P, Nadol JB, Galla RJ, et al., eds. *Surgical Anatomy of the Head and Neck.* Philadelphia, PA: Lippincott Williams & Wilkins; 2001.

Jansen DA, Murphy M, Kind GM, Sands K. Breast cancer in reduction mammaplasty: case reports and a survey of plastic surgeons. *Plast Reconstr Surg.* 1998;101:361–364.

Jaques B, Richter M, Arza A. Treatment of mandibular fractures with rigid osteosynthesis: using the AO system. *J Oral Maxillofac Surg.* 1997;55:1402–1406; discussion 1406–1407.

Jebson PJ, Engber WD. Radial tunnel syndrome: long-term results of surgical decompression. *J Hand Surg Am.* 1997;22:889–896.

Jebson PJ. Deep subfascial space infections. *Hand Clin.* 1998;14:557–566, viii.

Jebson PJ. Infections of the fingertip. Paronychias and felons. *Hand Clin.* 1998;14:547–555, viii.

Jelks G, et al. Blepharoplasty. In: Peck GC, ed. *Complications and Problems in Plastic Surgery.* New York, NY: Gower Medical Publishing; 1992:1–31.

Jelks GW, et al. Reconstruction of the eyelids and associated structures. In: McCarthy JG, ed. *Plastic Surgery.* Vol 2. Philadelphia, PA: WB Saunders; 1990:1671–1784.

Jelks GW, Jelks EB. The influence of orbital and eyelid anatomy on the palpebral aperture. *Clin Plast Surg.* 1991;18:183–195.

Jelks GW, Jelks EB. Preoperative evaluation of the blepharoplasty patient. Bypassing the pitfalls. *Clin Plast Surg.* 1993;20(2):213–223; discussion 224.

Jobe RP. A technique for lid loading in the management of the lagophthalmos of facial palsy. *Plast Reconstr Surg.* 1974;53:29–32.

Johnson IT, et al. Management of complications of head and neck surgery. In: Myers EM, Suen JY, eds. *Cancer of the Head and Neck.* Philadelphia, PA: WB Saunders; 1996:693–711.

Johnson MC, et al. Embryogenesis of cleft lip and palate. In: McCarthy JG, ed. *Plastic Surgery.* Vol 4. Philadelphia, PA: WB Saunders; 1990a:2525.

Johnson MC. Embryology of the head and neck. In: McCarthy JG, ed. *Plastic Surgery.* Vol 4. Philadelphia, PA: WB Saunders; 1990b:2451–2495.

Johnson TM, et al. Mohs' surgery for cutaneous basal cell and squamous cell carcinoma. In: Weber RS, Miller MJ, Goepfert H, eds. *Basal and Squamous Cell Cancers of the Head and Neck.* Baltimore, MD: Williams & Wilkins; 1996:147–155.

Jones I, Currie L, Martin R. A guide to biological skin substitutes. *Br J Plast Surg.* 2002;55:185–193.

Jones KJ, et al. Thoracic outlet syndrome. In: Green DP, Hotchkiss RN, Pederson WC, eds. *Operative Hand Surgery.* Vol 2. 4th ed. New York, NY: Churchill Livingstone; 1999:1448–1465.

Jones N. Orbit and eye injuries. In: Jones N, ed. *Craniofacial Trauma.* New York, NY: Oxford University Press; 1997:119–161.

Jones NF, et al. Free skin and composite flaps. In: Green DP, Hotchkiss RN, Pederson WC, eds. *Operative Hand Surgery.* Vol 1. 4th ed. New York, NY: Churchill Livingstone; 1999:1159–1200.

Jones NF. Intraoperative and postoperative monitoring of microsurgical free tissue transfers. *Clin Plast Surg.* 1992;19:783–797.

Jones NF. Ischaemia of the hand. In: Peimer CA, ed. *Surgery of the Hand and Upper Extremity.* Vol 2. New York, NY: McGraw-Hill; 1996:1705.

Jones NF. Ischemia of the hand in systemic disease. The potential role of microsurgical revascularization and digital sympathectomy. *Clin Plast Surg.* 1989;16:547–556.

Jonsson CE, Dalsgaard CJ. Early excision and skin grafting of selected burns of the face and neck. *Plast Reconstr Surg.* 1991;88:88–92; discussion 93–94.

Jordan RB, Daher J, Wasil K. Splints and scar management for acute and reconstructive burn care. *Clin Plast Surg.* 2000;27:71–85.

Juliano PT, Eglseder WA. Limited open-tendon-sheath irrigation in the treatment of pyogenic flexor tenosynovitis. *Ortho Res.* 1991;20:1065–1069.

Kaban LB, Pogrel MA, Perrot DH, eds. *Complications in Oral and Maxillofacial Surgery.* Philadelphia, PA: WB Saunders; 1997:209.

Kahout MP, Hansen M, Pribaz JJ, Mulliken JB. Arteriovenous malformations of the head and neck: natural history and management. *Plast Reconstr Surg.* 1998;102:643–654.

Kane WJ, Petty PM, Sterioff S, McCarthy JT, Crotty TB. The uremic gangrene syndrome: improved wound healing in spontaneously forming wounds following subtotal parathyroidectomy. *Plast Reconstr Surg.* 1996;98:671–678.

Kao CC, Garner WL. Acute burns. *Plast Reconstr Surg.* 2000;105:2482–2492; quiz 2493; discussion 2494.

Karabulut AB, Tümerdem B. Forehead lift: a combined approach using subperiosteal and subgaleal dissection planes. *Aesthetic Plast Surg.* 2001;25:378–381.

Karmo FR, et al. Blood loss in major liposuction procedures: a comparison study using suction-assisted versus ultrasonically assisted lipoplasty. *Plast Reconstr Surg.* 2001;108:241–247; discussion 248–249.

Karp NS, McCarthy JG, Schreiber JS, Sissons HA, Thorne CH. Membranous bone lengthening: a serial histological study. *Ann Plast Surg.* 1992;29:2–7.

Kasabian AK, Glat PM, Eidelman Y, et al. Salvage of traumatic below-knee amputation stumps utilizing the filet of foot free flap: critical evaluation of six cases. *Plast Reconstr Surg.* 1995;96:1145–1153.

Kasabian AK, McCarthy J, Karp N. Use of a multiplanar distracter for the correction of a proximal interphalangeal joint contracture. *Ann Plast Surg.* 1998;40:378–381.

Kasabian AK, Karp NS. Lower-extremity reconstruction. In: Thorne CH, Beasley RW, Aston SJ, et al., eds. *Grabb and Smith's Plastic Surgery.* 6th ed. Philadelphia, PA: Lippincott Williams & Wilkins; 2006:676–688.

Kasdan ML, Stallings SP, Leis VM, Wolens D. Outcomes of surgically treated mucous cysts of the hand. *J Hand Surg Am.* 1994;19: 504–507.

Kato T, Suetake T, Sugiyama Y, Tabata N, Tagami H. Epidemiology and prognosis of subungual melanoma in 34 Japanese patients. *Br J Dermatol.* 1996;134:383–387.

Katsaros J. Indications for free soft-tissue flap transfer to the upper limb and the role of alternative procedures. *Hand Clin.* 1992;8: 479–507.

Kaufman MR, Miller TA, Huang C, et al. Autologous fat transfer for facial recontouring: is there science behind the art? *Plast Reconstr Surg.* 2007;119(7):2287–2296.

Kawamoto HK Jr, et al. Atypical facial clefts. In: Bentz ML, ed. *Pediatric Plastic Surgery.* Stamford, CT: Appleton & Lange; 1998; 175–225.

Kawamoto HK Jr. Craniofacial clefts. In: Aston SJ, Beasley RW, Thorne CH, eds. *Grabb & Smith's Plastic Surgery.* 5th ed. Philadelphia, PA: Lippincott-Raven; 1997:349–63.

Kawamoto HK Jr. Rare craniofacial clefts. In: McCarthy JG, ed. *Plastic Surgery.* Vol 4. Philadelphia, PA: WB Saunders; 1990:2945–2951.

Kay SP, Wiberg M. Toe to hand transfers in children, part I: technical aspects. *J Hand Surg Br.* 1996;21:723–734.

Kay SP, Wiberg M, Bellew M, Webb F. Toe to hand transfers in children, part II: functional and psychological aspects. *J Hand Surg Br.* 1996;21:735–745.

Kay SP. Cleft hand. In: Green DP, Hotchkiss RN, Pederson WC, eds. *Operative Hand Surgery.* Vol 1. 4th ed. New York, NY: Churchill Livingstone; 1999:402–413.

Keeling CA. Range of motion measurement in the hand. In: Hunter JM, Mackin EJ, Callahan AD, eds. *Rehabilitation of the Hand: Surgery and Therapy.* Vol 1. St Louis, MO: Mosby-Year Book; 1995:93–107.

Keleher AJ, Langstein HN, Ames FC, et al. Breast cancer in reduction mammaplasty specimens: case reports and guidelines. *Breast J.* 2003;9:120–125.

Kelly KJ. Pediatric facial trauma. In: Vander Kolk CA, ed. *Plastic Surgery: Indications, Operations, and Outcomes.* Vol 2. St Louis, MO: Mosby-Year Book; 2000:941–969.

Kemp ED. Bites and stings of the arthropod kind. Treating reactions that can range from annoying to menacing. *Postgrad Med.* 1998;103:88–90, 93–6, 102 passim.

Kenny P. The management of platysmal bands. *Plast Reconstr Surg.* 1996;98:99.

Kessler I. Centralization of the radial club hand by gradual distraction. *J Hand Surg Br.* 1989;14:37–42.

Khairalla E. Epinephrine-induced digital ischemia relieved by phentolamine. *Plast Reconstr Surg.* 2001;108(6):1831–1832.

Kiefhaber TR. Phalangeal dislocations/periarticular trauma. In: Peimer CA, ed. *Surgery of the Hand and Upper Extremity.* New York, NY: McGraw-Hill; 1996:939–972.

Kikkawa DO, et al. Orbital and eyelid anatomy. In: Dortzbach RK, ed. *Ophthalmic Plastic Surgery: Prevention and Management of Complications.* New York, NY: Raven Press; 1994:1–29.

Kilmer SL, Lee MS, Grevelink JM, Flotte TJ, Anderson RR. The Q-switched Nd:YAG laser effectively treats tattoos. A controlled, dose–response study. *Arch Dermatol.* 1993;129:971–978, A607.

Kim JC, Choi YC. Regrowth of grafter human scalp hair after removal of the bulb. *Dermatol Surg.* 1995;21:312–313.

King GM. Microvascular ear transplantation. *Clin Plast Surg.* 2002;29:233–248, vii.

Kitay GS, et al. Compression neuropathies. In: Peimer CA, ed. *Surgery of the Hand and Upper Extremity.* Vol 2. New York, NY: McGraw-Hill; 1996:1339–1362.

Klatsky SA. Blepharoplasty. In: Cohen M, ed. *Mastery of Plastic Surgery.* Vol 2. Boston, MA: Little Brown & Co; 1994:1920–1940.

Klein AW. Skin filling. Collagen and other injectables of the skin. *Dermatol Clin.* 2001;19:491–508, ix.

Klein JA. Tumescent technique for local anesthesia improves safely in large-volume liposuction. *Plast Reconstr Surg.* 1993;92:1085–1098; discussion 1099–1100.

Klein JA. Tumescent technique for regional anesthesia permits lidocaine doses of 35 mg/kg for liposuction. *J Dermatol Surg Oncol.* 1990;16:248–263.

Klein L, Rudolph R. 3H-collagen turnover in skin grafts. *Surg Gynecol Obstet.* 1972;135:49–57.

Kleinert JM, Mehta S. Radial nerve entrapment. *Orthop Clin North Am.* 1996;27:305–315.

Kleinman WB, et al. Thumb reconstruction. In: Green DP, Hotchkiss RN, Pederson WC, eds. *Operative Hand Surgery.* Vol 2. 4th ed. New York, NY: Churchill Livingstone; 1999:2068–2170.

Kligman AM, Grove GL, Hirose R, Leyden JJ. Topical tretinoin for photoaged skin. *J Am Acad Dermatol.* 1986;15:836–859.

Klimo GF, Verma RB, Baratz ME. The treatment of trapeziometacarpal arthritis with arthrodesis. *Hand Clin.* 2001;17:261–270.

Kline DG, et al. *Atlas of Peripheral Nerve Surgery.* Philadelphia, PA: WB Saunders; 2001:135–144, 145–150.

Kline DG. Timing for exploration of nerve lesions and evaluation of neuroma-in-continuity. *Clin Orthop Relat Res.* 1982;(163):42–49.

Klinert HE, Kutz JE, Fishman JH, McCraw LH. Etiology and treatment of the so-called mucous cyst of the finger. *J Bone Joint Surg Am.* 1992;54:1455–1458.

Klingman AM, Grove GL, Hirose R, Leyden JJ. Topical tretinoin for photoaged skin. *J Am Acad Dermatol.* 1986;15:836–859.

Knize DM. A study of the supraorbital nerve. *Plast Reconstr Surg.* 1995;96:564–569.

Knize DM. An anatomically based study of the mechanism of eyebrow ptosis. *Plast Reconstr Surg.* 1996;97:1321–1333.

Knize DM. Limited incisions of mental lipectomy and platysmaplasty. *Plast Reconstr Surg.* 1998;101:473–481.

Knize DM. Limited-incision forehead lift for eyebrow elevation to enhance upper blepharoplasty. *Plast Reconstr Surg.* 1994;93:1392.

Knize DM. Reassessment of the coronal incision and subgaleal dissection for foreheadplasty. *Plast Reconstr Surg.* 1996;97:1334–1342.

Knoetgen J 3rd, Moran SL. Long-term outcomes and complications associated with brachioplasty: a retrospective review and cadaveric study. *Plast Reconstr Surg.* 2006;117(7):2219–2223.

Kobayashi S, Haramoto U, Ohmori K. Correction of the hypoplastic nasal ala using an auricular composite graft. *Ann Plast Surg.* 1996;37:490–494.

Kobayashi S, Hashimoto H. [Recent advance in vasculitis syndrome]. *Nippon Rinsho.* 1999;57:388–392.

Kobayashi MR, Miller TA. Lymphedema. *Clin Plast Surg.* 1987;14:303–313.

Koch BL. Cystic malformations of the neck in children. *Pediatr Radiol.* 2005;35(5):463–477.

Koh WL. When to worry about spider bites. Inaccurate diagnosis can have serious, even fatal, consequences. *Postgrad Med.* 1998;103:235–236, 243–244, 249–250.

Kohout MP, Hansen M, Pribaz JJ, Mulliken JB. Arteriovenous malformations of the head and neck: natural history and management. *Plast Reconstr Surg.* 1998;102:643–654.

Koman LA, Gelberman RH, Toby EB, Poehling GG. Cerebral palsy. Management of the upper extremity. *Clin Ortho Relat Res.* 1990;253:62–74.

Koman LA, et al. RSD after wrist injury. In: Levin LS, ed. *Problems in Plastic and Reconstructive Surgery: the Wrist.* Philadelphia, PA: JB Lippincott; 1992:300–321.

Koman LA, et al. Vascular disorders. In: Green DP, Hotchkiss RN, Pederson WC, eds. *Operative Hand Surgery.* Vol 2. 4th ed. New York, NY: Churchill Livingstone; 1999:2254–2302.

Koman LA, et al. Venous grafts for ulnar artery thrombosis. In: Blair WF, ed. *Techniques in Hand Surgery.* Baltimore, MD: Williams & Wilkins; 1996:1155–1163.

Koshima I, Endou T, Soeda S, Yamasaki M. The free or pedicled saphenous flap. *Ann Plast Surg.* 1988;21:369–374.

Kottke-Marchant K, Anderson JM, Umemura Y, Marchant RE. Effect of albumin coating on the in vitro blood compatibility of Dacron arterial prostheses. *Biomaterials.* 1989;10:147–155.

Koury ME, Perrott DH, Kaban LB. The use of rigid internal fixation in mandibular fractures complicated by osteomyelitis. *J Oral Maxillofac Surg.* 1994;52:1114–1119.

Koury ME. Complications of mandibular fractures. In: Kaban LB, Pogrel MA, Perrott DH, eds. *Complications in Oral and Maxillofacial Surgery.* Philadelphia, PA: WB Saunders; 1997:121–145.

Kozin SH. Congenital disorders: classification and diagnosis. In: Berger RA, Weiss A-PC, eds. *Hand Surgery.* Philadelphia, PA: Lippincott Williams & Wilkins; 2004:1027–1040.

Kramer GC, et al. Pathophysiology of burn shock and burn edema. In: Herndon DN, ed. *Total Burn Care.* 2nd ed. Philadelphia, PA: WB Saunders; 2002:79–85.

Kricker A, Armstrong BK, English DR, Heenan PJ. Does intermittent sun exposure cause basal cell carcinoma? Case–control study in Western Australia. *Int J Cancer.* 1995;60:489–494.

Kricker A, Armstrong BK, English DR, Heenan PJ. Pigmentary and cutaneous risk factors for nonmelanocytic skin cancer: a case–control study. *Int J Cancer.* 1991;48:650–662.

Kroll SS, Sharma S, Koutz C, et al. Postoperative morphine requirements of free TRAM and DIEP flaps. *Plast Reconstr Surg.* 2001;107:338–341.

Krueger J, Rohrich RJ. Clearing the smoke: the scientific rationale for tobacco abstention with plastic surgery. *Plast Reconstr Surg.* 2001;108(4):1063–1073; discussion 1074–1077.

Kulwin DR, et al. Blepharoplasty and brow elevation. In: Dortzbach RK, ed. *Ophthalmic Plastic Surgery: Prevention and Management of Complications.* New York, NY: Raven Press; 1994:91–112.

Kumagai N, Nishina H, Tanabe H, Hosaka T, Ishida H, Ogino Y. Clinical application of autologous cultured epithelia for the treatment of burn wounds and burn scars. *Plast Reconstr Surg.* 1988;82:99–110.

Kumar S, Sehgal V, Sharma RC. Cutis laxa. *J Dermatol.* 1996;23:721–722.

Kurihara K. Congenital deformities of the external ear. In: Cohen M, ed. *Mastery of Plastic and Reconstructive Surgery.* Vol 1. Boston, MA: Little Brown & Co; 1994:776–779.

Kurokawa M, Isshiki N, Taira T, Matsumoto A. The use of microsurgical planing to treat traumatic tattoos. *Plast Reconstr Surg.* 1994;94:1069–1072.

Kwa RE, Campana K, Moy RL. Biology of cutaneous squamous cell carcinoma. *J Am Acad Dermatol.* 1992;26(1):1–26.

Laclerca C, et al. Hand and wrist injuries in young athletes. *Hand Clin.* 2000;16:525–527.

Ladin DA. Understanding dressings. *Clin Plast Surg.* 1998;25:433–441.

Lambert PR, et al. Anatomy and embryology of the auditory and vestibular systems. In: Canalis RF, Lambert PR, eds. *The Ear: Comprehensive Otology.* Philadelphia, PA: Lippincott Williams & Wilkins; 2000:17–53.

Landau M, et al. Cutaneous manifestations of systemic diseases. In: Parish LC, Brenner S, Ramos-e-Silva M, eds. *Women's Dermatology— From Infancy to Maturity.* Pearl River, NY: The Parthenon Publishing; 2001:243–250.

Langstein HN, Chang DW, Robb GL. Coverage of skull base defects. *Clin Plast Surg.* 2001;28:375–387, x.

Larsen DL. Management of the recurrent, benign tumor of the parotid gland. *Plast Reconstr Surg.* 2001;108:734–740.

Larson PE. Traumatic injuries of the condyle. In: Peterson LJ, ed. *Oral and Maxillofacial Surgery.* Vol 1. Philadelphia, PA: JB Lippincott; 1992:435–469.

Laskawi R, Rohrbach S. Frey's syndrome. Treatment with botulinum toxin. *Curr Probl Dermatol.* 2002;30:170–177.

Lassus C. A 30-year experience with vertical mammaplasty. *Plast Reconstr Surg.* 1996;97:373–380.

Lawrence HJ, Walsh D, Zapotowski KA, Denham A, Goodnight SH, Gandara DR. Topical dimethylsulfoxide may prevent tissue damage from anthracycline extravasation. *Cancer Chemother Pharmacol.* 1989;23(5):316–318.

Lawrence WT. Physiology of the acute wound. *Clin Plast Surg.* 1998;25:321–340.

Lazova R, McNiff JM, Glusac EJ. Under the microscope: surgeons, pathologists, and melanocytic nevi. *Clin Plast Surg.* 2000;27:323–329, vii.

Le Roy JL Jr, Rees TD, Nolan WB 3rd. Infections requiring hospital readmission following face lift surgery: incidence, treatment, and sequelae. *Plast Reconstr Surg.* 1994;93:533–536.

Le TB, Hentz VR. Hand and wrist injuries in young athletes. *Hand Clin.* 2000;16:597–607.

Leana-Cox J, Pangkanon S, Eanet KR, Curtin MS, Wulfsberg EA. Familial DiGeorge/velocardiofacial syndrome with deletions of chromosome 22q11.2: report of five families with review of the literature. *Am J Med Genet.* 1996;65:309–316.

Leber D. Ear reconstruction. In: Georgiade GS, Riefkohl R, Levin LS, eds. *Textbook of Plastic, Maxillofacial and Reconstructive Surgery.* Baltimore, MD: Williams & Wilkins; 1997:497.

Leclercq C, et al. Treatment of fingertip amputations. In: Peimer CA, ed. *Surgery of the Hand and Upper Extremity.* Vol 1. New York, NY: McGraw-Hill; 1996:1069–1100.

Lee C, Mueller RV, Lee K, Mathes SJ. Endoscopic subcondylar fracture repair: functional, aesthetic, and radiographic outcomes. *Plast Reconstr Surg.* 1998;102:1434–1443; discussion 1444–1445.

Lee DH, Yang HN, Kim JC, Shyn KH. Sudden unilateral visual loss and brain infarction after autologous fat injection into nasolabial groove. *Br J Ophthalmol.* 1996;80:1026–1027.

Lee KJ. Thyroid and parathyroid glands. In: *Essential Otolaryngology Head & Neck Surgery.* 7th ed. Stamford, CT: Appleton & Lange; 1995:574–575.

Lee WP, et al. Transplant biology and applications to plastic surgery. In: Aston SJ, Beasley RW, Thorne CH, eds. *Grabb & Smith's Plastic Surgery.* 5th ed. Philadelphia, PA: Lippincott-Raven; 1997:27–38.

Lees M. Familial risks of oral clefts. *BMJ.* 2008;336(7641):399.

LeFlore I, Antoine GA. Keloid formation on palmar surface of hand. *J Natl Med Assoc.* 1991;83:463–464.

Lejour M. Applied anatomy for vertical mammaplasty. In: *Vertical Mammaplasty and Liposuction.* St Louis, MO: Quality Medical Publishing; 1994:53.

Lejour M. Evaluation of fat in breast tissue removed by vertical mammaplasty. *Plast Reconstr Surg.* 1997;99:386–393.

Lejour M. Vertical mammaplasty. *Plast Reconstr Surg.* 1993;92:985–986.

Lenert J, Viterbo F, Johnson PC. Pediatric facial paralysis syndromes. In: Bentz ML, ed. *Pediatric Plastic Surgery.* McGraw-Hill Professional; 1997:427–462.

Leslie BM. Rheumatoid extensor tendon ruptures. *Hand Clin.* 1989;5:191–202.

Lettieri S, et al. Craniofacial syndromes. In: Weinzweig J, ed. *Plastic Surgery Secrets.* Philadelphia, PA: Hanley & Belfus; 1999: 96–99.

Lettieri S. Facial trauma. In: Achauer BM, Eriksson E, Guyuron B, et al., eds. *Plastic Surgery: Indications, Operations, and Outcomes.* Vol 2. St Louis, MO: Mosby-Year Book; 2000:923–940.

Levine VJ, Geronemus RG. Tattoo removal with the Q-switched Nd:YAG laser: a comparative study. *Cutis.* 1995;55:291–296.

Levy HJ. Ring finger ray amputation: a 25-year follow-up. *Am J Orthop (Belle Mead NJ).* 1999;28:359–360.

Lewis VL Jr, Bailey MH, Pulawski G, Kind G, Bashioum RW, Hendrix RW. The diagnosis of osteomyelitis in patients with pressure sores. *Plast Reconstr Surg.* 1988;81:229–232.

Leyden JJ. Treatment of photodamaged skin with topical tretinoin: an update. *Plast Reconstr Surg.* 1998;102:1667–1671; discussion 1672–1675.

Li Z, Smith BP, Tuohy C, Smith TL, Andrew Koman L. Complex regional pain syndrome after hand surgery. *Hand Clin.*2010;26(2): 281–289.

Lie JT. Histopathologic specificity of systemic vasculitis. *Rheum Dis Clin North Am.* 1995;21:883–909.

Light TR, Ogden JA. The longitudinal epiphyseal bracket: implications for surgical correction. *J Pediatr Orthop.* 1981;1:299–305.

Light TR. Congenital anomalies: syndactyly, polydactyly, and cleft hand. In: Peimer CA, ed. *Surgery of the Hand and Upper Extremity.* New York, NY: McGraw-Hill; 1996;2:2111–2144.

Lim B, Tan BK, Peng YP. Digital replantations including fingertip and ring avulsions. *Hand Clin.* 2001;17:419–431, viii-ix.

Lin HW, Cooper K. The health impact of solar radiation and prevention strategies: report of the Environment Council, American Academy of Dermatology. *J Am Acad Dermatol.* 1999;41:81–99.

Lin TM, Tsai CC, Lin SD, Lai CS. Continuous intra-arterial infusion therapy in hydrofluoric acid burns. *J Occup Environ Med.* 2000;42:892–897.

Linares MD, Hardisson D, Perna C. Subungual malignant melanoma of the hand: unusual clinical presentation: case report. *Scand J Plast Reconstr Surg Hand Surg.* 1998;32:347–350.

Lineaweaver WC, Hill MK, Buncke GM. Aeromonas hydrophilia infections following use of medicinal leeches in replantation and flap surgery. *Ann Plast Surg.* 1992;29:238–244.

Linger TE, et al. Salivary tumors experience 30 years. *Clin Otolaryngol.* 1997;4:247.

Lisman RD, et al. Blepharoplasty: postoperative considerations and complications. In: Rees TD, LaTrenta GS, eds. *Aesthetic Plastic Surgery.* Vol 2. 2nd ed. Philadelphia, PA: WB Saunders; 1994:597–599.

Lisman RD, Hyde K, Smith B. Complication of blepharoplasty. *Clin Plast Surg.* 1988;15:309–335.

Liss FE, Green SM. Capsular injuries of the proximal interphalangeal joint. *Hand Clin.* 1992;8:755–768.

Lister G, ed. *The Hand: Diagnosis and Indications.* 3rd ed. Edinburgh, Scotland: Churchill Livingstone; 1993:43, 223, 288, 459–512, 520.

Lister GD, et al. Skin flaps. In: Green DP, Hotchkiss RN, Pederson WC, eds. *Operative Hand Surgery*. Vol 2. 4th ed. New York, NY: Churchill Livingstone; 1999:1783–1850, 1973–1976.

Lister GD. Skin flaps. In: Green DP, ed. *Operative Hand Surgery*. Vol 2. 3rd ed. New York, NY: Churchill Livingstone; 1993:1741–1822.

Liszka TG, Dellon AL, Manson PN. Iliohypogastric nerve entrapment following abdominoplasty. *Plast Reconstr Surg*. 1994;93:181–184.

Lockwood T. Brachioplasty with superficial fascial system suspension. *Plast Reconstr Surg*. 1995;96:912–920.

Lockwood T. Contouring of the arms, trunk, and thighs. In: Achauer BM, Eriksson E, Guyuron B, et al., eds. *Plastic Surgery: Indications, Operations, and Outcomes*. Vol 5. St Louis, MO: Mosby-Year Book; 2000:2839–2857.

Lockwood T. Lower body lift with superficial fascial suspension. *Plast Reconstr Surg*. 1993;92:1112-1122; discussion 1123–1125.

Lockwood T. Reduction mammaplasty and mastopexy with superficial fascial skin suspension. *Plast Reconstr Surg*. 1999;103:1411–1420.

Lockwood T. Superficial fascial system (SFS) of the trunk and extremities: a new concept. *Plast Reconstr Surg*. 1991;87:1009–1018.

Lockwood T. The role of excisional lifting in body contour surgery. *Clin Plast Surg*. 1996;23:695–712.

Longaker MT, Siebert JW. Microvascular free-flap correction of severe hemifacial atrophy. *Plast Reconstr Surg*. 1995;96:800–809.

Lorenz HP, Longaker MT, Kawamoto HK Jr. Primary and secondary orbit surgery: the transconjunctival approach. *Plast Reconstr Surg*. 1999;103:1124–1128.

Losken HW, et al. Craniosynostosis. In: Bentz ML, ed. *Pediatric Plastic Surgery*. Stamford, CT: Appleton & Lange; 1998:129–132.

Lou RB, Hickerson WL. The use of skin substitutes in hand burns. *Hand Clin*. 2009;25(4):497–509.

Louis DS, et al. Amputations. In: Green DP, ed. *Operative Hand Surgery*. 3rd ed. New York, NY: Churchill Livingstone; 1982:62–72.

Louis DS, et al. Amputations. In: Green DP, Hotchkiss RN, Pederson WC, eds. *Operative Hand Surgery*. Vol 1. 4th ed. New York, NY: Churchill Livingstone; 1999:48–94.

Low DW. Modified chondrocutaneous advancement flap for ear reconstruction. *Plast Reconstr Surg*. 1998;102:174–177.

Lowen RM, Rodgers CM, Ketch LL, Phelps DB. Aeromonas hydrophilia infection complicating digital replantation and revascularization. *J Hand Surg Am*. 1989;14:714–718.

Lubahn JD. Dupuytren's fasciectomy: open palm technique. In: Blair WF, ed. *Techniques in Hand Surgery*. Baltimore, MD: Williams & Wilkins; 1996.

Luce EA. Frontal sinus fractures: guidelines to management. *Plast Reconstr Surg*. 1987;80:500–510.

Lupo G. The history of aesthetic rhinoplasty: special emphasis on the saddle nose. *Aesthetic Plast Surg*. 1997;21:309–327.

Lutz BS, Wei FC. Microsurgical reconstruction of the buccal mucosa. *Clin Plast Surg*. 2001;28:339–347, ix.

Mackinnon SE, Dellon AL, eds. *Surgery of the Peripheral Nerve*. New York, NY: Thieme Medical Publishers; 1988:171, 197–216, 226, 289–303.

MacKinnon SE, Glickman LT, Dagum A. A technique for the treatment of neuroma-in-continuity. *J Reconstr Microsurg*. 1992;8: 379–383.

Mackinnon SE. Nerve injuries: primary repair and reconstruction. In: Cohen M, ed. *Mastery of Plastic and Reconstructive Surgery*. Vol 3. Boston, MA: Little Brown & Co; 1994:1598–1624.

MacLennan SE, Kitzmiller WJ, Yakuboff KP. Free tissue transfer for limb salvage in purpura fulminans. *Plast Reconstr Surg*. 2001;107:1437–1442.

Maddi R, Horrow JC, Mark JB, Concepcion M, Murray E. Evaluation of a new cutaneous topical anesthesia preparation. *Reg Anesth*. 1996;15:109–112.

Magee KL, Rapini RP, Duvic M, Adler-Storthz K. Human papilloma virus associated with keratoacanthoma. *Arch Dermatol*. 1989;125:1587–1589.

Manassa EH, Hertl CH, Olbrisch RR. Wound healing problems in smokers and nonsmokers after 132 abdominoplasties. *Plast Reconstr Surg*. 2003;111:2082–2087; discussion 2088–2089.

Mancoll JS, et al. Pressure sores. In: Aston SJ, Beasley RW, Thorne CH, eds. *Grabb & Smith's Plastic Surgery*. 5th ed. Philadelphia, PA: Lippincott-Raven; 1997:1083.

Manktelow RT, Zuker RM, Neligan PC. Facial paralysis reconstruction. In: Thorne CH, Beasley RW, Aston SJ, et al., eds. *Grabb and Smith's Plastic Surgery*. 6th ed. Philadelphia, PA: Lippincott Williams & Wilkins; 2006:417–427.

Mann RJ, Blount AL, Neaman KC, Korepta L. Mimix hydroxyapatite cement use in the reconstruction of the craniofacial skeleton. *J Craniofac Surg*. 2011;22(6):2144–2147.

Mannerfelt L, Oetker R, Ostlund B, Elbert B. Rupture of the extensor pollicis longus tendon after Colles' fracture and by rheumatoid arthritis. *J Hand Surg Br*. 1990;15:49–50.

Mannick JA, Rodrick ML, Lederer JA. The immunologic response to injury. *J Am Coll Surg*. 2001;193:237-244.

Manson P. Facial Fracture. In: Mathes SJ, Hentz VR, eds. *Plastic Surgery*. Vol 2. Philadelphia, PA: Saunders-Elsevier; 2006:77.

Manson P. Management of midfacial fractures. In: Georgiade GS, Riefkohl R, Levin LS, eds. *Plastic, Maxillofacial and Reconstructive Surgery*. Baltimore, MD: Williams & Wilkins; 1997:351–376.

Manson PN. Facial fractures. In: Aston SJ, Beasley RW, Thorne CH, eds. *Grabb & Smith's Plastic Surgery*. 5th ed. Philadelphia, PA: Lippincott-Raven; 1997:383–412.

Manson PN. Facial injuries. In: McCarthy JG, ed. *Plastic Surgery*. Philadelphia, PA: WB Saunders; 1990;2:867–1141.

Manson PN. Reoperative facial fracture repair. In: Grotting JC, ed. *Reoperative Aesthetic and Reconstructive Plastic Surgery*. Vol 1. St Louis, MO: Quality Medical Publishing; 1995:677–759.

Manson PN, Iliff N. Management of blow-out fractures of the orbital floor. II. Early repair for selected injuries. *Surg Ophthalmol*. 1991 35:280–292.

Manson PN, Clifford CM, Su CT, Iliff NT, Morgan R. Mechanisms of global support and posttraumatic enophthalmos: I. The anatomy of the ligament sling and its relation to intramuscular cone orbital fat. *Plast Reconstr Surg*. 1986;77:193–202.

Manson PN, Crawley WA, Yaremchuk MJ, Rochman GM, Hoopes JE, French JH Jr. Midface fractures: advantages of immediate extended open reduction and bone grafting. *Plast Reconstr Surg*. 1985;76:1–12.

Manson PN, Grivas A, Rosenbaum A, Vannier M, Zinreich J, Iliff N. Studies on enophthalmos II. The measurement of orbital injuries and their treatment by quantitative computed tomography. *Plast Reconstr Surg*. 1986;77:203–214.

Marchac D, et al. Craniosynostosis and craniofacial dysostosis. In: Cohen M, ed. *Mastery of Plastic and Reconstructive Surgery*. Vol 1. Boston, MA: Little Brown & Co; 1994:499–515.

Marchac D, Toth B. The axial frontonasal flap revisited. *Plast Reconstr Surg*. 1985;76:686–694.

Marieb EN, ed. Overview of the digestive system. In: *Human Anatomy and Physiology*. Redwood City, CA: Benjamin/Cummings Publishing; 1995.

Mark R, Sercarz JA, Tran L, Dodd LG, Selch M, Calcaterra TC. Osteogenic sarcoma of the head and neck: the UCLA experience. *Arch Otolaryngol Head Neck Surg*. 1991;117:761–766.

Markiewitz AD, et al. Carpal fractures and dislocations. In: Lichtman DM, Alexander AH, eds. *The Wrist and Its Disorders*. Philadelphia, PA: WB Saunders; 1997:206–211.

Markley JM Jr, et al. The composite neurovascular skin island graft in surgery of the hand. *Atlas Hand Clin*. 1998;59–76.

Marks R, Rennie G, Selwood TS. Malignant transformation of solar keratoses to squamous cell carcinoma. *Lancet*. 1998;1:795–797.

Marshall DR, Callan PP, Nicholson W. Breastfeeding after reduction mammaplasty. *Br J Plast Surg*. 1994;47:167–169.

Martin D, Bakhach J, Casoli V. Reconstruction of the hand with forearm island flaps. *Clin Plast Surg*. 1997;24:33–48.

Martin JJ Jr, Tenzel RR. Acquired ptosis: dehiscences and disinsertions. Are they real or iatrogenic? *Ophthal Plast Reconstr Surg*. 1992;8:130–132; discussion 133.

Mason ME, et al. Revision orthognathic surgery. In: Booth PW, Schendel SA, Hausamen JE, eds. *Maxillofacial Surgery*. Vol 2. London, UK: Churchill Livingstone; 1999:1321–1334.

Masquelet AC, et al. Skin island flaps supplied by the vascular axis of the sensitive superficial nerves: anatomic study and clinical experience in the leg. *Plast Reconstr Surg*. 1994;93:872.

Matarasso A. Buccal fat pad excision: aesthetic improvement of the midface. *Ann Plast Surg*. 1991;26:413–418.

Matarasso A. Abdominoplasty. In: Achauer BM, Eriksson E, Guyuron B, et al., eds. *Plastic Surgery: Indications, Operations, and Outcomes*. Vol 5. St Louis, MO: Mosby-Year Book; 2000a:2783–2821.

Matarasso A. Liposuction as an adjunct to a full abdominoplasty revisited. *Plast Reconstr Surg*. 2000b;106:1197–1202; discussion 1203–1205.

Matarasso A. Liposuction as an adjunct to a full abdominoplasty. *Plast Reconstr Surg*. 1995;95:829–836.

Matarasso A. Pseudoherniation of the buccal fat pad: a new clinical syndrome. *Plast Reconstr Surg*. 1997;100:723–730; discussion 731–736.

Matarasso A, Matarasso SL, Brandt FS, Bellman B. Botulinum A exotoxin for the management of platysma bands. *Plast Reconstr Surg*. 1999;103:645–652; discussion 653–655.

Matarasso SL. Comparison of botulinum toxin types A and B: a bilateral and double-blind randomized evaluation in the treatment of canthal rhytides. *Dermatol Surg*. 2003;29(1):7–13; discussion 13.

Matarasso SL. Complications of botulinum A exotoxin for hyperfunctional lines. *Dermatol Surg*. 1998;24:1249–1254.

Mathes DW, Thornton JF, Rohrich RJ. Management of posterior trunk defects. *Plast Reconstr Surg*. 2006;118(3):73e–83e.

Mathes SJ, Nahai F. Classification of the vascular anatomy of muscles: experimental and clinical correlation. *Plast Reconstr Surg*. 1981;67:177–187.

Mathes SJ, et al. Superficial inferior epigastric artery (SIEA) flap. In: *Reconstructive Surgery*. Vol 2. New York, NY: Churchill Livingstone; 1997:1095–1103.

Mathes SJ, et al. The principles of muscle and musculocutaneous flaps. In: McCarthy JG, ed. *Plastic Surgery*. Vol 1. Philadelphia, PA: WB Saunders; 1990:379–411.

Mathes SJ. Muscle flaps and their blood supply. In: Aston SJ, Beasley RW, Thorne CH, eds. *Grabb & Smith's Plastic Surgery*. 5th ed. Philadelphia, PA: Lippincott-Raven; 1997a:61–72.

Mathes SJ, Nahai F, eds. *Reconstructive Surgery: Principles, Anatomy and Technique*. St Louis, MO: Quality Medical Publishing; 1997b:29–31, 477–679, 617–642, 729–746, 965–984, 1005, 1043, 1161–1307, 1353–1370.

Mathes SJ, Nahai F. Lateral arm flap. In: Mathes SJ, Nahai F, eds. *Reconstructive Surgery: Principles, Anatomy and Technique*. Vol 1. New York, NY: Churchill Livingstone; 1997c:729–746.

Matsuo K, Hayashi R, Kiyono M, Hirose T, Netsu Y. Nonsurgical correction of congenital auricular deformities. *Clin Plast Surg*. 1990;17:383–395.

Matteucci BM, et al. Systemic arthritic conditions of the upper extremities—inflammatory. In: Peimer CA, ed. *Surgery of the Hand and Upper Extremity*. Vol 2. New York, NY: McGraw-Hill; 1996:1617–1631.

Mattison C. *The Encyclopedia of Snakes*. Blandford: UK; 1995.

Maxwell GP, et al. Management of complications following augmentation mammoplasty. In: Georgiade GS, Riefkohl R, Levin LS, eds. *Textbook of Plastic, Maxillofacial and Reconstructive Surgery*. Baltimore, MD: Williams & Wilkins; 1997:736.

May JW, et al. Micro neurovascular free transfer of the big toe. In: Strauch B, Vasconez LO, Hall-Findlay EJ, eds. *Grabb's Encyclopedia of Flaps*. 2nd ed. Philadelphia, PA: Lippincott-Raven; 1998:1013–1018.

Mayfield JK, Johnson RP, Kilcoyne RK. Carpal dislocations: pathomechanics and progressive perilunar instability. *J Hand Surg Am*. 1980;5:226–241.

McCarroll HR. Congenital anomalies: radial dysplasia. In: Peimer CA, ed. *Surgery of the Hand and Upper Extremity*. Vol 2. New York, NY: McGraw-Hill; 1996:2075–2093.

McCarroll HR. Congenital anomalies: a 25-year overview. *J Hand Surg Am*. 2000;25:1007–1037.

McCarthy JG, Coccaro PJ, Schwartz MD. Velopharyngeal function following maxillary advancement. *Plast Reconstr Surg*. 1979;64: 180–189.

McCarthy JG, Ruff GL, Zide BM. A surgical system for the correction of bony chin deformity. *Clin Plast Surg*. 1991;18:139–152.

McCarthy JG, et al. Craniofacial microsomia. In: McCarthy JG, ed. *Plastic Surgery*. Vol 4. Philadelphia, PA: WB Saunders; 1990a:2491, 3106, 3054–3055.

McCarthy JG, et al. Craniofacial syndromes. In: McCarthy JG, ed. *Plastic Surgery*. Philadelphia, PA: WB Saunders; 1990b;4:3101–3160.

McCarthy JG, et al. Craniosynostosis. In: McCarthy JG, ed. *Plastic Surgery*. Philadelphia, PA: WB Saunders; 1990c:3013–3055.

McCarthy JG. Introduction to plastic surgery. In: McCarthy JG, ed. *Plastic Surgery*. Vol 1. Philadelphia, PA: WB Saunders; 1990d:28, 68.

McCarthy JG, et al. Principles of craniofacial surgery. In: McCarthy JG, ed. *Plastic Surgery*. Vol 5. Philadelphia, PA: WB Saunders; 1990e:2974–3012.

McCarthy JG, et al. Rhinoplasty. In: McCarthy JG, ed. *Plastic Surgery*. Vol 3. Philadelphia, PA: WB Saunders; 1990f:1804.

McCarthy JG, et al. Surgery of the jaws. In: McCarthy JG, ed. *Plastic Surgery*. Vol 2. Philadelphia, PA: WB Saunders; 1990g:1187, 1188–1474.

McCarthy JG, Stelnicki EJ, Mehrara BJ, Longaker MT. Distraction osteogenesis of the craniofacial skeleton. *Plast Reconstr Surg*. 2001;107:1812–1827.

McCarthy JG, Coccaro PJ, Schwartz MD. Velopharyngeal function following maxillary advancement. *Plast Reconstr Surg*. 1979;64: 180–189.

McCarthy JG. Craniofacial microsomia. In: Aston SJ, Beasley RW, Thorne CH, eds. *Grabb & Smith's Plastic Surgery*. 5th ed. Philadelphia, PA: Lippincott-Raven; 1997:305–319.

McCauley RL. Correction of burn alopecia. In: Herndon DN, ed. *Total Burn Care*. Philadelphia, PA: WB Saunders; 1996:499–502.

McClinton MA. Tumors and aneurysms of the upper extremity. *Hand Clin*. 1993;9:151–169.

McComb H. Primary correction of unilateral cleft lip nasal deformity: a 10-year review. *Plast Reconstr Surg*. 1985;75:791–799.

McCord CD. *Eyelid Surgery: Principles and Techniques*. Philadelphia, PA: Lippincott-Raven; 1995.

McCord CD Jr. The evaluation and management of the patient with ptosis. *Clin Plast Surg*. 1988;15:169–184.

McCraw JB, Arnold PG, eds. *McCraw and Arnold's Atlas of Muscle and Musculocutaneous Flaps*. Norfolk, VA: Hampton Press; 1988: 89–91.

McCraw JB, Myers B, Shanklin KD. The value of fluorescein in predicting the viability of arterialized flaps. *Plast Reconstr Surg.* 1977;60:710–719.

McDowell CL, et al. Tetraplegia. In: Green DP, Hotchkiss RN, Pederson WC, eds. *Operative Hand Surgery.* Vol 2. 4th ed. New York, NY: Churchill Livingstone; 1999:1594.

McFarlane RM. Patterns of diseased fascia in the fingers of Dupuytren's contracture. Displacement of the neurovascular bundle. *Plast Reconstr Surg.* 1974;54:31–44.

McFarlane RM, Classen DA, Porte AM, Botz JS. The anatomy and treatment of camptodactyly of the small finger. *J Hand Surg Am.* 1992;17:35–44.

McFarlane RM. Dupuytren's contracture. In: Green DP, ed. *Operative Hand Surgery.* 3rd ed. New York, NY: Churchill Livingstone; 1982:563–591.

McFarlane RM. Dupuytren's disease. In: McCarthy JG, ed. *Plastic Surgery.* Vol 8. Philadelphia, PA: WB Saunders 1990:5061.

McFarlane RM. The anatomy of Dupuytren's disease. *Bull Hosp Jt Dis Orthop Inst.* 1984;44:318–337.

McGrath MH. Benign tumors of the teenage hand. *Plast Reconstr Surg.* 2000;105:218–222; quiz 223.

McGrath MH. Infections of the hand. In: McCarthy JG, ed. *Plastic Surgery.* Vol 8. Philadelphia, PA: WB Saunders; 1990:5229–5556.

McGregor IA. Major salivary glands. In: McGregor IA, Howard DJ, eds. *Rob & Smith's Operative Surgery: Head and Neck.* 4th ed. Oxford, UK: Butterworth-Heinemann; 1992:326–340.

McGrouther DA. Dupuytren's contracture. In: Green DP, Hotchkiss RN, Pederson WC, eds. *Operative Hand Surgery.* Vol 1. 4th ed. New York, NY: Churchill Livingstone; 1999:563–591.

McGuirt WF, Salisbury PL 3rd. Mandibular fractures. Their effect on growth and dentition. *Arch Otolaryngol Head Neck Surg.* 1987;113:257–261.

McKee NH. Amputation stump management and function preservation. In: McCarthy JG, ed. *Plastic Surgery.* Vol 7. Philadelphia, PA: WB Saunders; 1990:4329–4339.

McKinney P, Katrana DJ. Prevention of injury to the great auricular nerve during rhytidectomy. *Plast Reconstr Surg.* 1980;66:675–679.

McLeish WM, Anderson RL. Cosmetic eyelid surgery and the problem eyelid. *Clin Plast Surg.* 1992;19:357–368.

McMahon JD, Wolfe JA, Cromer BA, Ruberg RL. Lasting success in teenage reduction mammaplasty. *Ann Plast Surg.* 1995;35:227–231.

McNamara MG, Butler TE, Sanders WE, Pederson WC. Ischaemia of the index finger and thumb secondary to thrombosis of the radial artery in the anatomical snuffbox. *J Hand Surg Br.* 1998;23:28–32.

Meara JG, Kolker A, Bartlett G, Theile R, Mutimer K, Holmes AD. Tuberous breast deformity: principles and practice. *Ann Plast Surg.* 2000;45:607–611.

Medina JE, et al. Malignant melanoma of the head and neck. In: Myers EN, Suen JY, eds. *Cancer of the Head and Neck.* 3rd ed. Philadelphia, PA: WB Saunders; 1996:160–183.

Melone CP Jr, McLoughlin JC, Beldner S. Surgical management of the hand in scleroderma. *Curr Opin Rheumatol.* 1999;11(6):514–520.

Mendes D, et al. Traumatic deformities and reconstruction of the temporomandibular joint. In: Cohen M, ed. *Mastery of Plastic Surgery.* Vol 2. Boston, MA: Little Brown & Co; 1994:1220–1229.

Menick FJ. Anatomic reconstruction of the nasal tip cartilages in secondary and reconstructive rhinoplasty. *Plast Reconstr Surg.* 1999;104:2187–2198; discussion 2199–2201.

Mercer D, Brander P, Liddell K. Merkel cell carcinoma: the clinical course. *Ann Plast Surg.* 1990;25:136–141.

Messina A, Messina J. The contiguous elongation treatment by the TEC device for Dupuytren's contracture of the fingers. *Plast Reconstr Surg.* 1993;92:84–90.

Meyer K, et al. Secondary rhinoplasty. In: Daniel RK, ed. *Aesthetic Plastic Surgery: Rhinoplasty.* Boston, MA: Little Brown & Co; 1993:819–820.

Meyerson MD, Jensen KM, Meyers JM, Hall BD. Nager acrofacial dysostosis: early intervention and long-term planning. *Cleft Palate J.* 1977;14:35–40.

Michelow BJ, Clarke HM, Curtis CG, Zuker RM, Seifu Y, Andrews DF. The natural history of obstetrical brachial plexus palsy. *Plast Reconstr Surg.* 1994;93:675–680; discussion 681.

Michie DD, Hugill JV. Influence of occlusive and impregnated gauze dressings on incisional healing: a prospective, randomized, controlled study. *Ann Plast Surg.* 1994;32:57–64.

Millard DR Jr. Unilateral cleft lip deformities. In: McCarthy JG, ed. *Plastic Surgery.* Vol 4. Philadelphia, PA: WB Saunders; 1990:2627.

Miller E. The metabolism and pharmacology of 5-fluorouracil. *J Surg Oncol.* 1971;3(3):309–315.

Miller LM, Morgan RF. Vasospastic disorders. Etiology, recognition and treatment. *Hand Clin.* 1993;9:171–187.

Minamikawa Y. Extensor repair and rehabilitation. In: Peimer CA, ed. *Surgery of the Hand and Upper Extremity*. Vol 1. New York, NY: McGraw-Hill; 1996:1163.

Mitchnick MA, Fairhurst D, Pinnell SR. Microfine zinc oxide (Z-cote) as a photostable UVA/UVB sunblock agent. *J Am Acad Dermatol*. 1999;40:85–90.

Mladick RA. Body contouring of the abdomen, thighs, hips and buttocks. In: Georgiade GS, Riefkohl R, Levin LS, eds. *Textbook of Plastic, Maxillofacial and Reconstructive Surgery*. Baltimore, MD: Williams & Wilkins; 1997:674–684.

Moffat CJ, et al. Assessing a calcium alginate dressing in management of pressure sores. *J Wound Care*. 1992;1:22–44.

Moko SB, Mistry Y, Blandin de Chalain TM. Parry-Romberg syndrome: intracranial MRI appearances. J *Craniomaxillofac Surg*. 2003;31(5):321–324.

Molina F, Ortiz Monasterio F, de la Paz Aguilar M, Barrera J. Maxillary distraction: aesthetic and functional benefits in cleft lip-palate and prognathic patients during mixed dentition. *Plast Reconstr Surg*. 1998;101:951–963.

Monaco JL, Lawrence WT. Acute wound healing an overview. *Clin Plast Surg*. 2003;30:1–12.

Moore KE, Gooris PJ, Stoelinga PJ. The contributing role of condylar resorption to skeletal relapse following mandibular advancement surgery: report of five cases. *J Oral Maxillofac Surg*. 1991;49:448–460.

Moore KL, Dalley AF Jr. Head. In: Moore KL, Dalley AF Jr, eds. *Clinically Oriented Anatomy*. 5th ed. Philadelphia, PA: Lippincott Williams & Wilkins; 2006.

Moore KL, ed. *The Developing Human*. 6th ed. Philadelphia, PA: WB Saunders; 1998:170, 220.

Moran JF. Surgical treatment of pulmonary tuberculosis. In: Sabiston DC, ed. *Textbook of Surgery*. Philadelphia, PA: WB Saunders; 1991:1729–1737.

Moran SL, Steinmann SP, Shin AY. Adult brachial plexus injuries: mechanism, patterns of injury, and physical diagnosis. *Hand Clin*. 2005;21(1):13–24.

Morganroth GS, Leffell DJ. Nonexcisional treatment of benign and premalignant cutaneous lesions. *Clin Plast Surg*. 1993;20:91–104.

Morykwas MJ, Argenta LC, Shelton-Brown EI, McGuirt W. Vacuum-assisted closure: a new method for wound control and treatment: animal studies and basic foundation. *Ann Plast Surg*. 1997;38:553–562.

Moscona RR, Bergman R, Friedman-Birnbaum R. An unusual late reaction to Zyderm I injections: a challenge for treatment. *Plast Reconstr Surg*. 1993;92:331–334.

Motoki DS, Mulliken JB. The healing of bone and cartilage. *Clin Plast Surg*. 1990;17:527–544.

Mowlavi A, Lille S, Andrews K, et al. Psychiatric patients who desire aesthetic surgery: identifying the problem patient. *Ann Plast Surg*. 2000;44(1):97–106.

Mowlavi A, Neumeister MW, Wilhelmi BJ. Lower blepharoplasty using bony anatomical landmarks to identify and avoid injury to the inferior oblique muscle. *Plast Reconstr Surg*. 2002;110(5):1318–1322; discussion 1323–1324.

Moy OJ, et al. Microsurgical methods and replantation. In: Peimer CA, ed. *Surgery of the Hand and Upper Extremity*. New York, NY: McGraw-Hill; 1996:1845–1874.

Mubarak SJ, Hargens AR. Acute compartment syndromes. *Surg Clin North Am*. 1983;63:539–565.

Mueller BU, Mulliken JB. The infant with a vascular tumor. *Semin Perinatol*. 1999;23:332–340.

Muhling J. Surgical treatment of craniosynostosis. In: Booth PW, Schendel SA, Hausamen JE, eds. *Maxillofacial Surgery*. Vol 2. London, UK: Churchill Livingstone; 1999:877–888.

Mukund RP, Malaviya GN, Sugar AM. Chronic infections. In: Green DP, Hotchkiss RN, Pederson WC, et al., eds. *Green's Operative Hand Surgery*. 5th ed. Philadelphia, PA: Churchill Livingstone; 2005: 94–159.

Mullaney PB, Teichmann K, Huaman A, Heinz G. Corneal keloid from unusual penetrating trauma. *J Pediatr Ophthalmol Strabismus*. 1995;32:331–334.

Mulliken JB, Vander Woude DL, Hansen M, LaBrie RA, Scott RM. Analysis of posterior plagiocephaly: deformational versus synostotic. *Plast Reconstr Surg*. 1999;103:371–380.

Mulliken JB, Glowacki J. Hemangiomas and vascular malformations in infants and children: a classification based on endothelial characteristics. *Plast Reconstr Surg*. 1982;69:412–422.

Mulliken JB, Kaban LB, Glowacki J. Induced osteogenesis–the biological principle and clinical applications. *J Surg Res*. 1984;37: 487–496.

Mulliken JB, Pensler JM, Kozakewich HP. The anatomy of Cupid's bow in normal and cleft lip. *Plast Reconstr Surg*. 1993;92:395–403; discussion 404.

Mulliken JB, Young AE, eds. *Vascular Birthmarks: Hemangiomas and Malformations*. Philadelphia, PA: WB Saunders; 1988.

Mulliken JB. Cutaneous vascular anomalies. In: McCarthy JG, ed. *Plastic Surgery*. Vol 5. Philadelphia, PA: WB Saunders; 1990:3191–3274.

Mulliken JB. Cutaneous vascular lesions in children. In: Serafin D, Georgiade NG, eds. *Pediatric Plastic Surgery*. St Louis, MO: CV Mosby; 1984:137–154.

Mullins JB, Holds JB, Branham GH, Thomas JR. Complications of the transconjunctival approach: a review of 400 cases. *Arch Otolaryngol Head Neck Surg*. 1997;123:385–388.

Munro IR, et al. Craniofacial syndromes. In: McCarthy JG, ed. *Plastic Surgery*. Vol 4. Philadelphia, PA: WB Saunders; 1990:3101–3123.

Munro IR, Sinclair WJ, Rudd NL. Maxillonasal dysplasia (Binder's syndrome). *Plast Reconstr Surg*. 1979;63:657–663.

Munser AM. Alteration of the immune system in burns and implications for therapy. *Eur J Pediatr Surg*. 1994;4:231–242.

Murphy RX Jr, Alderman A, Gutowski K, et al. Evidence based practices for thromboembolism prevention: summary of the ASPS Venous Thromboembolism Task Force Report. *Plast Reconstr Surg*. 2012;130(1):168e–175e.

Murray J. Cold, chemical and irradiation injuries. In: McCarthy, ed. *Plastic Surgery*. Vol 7. Philadelphia, PA: WB Saunders; 1990:5431–5440.

Murray JF, Carman W, MacKenzie JK. Transmetacarpal amputation of the index finger: a clinical assessment of hand strength and complications. *J Hand Surg Am*. 1977;2:471–481.

Murray PM. Septic arthritis of the hand and wrist. *Hand Clin*. 1998;14:579–587.

Mustarde JC. The correction of prominent ears using mattress sutures. *Br J Plast Surg*. 1963;16:170–178.

Mustarde JC. The treatment of prominent ears by buried mattress sutures: a ten year survey. *Plast Reconstr Surg*. 1967;39:382–386.

Mustoe T, Upton J, Marcellino V, Tun CJ, Rossier AB, Hachend HJ. Carcinoma in chronic pressure sores: a fulminant disease process. *Plast Reconstr Surg*. 1986;77:116–121.

Myckatyn TM, Mackinnon SE. The surgical management of facial nerve injury. *Clin Plast Surg*. 2003;30(2):307–318.

Myers JN, Simental AA. Cancer of the oral cavity. In: Myers EN, Suen JY, Myers N, et al., eds. *Cancer of the Head and Neck*. 4th ed. Philadelphia, PA: WB Saunders; 2003;13:279–320.

Nagata S. Microtia: auricular reconstruction. In: Achauer BM, Eriksson E, Guyuron B, et al., eds. *Plastic Surgery: Indications, Operations, and Outcomes*. St Louis, MO: Mosby-Year Book; 1023–1056.

Nahas FX, Sterman S, Gemperli R, Ferreira MC. The role of plastic surgery in congenital cutis laxa: a 10-year follow-up. *Plast Reconstr Surg*. 1999;104:1174–1178.

Nakajima T, Yoshimura Y, Onishi K, Sakakibara A. One-stage repair of blepharophimosis. *Plast Reconstr Surg*. 1991;87:24–31.

Nath RK, Kwon B, Mackinnon SE, Jensen JN, Reznik S, Boutros S. Antibody to transforming growth factor beta reduces collagen production in injured peripheral nerve. *Plast Reconstr Surg*. 1998;102:1100–1108.

Natvig K, Søberg R. Relationship of intraoperative rupture of pleomorphic adenomas to recurrence: an 11–25 year follow-up study. *Head Neck*. 1994;16:213–217.

Naumann M. Evidence-based medicine: botulinum toxin in focal hyperhidrosis. *J Neurol*. 2001;248:31–33.

Nelson BR, Hamlet KR, Gillard M, Railan D, Johnson TM. Sebaceous carcinoma. *J Am Acad Dermatol*. 1995;33:1–15.

Nelson RD, Hasslen SR, Ahrenholz DH, Solem LD. Mechanisms of loss of human neutrophil chemotaxis following thermal injury. *J Burn Care Rehabil*. 1987;8:496–502.

Neovius E, Engstrand T. Craniofacial reconstruction with bone and biomaterials: review over the last 11 years. *J Plast Reconstr Aesthet Surg*. 2010;63(10):1615–1623.

Nesi FA, et al. Correction of traumatic ptosis of the eyelid and reconstruction of the lacrimal system. In: Cohen M, ed. *Mastery of Plastic and Reconstructive Surgery*. Vol 2. Boston, MA: Little Brown & Co; 1994:1105–1108.

Nesi FA. *Smith's Ophthalmic Plastic and Reconstructive Surgery*. St Louis, MO: Mosby-Year Book; 1998a:375, 511.

Nesi FA, et al. Instrumentation in ophthalmic plastic surgery. In: *Smith's Ophthalmic Plastic and Reconstructive Surgery*. 2nd ed. St Louis, MO: Mosby-Year Book; 1998b:117–118.

Netscher D, et al. Benign and premalignant skin conditions. In: Achauer BM, Eriksson E, Guyuron B, et al., eds. *Plastic Surgery: Indications, Operations, and Outcomes*. Vol 1. St Louis, MO: Mosby-Year Book; 2000:293–324.

Netscher DT, et al. Premalignant skin tumors, basal cell carcinoma, and squamous cell carcinoma. In: Cohen M, ed. *Mastery of Plastic and Reconstructive Surgery*. Vol 1. Boston, MA: Little Brown & Co; 1994:309–332.

Netscher DT. Congenital hand problems. *Hand Clin*. 1998;25:544.

Netter FH, ed. *Atlas of Human Anatomy*. 2nd ed. East Hanover, NJ: Novartis/Hoechstetter Printing Co; 1997:18–21, 47–49.

Netter FH, ed. *Atlas of Human Anatomy*. 3rd ed. New York, NY: Novartis Medical Education; 2003.

Netter FH, ed. *Atlas of Human Anatomy*. Summit, NJ: Ciba-Geigy Corporation; 1989:19, 34, 36–37, 113–115, A436122, 491, 506, 508, 510.

Neuman JF. Evaluation and treatment of gynecomastia. *Am Fam Physician*. 1997;55:1835–1844, 1849–1850.

Neumeister MW, Murray KA. Calcinosis of the hand in scleroderma: a case report. *Plast Surg.* 1999;7:241–244.

Neviaser RJ. Acute infections. In: Green DP, Hotchkiss RN, Pederson WC, eds. *Operative Hand Surgery.* Vol 2. 4th ed. New York, NY: Churchill Livingstone; 1999:1033–1047.

Nguyen PN, Sullivan P. Advances in the management of orbital fractures. *Clin Plast Surg.* 1992;19:87–98.

Niessen FB, Spauwen PH, Schalkwijk J, Kon M. On the nature of hypertrophic scars and keloids: a review. *Plast Reconstr Surg.* 1999;104:1435–1458.

Norris RL Jr. Envenomations. In: *Intensive Medicine.* Boston, MA: Little Brown & Co; 1996; 1585–1590.

Notani K, Yamazaki Y, Kitada H, et al. Management of osteoradionecrosis corresponding to the severity of osteoradionecrosis and the method of radiotherapy. *Head Neck.* 2003;25(3):181–186.

O'Brien CJ, et al. Neck dissection and parotidectomy. In: Balch CM, Houghton AN, Sober AJ, et al., eds. *Cutaneous Melanoma.* 3rd ed. St Louis, MO: Quality Medical Publishing; 1998:245–257.

O'Connor WJ, Brodland DG. Merkel cell carcinoma. *Dermatol Surg.* 1996;22:262–267.

O'Neal D, Sheppard JE. Transient compartment syndrome of the forearm resulting from venous congestion from a tourniquet. *J Hand Surg Am.* 1989;14:894–896.

O'Sullivan ST, O'Connor TP. Immunosuppression following thermal injury: pathogenesis of immunodysfunction. *Br J Plast Surg.* 1997;50:615–623.

Ogawa R, Mitsuhashi K, Hyakusoku H, Miyashita T. Postoperative electron-beam irradiation therapy for keloids and hypertrophic scars: retrospective study of 147 cases followed for more than 18 months. *Plast Reconstr Surg.* 2003;111:547–553.

Ogawa R. The most current algorithms for the treatment and prevention of hypertrophic scars and keloids. *Plast Reconstr Surg.* 2010;125(2):557–568.

Ogose A, Emura I, Iwabuchi Y, Hotta T, Inoue Y, Saito H. Malignant melanoma extending along ulnar, median, and musculocutaneous nerves: a case report. *J Hand Surg Am.* 1998;23:875–878.

Ohlms LA, Jones DT, McGill TJ, Healy GB. Interferon alfa-2a therapy for airway hemangiomas. *Ann Otol Rhinol Laryngol.* 1994;103: 1–8.

Ohmori K. Application of microvascular free flaps to burn deformities. *World J Surg.* 1978;2:193–202.

Ohtsuka H, Shioya N, Asano T. Clinical experience with nasolabial flaps. *Ann Plast Surg.* 1981;6:207–212.

Oikarinen KS. Clinical management of injuries of the maxilla, mandible, and alveolus. *Dent Clin N Am.* 1995;39:113–131.

Oishi SN, Luce EA. The difficult scalp and skull wound. *Clin Plast Surg.* 1995;22:51–59.

Olbricht SM. Treatment of malignant cutaneous tumors. *Clin Plast Surg.* 1993;20:167–180.

Olehnik WK, Manske PR, Szerzinski J. Median nerve compression in the proximal forearm. *J Hand Surg.* 1994;19:121–126.

Opperman LA, Nolen AA, Ogle RC. TGF-beta 1, TGF-beta 2, and TGF-beta 3 exhibit distinct patterns of expression during cranial suture formation and obliteration in vivo and in vitro. *J Bone Miner Res.* 1997;12:301–310.

Orentreich N, Durr NP. Biology of scalp hair growth. *Clin Plast Surg.* 1982;9:197–205.

Orentreich N, Orentreich DS. Dermabrasion: as a complement to dermatology. *Clin Plast Surg.* 1998;25:63–80.

Ortiz-Monasterio F, del Campo AF, Carrillo A. Advancement of the orbits and the midface in one piece, combined with frontal repositioning, for the correction of Crouzon's deformities. *Plast Reconstr Surg.* 1978;61:507–516.

Osburn K, Schosser RH, Everett MA. Congenital pigmented and vascular lesions in newborn infants. *J Am Acad Dermatol.* 1987;16: 788–792.

Osler T. Antiseptics in surgery. In: *Surgical Infections.* Boston, MA: Little Brown & Co; 1994:119.

Ostad A, Kageyama N, Moy RL. Tumescent anesthesia with a lidocaine dose of 35 mg/kg is safe. *Dermatol Surg.* 1996;22:921–927.

Owen C, et al. Keratoacanthoma. In: Lebwohol MG, ed. *Treatment of Skin Disease: Comprehensive Therapeutic Strategies.* Philadelphia, PA: Mosby-Year Book; 2002:315.

Owsley JQ, Weibel TJ, Adams WA. Does steroid medication reduce facial edema following face lift surgery? A prospective, randomized study of 30 consecutive patients. *Plast Reconstr Surg.* 1996;98:1-6.

Ozyazgan I, Tercan M, Melli M, Bekerecioğlu M, Ustün H, Günay GK. Eicosanoids and the inflammatory cells in frostbitten tissue: prostacyclin, thromboxane, polymorphonuclear leukocytes, and mast cells. *Plast Reconstr Surg.* 1998;101:1881–1886.

Padwa BL, Hayward PG, Ferraro NF, Mulliken JB. Cervicofacial lymphatic malformation: clinical course, surgical intervention, and pathogenesis of skeletal pathology. *Plast Reconstr Surg.* 1995;951–960.

Pakiam AI. Reversed dermis flap. In: Strauch B, Vasconez LO, Hall-Findlay EJ, eds. *Grabb's Encyclopedia of Flaps.* 2nd ed. Philadelphia, PA: Lippincott-Raven; 1998.

Pannucci CJ, Bailey SH, Dreszer G, et al. Validation of the Caprini risk assessment model in plastic and reconstructive surgery patients. *J Am Coll Surg.* 2011;212(1):105–112.

Park C, Lew DH, Yoo WM. An analysis of 123 temporoparietal fascial flaps: anatomic and clinical considerations in total auricular reconstruction. *Plast Reconstr Surg.* 1999;104:1295–1306.

Park C, Lineaweaver WC, Rumly TO, Buncke HJ. Arterial supply of the anterior ear. *Plast Reconstr Surg.* 1992;90:38–44.

Park CA, Defranzo AJ, Marks MW, Molnar JA. Outpatient reconstruction using Integra and subatmospheric pressure. *Ann Plast Surg.* 2009;62(2):164–169.

Parkes A. The "lumbrical plus" finger. *Hand.* 1970;2:164–165.

Parsa FD. How to avoid eyelid ptosis when injecting botulinum toxin into the corrugators. *Plast Reconstr Surg.* 2000;105:1564–1565.

Pasyayan HM, Lewis MB. Clinical experience with the Robin sequence. *Cleft Palate J.* 1984;21:270–276.

Pasyk KA, Austad ED, McClatchey KD, Cherry GW. Elecrton microscopic evaluation of guinea pig skin and soft tissues "expanded" with a self-inflating silicone implant. *Plast Reconstr Surg.* 1982;70:37–45.

Patel MR. Chronic infections. In: Green DP, Hotchkiss RN, Pederson WC, eds. *Operative Hand Surgery.* Vol 2. 4th ed. New York, NY: Churchill Livingstone; 1999:1783–1850.

Patipa M. The evaluation and management of lower eyelid retraction following cosmetic surgery. *Plast Reconstr Surg.* 2000;106:438–453.

Patrice SJ, Wiss K, Mulliken JB. Pyogenic granuloma (lobular capillary hemangioma): a clinicopathologic study of 178 cases. *Pediatr Dermatol.* 1991;8:267–276.

Peacock EE Jr, et al. Wound healing. In: McCarthy JG, ed. *Plastic Surgery.* Vol 1. Philadelphia, PA: WB Saunders; 1990:161–185.

Pearl RM. Treatment of enophthalmos. *Clin Plast Surg.* 1992;19:99–111.

Peck G. Nasal tip projection: goals and maintenance. In: Rees TD, ed. *Rhinoplasty: Problems and Controversies.* St Louis, MO; CV Mosby; 1988:10.

Peck GC, et al. Unfavorable results in rhinoplasty. In: Goldwyn RM, ed. *The Unfavorable Results in Plastic Surgery.* Vol 2. Boston, MA: Little Brown & Co; 1984:539–561.

Peck GC. *Complications and Problems in Aesthetic Plastic Surgery.* New York, NY: Gower; 1992.

Peck GP, et al. Secondary rhinoplasty. In: Georgiade GS, Riefkohl R, Levin LS, eds. *Plastic, Maxillofacial and Reconstructive Surgery.* Baltimore, MD: Williams & Wilkins; 1997:646–656.

Pederson E, Hogetveit AC, Andersen A. Cancer of respiratory origins among workers at a nickel refinery in Norway. *Int J Cancer.* 1973;12:32–41.

Pederson WC. Lymphedema of the extremities. In: Aston SJ, Beasley RW, Thorne CH, eds. *Grabb & Smith's Plastic Surgery.* 5th ed. Philadelphia, PA: Lippincott-Raven; 1997:1124–1130.

Peer LA. The fate of autogenous human bone grafts. *Br J Plast Surg.* 1950;3:233–243.

Pegington J. The side of the mouth and parapharynx. In: Pegington J, ed. *Clinical Anatomy in Action—The Head and Neck.* Vol 2. Edinburgh, Scotland: Churchill Livingstone; 1986:143–150.

Peimer CA, Wheeler DR, Barrett A, Goldschmidt PG. Hand function following single ray amputation. *J Hand Surg Am.* 1999;24:1245–1248.

Peimer CA, et al. Tumors of bone and soft tissue. In: Green DP, ed. *Operative Hand Surgery.* Vol 3. 3rd ed. New York, NY: Churchill Livingstone; 1993:2225–2250.

Pelc NJ, Nordlund JJ. Pigmentary changes in the skin: an introduction for surgeons. *Clin Plast Surg.* 1993;20:53–65.

Pellegrini VD Jr. The basal articulations of the thumb: pain, instability and osteoarthritis. In: Peimer CA, ed. *Surgery of the Hand and Upper Extremity.* New York, NY: McGraw-Hill; 1996:1019–1042.

Pellitteri PK, Takes RP, Lewis JS, et al. Merkel cell carcinoma of the head and neck. *Head Neck.* 2012;34(9):1346–1354.

Peng YP, Low CK, Looi KP. Comparison of first carpometacarpal joint arthrodesis with contralateral excision arthroplasty in a patient with bilateral saddle arthritis: a case report. *Ann Acad Med Singapore.* 1999;28:451–454.

Pensler JM, Ivescu AS, Ciletti SJ, Yokoo KM, Byrd SE. Craniofacial gliomas. *Plast Reconstr Surg.* 1996;98:27–30.

Perez CA, Devineni VR, Marcial-Vega V, Marks JE, Simpson JR, Kucik N. Carcinoma of the nasopharynx: factors affecting prognosis. *Int J Radiat Oncol Biol Phys.* 1992;23:271–280.

Perrott DH, Kaban LB. Acute management of orbitozygomatic fractures. *Oral Maxillofac Surg Clin North Am.* 1993;5:475–493.

Peterson KL, Wang M, Canalis RF, Abemayor E. Rhinocerebral mucormycosis: evolution of the disease and treatment options. *Laryngoscope.* 1997;107(7):855–862.

Peterson RA, Johnston DL. Facile identification of the facial nerve branches. *Clin Plast Surg.* 1987;14:785–788.

Petri WA. Antimicrobial agents. In: Hardman JG, Limbirg LE, Gilman AG, eds. *The Pharmacological Basis of Therapeutics*. New York, NY: McGraw-Hill; 2001:1171–1192.

Petricig P, Pepe E. First choice treatment of the pediatric wrist ganglia. *Minerva Pediatr.* 2006;58(4):379–383.

Phillips JW,de Camara DL, Lockwood MD, Grebner WC. Strength of silicone breast implants. *Plast Reconstr Surg.* 1996;97:1215–1225.

Phillips LG, et al. Pressure ulcerations. In: Jurkiewicz MJ, Krizek TJ, Mathes SJ, et al., eds. *Plastic Surgery: Principles and Practice*. St Louis, MO: CV Mosby; 2:1223–1251.

Physicians' Desk Reference. Montvale, NJ: Medical Economics Co; 2000:638.

Physicians' Desk Reference. Montvale, NJ: Medical Economics Co; 2003:2825.

Piccirillo JF, et al. Evaluation, classification, and staging. In: Myers EN, Suen JY, eds. *Cancer of the Head and Neck*. Philadelphia, PA: WB Saunders; 1996:33–49.

Pick TP, Howden R, eds. *Gray's Anatomy*. New York, NY: Bounty Books; 1977:77–80, 113–117, 884–886.

Pickford MA, Hogg FJ, Fallowfield ME, Webster MH. Sebaceous carcinoma of the periorbital and extraorbital regions. *Br J Plast Surg.* 1995;48:93–96.

Pinnell SR, Madey DL. New and improved daily photoprotection: microfine zinc oxide (Z-Cote). *Aesthet Surg J.* 1999;19:260–263.

Pinski JB. Hair transplantation and bald-scalp reduction. *Dermatol Clin.* 1991;9:151–168.

Pinzur MS, Bowker JH, Smith DG, Gottschalk F. Amputation surgery in peripheral vascular disease. *Instr Course Lect.* 1999;48:687–691.

Pitanguy I, Vaena M, Radwanski HN, Nunes D, Vargas AF. Relative implant volume and sensibility alterations after breast augmentation. *Aesthetic Plast Surg.* 2007;31(3):238–243.

Pittman GH. *Liposuction and Aesthetic Surgery*. St Louis, MO: Quality Medical Publishing; 1993:169.

Place MJ, et al. Basic techniques and principles in plastic surgery. In: Aston SJ, Beasley RW, Thorne CH, eds. *Grabb & Smith's Plastic Surgery*. 5th ed. Philadelphia, PA: Lippincott-Raven; 1997:13–26.

Pokrovsky AV, Dan VN, Chupin AV, Khorovets AG. Arterialization of the foot venous system in the treatment of the critical lower limb ischaemia and distal arterial bed occlusion. *Ang Vasc Surg.* 1996;4:73–93.

Pollard RL, Kennedy PJ, Maitz PK. The use of artificial dermis (Integra) and topical negative pressure to achieve limb salvage following soft-tissue loss caused by meningococcal septicaemia. *J Plast Reconstr Aesthet Surg.* 2008;61(3):319–322.

Polley JW, Figueroa AA. Management of severe maxillary deficiency in childhood and adolescence through distraction osteogenesis with an external, adjustable, rigid distraction device. *J Craniofac Surg.* 1997a;8:181–185.

Polley JW, Figueroa AA, Liou EJ, Cohen M. Longitudinal analysis of mandibular asymmetry in hemifacial microsomia. *Plast Reconstr Surg.* 1997b;99:328–339.

Polley JW, Figueroa AA. Rigid external distraction: its application in cleft maxillary deformities. *Plast Reconstr Surg.* 1998;102:1360–1372.

Polley JW. Bone grafts. In: Cohen M, ed. *Mastery of Plastic and Reconstructive Surgery*. Vol 1. Boston, MA: Little Brown & Co; 1994:102–112.

Popkin GL. Tumors of the skin: a dermatologist's viewpoint. In: McCarthy JG, ed. *Plastic Surgery*. Vol 5. Philadelphia, PA: WB Saunders; 1990:3560–3613.

Posner MA. Differential diagnosis of wrist pain: tendinitis, ganglia, and other syndromes. In: Peimer CA, ed. *Surgery of the Hand and Upper Extremity*. New York, NY: McGraw-Hill; 1996:837–851.

Posnick JC. Management of facial fractures in children and adolescents. *Ann Plast Surg.* 1994;33:442–457.

Posnick JC. Surgical correction of mandibular hypoplasia in hemifacial microsomia: a personal perspective. *J Oral Maxillofac Surg.* 1998;56:639–650.

Posnick JC. The craniofacial dysostosis syndromes. Current reconstructive strategies. *Clin Plast Surg.* 1994;21:585–598.

Posnick JC. Treacher Collins syndrome. In: Aston SJ, Beasley RW, Thorne CH, eds. *Grabb & Smith's Plastic Surgery*. 5th ed. Philadelphia, PA: Lippincott-Raven; 1997:313–319.

Posnick JC, Wells M, Pron GE. Pediatric facial fractures: evolving patterns of treatment. *J Oral Maxillofac Surg.* 1993;51:836–844.

Posnick JC, Zimbler AG, Grossman JA. Normal cutaneous sensibility of the face. *Plast Reconstr Surg.* 1990;86:429–433.

Posnick JC, et al. Surgical correction of temporomandibular joint ankylosis. *Clin Plast Surg.* 1989;16:725–732.

Press B. Thermal, electrical, and chemical injuries. In: Aston SJ, Beasley RW, Thorne CH, eds. *Grabb & Smith's Plastic Surgery*. 5th ed. Philadelphia, PA: Lippincott-Raven; 1997:161–191.

Preston DS, Stern RS. Nonmelanoma cancers of the skin. *N Engl J Med.* 1992;327:1649–1662.

Preuss S, et al. Prominent ears. In: Achauer BM, Eriksson E, Guyuron B, et al., eds. *Plastic Surgery: Indications, Operations, and Outcomes*. Vol 2. St Louis, MO: Mosby-Year Book; 2000:1057–1065.

Pribaz JJ, Weiss DD, Mulliken JB, Eriksson E. Prelaminated free flap reconstruction of complex central facial defects. *Plast Reconstr Surg.* 1999;104:357–365.

Price CI, Eaves FF 3rd, Nahai F, Jones G, Bostwick J 3rd. Endoscopic transaxillary subpectoral breast augmentation. *Plast Reconstr Surg.* 1994;94:612–619.

Price HN, Zaenglein AL. Diagnosis and management of benign lumps and bumps in childhood. *Curr Opin Pediatr.* 2007; 19(4):420–424.

Price VH. Treatment of hair loss. *N Engl J Med.* 1999;341:964–973.

Prockop DJ, Kivirikko KI, Tuderman L, Guzman NA. The biosynthesis of collagen and its disorders. *N Engl J Med.* 1979;301:13–23.

Proffit WR. Treatment planning: the search for wisdom. In: Proffit WR, White RP, eds. *Surgical Orthodontic Treatment.* St Louis, MO: Mosby-Year Book; 1991:158–161.

Proffitt WR, Vig KW, Turvey TA. Early fracture of the mandibular condyles: frequently and unsuspected cause of growth disturbances. *Am J Orthod.* 1980;78:1–24.

Prosser R. Splinting in the management of proximal interphalangeal joint flexion contracture. *J Hand Ther.* 1996;9:378–386.

Puckett CL. Lymphedema of the upper extremity. In: McCarthy JG, ed. *Plastic Surgery.* Vol 7. Philadelphia, PA: WB Saunders; 1990:5023–5031.

Putnam MD, Cohen M. Malignant bony tumors of the upper extremity. *Hand Clin.* 1995;11:265–286.

Putterman AM. *Cosmetic Oculoplastic Surgery: Eyelid, Forehead, and Facial Techniques.* Philadelphia, PA: WB Saunders; 1999:429–256.

Putz R, Pabst R, eds. *Sobatta's Atlas of Human Anatomy.* Vol 1. Baltimore, MD: Williams & Wilkins; 1997:43.

Pyo DJ, et al. Craniosynostosis. In: Aston SJ, Beasley RW, Thorne CH, eds. *Grabb & Smith's Plastic Surgery.* 5th ed. Philadelphia, PA: Lippincott-Raven; 1997:281–293.

Quinn MJ, et al. Subungual melanoma of the hand. *J Hand Surg.* 1998;21:506–511.

Rae V, Falanga V. Wrinkling due to middermal elastolysis: report of a case and review of the literature. *Arch Dermatol.* 1989;125:950–951.

Ramakrishnan MK, Sankar J, Venkatraman J, Ramesh J. Infections in burn patients—experience in a tertiary care hospital. *Burns.* 2006;32:594–596.

Ramasastry SS. Chronic problem wounds. *Clin Plast Surg.* 1998;25:367–396.

Ramasastry SS, Conklin WT, Granick MS, Futrell JW. Surgical management of massive perianal hidradenitis suppurativa. *Ann Plast Surg.* 1985;15:218–223.

Ramirez O. Abdominoplasty and abdominal wall rehabilitation: a comprehensive approach. *Plast Reconstr Surg.* 2000;105:425–435.

Ramirez OM, Orlando JC, Hurwitz DJ. The sliding gluteus maximus myocutaneous flap: its relevance in ambulatory patients. *Plast Reconstr Surg.* 1984;74:68–75.

Ramirez OM, Ruas E, Dellon AL. "Component separation" method for closure of abdominal-wall defects: an anatomic and clinical study. *Plast Reconstr Surg.* 1990;86(3):519–526.

Rao RB, Ely SF, Hoffman RS. Deaths related to liposuction. *N Engl J Med.* 1999;340:1471–1475.

Rao SB, et al. Traumatic and acquired wrist disorders in children. In: Lichtman DM, Alexander AH, eds. *The Wrist and Its Disorders.* Philadelphia, PA: WB Saunders; 1997:540.

Rapaport DP, Bass LS, Aston SJ. Influence of steroids on postoperative swelling after facialplasty: a prospective, randomized study. *Plast Reconstr Surg.* 1995;96:1547–1552.

Raulin C, Schönermark MP, Greve B, Werner S. Q-switched ruby laser treatment of tattoos and benign pigmented skin lesions: a critical review. *Ann Plast Surg.* 1998;41:555–565.

Rayan GM. Clinical presentation and types of Dupuytren's disease. *Hand Clin.* 1999a;15:87–96.

Rayan GM. Palmar fascial complex anatomy and pathology in Dupuytren's disease. *Hand Clin.* 1999b;15:73–86.

Raymond GV. Craniofacial genetics and dysmorphology. In: Achauer BM, Eriksson E, Guyuron B, et al., eds. *Plastic Surgery: Indications, Operations, and Outcomes.* Vol 2. St Louis, MO: Mosby-Year Book; 2000:614–615.

Rayner CR, Towers JF, Wilson JS. What is Gorlin's syndrome? The diagnosis and management of the basal cell naevus syndrome, based on a study of thirty-seven patients. *Br J Plast Surg.* 1977;30:62–67.

Rees TD. *Aesthetic Plastic Surgery.* Vol 2. Philadelphia, PA: WB Saunders; 1980:525–580, 601–606.

Rees TD. Chemabrasion and dermabrasion. In: Rees TD, LaTrenta GS, eds. *Aesthetic Plastic Surgery.* 2nd ed. Philadelphia, PA: WB Saunders; 1994:757.

Rees TD. Unique problems associated with the lip–columella–tip complex. In: Rees TD, Baker DC, Tabbal N, eds. *Rhinoplasty: Problems and Controversies.* St Louis, MO: 1998:118–123.

Rees TD, et al. Blepharoplasty and facialplasty. In: McCarthy JG, ed. *Plastic Surgery*. Vol 3. Philadelphia, PA: WB Saunders; 1990:2320–2414.

Rees TD, LaTrenta GS. The role of the Schirmer's test and orbital morphology in predicting dry-eye syndrome after blepharoplasty. *Plast Reconstr Surg*. 1988;82:619–625.

Regnault P. Breast ptosis: definition and treatment. *Clin Plast Surg*. 1976;3:193–203.

Reiger RA. A local flap for repair of the nasal tip. *Plast Reconstr Surg*. 1967;40:147–149.

Reintgen DS, et al. Lymphatic mapping and sentinel lymphadenectomy. In: Balch CM, Houghton AN, Sober AJ, et al., eds. *Cutaneous Melanoma*. 3rd ed. St Louis, MO: Quality Medical Publishing; 1998:227–244.

Renehan A, Gleave EN, McGurk M. An analysis of the treatment of 114 patients with recurrent pleomorphic adenomas of the parotid gland. *Am J Surg*. 1996;172:710–714.

Restifo RJ, Ward BA, Scoutt LM, Brown JM, Taylor KJ. Timing, magnitude, and utility of surgical delay in the TRAM flap: II: clinical studies. *Plast Reconstr Surg*. 1997;99:1217–1223.

Rettig AC. Management of acute scaphoid fractures. *Hand Clin*. 2000;16:381–394.

Rettig ME, et al. Fractures of the distal radius. In: Lichtman DM, Alexander AH, eds. *The Wrist and Its Disorders*. Philadelphia, PA: WB Saunders; 1997;347–372.

Reus WF 3rd, Colen LB, Straker DJ. Tobacco smoking and complications in elective microsurgery. *Plast Reconstr Surg*. 1992;89:490–494.

Reus WF, Robson MC, Zachary L, Heggers JP. Acute effects of tobacco smoking on blood flow and cutaneous micro circulation. *Br J Plast Surg*. 1994;37:213–215.

Ricciardelli E, et al. Anatomy/physiology/embryology. In: Ruberg RL, Smith DJ, eds. *Plastic Surgery: A Core Curriculum*. St Louis, MO: CV Mosby; 1994:251–259.

Rice DH. Diseases of the salivary glands—nonneoplastic. In: Bailey BJ, Calhoun KH, Deskin RW, et al., eds. *Head and Neck Surgery—Otolaryngology*. Vol 1. 2nd ed. Philadelphia, PA: Lippincott-Raven; 1998:561–570.

Richmond JD, Davie RM. The significance of incomplete excision in patients with basal cell carcinoma. *Br J Plast Surg*. 1987;40:63–67.

Ridenour BD. The nasal septum. In: Cummings CW, Fredrickson JM, Harker LA, eds. *Otolaryngology Head & Neck Surgery*. Vol 2. 3rd ed. St Louis, MO: Mosby-Year Book; 1998:921–848.

Riefkohl R, et al. Gynecomastia. In: Georgiade GS, Riefkohl R, Levin LS, eds. *Textbook of Plastic, Maxillofacial and Reconstructive Surgery*. Baltimore, MD: Williams & Wilkins; 1997:820–828.

Ritchie JM, et al. Local anesthetics. In: Goodman G, Gilman AG, eds. *Goodman & Gilman's The Pharmacological Basis of Therapeutics*. 6th ed. New York, NY: Macmillan; 1980:300–322.

Rizio L, Belsky MR. Finger deformities in rheumatoid arthritis. *Hand Clin*. 1996;12:531–540.

Robb GL. Free scapular flap reconstruction of the head and neck. *Clin Plast Surg*. 1994;21:45–58.

Robbins KT. Neck dissection. In: Cummings CW, Fredrickson JM, Harker LA, et al., eds. *Otolaryngology Head Neck Surgery*. Vol 3. 3rd ed. St Louis, MO: Mosby-Year Book; 1998:1787–1810.

Roberts TL, et al. Aesthetic laser surgery. In: Achauer BM, Eriksson E, Guyuron B, et al., eds. *Plastic Surgery: Indications, Operations, and Outcomes*. Vol 5. St Louis, MO: Mosby-Year Book; 2000:2457–2486.

Robertson B, et al. Orthognathic surgery. In: Evans GR, ed. *Operative Plastic Surgery*. New York, NY: McGraw-Hill; 2000:585–593.

Robson MC, Barnett RA, Leitch IO, Hayward PG. Prevention and treatment of post burn scars and contracture. *World J Surg*. 1992;16:87–96.

Robson MC, et al. Cold injuries. In: McCarthy JG, ed. *Plastic Surgery*. Vol 1. Philadelphia, PA: WB Saunders; 1990:849–866.

Robson MC, et al. Wound repair: principles and applications. In: Ruberg RL, Smith DL, eds. *Plastic Surgery—A Core Curriculum*. Vol 1. St Louis, MO: Mosby-Year Book; 1994:5–6.

Rockwell WB, Butler PN, Byrne BA. Extensor tendon: anatomy, injury, and reconstruction. *Plast Reconstr Surg*. 2000;106:1592–1603.

Rockwell WB, Cohen IK, Ehrlich HP. Keloids and hypertrophic scars: a comprehensive review. *Plast Reconstr Surg*. 1989;84:827–837.

Rockwell WB, et al. Nail bed injuries and reconstruction. In: Peimer CA, ed. *Surgery of the Hand and Upper Extremity*. Vol 2. New York, NY: McGraw-Hill; 1996:1101–1111.

Rodeheaver GT, Pettry D, Thacker JG, Edgerton MT, Edlich RF. Wound cleansing by high pressure irrigation. *Surg Gynecol Obstet*. 1975;141:357–362.

Roenigk HH Jr. Dermabrasion: state of the art. *J Dermatol Surg Oncol*. 1985;11:306–314.

Rohrich R, Coberly D, Fagien S, Stuzin JM. Current concepts in aesthetic upper blepharoplasty. *Plast Reconstr Surg*. 2004;113:32e–42e.

Rohrich RJ, Adams WP Jr. Nasal fracture management: minimizing secondary nasal deformities. *Plast Reconstr Surg*. 2000;106:266–273.

Rohrich RJ, Adams WP Jr, Beran SJ, et al. An analysis of silicone gel-filled breast implants: diagnosis and failure rates. *Plast Reconstr Surg.* 1998a;102:2304–2308.

Rohrich RJ, Beran SJ, Restifo RJ, Copit SE. Aesthetic management of the breast following explantation: evaluation and mastopexy options. *Plast Reconstr Surg.* 1998b;101:827–837.

Rohrich RJ, Kenkel JM, Janis JE, Beran SJ, Fodor PB. An update on the role of subcutaneous infiltration in suction-assisted lipoplasty. *Plast Reconstr Surg.* 2003;111:926–927,

Rohrich RJ, Reagan BJ, Adams WP Jr, Kenkel JM, Beran SJ. Early results of vermilion lip augmentation using acellular allogenic dermis: an adjunct in facial rejuvenation. *Plast Reconstr Surg.* 2000;105:409–416.

Rohrich RJ, Hollier LH. Management of frontal sinus fractures: changing concepts. *Clin Plast Surg.* 1992a;19:219–232.

Rohrich RJ, Shewmake KB. Evolving concepts of craniomaxillofacial fracture management. *Clin Plast Surg.* 1992b;19:1–10.

Rohrich RJ, Zbar RI. A simplified algorithm for the use of Z-plasty. *Plast Reconstr Surg.* 1999; 103:1513–1517.

Rohrich RJ, et al. Nasal aesthetics. In: Aston SJ, Beasley RW, Thorne CH, eds. *Grabb & Smith's Plastic Surgery.* 5th ed. Philadelphia, PA: Lippincott-Raven; 1997:513.

Rohrich RJ, et al. Secondary rhinoplasty. In: Grotting JC, ed. *Reoperative Aesthetic and Reconstructive Surgery.* St Louis, MO: Quality Medical Publishing; 1995a;401–510.

Rohrich RJ, Gunter JP, Friedman RM. Nasal tip blood supply: an anatomic study validating the safety of the transcolumellar incision in rhinoplasty. *Plast Reconstr Surg.* 1995b;95:795–799.

Rohrich RJ, Hollier LH, Watumull D. Optimizing the management of orbitozygomatic fractures. *Clin Plast Surg.* 1992;19:149–165.

Rohrich RJ, Hochstein LM, Millwee RH. Subungual glomus tumors: an algorithmic approach. *Ann Plast Surg.* 1994;33:300–304.

Rohrich RJ, Krueger JK, Adams WP Jr, Marple BF. Rationale for submucous resection of hypertrophied inferior turbinates in rhinoplasty: an evolution. *Plast Reconstr Surg.* 2001; 108(2):536–544.

Rohrich RJ, Raniere J, Ha RY. The alar contour graft: correction and prevention of alar rim deformities in rhinoplasty. *Plast Reconstr Surg.* 2002;109(7):2495–2505.

Rosen HM. When osteotomies should be considered. *Clin Plast Surg.* 1991;18:205–212.

Rosen HM. Chin surgery. In: Rosen HM, ed. *Aesthetic Perspectives in Jaw Surgery.* New York, NY: Springer-Verlag; 1999:248–249.

Rosenthal JS. The thermally injured ear: a systematic approach to reconstruction. *Clin Plast Surg.* 1992;19:645–661.

Ross JJ, Granick MS. Squamous cell and adnexal carcinomas of the skin. *Clin Plast Surg.* 1997;24:687–703.

Rosse C, Gaddum-Rosse P, eds. *Hollinshead's Textbook of Anatomy.* 5th ed. Philadelphia, PA: Lippincott-Raven; 1997:359, 767-793.

Rosson JW, Walker G. The natural history of ganglia in children. *J Bone Joint Surg Br.* 1989;71(4):707–708.

Roth DA, Gold LI, Han VK, et al. Immunolocalization of transforming growth factor beta 1, beta 2, and beta 3 and insulin-like growth factor I in premature cranial suture fusion. *Plast Reconstr Surg.* 1997a;99:300–309.

Roth DA, Longaker MT, McCarthy JG, et al. Studies in cranial suture biology: part I. Increased immunoreactivity for TGF-beta isoforms (beta 1, beta 2, and beta 3) during rat cranial suture fusion. *J Bone Miner Res.* 1997b;12:311–321.

Rowe NL. Fractures of the jaws in children. *J Oral Surg.* 1969;27:497–507.

Rowland LP. Stroke, spasticity, and botulinum toxin. *N Engl J Med.* 2002;347:382–383.

Rowland SA. Fasciotomy: the treatment of compartment syndrome. In: Green DP, ed. *Operative Hand Surgery.* Vol 2. 3rd ed. New York, NY: Churchill Livingstone; 1993:661–710.

Rowland SA. Fasciotomy: the treatment of compartment syndrome. In: Green DP, Hotchkiss RN, Pederson WC, eds. *Operative Hand Surgery.* Vol 1. 4th ed. New York, NY: Churchill Livingstone; 1999:689–710.

Ruan CM, Escobedo E, Harrison S, Goldstein B. Magnetic resonance imaging of nonhealing pressure ulcers and myocutaneous flaps. *Arch Phys Med Rehabil.* 1998;79:1080–1088.

Rubenstein R, Roenigk HH Jr, Stegman SJ, Hanke CW. Atypical keloids after dermabrasion of patients taking isotretinoin. *J Acad Dermatol Surg Oncol.* 1986;15:280–285.

Ruberg R, et al. *Plastic Surgery: A Core Curriculum.* St Louis, MO: CV Mosby; 1994:251.

Rubin MG, ed. *Manual of Chemical Peels: Superficial and Medium Depth.* Philadelphia, PA: JB Lippincott; 1995:3.

Rubin MG. Trichloroacetic acid and other non-phenol peels. *Clin Plast Surg.* 1992;19:525–536.

Rudolph R, et al. Skin grafts. In: McCarthy JG, ed. *Plastic Surgery.* Vol 1. Philadelphia, PA: WB Saunders; 1990:221–274.

Ruff GL. Progressive hemifacial atrophy: Romberg's disease. In: McCarthy JG, ed. *Plastic Surgery.* Vol 5. Philadelphia, PA: WB Saunders; 1990:3135–3143.

Ruggles G. Coincidence of palmaris longus and plantaris muscles. *Anat Rec.* 1953;116(4):521-523.

Rusby JE, Smith BL, Gui GP. Nipple-sparing mastectomy. *Br J Surg.* 2010;97(3):305–316.

Rushton DH. Management of hair loss in women. *Dermatol Clin.* 1993;11:47–53.

Sadler TW, ed. *Langman's Medical Embryology.* Baltimore, MD: Williams & Wilkins; 1990:328–337.

Sakar M, Mulliken JB, Kozakewich HP, Robertson RL, Burrows PE. Thrombocytopenic coagulopathy (Kasabach-Merritt phenomenon) is associated with Kaposiform hemangioendothelioma and not with common infantile hemangioma. *Plast Reconstr Surg.* 1997; 100:1377–1386.

Salisbury RE. Thermal burns. In: McCarthy JG, ed. *Plastic Surgery.* Vol 2. Philadelphia, PA: WB Saunders; 1990:787–813.

Salmerk L, Wieslander JB, Dougan P, Arnljots B. Studies of antithrombotic effects of Dextran 40 following microarterial trauma. *Br J Plast Surg.* 1991;44:15–22.

Salmerk L, Knudsen F, Dougan P. The effect of Dextran 40 on patency following severe trauma in small arteries and veins. *Br J Plast Surg.* 1995;48:121–126.

Salmons S. Muscles and fasciae of the head. In: *Gray's Anatomy.* 38th ed. New York, NY: Churchill Livingstone; 1995:796–802.

Salyer KE. Primary correction of the unilateral cleft lip nose: a 15-year experience. *Plast Reconstr Surg.* 1986;77:558–568.

Samuels TH, Haider MA, Kirkbride P. Poland's syndrome: a mammographic presentation. *AJR Am J Roentgenol.* 1996;347–348.

Sanders GH, Miller TA. Are keratoacanthomas really squamous cell carcinomas? *Ann Plast Surg.* 1982;9:306–309.

Sandow MJ, et al. Single-cross grasp six-strand repair for acute flexor tenorrhaphy: modified Savage technique. In: Taras SJ, Schneider LH, eds. *Atlas of the Hand Clinics.* Philadelphia, PA: WB Saunders; 1996:65–77.

Sanz-Gallen P, Nogué S, Munné P, Faraldo A. Hypocalcemia and hypomagnesemia due to hydrofluoric acid. *Occup Med (Lond).* 2001;51:294–295.

Sarhadi NS, Shaw Dunn J, Lee FD, et al. An anatomical study of the nerve supply of the breast, including the nipple and areola. *Br J Plast Surg.* 1996;49(3):156–164.

Sasaki GH, Pang CY. Pathophysiology of skin flaps raised on expanded pig skin. *Plast Reconstr Surg.* 1984a;74:59–67.

Sasaki GH, Pang CY, Wittliff JL. Pathogenesis and treatment of infant skin strawberry hemangiomas: clinical and in vitro studies of hormonal effects. *Plast Reconstr Surg.* 1984b;73:359–370.

Sauerland S, Korenkov M, Kleinen T, Arndt M, Paul A. Obesity is a risk factor for recurrence after incisional hernia repair. *Hernia.* 2004;8(1):42–46.

Saulis AS, Dumanian GA. Periumbilical rectus abdominis perforator preservation significantly reduces superficial wound complications in "separation of parts" hernia repairs. *Plast Reconstr Surg.* 2002;109(7):2275–2280; discussion 2281–2282.

Schaffer JV, Bolognia JL. The clinical spectrum of pigmented lesions. *Clin Plast Surg.* 2000;27:391–408.

Schall SB, Vu-Rose T, Holtom PD, Doyle B, Stevanovic M. Tissue pressures in pyogenic flexor tenosynovitis of the finger. *J Bone Joint Surg Br.* 1996;78:793–795.

Schenck RE. Full thickness skin grafts to the hand. In: Blair WF, ed. *Techniques in Hand Surgery.* Baltimore, MD: Williams & Wilkins; 1996:13–18.

Schenck RR. Dynamic traction and early passive movement for fractures of the proximal interphalangeal joint. *J Hand Surg Am.* 1986;11:850–858.

Schendel SA. Cephalometrics and orthognathic surgery. In: Bell WH, ed. *Modern Practice in Orthognathic and Reconstructive Surgery.* Vol 1. Philadelphia, PA: WB Saunders; 1992:85–99.

Schendel SA. Orthognathic surgery. In: Achauer BM, Eriksson E, Guyuron B, et al., eds. *Plastic Surgery: Indications, Operations, and Outcomes.* Vol 2. St Louis, MO: Mosby-Year Book; 2000:871–895.

Schendel SA. Vertical maxillary deformities. In: Ferraro JW, ed. *Fundamentals in Maxillofacial Surgery.* New York, NY: Springer-Verlag; 1997:284–286.

Schenkler JD, et al. The abdominohypogastric skin flap for hand and forearm coverage. In: Strauch B, Vasconez LO, eds. *Grabb's Encyclopedia of Flaps.* Vol 2. Boston, MA: Little Brown & Co; 1990:1158–1160.

Schierle C, Winograd JM. Radiation-induced brachial plexopathy: review. Complication without a cure. *J Reconstr Microsurg.* 2004;20(2):149–152.

Schlenz I, Kuzbari R, Gruber H, Holle J. The sensitivity of the nipple–areolar complex: an anatomic study. *Plast Reconstr Surg.* 2000;105:905–909.

Schmitz JP, Hollinger JO, Milam SB. Reconstruction of bone using calcium phosphate bone cements: a critical review. *J Oral Maxillofac Surg.* 1999;57:1122–1126.

Schneider JM, Roger DJ, Uhl RL. Bilateral forearm compartment syndrome resulting from neuroleptic malignant syndrome. *J Hand Surg Am.* 1996;21:287–289.

Schneider LH. Flexor tendons—late reconstruction. In: Green DP, Hotchkiss RN, Pederson WC, eds. *Operative Hand Surgery*. Vol 2. 4th ed. New York, NY: Churchill Livingstone; 1999:1898–1949.

Schneider MS, Borkow JE, Cruz IT, Marangoni RD, Shaffer J, Grove D. The tensiometric properties of expanded guinea pig skin. *Plast Reconstr Surg*. 1988;81:398–405.

Schon MP, Schon M. Imiquimod: mode of action. *Br J Dermatol*. 2007;157(Suppl 2):8–13.

Schuller DE, Dankle SD, Strauss RH. A technique to treat wrestlers' auricular hematoma without interrupting training or competition. *Arch Otolaryngol Head Neck Surg*. 1989;15:202–206.

Schwartz RA. The actinic keratoses: a prospective and update. *Dermatol Surg*. 1997;23:1009–1019.

Schwartz SI, ed. *Principles of Surgery*. New York, NY: McGraw-Hill; 1999.

Sclafani AP, Gordon L, Chadha M, Romo T 3rd. Prevention of earlobe keloid recurrence with postoperative corticosteroid injections versus radiation therapy: a randomized, prospective study and review of the literature. *Dermatol Surg*. 1996;22:569–574.

Scott SM. Pulmonary infections. In: Sabiston DC, ed. *Textbook of Surgery*. Philadelphia, PA: WB Saunders; 1991:1701–1717.

Searles JM Jr, Colen LE. Foot reconstruction in diabetes mellitus and peripheral vascular insufficiency. *Clin Plast Surg*. 1991;18:467–483.

Seckel BR. *Facial Danger Zones: Avoiding Nerve Injury in Facial Plastic Surgery*. St Louis, MO: Quality Medical Publishing; 1994.

Seibert JW, Angrigiani C, McCarthy JG, Longaker MT. Blood supply of the Le Fort I maxillary segment: an anatomic study. *Plast Reconstr Surg*. 1997;100:843–851.

Seitz A, Papp S, Papp C, Maurer H. The anatomy of the angular branch of the thoracodorsal artery. *Cells Tissues Organs*. 1999;164: 227–236.

Seitz WH Jr. Complications and problems in the management of distal radius fractures. *Hand Clin*. 1994;10:117–123.

Selber JC, Samra F, Bristol M, et al. A head-to-head comparison between the muscle-sparing free TRAM and the SIEA flaps: is the rate of flap loss worth the gain in abdominal wall function? *Plast Reconstr Surg*. 2008;122(2):348–355.

Semple JL, Lugowski SJ, Baines CJ, Smith DC, McHugh A. Breast milk contamination and silicone implants: preliminary results using silicon as a proxy measurement for silicone. *Plast Reconstr Surg*. 1998;102:528–533.

Senturk S, HoSnuter M, Tosun Z, Savaci N. Calciphylaxis: cutaneous necrosis in chronic renal failure. *Ann Plast Surg*. 2002;48:104–105.

Serafin D. Radial forearm flap. In: *Atlas of Microsurgical Composite Tissue Transplantation*. Philadelphia, PA: WB Saunders; 1996:389.

Servelle M. Klippel and Trenaunay's syndrome: 768 operated cases. *Ann Surg*. 1985;201:365–373.

Seyfer AE, Icochea R, Graeber GM. Poland's anomaly: natural history and long-term results of chest wall reconstruction in 33 patients. *Ann Surg*. 1988;208:776–782.

Shack RB, Barton RM, DeLozier J, Rees RS, Lynch JB. Is aggressive surgical management justified in the treatment of Merkel cell carcinoma? *Plast Reconstr Surg*. 1994;94:970–975.

Shah JP. Cervical lymph nodes. In: Shah JP, ed. *Head and Neck Surgery*. London, UK: Mosby-Wolfe; 1996:355–392.

Shankar R, et al. Hematologic, hematopoietic, and acute phase response. In: Herndon DN, ed. *Total Burn Care*. 2nd ed. Philadelphia, PA: WB Saunders; 2002:334–335.

Shapiro PS, Seitz WH Jr. Non-neoplastic tumors of the hand and upper extremity. *Hand Clin*. 1995;11:133–160.

Shaw JH, Rumball E. Merkel cell tumour: clinical behaviour and treatment. *Br J Surg*. 1991;78:138–142.

Sheen JH. Closed versus open rhinoplasty–and the debate goes on. *Plast Reconstr Surg*. 1997;99:859–862.

Sheen JH, et al. Applied anatomy and physiology. In: *Aesthetic Rhinoplasty*. St Louis, MO: Quality Medical Publishing; 1998a:14.

Sheen JH, et al. Problems in secondary rhinoplasty. In: *Aesthetic Rhinoplasty*. St Louis, MO: Quality Medical Publishing; 1998b:1135–1408.

Sheen JH. Spreader graft: a method of reconstructing the roof of the middle nasal vault following rhinoplasty. *Plast Reconstr Surg*. 1984;73:230–239.

Sheen JH. Tip graft: a 20 year retrospective. *Plast Reconstr Surg*. 1993;91:48–63.

Shenaq SM, et al. Principles of microvascular surgery. In: Aston SJ, Beasley RW, Thorne CH, eds. *Grabb & Smith's Plastic Surgery*. 5th ed. Philadelphia, PA: Lippincott-Raven; 1997:73.

Shepard DD. Betadine: ophthalmic preparation and intraocular lens surgery. In: *Proceedings of the World Congress on Antiseptics*. Lahn, Germany: Mundipharma Limberg; 1979.

Shepard GH. Nail grafts for reconstruction. *Hand Clin*. 1990;6:79–102.

Sheridan RL, Schulz JT, Ryan CM, et al. Long-term consequences of toxic epidermal necrolysis in children. *Pediatrics*. 2002;109:74–78.

Sheridan RL, Hurley J, Smith MA, et al. The acute burned hand: management and outcome based on 10-year experience with 1047 acute hand burns. *J Trauma*. 1995;38:406–411.

Shermak MA, Wong L, Inoue N, Chao EY, Manson PN. Butyl-2-cyanoacrylate fixation of mandibular osteotomies. *Plast Reconstr Surg.* 1998;102:319–324.

Sherman R, et al. Lower extremity reconstruction. In: Achauer BM, Eriksson E, Guyuron B, et al., eds. *Plastic Surgery: Indications, Operations, and Outcomes.* Vol 1. St Louis, MO: Mosby-Year Book; 2000:475–496.

Shiffman MA, Mirrafati S. Fat transfer techniques: the effect of harvest and transfer methods on adipocyte viability and review of the literature. *Dermatol Surg.* 2001;27:819–826.

Shprintzen RJ. Velocardiofacial syndrome. *Otolaryngol Clin North Am.* 2000;33:1217–1240.

Shulman O, Badani E, Wolf Y, Hauben DJ. Appropriate location of the nipple–areola complex in males. *Plast Reconstr Surg.* 2001;108(2):348–351.

Sidoti EJ Jr, Marsh JL, Marty-Grames L, Noetzel MJ. Long-term studies of metopic synostosis: frequency of cognitive impairment and behavioral disturbances. *Plast Reconstr Surg.* 1996;97:276–281.

Siegel RJ, McCoy JP Jr, Schade W, Swanson NA. Intradermal implantation of bovine collagen: humoral immune responses associated with clinical reactions. *Arch Dermatol.* 1984;120:183–187.

Siftan DW, ed. *Physicians' Desk Reference.* 54th ed. Montvale, NJ: Medical Economics Co; 2000.

Siftan DW, ed. *Physicians' Desk Reference.* Montvale, NJ: Medical Economics Co; 2002.

Silkiss RZ, Carroll RP. Transconjunctival surgery. *Ophthalmic Surg.* 1992;23:288–291.

Silverstein MJ, Handel N, Gamagami P, Waisman E, Gierson ED. Mammographic measurements before and after augmentation mammaplasty. *Plast Reconstr Surg.* 1990;86:1126–1130.

Simmons BP, Nutting JT. Juvenile rheumatoid arthritis. *Hand Clin.* 1989;5:157–168.

Simmons KE. Orthodontic role in clefts. In: Booth PW, Schendel SA, Hausamen JE, eds. *Maxillofacial Surgery.* Vol 2. London, UK: Churchill Livingstone; 1999:1101–1111.

Simon BE, Hoffman S, Kahn S. Classification and surgical correction of gynecomastia. *Plast Reconstr Surg.* 1973;51:48–52.

Simon MS, Cody RL. Cellulitis after axillary lymph node dissection for carcinoma of the breast. *Am J Med.* 1992;93:543–548.

Simon RR, Wolgin M. Subungual hematoma: association with occult laceration requiring repair. *Am J Emerg Med.* 1987;5:302–304.

Sims NM. Upper extremity anesthesia. In: McCarthy JG, ed. *Plastic Surgery.* Vol 8. Philadelphia, PA: WB Saunders; 1990:4302–4328.

Singleton GT, Cassisi NJ. Frey's syndrome: incidence related to skin flap thickness in parotidectomy. *Laryngoscope.* 1980;90:1636–1639.

Skandalakis JE, et al. The anterior body wall. In: Skandalakis JE, ed. *Embryology for Surgeons.* Baltimore, MD: Williams & Wilkins; 1994:540–593.

Slade DE, Powell BW, Mortimer PS. Hidradenitis suppurativa: pathogenesis and management. *Br J Plast Surg.* 2003;56(5):451–461.

Smeltzer DM, Stickler GB, Schirger A. Primary lymphedema in children and adolescents: a follow-up study and review. *Pediatrics.* 1985;79(2):206–218.

Smith B. Superior oblique paresis after blepharoplasty. *Plast Reconstr Surg.* 1980;66:287.

Smith DG. Principles of partial foot amputations in the diabetic. *Instr Course Lect.* 1999;48:321–329.

Smith DJ Jr, Thomson PD, Bolton LL, Hutchinson JJ. Microbiology and healing of the occluded skin-graft donor site. *Plast Reconstr Surg.* 1993;91:1094–1097.

Smith MA, Munster AM, Spence RJ. Burns of the hand and upper limb—a review. *Burns.* 1998;24:493–505.

Smith ML, et al. Management of orbital fractures. *Oper Tech Plast Reconstr Surg.* 1998;5:312–324.

Smith P, et al. Syndactyly. In: Gupta A, Kay SP, Scheker LR, eds. *The Growing Hand.* London, UK: Mosby-Year Book; 2000:225–230.

Smith RJ. Intrinsic contracture. In: Green DP, Hotchkiss RN, Pederson WC, eds. *Operative Hand Surgery.* Vol 1. 4th ed. New York, NY: Churchill Livingstone; 1999:611.

Smith RJ. Tendon transfers following injuries about the elbow. In: *Tendon Transfers of the Hand and Forearm.* Boston, MA: Little Brown & Co; 1987.

Smoot EC, Marx A, Weiman D, Deitcher SR. Recognition, diagnosis, and management of heparin-induced thrombocytopenia and thrombosis. *Plast Reconstr Surg.* 1999;103(2):559–565.

Snell RS, ed. *Clinical Anatomy for Medical Students.* 5th ed. Boston, MA: Little Brown & Co; 1995:671–682.

Snyder MC, Johnson PJ, Moore GF, Ogren FP. Early versus late gold weight implantation for rehabilitation of the paralyzed eyelid. *Laryngoscope.* 2001;111:2109–2113.

Sommer NZ, Brown RE, Zook EG. Surgery of the perionychium. In: Mathes SJ, Hentz VR, eds. *Plastic Surgery.* Vol 7. 2nd ed. Philadelphia, PA: WB Saunders; 2006:201–203.

Sommer NZ, Brown RE. The perionychium. In: Green DP, Hotchkiss RN, Pederson WC, et al., eds. *Green's Operative Hand Surgery.* 5th ed. Philadelphia, PA: Elsevier Churchill Livingstone; 2005; 10:389.

Sood S, Quraishi MS, Bradley PJ. Frey's syndrome and parotid surgery. *Clin Otolaryngol.* 1998;23:291–301.

Sotereanos DG, et al. Hand and digital amputations. In: Peimer CA, ed. *Surgery of the Hand and Upper Extremity.* Vol 2. New York, NY: McGraw-Hill; 1996:1000–1002.

Souba WW. Evaluation and treatment of benign breast disorders. In: Bland KI, Copeland EM, eds. *The Breast: Comprehensive Management of Benign and Malignant Diseases.* Philadelphia, PA: WB Saunders; 1991:715.

Soucacos PN, Diznitsas LA, Beris AE, Xenakis TA, Malizos KN. Reflex sympathetic dystrophy of the upper extremity. *Hand Clin.* 1997;13:339–354.

Soucacos PN. Indications and selection for digital amputation and replantation. *J Hand Surg Br.* 2001;26:572–581.

Soutar DS, Tanner NS. The radial forearm flap in the management of soft tissue injuries of the hand. *Br J Plast Surg.* 1984;37:18–26.

Souza JM, Dumanian GA. An evidence-based approach to abdominal wall reconstruction. *Plast Reconstr Surg.* 2012;130(1):116–124.

Soxanas MT. Surgical anatomy of the eyelids and orbit. In: Wright DW, ed. *Color Atlas of Ophthalmic Surgery.* Philadelphia, PA: JB Lippincott; 1992;1–16.

Sparkes BG. Immunological responses to thermal injury. *Burns.* 1997;23:106–113.

Spear SL, Giese SY, Ducic I. Concentric mastopexy revisited. *Plast Reconstr Surg.* 2001;107:1294–1299.

Spear SL, Burke JB, Forman D, Zuurbier RA, Berg CD. Experience with reduction mammaplasty following breast conservation and radiation therapy. *Plast Reconstr Surg.* 1998;102:1913–1916.

Spear SL, Kassan M, Little JW. Guidelines in concentric mastopexy. *Plast Reconstr Surg.* 1990;85:961–966.

Spear SL, et al. Reduction mammoplasty and mastopexy. In: Aston SJ, Beasley RW, Thorne CH, eds. *Grabb & Smith's Plastic Surgery.* 5th ed. Philadelphia, PA: Lippincott-Raven; 1997:742–751.

Spear SL, Onyewu C. Staged breast reconstruction with saline-filled implants in the irradiated breast: recent trends and therapeutic implications. *Plast Reconstr Surg.* 2000;105:930–942.

Spear SL, Hannan CM, Willey SC, Cocilovo C. Nipple-sparing mastectomy. *Plast Reconstr Surg.* 2009;123(6):1665–1673.

Spear SL, Pelletiere CV. Augmentation mammoplasty in women with thoracic hypoplasia. In: Spear SL, ed. *Surgery of the Breast: Principles and Art.* 2nd ed. Philadelphia, PA: Lippincott Williams & Wilkins; 2005:1377–1382.

Spencer JM, Amonette RA. Indoor tanning: risks, benefits, and future trends. *J Am Acad Dermatol.* 1995;33:288–298.

Spira M, Rosen T. Injectable soft tissue substitutes. *Clin Plast Surg.* 1993;20:181–188.

Spira M. Otoplasty: what I do now—a 30-year perspective. *Plast Reconstr Surg.* 1999;104:834–840.

Spiro RH, Thaler HT, Hicks WF, Kher UA, Huvos AH, Strong EW. The importance of clinical staging of minor salivary gland carcinoma. *Am J Surg.* 1991;162:330–336.

Spiro RH. Salivary neoplasms: overview of 35-year experience with 2,807 patients. *Head Neck Surg.* 1986;8:177–184.

Sporn MB, Roberts AB, Wakefield LM, Assoian RK. Transforming growth factor-beta: biologic function and chemical structure. *Science.* 1986;233:532–534.

Sriprachya-Anunt S, Fitzpatrick RE, Goldman MP, Smith SR. Infectious complications of pulsed carbon dioxide laser resurfacing for photoaged skin. *Dermatol Surg.* 1997;23:527–536.

Stal GH, Hamilton S, Spira M. Hemangiomas, lymphangiomas, and vascular malformations of the head and neck. *Otolaryngol Clin North Am.* 1986;19:769–796.

Stal S, et al. Basal and squamous cell carcinoma of the skin. In: Aston SJ, Beasley RW, Thorne CH, eds. *Grabb & Smith's Plastic Surgery.* 5th ed. Philadelphia, PA: Lippincott-Raven; 1997:107–120.

Stal S, Hollier L. Correction of secondary cleft lip deformities. *Plast Reconstr Surg.* 2002;109:1672–1681.

Stanton RA, Billmire DA. Skin resurfacing for the burned patient. *Clin Plast Surg.* 2002;29:29–51.

Stark HH, Gainor BJ, Ashworth CR, Zemel NP, Rickard TA. Operative treatment of intra-articular fractures of the dorsal aspect of the distal phalanx of digits. *J Bone Joint Surg Am.* 1987;69:892–896.

Stark WJ, Kaltman SI. Current concepts in the surgical management of traumatic auricular hematoma. *J Oral Maxillofac Surg.* 1992;50:800–802.

Starkweather KD, Lattuga S, Hurst LC, et al. Collagenase in the treatment of Dupuytren's disease: an in vitro study. *J Hand Surg Am.* 1996;21:490–495.

Steinmann SP, Bishop AT, Berger RA. Use of the 1,2 intercompartmental supraretinacular artery as a vascularized pedicle bone graft for difficult scaphoid union. *J Hand Surg Am.* 2002;27:391–401.

Stern PJ, et al. Evaluation, staging, and principles of tumor surgery. In: Peimer CA, ed. *Surgery of the Hand and Upper Extremity.* Vol 2. New York, NY: McGraw-Hill; 1996:2221–2263.

Stern PJ. Fractures of the metacarpals and phalanges. In: Green DP, Hotchkiss RN, Pederson WC, eds. *Operative Hand Surgery*. Vol 1. 4th ed. New York, NY: Churchill Livingstone; 1999:711–771.

Stevens DL. Invasive streptococcal infections. *J Infect Chemother*. 2001;7:69–80.

Stewart DA, Smitham PJ, Gianoutsos MP, Walsh WR. Biomechanical influence of the vincula tendinum on digital motion after isolated flexor tendon injury: a cadaveric study. *J Hand Surg Am*. 2007;32(8):1190–1194.

Stoelinga P. Orthognathic surgery: maxilla, Le Fort I, II, and III. In: Langdon J, Patel M, eds. *Operative Maxillary Facial Surgery*. New York, NY: Chapman and Hall; 1998:447–461.

Stokes MC, Bennett J, Beech DJ, Ballard B. Angiosarcoma of the scalp. *Am Surg*. 2008;74(12):1228–1230.

Stokes RB, Whetzel TP, Sommerhaug E, Saunders CJ. Arterial vascular anatomy of the umbilicus. *Plast Reconstr Surg*. 1998;102: 761–764.

Stratoudakis AC. Craniofacial anomalies and principles of their correction. In: Georgiade GS, Riefkohl R, Levin LS, eds. *Textbook of Plastic, Maxillofacial and Reconstructive Surgery*. 3rd ed. Baltimore, MD: Williams & Wilkins; 1992a:273–296.

Stratoudakis AC. Principles of bone transplantation. In: Georgiade GS, Riefkohl R, Levin LS, eds. *Textbook of Plastic, Maxillofacial and Reconstructive Surgery*. 3rd ed. Baltimore, MD: Williams & Wilkins; 1992b:39–46.

Strauch B, Vasconez LO, Hall-Findlay EJ, eds. *Grabb's Encyclopedia of Flaps*. 2nd ed. Philadelphia, PA: Lippincott-Raven; 1998.

Strauch B, Yu HL, eds. *Atlas of Microvascular Surgery: Anatomy and Operative Approaches*. New York, NY: Thieme Medical Publishers; 1993.

Strauch B. User of nerve conduits in peripheral nerve repair. *Hand Clin*. 2000;16:123–130.

Strickland JW, Leibovic SJ. Anatomy and pathogenesis of the digital cords and nodules. *Hand Clin*. 1991;7:645–657.

Strickland JW. Flexor tendons—acute injuries. In: Green DP, Hotchkiss RN, Pederson WC, eds. *Operative Hand Surgery*. Vol 2. 4th ed. New York, NY: Churchill Livingstone; 1999:1851–1897.

Stromberg BV, Knibbe M. Anisocoria following reduction of bilateral orbital wall fractures. *Ann Plast Surg*. 1988;2:486–488.

Struewing JP, Hartge P, Wacholder S. The risk of cancer associated with specific mutations of *BRCA1* and *BRCA2* among Ashkenazi Jews. *N Engl J Med*. 1997;336:1401–1408.

Stuzin JM, Wagstrom L, Kawamoto HK, Wolfe SA. Anatomy of the frontal branch of the facial nerve: the significance of the temporal fat pad. *Plast Reconstr Surg*. 1989;83:265–271.

Stuzin JM, et al. Reoperative rhytidectomy. In: Grotting JC, ed. *Reoperative Aesthetic & Reconstructive Surgery*. St Louis, MO: Quality Medical Publishing; 1995; 205–244.

Stuzin JM. Phenol peeling and the history of phenol peeling. *Clin Plast Surg*. 1998;25:1–19.

Su CW, Lohman R, Gottlieb LJ. Frostbite of the upper extremity. *Hand Clin*. 2000;16:235–247.

Suen JY, et al. Cancer of the neck. In: Myers EN, Suen JY, eds. *Cancer of the Head and Neck*. Philadelphia, PA: WB Saunders; 1996:462–484.

Sugino H, Tsuzuki K, Bandoh Y, Tange I. Surgical correction of Stahl's ear using the cartilage turnover and rotation method. *Plast Reconstr Surg*. 1989;83:160–164.

Sunderland S. *Nerve and Nerve Injuries*. Baltimore, MD: Williams & Wilkins; 1968:758–762.

Suzuki H. Treatment of traumatic tattoos with the Q-switched neodymium: YAG laser. *Arch Dermatol*. 1996;132:1226–1229.

Swanson AB, de Groot Swanson G. Evaluation and treatment of the upper extremity in the stroke patient. *Hand Clin*. 1989;5:75–96.

Swartz WM, Banis JC, Newton ED, Ramasastry SS, Jones NF, Acland R. The osteocutaneous scapular flap for mandibular and maxillary reconstruction. *Plast Reconstr Surg*. 1986;77:530–545.

Swartz WM, Ramasastry SS, McGill JR, Noonan JD. Distally based vastus lateralis muscle flap for coverage of wounds about the knee. *Plast Reconstr Surg*. 1987;80:255–265.

Szabo RM, et al. Acute carpal fractures and dislocations. In: Peimer CA, ed. *Surgery of the Hand and Upper Extremity*. New York, NY: McGraw-Hill; 1996:711–726.

Szabo RM. Entrapment and compression injuries. In: Green DP, Hotchkiss RN, Pederson WC, eds. *Operative Hand Surgery*. Vol 2. 4th ed. New York, NY: Churchill Livingstone; 1999:1404–1447.

Tai YC, Domchek S, Parmigiani G, Chen S. Breast cancer risk among male *BRCA1* and *BRCA2* mutation carriers. *J Natl Cancer Inst*. 2007;99(23):1811–1814.

Taira N, Takabatake D, Aogi K, et al. Phyllodes tumor of the breast: stromal overgrowth and histological classification are useful prognosis-predictive factors for local recurrence in patients with a positive surgical margin. *Jpn J Clin Oncol*. 2007;37(10): 730–736.

Tanaka E, Detamore MS, Mercuri LG. Degenerative disorders of the temporomandibular joint: etiology, diagnosis, and treatment. *J Dent Res*. 2008;87(4):296–307.

Tang CL, Brown MH, Levine R, Sloan M, Chong N, Holowaty E. A follow-up study of 105 women with breast cancer following reduction mammaplasty. *Plast Reconstr Surg.* 1999a;103:1687–1690.

Tang CL, Brown MH, Levine R, Sloan M, Chong N, Holowaty E. Breast cancer found at the time of breast reduction. *Plast Reconstr Surg.* 1999b:103:1682–1686.

Tang L, Eaton JW. Fibrin(ogen) mediates acute inflammatory responses to biomaterials. *J Exp Med.* 1993;178:2147–2156.

Tang L, Eaton JW. Natural responses to unnatural materials: a molecular mechanism for foreign body reactions. *Molec Med.* 1999;5: 351–358.

Tanzer RC. The constricted (cup and lop) ear. *Plast Reconstr Surg.* 1975;55:406–415.

Tanzer RC. Microtia: a long-term follow-up of 44 reconstructed auricles. *Plast Reconstr Surg.* 1978;61:161–166.

Tardy ME Jr, Walter MA, Patt BS. The overprojecting nose: anatomic component analysis and repair. *Facial Plast Surg.* 1993;9:306–316.

Taylor CR. Laser ignition of traumatically embedded firework debris. *Lasers Surg Med.* 1998;22:157–158.

Taylor RS, Belli AM, Jacob S. Distal venous arterialisation for salvage of critically ischaemic inoperable limb. *Lancet.* 1999;354:1962–1965.

Tebbetts JB. Axillary endoscopic breast augmentation: processes derived from a 28-year experience to optimize outcomes. *Plast Reconstr Surg.* 2006;118(7 suppl):53S–80S.

Tebbetts JB. Blepharoplasty: a refined technique emphasizing accuracy and control. *Clin Plast Surg.* 1992;19:329–349.

Teimourian B. Blindness following fat injections (letter). *Plast Reconstr Surg.* 1988a;82:361.

Teimourian B, Malekzadeh S. Rejuvenation of the upper arm. *Plast Reconstr Surg.* 1998b;102:545–553.

Tellioglu AT, Tekdemir I, Erdemli EA, Tüccar E, Ulusoy G. Temporoparietal fascia: an anatomic and histologic reinvestigation with new potential clinical applications. *Plast Reconstr Surg.* 2000;105:40–45.

Tenenhaus M, Rennekampff HO. Burn surgery. *Clin Plast Surg.* 2007;34(4):697–715.

Terenzi V, Leonardi A, Covelli E, et al. Parry-Romberg syndrome. *Plast Reconstr Surg.* 2005;116:97e–102e.

Terino EO. Alloplastic facial contouring by zonal principles of skeletal anatomy. *Clin Plast Surg.* 1992;19:487–510.

Tessier P. Anatomical classification of facial, craniofacial and latero-facial clefts. *J Maxillofac Surg.* 1969;4:69–92.

Thomas JM. Premalignant and malignant epithelial tumors. In: Sams WM Jr, Lynch PJ, eds. *Principles and Practice of Dermatology.* New York, NY: Churchill Livingstone; 1996:225–239.

Thomas WO, Moses MH, Craver RD, Galen WK. Congenital cutis laxa: a case report and review of loose skin syndromes. *Ann Plast Surg.* 1993;30:252–256.

Thompson H. Cutaneous hemangiomas and lymphangiomas. *Clin Plast Surg.* 1987;13:341–356.

Thomson HG, Winslow J. Microtia reconstruction: does the cartilage framework grow? *Plast Reconstr Surg.* 1989;84:908–915.

Thorne CH, et al. Aesthetic surgery of the aging face. In: Aston SJ, Beasley RW, Thorne CH, eds. *Grabb & Smith's Plastic Surgery.* 5th ed. Philadelphia, PA: Lippincott-Raven; 1997a:633–649.

Thorne CH, et al. Aesthetic surgery of the face. In: Aston SJ, Beasley RW, Thorne CH, eds. *Grabb & Smith's Plastic Surgery.* 5th ed. Philadelphia, PA: Lippincott-Raven; 1997b:617.

Thorne CH, et al. Reconstructive surgery of the lower extremity. In: McCarthy JG, ed. *Plastic Surgery.* Vol 6. Philadelphia, PA: WB Saunders; 1990:4029–4092.

Thorne CH. Otoplasty and ear reconstruction. In: Thorne CH, Beasley RW, Aston SJ, et al., eds. *Grabb and Smith's Plastic Surgery.* 6th ed. Philadelphia, PA: Lippincott Williams & Wilkins; 2006:304–310.

Titus-Ernstoff L. An overview of the epidemiology of cutaneous melanoma. *Clin Plast Surg.* 2000;27:305–316.

Tobin HA, Karas ND. Lip augmentation using an AlloDerm graft. *J Oral Maxillofac Surg.* 1998;56:722–727.

Tomaino MM, et al. Arthroplasty. In: Herndon JH, ed. *Surgical Reconstruction of the Upper Extremity.* Stamford, CT: Appleton & Lange; 1999:963–995.

Tomaino MM. Treatment of Eaton stage I trapeziometacarpal disease: ligament reconstruction or thumb metacarpal extension osteotomy? *Hand Clin.* 2001;17:197–205.

Tonnard P, Verpaele A. The MACS-lift short scar rhytidectomy. *Aesthet Surg J.* 2007;27(2):188–198.

Tortora GJ, Grabowski SR, eds. The special senses. In: Tortora GJ, Grabowski SR, eds. *Principles of Anatomy and Physiology.* 9th ed. New York, NY: John Wiley & Sons; 2000:512–529.

Tran N, Chang DW, Gupta A, Kroll SS, Robb GL. Comparison of immediate and delayed free TRAM flap breast reconstruction in patients receiving postmastectomy radiation therapy. *Plast Reconstr Surg.* 2001;108:78–82.

Trent JT, Kirsner RS. Diagnosing necrotizing fasciitis. *Adv Skin Wound Care.* 2002;15:135–138.

Troilius AM. Effective treatment of traumatic tattoos with a Q-switched Nd:YAG laser. *Lasers Surg Med.* 1998;22:103–108.

Trott SA, Beran SJ, Rohrich RJ, Kenkel JM, Adams WP Jr, Klein KW. Safety considerations and fluid resuscitation in liposuction: an analysis of 53 consecutive patients. *Plast Reconstr Surg.* 1998;102:2220–2229.

Trumble TE, McCallister WV. Repair of peripheral nerve defects in the upper extremity. *Hand Clin.* 2000;16:37-52.

Truppman ES, Ellenby JD. Major electrocardiographic changes during chemical face peeling. *Plast Reconstr Surg.* 1979;63:44–48.

Tsuge K. Management of established Volkmann's contracture. In: Green DP, Hotchkiss RN, Pederson WC, eds. *Operative Hand Surgery.* Vol 1. 4th ed. New York, NY: Churchill Livingstone; 1999:591–603.

Tsuge K. Tendon transfers for radial nerve palsy. *Aust NZ J Surg.* 1980;50:267–272.

Tubiana R, Gilbert A, Masquelet AC, eds. *An Atlas of Surgical Techniques of the Hand and Wrist.* Baltimore, MD: Williams & Wilkins; 1999:38–39.

Tuerk M. Medications that cause gynecomastia. *Plast Reconstr Surg.* 1993;92:1411.

Tung TC, Wang KC, Fang CM, Lee CM. Reverse pedicled lateral arm flap for reconstruction of posterior soft-tissue defects of the elbow. *Ann Plast Surg.* 1997;38(6):635–641.

Tung TC. Endoscopic shaver with liposuction for treatment of axillary osmidrosis. *Ann Plast Surg.* 2001;46:400–404.

Turpin IM. Microsurgical replantation of the external ear. *Clin Plast Surg.* 1990;17:397–404.

Tuttle HG, Olvey SP, Stern PJ. Tendon avulsion injuries of the distal phalanx. *Clin Orthop Relat Res.* 2006;445:157–168.

Uebel CO. Micrografts and minigrafts: a new approach for baldness surgery. *Ann Plast Surg.* 1991;27:476–487.

Ueda K, Furuya E, Yasuda Y, Oba S, Tajima S. Keloids have continuous high metabolic activity. *Plast Reconstr Surg.* 1999;104:694–698.

Upton J, et al. Congenital anomalies: shoulder region. In: Peimer CA, ed. *Surgery of the Hand and Upper Extremity.* Vol 3. New York, NY: McGraw-Hill; 1996:2001–2048.

Upton J, Coombs CJ, Mulliken JB, Burrows PE, Pap S. Vascular malformations of the upper limb: a review of 270 patients. *J Hand Surg Am.* 1999;24:1019–1035.

Upton J. Congenital anomalies of the hand and forearm. In: McCarthy JG, ed. *Plastic Surgery.* Vol 8. Philadelphia, PA: WB Saunders; 1990:5213–5398.

Upton J. Congenital anomalies of the hand. In: Cohen M, ed. *Mastery of Plastic and Reconstructive Surgery.* Vol 3. Boston, MA: Little Brown & Co; 1994:1424–1453.

Upton J. Hypoplastic or absent thumb. In: Mathes SJ, Hentz VR, eds. *Plastic Surgery.* Vol 8. 2nd ed. Philadelphia, PA: WB Saunders; 2005:332–338.

Urban MA, Osterman AL. Management of radial dysplasia. *Hand Clin.* 1990;6:589–605.

Urken ML, et al. Lateral thigh. In: Urken ML, Cheney ML, Sullivan MJ, eds. *Atlas of Regional and Free Flaps for Head and Neck Reconstruction.* New York, NY: Raven Press; 1995:169–182.

Vallis CP. Hair replacement surgery. In: McCarthy JG, ed. *Plastic Surgery.* Vol 2. Philadelphia, PA: WB Saunders; 1990:1514–1537.

Van Adrichem LN, Hoegen R, Hovius SE, et al. The effect of cigarette smoking on the survival of free vascularized and pedicled epigastric flaps in the rat. *Plast Reconstr Surg.* 1996; 97:86–96.

van der Velden EM, van der Walle HB, Groote AD. Tattoo removal: tannic acid method of Variot. *Int J Dermatol.* 1993;32:276–180.

Van Hoest AE, House JH, Cariello C. Upper extremity surgical treatment of cerebral palsy. *J Hand Surg.* 1999;24:323–330.

Van Hoest AE. Congenital disorders of the hand and upper extremity. *Pediatr Clin North Am.* 1996;43:1123–1124.

Van Uchelen J, Werker PM, Kon M. Complications of abdominoplasty in 86 patients. *Plast Reconstr Surg.* 2001;107:1869–1873.

VanderKolk CA. Craniofacial surgery. *Clin Plast Surg.* 1994;21:481-631.

Vedder NB. Flap physiology. In: Mathes SJ, ed. *Plastic Surgery.* Philadelphia, PA: Saunders Elsevier; 2006; 17:483–506.

Verpaele AM, Blondeel PN, Van Landuyt K. The superior gluteal artery perforator flap: an additional tool in the treatment of sacral pressure sores. *Br J Plast Surg.* 1999;52:385–391.

Verwoerd CD. Present day treatment of nasal fractures: closed versus open reduction. *Facial Plast Surg.* 1992;8:220–223.

Villafane O, Garcia-Tutor E, Taggart I. Endoscopic transaxillary subglandular breast augmentation using silicone gel textured implants. *Aesthetic Plast Surg.* 2000;24:212–215.

Vlachos CC. Orthodontic treatment for the cleft palate patient. *Semin Orthod.* 1996;2:197–204.

Von Heimburg HD, Exner K, Kruft S, Lemperle G. The tuberous breast deformity: classification and treatment. *Br J Plast Surg.* 1996;49:339–345.

Vu HL, Panchal J, Parker EE, Levine NS, Francel P. The timing of physiologic closure of the metopic suture: a review of 159 patients using reconstructed 3D CT scans of the craniofacial region. *J Craniofac Surg.* 2001;12(6):527–532.

Wagner JD, et al. Salivary gland disorders. In: Achauer BM, Eriksson E, Guyuron B, et al., eds. *Plastic Surgery: Indications, Operations, and Outcomes.* Vol 3. St Louis, MO: Mosby-Year Book; 2000:1355–1395.

Wallace JF. Disorders caused by venoms, bites, and stings. In: Isselbacher KJ, Braunwald E, Wilson JD, et al., eds. *Harrison's Principles of Internal Medicine.* Vol 2. 13th ed. New York, NY: McGraw-Hill; 1994:2467–2473.

Walton RL, et al. Pedicled flaps and grafts. In: Achauer BM, Eriksson E, Guyuron B, et al., eds. *Plastic Surgery: Indications, Operations, and Outcomes.* Vol 4. St Louis, MO: Mosby-Year Book; 2000:1793–1817.

Wang AA, Hutchinson DT. Longitudinal observation of pediatric hand and wrist ganglia. *J Hand Surg Am.* 2001;26(4):599–602.

Wang KC, Hsu KY, Shih CH. Irreducible volar rotary dislocation of the proximal interphalangeal joint. *Orthop Rev.* 1994;23:886–888.

Wang TY, Serletti JM, Cuker A, et al. Free tissue transfer in the hypercoagulable patient: a review of 58 flaps. *Plast Reconstr Surg.* 2012;129(2):443–453.

Warpeha RL. Resurfacing the burned face. *Clin Plast Surg.* 1981;8:255–267.

Warren AG, Brorson H, Borud LJ, Slavin SA. Lymphedema: a comprehensive review. *Ann Plast Surg.* 2007;59(4):464–472.

Warso M, Gray T, Gonzalez M. Melanoma of the hand. *J Hand Surg Am.* 1997;22:354–360.

Warwick R, Williams P, eds. *Gray's Anatomy.* Philadelphia, PA: WB Saunders; 1993:1050.

Watson HK, Paul H Jr. Pathologic anatomy. *Hand Clin.* 1991;7:661–668.

Watson JD. Hidradenitis suppurativa: a clinical review. *Br J Plast Surg.* 1985;38:567–569.

Watson KH, et al. Intercarpal arthrodesis. In: Green DP, Hotchkiss RN, Pederson WC, eds. *Operative Hand Surgery.* Vol 1. 4th ed. New York, NY: Churchill Livingstone; 1999a:122–216.

Watson KH, et al. Stiff joints. In: Green DP, Hotchkiss RN, Pederson WC, eds. *Operative Hand Surgery.* Vol 1. 4th ed. New York, NY: Churchill Livingstone; 1999b:552–561.

Watson S. The principles of management of congenital anomalies of the upper limb. *Arch Dis Child.* 2000;83:10–17.

Watson WL, McCarthy WD. Blood vessel and lymph vessel tumors: a report of 1056 cases. *Surg Gynecol Obstet.* 1940;71:569–588.

Weber ER, et al. Chronic wrist instability. In: Peimer CA, ed. *Surgery of the Hand and Upper Extremity.* New York, NY: McGraw-Hill; 1996:727–758.

Weber RA, Breidenbach WC, Brown RE, Jabaley ME, Mass DP. A randomized prospective study of polyglycolic acid conduits for digital nerve reconstructions in humans. *Plast Reconstr Surg.* 2000;106:1036–1045; discussion 1046–1048.

Weber RS, et al. Clinical assessment and staging. In: Weber RS, Miller MJ, Goepfert H, eds. *Basal and Squamous Cell Skin Cancers of the Head and Neck.* Baltimore, MD: Williams & Wilkins; 1996a:65–77.

Weber RS, et al. Surgical principles. In: Weber RS, Miller MJ, Goepfert H, eds. *Basal and Squamous Cell Skin Cancers of the Head and Neck.* Baltimore, MD: Williams & Wilkins; 1996b:115–132.

Weber RV, MacKinnon SE. Nerve transfers in the upper extremity. *J Am Soc Surg Hand.* 2004;4(3):200–213.

Weedon D. The granulomatous reaction pattern. In: Weedon D, ed. *Skin Pathology.* 2nd ed. London, UK: Churchill Livingstone; 2002:193–209.

Wei FC, Jain V, Celik N, Chen HC, Chuang DC, Lin CH. Have we found an ideal soft-tissue flap? An experience with 672 anterolateral thigh flaps. *Plast Reconstr Surg.* 2002;109(7):2219–2226; discussion 2227–2230.

Wei W, Zuoliang Q, Xiaoxi L. Free split and segmental latissimus dorsi transfer in one stage for facial reanimation. *Plast Reconstr Surg.* 1999;103:473–480; discussion 481–482.

Weiland AJ, et al. Vascularized bone transfers. In: Yaremchuk MJ, Burgess AR, Brumback RJ, eds. *Lower Extremity Salvage and Reconstruction: Orthopedic and Plastic Surgical Management.* Stamford, CT: Appleton & Lange; 1989.

Weinstein C, Roberts TL 3rd. Aesthetic skin resurfacing with the high-energy ultrapulsed CO2 laser. *Clin Plast Surg.* 1997;24:379–405.

Weinstein C, Scheflan M. Simultaneously combined ER:YAG and carbon dioxide laser (derma K) for skin resurfacing. *Clin Plast Surg.* 2000;27:273–285, xi.

Weinstein C. Erbium laser resurfacing: current concepts. *Plast Reconstr Surg.* 1999;103:602–616; discussion 617–618.

Weisberg NK, Becker DS. Repair of nasal ala defects with conchal bowl composite grafts. *Dermatol Surg.* 2000;26:1047–1051.

Weiss JS, Ellis CN, Headington JT, Tincoff T, Hamilton TA, Voorhees JJ. Topical tretinoin improves photoaged skin. A double-blind vehicle-controlled study. *JAMA.* 1988;259:527–532.

Wellisz T. Reconstruction of the burned external ear using a Medpor porous polyethylene pivoting helix framework. *Plast Reconstr Surg.* 1993;91:811–818.

Wells MD, Manktelow RT. Surgical management of facial palsy. *Clin Plast Surg.* 1990;17:645–653.

Wesley RE, Pollard ZF, McCord CD Jr. Superior oblique paresis after blepharoplasty. *Plast Reconstr Surg.* 1980;66:283–286.

West BR, Nichter LS, Halpern DE, Nimni ME, Cheung DT, Zhou ZY. Ultrasound debridement of trabeculated bone: effective and atraumatic. *Plast Reconstr Surg.* 1994;93:561–566.

Westesson P. Magnetic resonance imaging of the temporomandibular joint. *Oral Maxillofac Surg Clin North Am.* 1992;4:183–206.

Westfall CT, Shore JW, Nunery WR, Hawes MJ, Yaremchuk MJ. Operative complications of the transconjunctival inferior fornix approach. *Ophthalmology.* 1991;98:1525–1528.

Wexler A, Harris M, Lesavoy M. Conservative treatment of cutis aplasia. *Plast Reconstr Surg.* 1990;86:1066–1071.

Wexler A. Anatomy of the head and neck. In: Ferraro JW, ed. *Fundamentals in Maxillofacial Surgery.* New York, NY: Springer-Verlag; 1997:53–113.

Wheatley MJ, Marx MV. The use of intra-arterial urokinase in the management of hand ischaemia secondary to palmar and digital arterial occlusion. *Ann Plast Surg.* 1996;37:356–362; discussion 362–363.

Wheeler DR. Reconstruction for radial nerve palsy. In: Peimer CA, ed. *Surgery of the Hand and Upper Extremity.* New York, NY: McGraw-Hill; 1996:1363–1379.

White B, Adkins WY. The use of the carbon dioxide laser in head and neck lymphangioma. *Laser Surg Med.* 1986;6:293–295.

White CW, Wolf SJ, Korones DN, Sondheimer HM, Tosi MF, Yu A. Treatment of childhood angiomatous diseases with recombinant interferon alfa-2a. *J Pediatr.* 1991;118:59–66.

Wider TM, Spiro SA, Wolfe SA. Simultaneous osseous genioplasty and meloplasty. *Plast Reconstr Surg.* 1997;99:1273–1281.

Wiedrich TA. Congenital constriction band syndrome. *Hand Clin.* 1998;14:29–38.

Wieland U, Jurk S, Weissenborn S, Krieg T, Pfister H, Ritzkowsky A. Erythroplasia of Queyrat: coinfection with cutaneous carcinogenic human papillomavirus type 8 and genital papillomaviruses in a carcinoma in situ. *J Invest Dermatol.* 2000;115:396–401.

Wilgis EF. Evaluation and treatment of chronic digital ischemia. *Ann Surg.* 1981;193:693–698.

Wilhelmi BJ, Mowlavi A, Neumeister MW. Upper blepharoplasty with bony anatomical landmarks to avoid injury to trochlea and superior oblique muscle tendon with fat resection. *Plast Reconstr Surg.* 2001;108:2137–2140; discussion 2141–2142.

Williams CN Jr, et al. Fingernail and fingertip injuries. In: Cohen M, ed. *Mastery of Plastic and Reconstructive Surgery.* Vol 3. Boston, MA: Little Brown & Co; 1994:1493–1507.

Williams CW. Silicone gel granuloma following compressive mammography. *Aesthet Plast Surg.* 1991 Winter;15:49–51.

Williams HB. Vascular neoplasms. *Clin Plast Surg.* 1980;7:397–411.

Williams JK, et al. Nonsyndromic craniosynostosis. In: Achauer BM, Eriksson E, Guyuron B, et al., eds. *Plastic Surgery: Indications, Operations, and Outcomes.* Vol 2. St Louis, MO: Mosby-Year Book; 2000:683–706.

Williams PL, Warwick R, Dyson M, et al., eds. *Gray's Anatomy.* 37th ed. Edinburgh, Scotland: Churchill Livingstone; 1989:337–367, 570–575, 1098–1107, 1564.

Williams WG, et al. Pathophysiology of the burn wound. In: Herndon DN, ed. *Total Burn Care.* Philadelphia, PA: WB Saunders; 1996:63–67.

Wilson BC, Davidson B, Corey JP, Haydon RC 3rd. Comparison of complications following frontal sinus fractures managed with exploration with or without obliteration over 10 years. *Laryngoscope.* 1988;98:516–520.

Wilson M, et al. Complications of upper blepharoplasty. In: Putterman A, ed. *Cosmetic Oculoplastic Surgery.* Philadelphia, PA: WB Saunders; 1993:342.

Wilson MR, Louis DS, Stevenson TR. Poland's syndrome: variable expression and associated anomalies. *J Hand Surg Am.* 1988;13: 880–882.

Wind GG, Valentine RJ. *Anatomic Exposures in Vascular Surgery.* Baltimore, MD: Williams & Wilkins; 1991.

Wise JB, Cryer JE, Belasco JB, Jacobs I, Elden L. Management of head and neck plexiform neurofibromas in pediatric patients with neurofibromatosis type 1. *Arch Otolaryngol Head Neck Surg.* 2005;131(8):712–718.

Wisnicki JL. Hemangiomas and vascular malformations. *Ann Plast Surg.* 1984;12:41–59.

Witt PD. Velopharyngeal insufficiency. In: Achauer BM, Eriksson E, Guyuron B, et al., eds. *Plastic Surgery: Indications, Operations, and Outcomes.* Vol 2. St Louis, MO: Mosby-Year Book. 2000:819–933.

Wolfe SA, Davidson J. Avoidance of lower-lid contraction in surgical approaches to the inferior orbit. *Oper Tech Plast Reconstr Surg.* 1998;5:201–212.

Wolfe SA, et al. *Facial Fractures.* New York, NY: Thieme Medical Publishers; 1993:41–61.

Wolfe SA, Johnson P. Frontal sinus injuries: primary care and management of late complications. *Plast Reconstr Surg.* 1988;82:781–791.

Wolfe SA, Spiro SA, Wider TM. Surgery of the jaws. In: Aston SJ, Beasley RW, Thorne CHM, eds. *Grabb & Smith's Plastic Surgery.* 5th ed. Philadelphia, PA: Lippincott-Raven; 1997:321–333.

Wolfe SW, et al. Metacarpal and carpometacarpal trauma. In: Peimer CA, ed. *Surgery of the Hand and Upper Extremity.* Vol 1. New York, NY: McGraw-Hill; 1996:883.

Wolfe SW. Tenosynovitis. In: Green DP, Hotchkiss RN, Pederson WC, eds. *Operative Hand Surgery.* Vol 2. 4th ed. New York, NY: Churchill Livingstone; 1999:2022–2044.

Wolford LM, et al. Surgical planning. In: Booth PW, Schendel SA, Hausamen JE, eds. *Maxillofacial Surgery.* Vol 2. London, UK: Churchill Livingstone; 1999:1205–1257.

Wolfort FG, et al. Pearls and pitfalls: how to avoid and manage complications. In: Wolfort FG, Kanter WR, eds. *Aesthetic Blepharoplasty.* Boston, MA: Little Brown & Co; 1995; 189–218.

Wolfort FG, Vaughan TE, Wolfort SF, Nevarre DR. Retrobulbar hematoma and blepharoplasty. *Plast Reconstr Surg.* 1999;104:2154–2162.

Wolfort FG, Cetrulo CL Jr, Nevarre DR. Suction-assisted lipectomy for lipodystrophy syndromes attributed to HIV-protease inhibitor use. *Plast Reconstr Surg.* 1999;104:1814–1820.

Wong RJ, et al. Cancer of the nasal cavity in the paranasal sinuses. In: Shah JP, ed. *Cancer of the Head and Neck.* Hamilton, Ontario: BC Decker; 2001.

Woo KI, Yi K, Kim YD. Surgical correction for lower lid epiblepharon in Asians. *Br J Ophthalmol.* 2000; 84(12):1407–1410.

Wray CR. Fractures and joint injuries of the hand. In: McCarthy JG, ed. *Plastic Surgery.* Philadelphia, PA: WB Saunders; 1990;7:4617–4627.

Wray RD, Holtmann B, Ribaudo JM, Keiter J, Weeks PM. A comparison of conjunctival and subciliary incisions for orbital fractures. *Br J Plast Surg.* 1977;30:142–145.

Wright SW, Wrenn KD, Murray L, Seger D. Clinical presentation and outcome of brown recluse spider bite. *Ann Emerg Med.* 1997;30:28–32.

Wright T. Anatomy and development of the ear and hearing. In: Ludman H, Wright T, eds. *Diseases of the Ear.* 6th ed. London, UK: Arnold; 1998:8–13.

Wrobel JS, Connolly JE. Making the diagnosis of osteomyelitis: the role of prevalence. *J Am Podiatr Med Assoc.* 1998;88:337–343.

Wuring E. Refinement of central pedicle reconstruction by application of the ligamentous suspension. *Plast Reconstr Surg.* 1999;103:1400–1409.

Wyrick JD, Stern PJ. Secondary nerve reconstruction. *Hand Clin.* 1992;8:587–598.

Yaghoubian R, Goebel F, Musgrave DS, Sotereanos DG. Diagnosis and management of acute fracture-dislocations of the carpus. *Ortho Clin North Am.* 2001;32:295–305.

Yajima H, Tamai S, Yamauchi T, Mizumoto S. Osteocutaneous radial forearm flap for hand reconstruction. *J Hand Surg Am.* 1999;24:594–603.

Yamaguchi Y, Yu YM, Zupke C, et al. Effect of burn injury on glucose and nitrogen metabolism in the liver: preliminary studies in a perfused liver system. *Surgery.* 1997;121:295–303.

Yap LH, Butler CE. Principles of microsurgery. In: Thorne CH, Beasley RW, Aston SJ, et al., eds. *Grabb and Smith's Plastic Surgery.* 6th ed. Philadelphia, PA: Lippincott Williams & Wilkins; 2006:66–72.

Yaremchuk MJ, Kim WK. Soft tissue alterations associated with acute extended open reduction and internal fixation of orbital fractures. *J Craniofac Surg.* 1992;3:134–140.

Yaremchuk MJ. Fractures of the maxilla. In: Cohen M, ed. *Mastery of Plastic and Reconstructive Surgery.* Boston, MA: Little Brown & Co; 1994:1156–1165.

Yin HQ, Langford R, Burrell RE. Comparative evaluation of antimicrobial activity of Acticoat antimicrobial barrier dressing. *J Burn Care Rehab.* 1999;20:195–200.

Yotsuyanagi T, Yokoi K, Sawada Y. Nonsurgical treatment of various auricular deformities. *Clin Plast Surg.* 2002;29:327–332.

Young AE. Venous and arterial malformations. In: Mulliken JB, Young AE, eds. *Vascular Birthmarks: Hemangiomas and Malformations.* Philadelphia, PA: WB Saunders; 1988:196–214.

Yowler CJ, Fratianne RB. Current status of burn resuscitation. *Clin Plast Surg.* 2000;27(1):1-10.

Yu GY, Ma DQ. Carcinoma of the salivary gland: a clinicopathologic study of 405 cases. *Semin Surg Oncol.* 1987;3:240–244.

Zaias N, ed. *The Nail in Health and Disease.* 2nd ed. Stamford, CT: Appleton & Lange; 1990:67–85.

Zampino G, Di Rocco C, Butera G, et al. Opitz C trigonocephaly syndrome and midline brain anomalies. *Am J Med Genet.* 1997;73:484–488.

Zancolli E, ed. *Structural and Dynamic Bases of Hand Surgery.* 2nd ed. Philadelphia, PA: JB Lippincott; 1979;19–20.

Zancolli E. Surgery for the quadriplegic hand with active, strong wrist extension preserved: a study of 97 cases. *Clin Orthop Relat Res.* 1975;112:101–113.

Zarem HA, Lowe NJ. Benign growths and generalized skin disorders. In: Thorne CH, Beasley RW, Aston SJ, et al., eds. *Grabb and Smith's Plastic Surgery*. 5th ed. Philadelphia, PA: Lippincott Williams & Wilkins; 1997.

Zawacki BE. The natural history of reversible burn injury. *Surg Gynecol Obstet*. 1974;139:867–872.

Zbar RIS, Canady JW. Cold injuries. In: Mathes SJ, Hentz VR, eds. *Plastic Surgery*. Vol 1. 2nd ed. Philadelphia, PA: WB Saunders; 2005:858–861.

Zeineh L, Wilhelmi BJ, Zook EG. Managing acute nerve injuries in extremities. *Oper Tech Plast Reconstr Surg*. 2003;9(3):111–116.

Zempsky WT, Karasic RB. EMLA versus TAC for topical anesthesia of extremity wounds in children. *Ann Emerg Med*. 1997;30: 163–166.

Zhang B, Wieslander JB. Dextran's antithrombotic properties in small arteries are not altered by low-molecular-weight heparin or the fibrinolytic inhibitor tranexamic acid: an experimental study. *Microsurgery*. 1993;14:289–295.

Zide B, Grayson B, McCarthy JG. Cephalometric analysis: part I. *Plast Reconstr Surg*. 1981a;68:816–823.

Zide B, Grayson B, McCarthy JG. Cephalometric analysis for upper and lower midface surgery: part II. *Plast Reconstr Surg*. 1981b;68:961–968.

Zide B, Jelks G. Medial canthus. In: Zide B, Jelks G, eds. *Surgical Anatomy of the Orbit*. New York, NY: Raven Press; 1985:41.

Zide BM. Nasal anatomy: the muscles and tip sensation. *Aesthetic Plast Surg*. 1985;9:193–196.

Zide BM. The temporomandibular joint. In: McCarthy JG, ed. *Plastic Surgery*. Vol 2. Philadelphia, PA: WB Saunders; 1990:1475–1513.

Zide MF, Kent JN. Indications for open reduction of mandibular condyle fractures. *J Oral Maxillofac Surg*. 1983;41:89–98.

Zide BM, Longaker MT. Chin surgery II: submental ostectomy and soft-tissue excision. *Plast Reconstr Surg*. 1999a;104:1854–1860.

Zide BM, Pfeifer TM, Longaker MT. Chin surgery I: augmentation—the allures and the alerts. *Plast Reconstr Surg*. 1999b;104:1843-1862.

Zide BM, Boutros S. Chin surgery III: revelations. *Plast Reconstr Surg*. 2003;111:1542–1550.

Zide BM, Swift R. How to block and tackle the face. *Plast Reconstr Surg*. 1998;101:840–851.

Zollinger PE, Tuinebreijer WE, Breederveld RS, Kreis RW. Can vitamin C prevent complex regional pain syndrome in patients with wrist fractures? A randomized, controlled, multicenter dose-response study. *J Bone Joint Surg Am*. 2007;89(7):1424–1431.

Zook EG, Guy RJ, Russell RC. A study of nail bed injuries: causes, treatment, and prognosis. *J Hand Surg Am*. 1984;9:247–252.

Zook EG, Van Beek AL, Russell RC, Beatty ME. Anatomy and physiology of the perionychium: a review of the literature and anatomic study. *J Hand Surg Am*. 1980;5:528–536.

Zook EG, et al. The perionychium. In: Green DP, Hotchkiss RN, Pederson WC, eds. Operative *Hand Surgery*. Vol 1. 4th ed. New York, NY: Churchill Livingstone; 1999:1353–1380.

Zook EG. Anatomy and physiology of the perionychium. *Hand Clin*. 2002;18:553–559.

Zook EG. Surgically treatable problems of the perionychium. In: McCarthy JG, ed. *Plastic Surgery*. Vol 8. Philadelphia, PA: WB Saunders; 1990;8:4499–4515.

Zook N, Hussmann J, Brown R, et al. Microcirculatory studies of frostbite injury. *Ann Plast Surg*. 1998;40(3):246–253.

INDEX

Printed in the USA
CPSIA information can be obtained
at www.ICGtesting.com
JSHW05082608I124
73105JS00003B/14